Neoplasms of the Larynx

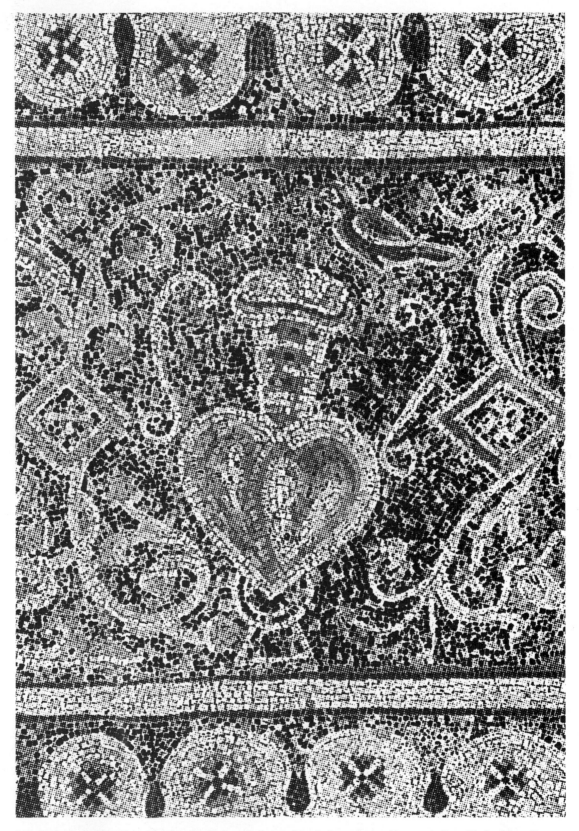

Mosaic illustrating the voice originating directly from the heart, through the trachea and larynx, in line with the Aristotelian concept (Basilica of S. Apollinare in Classe, Ravenna, 6th century). It is the emblem of The Laryngeal Cancer Association.

Neoplasms of the Larynx

Edited by

Alfio Ferlito MD
Professor of Otolaryngology at the University of Padua School of Medicine,
Padua, Italy

CHURCHILL LIVINGSTONE
EDINBURGH LONDON MADRID MELBOURNE NEW YORK AND TOKYO 1993

CHURCHILL LIVINGSTONE
Medical Division of Longman Group UK Limited

Distributed in the United States of America by Churchill
Livingstone Inc., 650 Avenue of the Americas, New York, N.Y. 10011, and
by associated companies, branches and representatives
throughout the world.

First published 1993

0 443 04571 2

British Library Cataloguing in Publication Data
A catalogue record for this book is available from the British Library.

Library of Congress Cataloging in Publication Data
Neoplasms of the larynx/edited by Alfio Ferlito.
     p.   cm.
  Includes index.
  ISBN 0-443-04571-2
  1. Larynx-Cancer. I. Ferlito, Alfio.
  [DNLM: 1. Laryngeal Neoplasms. WV520 N438]
RC280.T5N46   1993
616.99'322-dc20
DLC
for Library of Congress   92-49877
                                                           CIP

The
publisher's
policy is to use
paper manufactured
from sustainable forests

Printed in Hong Kong
WC/01

About the Editor

Alfio Ferlito is Professor of Otolaryngology at the University of Padua School of Medicine. He graduated in medicine at the University of Bologna in 1968. He worked in the Pathology Department of Trieste University for two years. Since 1970, he has been working at the ENT Department of Padua University.

His contributions to the literature cover all fields of otolaryngology. He is author of about 200 scientific papers and chapters, the majority of which have been published in English, in the UK and in the USA. He has already edited a three-volume book entitled *Cancer of the Larynx* (CRC Press, Boca Raton, 1985) and is co-author of a book entitled *Granulomas and Neoplasms of the Larynx* (Churchill Livingstone, Edinburgh, 1988). He is an editor for the Journal for Oto-Rhino-Laryngology and its Related Specialties, for which he edited a special issue on Neuroendocrine Neoplasms of the Larynx (1991).

He is also on the Editorial Board of other international journals, such as: Annals of Otology, Rhinology and Laryngology; The Journal of Otolaryngology; Ear, Nose and Throat Journal; Advances in Therapy; Operative Techniques in Otolaryngology–Head and Neck Surgery; ORL Digest.

He is founder member and president of The Laryngeal Cancer Association and is also a member of various scientific societies, i.e. the American Laryngological Association, the Royal Society of Medicine of London, the Collegium Oto-Rhino-Laryngologicum Amicitiae Sacrum, the Japan Laryngological Association, the American Laryngological Rhinological and Otological Society, the American Society for Head and Neck Surgery, the American Broncho-Esophagological Association, the Association for Research in Otolaryngology, the American Academy of Otolaryngology–Head and Neck Surgery, the International Broncho-Esophagological Society, the Oto-Rhino-Laryngological Society of Japan, the New York Academy of Science, the American Association for the Advancement of Science and the International Academy of Pathology.

He was consultant in laryngeal pathology to Yale University. He was visiting professor at the Departments of Otolaryngology of the Universities of Yale (1985, 1987, 1988) and Pittsburgh (1988).

He has collaborated as a member of the World Health Organization's Committee on *Histological Typing of Tumours of the Upper Respiratory Tract and Ear* (whose findings were published in 1991) and is a member of The Laryngeal Cancer Association's Committee on the Classification of Laryngeal Cancer.

One of his chief interests is the promotion of international co-operation in cancer research.

For Churchill Livingstone

Publisher: Miranda Bromage
Project Editor: Lucy Gardner
Copy Editor: Paul Singleton
Indexer: Laurence Errington
Production Controllers: Nancy Arnott, Mark Sanderson
Sales Promotion Executive: Caroline Boyd

Contents

Contributors

Byron J. Bailey MD FACS
Wiess Professor and Chairman, Department of
Otolaryngology, University of Texas Medical Branch,
Galveston, Texas, USA

Leon Barnes MD
Professor of Pathology and Otolaryngology and Director,
Division of Anatomic Pathology, University of Pittsburgh
Medical Center, Pittsburgh, Pennsylvania, USA

Barry K. B. Berkovitz BDS MSc PhD
Reader in Anatomy, Biomedical Sciences Division,
Anatomy and Human Biology Group, King's College,
London, UK

Nicholas J. Cassisi DDS MD
Professor and Chairman, Department of
Otolaryngology–Head and Neck Surgery, University of
Florida College of Medicine, Gainesville, Florida, USA

Joseph N. El-Jabbour MD MRCPath
Senior Registrar, Department of Histopathology, Charing
Cross and Westminster Medical School, London, UK

Alfio Ferlito MD
Professor of Otolaryngology, University of Padua Medical
School, Padua, Italy

Michael Friedman MD
Associate Professor, Department of Otolaryngology and
Bronchoesophagology, Rush Medical College of Rush
University, Rush–Presbyterian–St Luke's Medical
Center, Chicago; Director, Head and Neck Treatment
Center, Illinois Masonic Medical Center, Chicago,
Illinois, USA

Imrich Friedmann MD DSc FRCS FRCPath DCP
Professor Emeritus of Pathology, University of London;
Formerly Director, Department of Pathology, Institute of
Laryngology and Otology and Consultant Pathologist,
Royal National Throat, Nose and Ear Hospital, London,
UK

Geerten J. Gerritsen MD PhD
Otolaryngologist/Head and Neck Surgeon, Red Cross
Hospital, The Hague, The Netherlands

William E. Golden MD
Director, Division of General Internal Medicine,
University of Arkansas for Medical Sciences, Little Rock,
Arkansas, USA

Sir Donald F. N. Harrison MD MS PhD FRCS
Professor Emeritus of Laryngology and Otology,
University of London; ENT Surgeon Emeritus,
Moorfields Eye Hospital, London, UK

Simon A. Hickey MA FRCS
Senior ENT Registrar, Charing Cross, Westminster and
Mayday Hospitals, London, UK

Haskins K. Kashima MD
Professor, Departments of Otolaryngology–Head and
Neck Surgery and of Oncology, Johns Hopkins Medical
Institutions, Baltimore, Maryland, USA

Robert C. Lavender MD
Associate Professor of Medicine, University of Arkansas
for Medical Sciences; Director, General Medicine Clinic,
Little Rock, Arkansas, USA

Brigid G. Leventhal MD
Director, Clinical Research Administrator, Associate
Professor of Pediatrics and Associate Professor of
Oncology, Johns Hopkins University School of Medicine,
Baltimore, Maryland, USA

Frank E. Lucente MD FACS
Chairman, Department of Otolaryngology, State
University of New York–Health Science Center at
Brooklyn; Chairman, Department of Otolaryngology,
Long Island College Hospital, Long Island, New York,
USA

Kenneth A. MacLennan DM MRCPath
Consultant Histopathologist, Royal Marsden Hospital;
Honorary Senior Lecturer, Institute of Cancer Reseach,
London, UK

Amy D. Mayer MD
Manhattan Eye, Ear and Throat Hospital, New York,
USA

Martyn S. Mendelsohn MB BS FRACS
Clinical and Research Fellow, Department of
Otolaryngology, Mount Sinai Hospital, University of
Toronto, Toronto, Ontario, Canada

William M. Mendenhall MD
Associate Professor, Department of Radiation Oncology,
University of Florida College of Medicine, Gainesville,
Florida, USA

Rodney R. Million MD
Professor and Chairman, Department of Radiation
Oncology, University of Florida College of Medicine,
Gainesville, Florida, USA

Idel I. Moisa MD
Attending Otolaryngologist, North Shore University,
Manhasset; Assistant Attending Otolaryngologist,
Department of Otolaryngology, Montefiore Medical
Center, The Albert Einstein College of Medicine, New
York, USA

Bernard J. Moxham BSc BDS PhD
Professor and Head of Department of Anatomy,
University of Wales College of Cardiff, UK

Yasushi Murakami MD
Professor and Chairman, Department of Otolaryngology,
Kyoto Prefectural University School of Medicine, Kyoto,
Japan

Eugene N. Myers MD FACS
Professor and Chairman, Department of Otolaryngology,
University of Pittsburgh School of Medicine, The Eye
and Ear Institute of Pittsburgh, Pittsburgh, Pennsylvania,
USA

Arnold M. Noyek MD FRCS(C) FACS
Otolaryngologist-in-Chief, Professor of Otolaryngology
and of Radiology, University of Toronto, Toronto,
Ontario, Canada

Jan Olofsson MD PhD
Professor and Head of Department of
Otolaryngology/Head and Neck Surgery, Haukeland
University Hospital, Bergen, Norway

James T. Parsons MD
Associate Professor, Radiation Oncology Department,
University of Florida Health Science Center, Gainesville,
Florida, USA

Loring W. Pratt MD FACS
Formerly Visiting Professor, Department of
Otolaryngology, Johns Hopkins School of Medicine,
Baltimore, Maryland, USA

Elie E. Rebeiz MD
Assistant Professor of Otolaryngology, Lahey Clinic
Medical Center, Burlington, Massachusetts, USA

Umberto Saffiotti MD
Chief, Laboratory of Experimental Pathology, Division of
Cancer Etiology, National Cancer Institute, Bethesda,
Maryland, USA

John B. Schofield MB BS MRCPath
Senior Registrar in Histopathology, Hammersmith
Hospital and Royal Postgraduate Medical School,
London, UK

Stanley M. Shapshay MD FACS
Chairman, Department of Otolaryngology-Head and
Neck Surgery, Lahey Clinic Medical Center, Burlington,
Massachusetts; Professor of Otolaryngology, Boston
University School of Medicine, Boston, Massachusetts,
USA

Harry S. Shulman MD FRCP(C)
Professor of Radiology, University of Toronto;
Radiologist-in-Chief, Sunnybrook Health Science Centre,
Toronto, Ontario, Canada

Carl E. Silver MD FACS
Professor of Surgery, Albert Einstein College of
Medicine; Director, Head and Neck Surgery, Montefiore
Medical Center, Bronx, New York, USA

Mark I. Singer MD
Professor, Department of Otolaryngology, University of
California at San Francisco; Chief, Head and Neck
Surgery, Mount Zion Medical Center of UCSF; Vice-
Chairman, Department of Otolaryngology, UCSF, San
Francisco, USA

Gordon B. Snow MD PhD
Professor and Head of Department of
Otolaryngology/Head and Neck Surgery, Free University
Hospital, Amsterdam, The Netherlands

Philip M. Stell ChM FRCS
Former Professor of Otolaryngology, University of
Liverpool, Liverpool, UK

Wendy B. R. Stern MD
Fellow in Head and Neck Surgery, Albert Einstein
College of Medicine, New York; Clinical Associate
Professor of Otolaryngology, University of Utah Medical
Center, Salt Lake City, Utah, USA

Scott P. R. Stringer MD
Associate Professor and Vice Chairman, Department of
Otolaryngology, University of Florida College of
Medicine, Gainesville, Florida, USA

Andrew C. Urquhart MB ChB FCS(SA)
Fellow, Head and Neck Oncologic Surgery, Department
of Otolaryngology, University of Pittsburgh School of
Medicine, Pittsburgh, Pennsylvania, USA

John A. H. Waterhouse MA PhD FFOM
Honorary Senior Research Fellow, Institute of
Occupational Health, University of Birmingham;
Formerly Director, Cancer Epidemiology Research Unit
and Director, Birmingham and West Midland Regional
Cancer Registry, Birmingham, UK

Bruce M. Wenig MD
Assistant Chairman, Department of Otolaryngic-
Endocrine Pathology and Chief, Otolaryngic Division,
Armed Forces Institute of Pathology, Washington, DC,
USA

Eiji Yanagisawa MD FACS
Clinical Professor of Otolaryngology, Yale University
School of Medicine, New Haven, Connecticut, USA

Dedication

This text is dedicated to the memory of my father, Mario Ferlito (1914–1990), to my wife Gianna, whose unfailing support and hard work have made the book possible, to my sons Mario and Giuseppe for accepting weekends at home while it was being written and to my brother Salvatore for his continual help.

A.F.

Preface

The larynx plays an important role as a site of neoplastic disease. This book presents an all-round account of the subject, starting from historical aspects of laryngeal cancer, embryology and anatomy of the normal larynx, epidemiology, considerations on prevention and experimental carcinogenesis. The majority of the text is devoted to the pathological and clinical aspects of all benign and malignant neoplasms of the larynx, dealing with classification (according to the WHO), diagnosis, treatment modalities, complications, rehabilitation and prognosis, and concluding with a discussion of psychological implications.

The essential function of this book is to record the present state of our knowledge on all aspects of laryngeal neoplasms. The contributors have been selected in view of their high stature in their respective specialist fields, which has meant involving experts from countries all over the globe. It has been a pleasure to collaborate with these distinguished authorities and there has been a valid and continuous exchange of opinions and information during preparation of the text.

Our hope is that this book will prove a useful tool for all physicians particularly involved in the pathology, diagnosis, treatment and prognosis of laryngeal neoplasms.

Padua, 1993   **A.F.**

Acknowledgements

I would like to thank the editors and publishers of the medical journals mentioned in the figure captions for allowing me to reproduce their illustrations.

Sincere thanks are also due to those colleagues whose illustrations and specimens have enhanced the quality of various chapters.

My grateful thanks also go to Frances Coburn for her help in shaping the English of the chapters assigned to myself.

Finally, I am indebted to my publishers, Churchill Livingstone, for making this book possible and particularly to Yvonne O'Leary, Lucy Gardner and Elspeth Masson for their patient and efficient assistance.

The generous financial support of The Laryngeal Cancer Association has been very helpful in the production of this book.

A.F.

1. Historical perspective

L.W. Pratt

The early history of laryngeal cancer is shrouded by the mists of time and obscured by the fact that medical workers in prehistoric and early historic times were lacking in the sophistication and knowledge necessary to make an accurate diagnosis by modern standards and prescribe adequate treatment for this disease.

Although the 'record in the rocks' has been helpful in determining skeletal characteristics in animals and in man, the larynx is composed chiefly of cartilage and lightly calcified cartilage, and is not preserved in the specimens which have been found. Those tumours which produce characteristic metastatic patterns of bone destruction may be suspected when the bony remains are studied, but laryngeal cancer does not usually spread by this route.[51] Even where laryngeal cartilages may have been found, the soft tissues associated with them are gone and identification of malignant changes have not been made. Several reports of autopsy studies on Egyptian and other mummies — and CT and MRI studies of mummies — have been made, but no indication of laryngeal malignancy has been found. One must take into account the fact that there have been a relatively small group of mummies so studied, although it is said that 'tens of thousands' of early Egyptian bodies have been studied in general. We know of reports of three osteogenic sarcomas, three carcinomas of the nasopharynx[146] and two melanomas from Peru, described by Urteaga and Pack in 1966.[140] It would be a fortuitous finding if, from such a small series, a malignancy of the larynx were identified, as these occur today at a rate of 2.5 per 100 000 population in males and 0.5 per 100 000 in females. Although laryngeal cancer does occur in children, it is uncommon to find it in children under fifteen years of age. Those so afflicted often have a history of laryngeal papilloma or previous radiation treatment, a therapeutic modality not available until the recent past.[48, 142] Although the current rate in males is nearly constant, the rate in females has increased by 150% in the past 30 years.[8,21,33,51,69,70,83,95,96,146]

Those unfortunates who did develop malignancies in their larynges in yesteryear must have died of asphyxiation, as tracheotomy was unknown to the ancients and adequate procedures for relief of airway obstruction were unknown. It is most likely that those cases of terminal upper airway obstruction secondary to malignancies were mingled with other diseases which also produced upper airway obstruction, such as croup, diphtheria, foreign bodies, trauma, and any other disease which produced severe respiratory obstruction.

Thus, study of the history of laryngeal cancer must be largely confined to more recent times during which there has been written evidence and historical data with which to confirm the presence and the diagnosis of this disease.

Aretaeus the Cappadocian referred to cancer of the larynx,[3] but there is little detail about the problem in his reports. Galen referred to a 'malignant ulceration of the throat' which could have been a report of laryngeal cancer, or it could have been some other part of the throat, or even some other disease.

Giulio Casserius described tracheotomy in 1601, in his text on speech and hearing. This text is illustrated with a dramatic plate showing the insertion of a tracheostomy tube into a patient who is obviously unanaesthetized and is completely terrorized.

Boerhave, in the 17th century, described a 'cancerous angina'.

In early times, infectious disease ran rampant and it seems logical to assume that in a population whose life expectancy was no more than an average of 20–30 years the most common causes of airway obstruction would be inflammatory diseases and foreign bodies. Historians tell us that life expectancy in ancient Rome and Greece was 20 years. It is hypothesized that, in medieval Europe, this had extended to 30 years, and, by 1850, life expectancy in the United States of America, had lengthened to 40 years. Currently, life expectancy in the United States exceeds 73 years, according to the Encyclopedia Americana. After 1900, both the population of the world and the life expectancy of the individual increased greatly, so one would logically anticipate that the incidence of laryngeal cancer would also increase significantly in the twentieth century.[129]

In general commentary, Hippocrates in Aphorism number 38. said 'It is better not to apply any treatment in cases of occult cancer; for, if treated, the patients die quickly; but if not treated, they hold out for a long time.'[2].

'All the ancient commentators explain that by "occult" may be meant either "not ulcerated" or "deep seated" . . . "when the disease is deep seated it is better to leave it alone.".'[2]

Ancient physicians made their examination and diagnosis of laryngeal lesions by intraoral palpation of the larynx, prior to the 19th century. Trousseau is said to have declared that visualization of the living larynx was impossible.[137]

It is now clear that laryngeal cancer is most commonly a disease of the elderly. The average age of onset is 59 years;[106] it is most common in those who smoke, and still more common among those who both smoke and drink alcohol regularly. Although the use of alcohol has long been a part of human culture, heavy smoking is a relatively recent addition to the social activity of man. In 1584 Sir Walter Raleigh visited America, and on his return to England he introduced smoking to the court — where its use became very popular.[144] In early times, life expectancy was short, and the average life of a man was less than thirty-five years. Even with the added carcinogenic effect of alcohol, the development of cancer at an early age is not common today.[48] It seems that synergism between alcohol and tobacco is a major factor in producing laryngeal cancer. Exposure to these two agents must usually be present for several years before their carcinogenic potential is realized.[75, 149–151]

When Columbus discovered America he found the American Indians used tobacco, smoking it much as we do today. This turned out to be one of the most important economic finds in the New World. Sir John Hawkins has been credited by some with bringing tobacco from Florida to England in 1565. Others believe that Sir Francis Drake brought tobacco back to England after sailing around the world in 1580. Other report that Roger Lane, Governor of Raleigh's colonizing effort in what has become North Carolina brought tobacco home to England with him in 1586. The gist of this indicates that by the middle of the 16th century tobacco had been introduced into England and may have come by a number of different routes. Tobacco is reported to have been growing in England by 1570. European settlers began to grow tobacco in Santa Domingo in 1531, Cuba in 1580, Brazil in 1600, Jamestown, Virginia, in 1612, and Maryland in 1631, according to the Encyclopaedia Britannica. This crop soon became the most important item of trade between the colonists and Europe. It is clear that Sir Walter Raleigh used tobacco at court in England,

and this undoubtedly enhanced its popularity and use among the general population at that time — so the complications of old age had little opportunity to wreak their havoc on the general population.[129–131]

Before 1600 there was no significant general exposure of European populations to the deleterious effects of tobacco. King James I of England was among the first to condemn the use of tobacco, in his *A Counterblaste to Tobacco*.[131] Cancer of the nose and lip was related to the use of snuff by John Hill in 1761 when he published his paper *Cautions against the immoderate use of Snuff*, and by Samuel Thomas von Soemmering in 1795 who pointed to the association of lip cancer with pipe smoking. In 1839 a report was published in France which showed that 66 out of 68 patients with cancer of the lips or other parts of the oral cavity, hospitalized in Montpelier, France, smoked short-stemmed clay pipes, and that all were pipe smokers.[131] In 1912 Adler suggested a relationship between smoking and lung tumours,[4] and in 1932 McNally suggested that tar in cigarette smoke could be responsible, by its irritating effect, for stimulating the growth of these malignancies.[86]

In May 1950, Wynder and Graham of the United States,[149] — followed in September of that year by Doll and Hill of Great Britain[31] — reported a definite aetiological association between smoking and the development of lung cancer.[5,31,150]

Prior to World War I, women in America rarely smoked in public, and they smoked much less in private than is the case today. The mores gradually changed, and by the close of World War II, women, in increasing numbers, were smoking both publicly and privately. It appears that these cancers are dose-related to smoking, and that 20 cigarettes per day for 20 years is the quantity of cigarettes beyond which the incidence of malignancy is more commonly a consequence. By 1965 many women had been smoking heavily for 20 years, and increasing numbers of tobacco-related malignancies made their appearance, in this previously favoured group; these malignancies are approaching the incidence of tobacco-related cancers in men. In 1963 the Royal College of Physicians of London pronounced cigarette smoking as a serious hazard to health. In 1964 the Surgeon General's Committee reported that there was a definite connection between lung cancer and smoking,[141] and in 1965 Federal legislation was passed which required a health hazard warning to be placed on all cigarette packages sold after 1 January 1966. In 1971, cigarette advertising was banned from television, and the American Cancer Society mounted a vigorous campaign calculated to deter smokers from continuing their habit and non-smokers from beginning. In the course of these developments, and changes in the social view of smoking, it became clear that cancer of the oropharynx and larynx was also intimately related to the use of tobacco and that this risk was increased if alcohol was also consumed on a regular basis.[34,90]

Although Janssen used lenses to magnify in 1590, the microscope, invented by van Leeuwenhoek in the 17th century, gave the first opportunity for detailed study of the structure of plants, tissues and otherwise invisible structures. Accurate tissue diagnosis of malignancy was dependent upon further development of the compound microscope. Morgagni, who died in 1771, described the gross findings in two cases of laryngeal cancer.[5]

In about 1850 Gehrlach demonstrated that tissues could be stained differentially with natural dyes; improvements in this process were subsequently made by the use of aniline dyes. With the added help of differential staining, medical diagnosis of tissue abnormalities was improved. Henle, Schwann and Kölliker developed the science of histology — to be followed by Malpighi, who was among the first of the biological scientists to utilize the microscope for the study of tissue architecture.[108] Müller, teacher of Virchow, developed the concept of the cell in normal and pathological anatomy, a concept which evolved with Virchow's teaching. It is paradoxical that Müller, who taught Virchow concluded wrongly that 'microscopical and chemical analyses can never become the means of surgical diagnosis'. Improved ability to make accurate microscopic diagnoses of tumour type and potential biological activity has come with years of studying the natural history of these tumours, and relating these studies to cellular architecture. Most laryngeal tumours are of epidermoid origin. Of Cady's 1968 series,[20] 55% of the non-epidermoid tumours were adenocarcinomas and 45% were sarcomas.[36,37,74,117,118,143]

Saffrey described, in detail, the lymphatic drainage of the supraglottic larynx. Hajek added a new dimension to this work when he identified anatomic compartments of the larynx by injecting dyes into different regions and then describing the limits within which the dye was permitted to spread by these membranes and bands of fibro-elastic tissue. His study was made to confirm his astute clinical observation that laryngeal oedema remained confined in compartments. He determined that even high injection pressures would not cause the dye to cross the ventricle. This work was corroborated by studies made by Pressman, who injected the dog, pig, human cadaver and some human volunteer larynges with dyes, and with radioactive isotopes, and identified both submucosal compartments and pathways of lymphatic vessels through which tumours spread. Tucker later demonstrated that elastic tissue formed the membranous boundaries separating the intralaryngeal compartments. The landmark work with whole organ sections and their interpretation was done by Kirchner, who combined the knowledge of biological activity with the anatomical complexities of the compartments of the larynx to produce a basic fund of knowledge upon which surgeons

rely when deciding on the most appropriate procedure for the particular patient.[109, 138] It is utilization of these concepts that has enabled surgeons to develop the concept of partial laryngectomy, improved their ability to interpret CT and MRI scans and to more precisely stage their patient's disease.[12,59–61,109,138]

The first real progress in visualization of the larynx came as a result of the work of Manuel Garcia, a singing teacher. Prior to this time, examination of the larynx was accomplished by palpation, externally, of the neck and intraorally of the glottis. It is said that some who were expert in this technique could diagnose palsies and tumours of the larynx. His report is of special interest:

'Presented with the ever recurring wish too often repressed as unrealizable, suddenly I saw two mirrors of the laryngoscope in their respective positions as if before my eyes. I went straight to Charriers, the surgical instrument maker, and asking if he possessed a small mirror with a long handle, was informed that he had a little dentist's mirror which had been one of the failures of the London Exhibition of 1851. I bought it for 6 francs. Having also obtained a hand mirror, I returned home at once, very impatient to begin my experiments. I placed against the uvula the little mirror (which I heated in warm water and carefully dried); then flashing upon its surface a ray of sunlight, I saw at once to my great joy, the glottis wide open before me, and so fully exposed that I could see a portion of the trachea. When my excitement had somewhat subsided I began to examine what was passing before my eyes. The manner in which the glottis opened and shut, and moved in the act of phonation, filled me with wonder.'

It is fortunate that Garcia was a singer, as his musical training had given him the ability to control his larynx and make such an examination more likely to succeed than had he been an individual untrained in such control of his voice mechanism. It was this contribution made by a singing teacher, not a physician, that opened the way for scientific progress in the field of laryngology as this made it possible to observe, record and compare findings in laryngeal disorders.[62,63,152] From today's viewpoint, one unbelievable technique was that of using a camel-hair brush and a retronasal syringe for applying materials to the larynx. These brushes were not sterilized, as this was before the time of Koch and Pasteur and practitioners in those days did not realize the very good possibility of passing tuberculosis, syphilis and other infectious diseases from one patient to another by this means. Further improvement in the techniques and instrumentation for visualization of the larynx came with the development of the laryngoscope, the use of electric illumination, the addition of the microscope to the viewing mechanism, the use of both optical and fibre-optic telescopes, and, finally, the application of photographic and video recordings with which to visualize and record for later study the vocal cords and their movements.[11,49,55]

EARLY HISTORY OF LARYNGEAL CANCER

Bronchotomy was the term first used to describe an opening into either the larynx or the trachea. This alternative approach to the airway was first described by Asclepiades, 'the restorer of medicine in Rome', as a means of providing an airway for those with obstruction to the passage of air through the larynx. It is reported that even in early Rome and Greece, intubation as a method of relieving respiratory distress was practiced in spite of the limited instrumentarium available to physicians at that time. The concept was opposed by great authorities such as Caelius Aurelaneus, Celsus and Areteus. It would appear that the operation was performed occasionally, and sometimes with success, even in those years. The Arab physicians Rhasis, Albucasis and Avenzoar never performed the procedure because of their fear of the results of the operation. It was not until early in the seventeenth century when Casserius, Fabricius ab Aquapendente[108] and a Parisian surgeon, Habicot, lent their enthusiasm to this subject.[112] Although most openings into the airway were thought to be adequate, Casserius first suggested the use of a tube to fix and maintain the airway. Laryngotomy was thought to be the most practical approach to maintaining an airway, due to the more superficial location of the larynx and the smaller amount of dissection necessary to provide the patient with an artificial airway than that required to open the trachea. Trousseau performed the first documented tracheostomy for carcinoma of the larynx in 1833.[137]

There is ample description of the usefulness of these procedures in the face of foreign body airway obstruction or acute oedematous change in the larynx, but relatively little specific attention was paid to chronic progressive obstruction lesions of the upper airway, into which group most laryngeal malignancies would fall. Liston, in 1837, discussed the usefulness of tracheostomy in the treatment of upper airway obstruction and included in that discourse chronic ulcerative lesions of the larynx, which he declared could be diagnosed *either* by palpation, or by the use of the dentist's mirror.[73]

As late as 1837, Ryland discussed tumours of the larynx and described cartilaginous tumours. The more interesting commentary is 'other tumours, which were probably of the same character, have occasionally been described as scirrhous or carcinomatous affections of the larynx have seldom, or perhaps never, been found, except when the disease has been propagated from the pharynx or oesophagus'.[112]

In 1837 Trousseau and Belloc published a monograph on 'Phthisie Laryngee' in which he says that phthisis is not a single disease, but rather a combination of disorders of different origins. He states that death due to these diseases is extremely rare and that more often death ensues from pulmonary complications. The term phthisis, today, is usually associated with tuberculosis, but Trousseau classified laryngeal phthisis in four groups,[137] as follows:

> 1° Phthisie Laryngee simple
> 2° Phthisie Laryngee syphilitique
> 3° Phthisie Laryngee cancereuse
> 4° Phthisie Laryngee tuberculeuse

It is clear from this classification that he recognized cancer of the larynx as a distinct entity, a fact substantiated by illustrations in his monograph which show drawings typical of cancer.[137]

SURGERY

The superb texts by Cummings, Loré, Montgomery, Silver and others have provided factual material on the techniques available to the surgeon which make it possible for one interested in surgery in this field to make fine distinctions with regard to indications and surgical techniques which will work to the benefit of their patients.[28,74,88a,118]

Total laryngectomy

The first total laryngectomy has been credited to Watson and was performed for syphilis of the larynx. Stell reports that, according to Watson's own account of the event, the patient, who had previously had a tracheostomy performed, died, and his larynx was removed post mortem. The confusion results from a misinterpretation of an ambiguous statement by Foulis fifteen years after the event.[28,32,126,127]

Billroth is credited with doing the first laryngectomy for cancer of the larynx seven years later.[1] The report of this case was not made by Billroth, but was made by his surgical assistant, Gussenbauer,[52] in 1874. This first patient to undergo total laryngectomy was a 36-year-old teacher of theology. He had a subglottic tumour which had produced hoarseness for about three years. The lesion had been treated by topical applications of silver nitrate and injections of liquor ferri, and was thought to be confined to the left side of the larynx — the right side being thought free of disease. A preoperative tracheostomy was performed, and the operation, facilitated by the use of a Trendelenburg (1871) tampon canula,[133] was performed on 27 November 1873; however, in spite of this, great trouble was encountered by aspiration of blood and the coughing which ensued. The left thyroid ala and the cricoid were split, and the tumour was removed by scissors and by curette. The base of the wound was cauterized and the wound irrigated with liquor ferri.

Closure was with plaster to approximate the wound edges. Examination on 16 December revealed that the left side of the larynx was filled with granulation tissue, and on 29 December the patient had increasing trouble breathing, to the extent that it was necessary to re-open the original tracheostomy during the night and re-insert the tracheal cannula. Repeat laryngofissure was recommended, and when the larynx was re-opened on 31 December it was found that the tumour had involved the perichondrium of the larynx and that further attempts at removal by laryngofissure would be hopeless. Anaesthesia was therefore lightened, and the patient was wakened and told of the surgical findings. Billroth recommended that total laryngectomy be performed. The patient agreed, was re-anaesthetized, and dissection was carried out through a vertical incision which was extended up to the hyoid bone. Scar tissue from the previous surgery, and much bleeding from the superior thyroid artery, complicated the surgical procedure. Hook retractors repeatedly tore out of the thyroid cartilage which was softened due to the 'granulation tissue'.* The patient became light and strained, increasing the problem with haemostasis. The trachea was divided and the tracheostomy cannula was put in place. The lower edge of the cricoid cartilage was dissected free of the anterior wall of the oesophagus, and the thyroid cartilage separated from the hypopharynx. The thyrohyoid ligament was cut as a final part of the separation and was associated with more bleeding — which was controlled by pressure of sponges. The base of the epiglottis and the upper two tracheal rings were removed. Both the tracheal stump and the pharyngeal opening were stitched to the skin with button threads. The 'edges of the esophagus' were brought 'in contact with one another to reduce the size of the wound'.[145] Neither the epiglottis nor hyoid bone were removed with the larynx. The patient's postoperative course was marred by haemorrhage from the superior laryngeal artery four hours after the surgery had been completed. This was controlled with some difficulty and, although the patient lost consciousness during this part of the procedure, he was revived and was able to cough large blood clots from his tracheobronchial tree. A postoperative fistula did develop, but the patient was taught how to cough secretion and food from the tracheostomy as well as how to introduce an oesophageal tube prior to eating. This fistula gradually decreased, and by the eighteenth day he was encouraged to eat solid food.[52]

It is of particular interest that this first laryngectomy patient was taught to use an artificial larynx, developed in 1874 by Gussenbauer,[52] with which he was able to be heard from one end of the ward to the other[126] — the instrument generating a dull, monotonous voice which

was loud and clear. The artificial larynx was made by substituting a device the general principles of which were suggested by Billroth, the mechanism of which was constructed by Gussenbauer. 'The vocal cords with a vibrating whistle tongue' were incorporated into a tracheostomy tube that connected to the resonating chamber of the nasopharynx, mouth and the adjacent cavities. Leiter and Thurriegl, instrument makers, manufactured the instrument. The patient was discharged from the hospital on 3 March 1874, swallowing well, free of cancer and able to communicate. The tumour recurred in four months and the patient died seven months after surgery.[53,54,145]

Mackenty, in 1926, selected his cases with great care, and as a result of this prudent selection he eliminated all but the most favourable intrinsic cases. Meticulous attention to the details of the surgery, postoperative care, surgical technique and the use of a tracheal tube, designed by the surgeon, which protected the airway during the surgical procedure were all essential factors in his considerable success. He used a combination of general and local innovations which provided the patient with intrinsic cancer a greatly improved outlook, but left those with extrinsic cancer little help as he considered that extrinsic was, and ever would be, inoperable.[77] New, in 1928, introduced the two-stage laryngectomy calculated to reduce the incidence of infectious complication and to reduce the incidence of postoperative complications associated with fistulas.[91] The narrow-field approach embodied the Crowe–Broyles technique of laryngectomy, and it accomplished many of the desirable features of such surgery, i.e., little disturbance of fascial planes and support of wound closure by preservation of the perichondrium of the larynx, thus reducing the problem of postoperative fistulization. These narrow-field procedures were applicable only to intrinsic lesions of the larynx and were useless in disease which had extended beyond the confines of the larynx, or which had arisen on extracordal sites.[27,33,35]

The introduction of antibiotics in the early 1940s contributed significantly to improvement in the results of laryngectomy, and to some extent obviated the need for narrow-field procedures as more extensive dissections could now be accomplished with less risk of devastating infection producing wound breakdown, fistulas and secondary haemorrhage from major vessels.

The more rational approach then made to carcinoma of the larynx was that of radical resection, based on the pathological nature and extent of the disease. Even in the pre-antibiotic era, Schall advocated the use of wide exposure which included the area of primary disease and all of its extensions. His construction of the tracheal stoma, following removal of the strap muscles, made the use of a tracheostomy tube a rare necessity. This approach led to the development of wide field procedures

---

* The author feels that this was most likely caused by invasion of the laryngeal cartilages by cancer.

to remove the lymphatic channels and nodes in the cervical region as part of the laryngectomy. With the advent of antibiotics, these procedures became safer and there was a marked decrease in postoperative morbidity.[14,25,30,56,57,92,97–99,110,113–115]

Stomal recurrences have been one of the serious complications associated with total laryngectomy. These recurrences are more commonly associated with subglottic cancers, and it has been well demonstrated that they are more common in patients who have had preoperative tracheostomies. For many years, radiotherapy was used in an effort to control or palliate these metastatic lesions, but without significant success. The use of preoperative or immediate postoperative radiation has been found of help in reducing the number of these recurrences. In 1975 Sisson reported a series of 28 patients treated surgically with 48% survival for one year and 32% for three years. This technique has been a significant contribution to the control of this ominous complication.[43,44,111,117,118,121,122,148]

It has been suggested that perhaps we make too much of the difficulty of the technical procedure of total laryngectomy — in view of a patient who was admitted to an army hospital with a large wound in his neck and a specimen, carried in a paper bag, made up of his larynx, including hyoid bone, thyroid gland, three parathyroid glands, trachea to the third ring and about one-half inch of the oesophagus. He is reported to have written that he did this with a single-edge razor blade, putting his fingers in the trachea, and with traction on the specimen, cutting it off. Repair was done and he survived.[116] Not all self-performed laryngectomies survive the immediate post-surgical period.[47]

Kaiser Frederick Wilhelm III and Morell Mackenzie

Perhaps the most discussed laryngeal cancer in all history is that of Prince Frederick Wilhelm III of Germany. When he developed hoarseness and difficulty with his throat in January, 1887, the German laryngologists were called to see him and pronounced his lesion to be a malignancy of the vocal cord. Biopsy was attempted but the procedure was unsuccessful because the lesion was hard and flat. A series of thirteen treatments with galvano-cautery were given without improvement in the lesion, and a panel of six German physicians agreed that the lesion had recurred and was growing larger. This group was unanimously of the opinion that the lesion was cancer and that it should be removed via thyrotomy. Erndt von Bergmann, Professor of Surgery at Berlin, planned to operate without telling Frederick either the nature of his disease or the planned procedure until just before the time of surgery. Objection was raised by both Bismark and Princess Victoria. Bismark insisted on consultation with the 'best' laryngologist in Europe

(Massey).[84] Frederick's wife, Princess Imperial, daughter of Queen Victoria, communicated to her mother the problem with which her husband was confronted, and the Queen, distrusting the knowledge and skill of the German physicians, insisted that Morell Mackenzie be called to see the Prince. Mackenzie was the leading British laryngologist; he responded promptly to the summons of his Queen and travelled to Germany to see the ailing Frederick. There he found a lesion which was sessile: 'a growth about the size of a split pea at the posterior part of the left vocal cord ... pale pink, slightly rough on the surface, but not lobulated ... a portion of the growth disappeared from view ... it was partly attached to the undersurface as well as the side of the vocal cord ... there was no trace of ulceration ... to the naked eye (it) bore the look of a simple wart or papilloma'.[76,96] Mackenzie insisted that it was wrong to perform a total laryngectomy before establishing a tissue diagnosis of malignancy and proceeded to take a total of three biopsies over the course of time. As the disease progressed, inexorably, it became clear clinically that the lesion was malignant, and in spite of the absence of a positive biopsy report, Mackenzie, von Schrötter and others ultimately signed a statement saying that they had established the fact that the Crown Prince's disease was due to a malignant new growth. The Crown Prince refused laryngectomy, although he eventually consented to tracheostomy to relieve his airway obstruction. One month after his tracheostomy, his father, the Emperor, died, and he was crowned Emperor. He died miserably on 15 June 1888, 99 days following his coronation, after many complications of tracheostomy, metastases, aspiration pneumonia and pulmonary gangrene. Post mortem examination confirmed the diagnosis of subglottic laryngeal carcinoma, with complete destruction of the larynx, except for the epiglottis, and its replacement by a large gangrenous ulcer.[78–81]

It has been suggested by Minnegerode[88] that Frederick's underlying disease was syphilis, producing its tertiary lesion in the larynx, and that it was often noted in such cases that neoplasia developed from the underlying luetic lesion. He indicates the political problems associated with such a diagnosis, and credits Mackenzie with willingly accepting the opprobrium associated with an erroneous diagnosis rather than revealing the true nature of Frederick's illness.

A lamentable consequence of the Kaiser's death was recrimination between German and British physicians about the management of the case. Mackenzie, citing hostility and jealousy on the part of the German physicians as the motive for their recrimination, finally responded to the controversy by the publication of a book, *The Fatal Illness of Fredrich the Noble*, which detailed the illness and suffering of the monarch, in addition to the clumsiness of the German physicians. He subsequently resigned from the Royal College of Surgeons, when it was broadly hinted that his resignation would be welcomed because of what were considered to be his unprofessional revelations concerning the illness of Frederick and the German physicians who assisted in his care. Only Virchow remained aloof from the controversy, thus preserving his dignity and reputation in this most unseemly storm of vindictive vituperation.

The stress associated with this regrettable situation has been credited with aggravating Mackenzie's asthma, which had been a significant problem for him over the years but which worsened during the time of these controversies. This, associated with cardiac problems and the depression, which reasonably followed such a series of confrontations leading to his resignation from the Royal College of Physicians, is thought to have contributed to his premature demise at the age of 55 in 1892.[23,45,46,53,54,71,72,76,81,84,85]

Rudolph Virchow, the world's foremost pathologist at that time, examined the three biopsies taken from Frederick's larynx by Mackenzie. None of these minute ($3 \times 2.5 \times 2.5$ mm; 2 mm in diameter; $5 \times 3 \times 2$ mm) biopsies contained tissue which would permit him to make the diagnosis of malignancy. The larynx had been biopsied repeatedly and treated with electrocautery thirteen times before these specimens were taken by Mackenzie. His diagnosis was verrucous pachydermia. A fourth specimen, which was expectorated, was described by Virchow as suggesting 'imperfectly masticated meat, ... or gangrene'. In each of his reports, Virchow made special note of the small size of the biopsy specimens with which he had been presented, and the limited value of his diagnostic and prognostic efforts because of the tiny size of the specimens from which he was forced to work. In those days the value of biopsy was not uniformly accepted by all surgeons, and it was the custom to send material for microscopic evaluation only if the surgeon was unsure of his gross diagnosis of the problem at hand.[99] The last specimen expectorated by Frederick was not reviewed by Virchow but was studied by Waldeyer (who first described the hypopharyngeal and pharyngeal lymphoid tissue now known as Waldeyer's ring) who stated that 'although there was no alveolar structure, he considered that from the relation of the nest cells to one another, he thought they could not have been produced superficially, but were evidently the result of a deep-seated destructive process'. On the basis of the extensive proliferation of the tumour, Waldeyer, for the first time, made the diagnosis of malignancy, nine months after the first negative biopsy had been reported.

The presumption, which has been made repeatedly in the ensuing years, that early correct diagnosis of Prince Frederick's cancer would have altered the course of world events, assumes that a cure of his tumour and longevity would have been the inevitable result. As a matter of fact, in those years, total laryngectomy carried with it nearly a 40% operative mortality. Some 25% of the patients developed recurrence of their cancers within six months, and only 8.5% lived free of disease for more than twelve months. Had Frederick been within that fortunate group, the course of world history might well have been changed if one believes that the influence of one individual on the course of world affairs could have been that significant; however, the likelihood that he would have been so fortunate is very small (8.5% or less) considering the fact that he had numerous previous biopsies and treatments with cautery which had delayed his treatment for some time before Mackenzie saw him for the first time. The growth was subglottic to begin with. Although subsequent delays were certainly contributing factors to the spread of his disease, there is significant doubt in this author's mind that the course of world history would have been significantly altered had he agreed to total laryngectomy.

Partial laryngectomy

Partial laryngectomy preceded total laryngectomy, as surgeons, for many years prior to the time of Billroth, performed less aggressive — and also less effective — procedures in their attempts to eliminate cancers of the larynx. In 1851 Buck performed a tracheostomy for an extensive intralaryngeal malignancy, with death resulting fifteen months later. Although Langenbeck recommended laryngectomy in 1854, Buck excised a cancer of the larynx via thyrotomy in 1855. In 1863, Sands obtained the first long-term control of cancer via laryngofissure. The use of laryngofissure continued over the years for the control of smaller and intrinsic lesions of the larynx, but was not thought to be applicable to extrinsic tumours. After Billroth's first successful total laryngectomy, more attention was paid to the use of total extirpative surgery, and this continued to the inclusion of total laryngectomy with en bloc radical neck dissection. Brunschwig continued this progression and reported five cases of radiation failure treated successfully by total laryngectomy combined with radical neck dissection, which he designated as panlaryngectomy.[17]

Once surgeons learned that it was both possible and practicable to remove successfully both larynx and tumour-bearing lymph nodes, they began to study the possibility of performing smaller operations in the form of partial laryngectomy, in selected cases. Criteria were developed, and a variety of procedures were refined to meet the needs of this new concept. In some instances it was necessary only to adapt procedures which had been previously used in order to apply them to the treatment of laryngeal malignancy. All agree that there is no sense in doing a smaller procedure unless it provides reasonable hope that total removal of the tumour can be accomplished and that the patient will live free of disease.

Techniques developed by Trotter, Wookey, Orton and Alonso, among others, became useful in utilizing vertical partial laryngectomy which made possible the removal of lesions primary in the pyriform sinus which had invaded only the lateral portion of the larynx.[6,10,11,15,104,105,134,135,147]

Laryngofissure

In order to remove a foreign body, Pelletan opened the larynx in 1778, and a variant of this procedure was performed by Desault in 1820. Brauers, in 1833 coupled thyrotomy with actual cautery to remove a growth from the larynx, with patient survival for 20 years. In 1844, Ehrman removed a laryngeal polyp via thyrotomy following a previously done tracheostomy. In 1851, the first laryngofissure for cancer was performed by Buck, without the benefit of anaesthesia. In 1863, using this technique, Sands operated for carcinoma and the patient lived for two years to die of an unrelated cause. The first successful laryngofissure in Great Britain was performed by Gibb, using chloroform for anaesthesia. It was not until 1867 that Solis-Cohen was able to report a permanent cure of cancer of the larynx following laryngo-fissure, when he reported a 20-year postoperative survival, free of cancer. In 1878, von Bruns reported 19 thyrotomies in 15 patients. Of this entire group, only two lived more than one year, and, of these two, one died at 22 months of an unrelated disease. Because the removal of malignant tumours by this approach was usually a piecemeal procedure, it was not usual to accomplish a complete removal of the tumour. In its early days, this procedure did not meet with approval because of the dismal results and associated high mortality rate. As anaesthetic technique and postoperative care improved, mortality became less of a problem, and in 1894 Semon reported eight cases with two operative deaths; in 1895 Butlin reported 14 cases with one operative death, and in 1938 St Claire Thomson was able to report 38 cases without a single operative death. Part of the success of St Claire Thomson's surgery was attributed to elimination of the sedative medications usually associated with the administration of chloroform, and improvement in attention to removal of tracheal secretions in the post-operative period.[132]

Concurrent with improvement in surgical technique and postoperative management of the patient, there came about improvement in the statistics of patient survival. In the ten-year period between 1897 and 1907, Semon was able to report an increased three-year survival rate which rose from 8.7% to 60%. Schmieglow in 1920 reported operative mortality of seven out of thirty-nine laryngofissure operations. In 1923, Fraser reported three mortalities from a group of fourteen patients. The statistics continued to soar, with Thomson reporting 51

patients of whom 11 died of causes other than cancer (eight cases with local recurrence) — representing 80% of the cases with 'enduring cure.' Jackson, in 1927 was able to report 29 three-year cures out of a group of 45 patients, and in 1928 Thomson reported 76% three-year cures. In 1930, Gluck and Sorenson reported 110 'long-term' cures out of a group of 125 patients, with the additional salvage of four patients by total laryngectomy.[132]

Thus we have been able to follow the course of laryngofissure from its early days when the procedure was poorly understood, anaesthesia was either inadequate or not used at all, and the postoperative care of the patient was less than desirable. As time passed and adequate anaesthetic techniques were developed (which permitted more deliberate and accurate surgical removal of tumours), coupled with more meticulous attention to tracheal toilet in the postoperative period, both the operative mortality statistics and the postoperative survival statistics improved remarkably. The procedure of laryngofissure became an accepted and acceptable method of managing cancer of the larynx and is used today in certain specific situations.[15,30,58,65,66,123]

Vertical laryngectomy

The first vertical hemilaryngectomy was performed by Billroth in 1878, five years following his first total laryngectomy. Although he was the leader in inaugurating this field of surgery, Gluck enhanced the procedure by developing a technique for removal of half of the larynx, removing half of the thyroid and cricoid cartilages and one arytenoid. The surgical defect was surfaced by rotation of a large skin flap into the defect and leaving a large laryngostomy, which was closed as a secondary procedure. The selection of tumours for this surgery was not made according to modern standards, and tumours with both fixed vocal cords and subglottic extension were treated by this technique, with resulting high rates of recurrence. For this reason, the operation fell into bad favour until more definite criteria for its application were developed. The laryngostomy was a bothersome part of the procedure which contributed to postoperative morbidity for the patient, and it was not until primary closure of the larynx (facilitated by preservation of the cricoid cartilage) was accomplished that this became an acceptable and useful procedure in the management of patients. The important workers in this field were Clerf (1940), Leroux-Robert (1956), Kemler (1947) and Norris (1958). Methods of closing the wound were improved by Figi (1950), Meurman (1953) and Som (1959). These technical improvements made the procedure much more useful, and it is now a standard part of the laryngeal surgeon's armamen-tarium.[24,39,40,58, 67,68,87,93,94,100,125]

Pharyngotomy and supraglottic partial laryngectomy

Astley Cooper is reported to have removed a large epiglottic tumour with his fingers in the early 19th century. Pratt, a French naval surgeon, is credited with the removal of an epiglottic tumour by way of a subhyoid pharyngotomy, and others were reported to have developed techniques for the supra-, sub- and transhyoid approaches to the hypopharynx. This approach provided limited exposure of the lesion and made removal of a tumour both difficult and often incomplete.

Kronlein was the first to plan and utilize a lateral subhyoid or suprahyoid approach to expose tumours of the lateral part of the base of the tongue, the pyriform sinus and the hypopharynx. The major problem with his procedure was that adequate closure of the defect produced by the removal of a large tumour was not possible. The first really practical approach to this region was made by Trotter who devised a practical approach to the lateral pharyngotomy associated with partial laryngectomy. His technique provided good access to the epiglottis, aryepiglottic fold, lateral pharyngeal wall and the pyriform sinus. This technique was utilized and improved by Colledge and by Orton, to the extent that a 1938 paper by Colledge reported a 29% cure in 55 cases of lateral pharyngotomy and pharyngolaryngectomy. As useful as these procedures were, there was still considerable morbidity associated with them and they were not commonly used until Alonso combined this approach with partial horizontal laryngectomy, refining the indications for the exact procedure to be accomplished dependent upon the precise size and location of the malignancy. The anatomical fact which made this type of surgery possible was that there is no connection between the lymphatics above and below the true vocal cords. This formed the anatomical and logical basis for conservation surgery. By applying this advancement in knowledge, Ogura, Som and Bocca continued to delineate the details of these procedures and developed specific techniques for each laryngeal compartment.[13,15,100–103,134–136]

It was the additional contributions of Kirchner to knowledge of the compartments of the larynx and the behaviour of tumours located in different parts of the larynx that made possible the surgical decisions regarding the location and extent of tumour to be removed. With these new approaches, it has been possible to achieve a high rate of cure with a minimum amount of postoperative disability. As Thomson said in 1925, 'Removal should be planned in regard to the location of the disease and not in reference to the removal of an organ.' He predicted that the use of laryngofissure would increase, and the utilization of total laryngectomy would decrease as the years pass and public education concerning the importance of hoarseness is improved.[59–61,109,132]

RADIATION THERAPY

Radiation therapy has long been an integral part of the treatment of malignancies. It has met two especially important necessities in the care of the patient. It has been used in the treatment of early, small malignancies, and in attempts to palliate large tumours which were beyond the scope of surgical removal. Since the discovery of X-rays, announced by Röentgen on 30 November 1895, gradual progress has been made over the years to determine the parameters within which this agent has become an important source of therapeutic help in the management of malignancies of all sorts. This is true also of laryngeal cancer. Laryngeal cancer has been one of the sites treated over the years, but its location where the airway and digestive tract cross has provided the site for debilitating, severe reactions which interfered with both nutrition and patency of airway. The lack of effectiveness of therapy, and the long-term complications of external irradiation, were in part related to poor penetration of early X ray beams; additionally, the osteocartilaginous framework of the larynx is highly susceptible to perichondritis. As with any new modality, due to the lack of understanding of the many ramifications of its potential, there was at first no real control of the amount of radiation administered, and the selection of cases was often improper, by present day standards. Treatment was given for many cases of widespread disease which we know today cannot be satisfactorily managed by such therapy. It was not until 1919 that the roentgen was accepted as the standard unit of dose, common to both X-irradiation and gamma radiation, and only after that time could adequate control of dosage be provided to permit accurate repetitive treatment and the exchange of data between different facilities. X-rays were the prime modality until 1905, but after that, radium and its emanations became the more popular method for treating laryngeal cancer. In 1909, Finzi applied radium externally, and ultimately telecurie therapy became the method of choice in the form of the cobalt bomb. Currently, use of the linear accelerator has replaced most of the other radiation sources because of its greater accuracy in isolating a field for treatment, and its ability to treat properly the desired area of the tumour-bearing organ.

Radioactivity was discovered by Becquerel in 1895; its use was enhanced when, in 1898, the Curies discovered radium. It was not long before the therapeutic potential of radium was recognized, and experimentation with both X-ray and radium therapy, and with the combination of both modalities, was begun. It was true that X-radiation could be applied to a wide area, but the damage to the skin and superficial tissues, and the difficulty of delivering a dose in depth to lesions in the body cavities, made the application of radiotherapy by encapsulated radium irradiation more desirable as those carriers could be inserted directly into the tumour and adequate radiation delivered directly to the tumour site without exposing the overlying skin to the full dose. As one would expect, there were many complications and accidents as a result of the early experimentation with the therapeutic use of radiotherapy. Laryngeal cancer was treated by the application of radium tubes, loaded into a catheter and inserted into the lumen of the larynx. The advent of radon gas provided one more source for radio-emanation, and capsules containing radon gas were utilized as sources for emanation in the treatment of laryngeal cancer. Finzi and Harmer were the first to demonstrate that laryngeal cancer could be cured by radium therapy, without also producing severe complications. Their treatment plan was useful only in the treatment of early lesions of the true vocal cord.[41]

Telecurie therapy was an important advance in which a source of radium, providing significant doses of gamma radiation, was placed near the tumour site and the emanations directed to the area in need of treatment. There were a variety of applicators which were devised to improve the application and control of therapy from these sources, and which improved from radium and radon gas to cobalt-60 (known as the cobalt bomb). In 1933, Seivert designed an apparatus which allowed treatment of cancer of the head and neck with greater accuracy than any previously developed equipment. This was followed by improvements and modifications made by Grimmett in 1936 who designed a safer and more convenient radium beam therapy unit which was especially useful in the treatment of cancer of the larynx. This evolved into the cobalt bomb which utilized Co^{60} as its source of radioactivity. Currently, the most desirable form of radiotherapy is derived from the use of the linear accelerator, which is able to deliver tumorocidal doses of radiation to precise targets, sparing the skin and superficial tissues from the full effect of the treatment dosage.[9,18,19,29,38,41, 42,49,50,64,118]

LASER THERAPY

Development of the surgical laser depended upon fundamental principles of stimulated emissions formulated by Lord Rayleigh in the latter part of the 19th century. Einstein, in 1917, laid the foundation for the development of a practical laser, which was constructed by Patel in 1964. He used CO_2 as the active medium and produced a beam in the infrared spectrum. This instrument has been of great use in laryngeal surgery. Its use was studied and developed by Jako and Strong, and it has become an important adjunct to the surgical armamentarium for laryngeal surgery. Although its use is not without some hazard of fire, this may be managed by standard safety procedures. The ability to vaporize premalignant lesions, small malignancies — and especially the ability to remove, en bloc, small laryngeal malignancies — has made it a popular instrument. It is of special use in the tiny larynx of the infant.[22] Laser energy is also useful in debulking large tumours, so that preoperative tracheostomy may be avoided and the likelihood of stomal recurrence thereby reduced.[124-128]

COMBINED THERAPY

The use of combinations of types of therapy has been of interest to many head and neck surgeons. Because it is difficult to accept failure in any particular case, many surgeons have endeavoured to improve their statistical survival results by using preoperative radiation, intraoperative radiation, and postoperative radiation. These modalities, in recent years, have been combined with chemotherapeutic agents used either for induction therapy or for definitive therapy. It has been well demonstrated that early tumours of the vocal cord can be cured in about the same statistical numbers by radiation as can be cured with surgery. The more advanced tumours respond better to surgery, with radiation administered as a postoperative measure. Although Goldman in 1967 and LeRoux-Robert in 1956 utilized radiation preoperatively, it has been well demonstrated that more postoperative fistulae and problems with wound healing result than with those patients given postoperative radiation. Radiotherapy is often of great help in palliating the patient with extensive disease.[48,50,67]

Some chemotherapeutic agents give startlingly good temporary palliation, but long-term cures of the squamous cell lesions which are encountered in the head and neck, as represented by the larynx, do not in general make long-term favourable response to such agents.

VOCAL REHABILITATION

The need for some method of providing speech for the alaryngeal patient apparently originated with Czermak in 1859 when he attended a patient who was voiceless because of a completely stenotic larynx. At that time he envisaged an artificial larynx as the solution to this problem. This need was considered important on the very first total laryngectomy done for cancer. Billroth suggested some possibilities by way of constructing a speaking tube, and Gussenbauer implemented them by making a tube with a vibrating reed and an air connection to the pharynx which permitted speech, so that the first patient with a total laryngectomy also had a practical speaking device which worked well. As more cases of total laryngectomy were done, the use of a pseudovoice became part of almost every patient's life. Four different types of pseudovoice were identified by Stern in 1923:

pseudowhispered speech or buccal speech, pharyngeal pseudospeech, oesophageal pseudospeech and 'stomach' pseudospeech. Many of the criteria for surgical procedures, calculated to provide improved pseudovoice capability were detailed by Stern and reiterated with embellishment by Morrison. Schall was among those to popularize the instruction of the patient in the use of oesophageal speech with which he was able to return almost all of his patients to a useful, functioning life. The need to swallow air and then use it by regurgitation for the production of voice has produced an intermittent and sometimes staccato type of speech. To improve on this situation, a number of devices have been employed to introduce air into the pharynx. The vibrating reed of the artificial larynx which utilizes air from the tracheostomy, passing it over a vibrating reed which produces a tone and introducing it into the mouth where movements of the tongue and pharynx may modify it, thus forming understandable words, was superseded by the electronic larynx which, by mechanical vibration of the outside of the neck, caused vibratory motion in the pharyngeal air and gave the opportunity to speak with this vibrating column of air. Both of these methods required external devices and were never adjudged wholly satisfactory, although they did permit easy communication between patient and others and were relatively easy to master. One of their best features was that they could often be utilized by those unable to learn oesophageal speech. The quest for an internally located fistula from trachea to pharynx was stimulated by the patient who made himself such a fistula by the application of a red hot poker, following which speech was possible. One of the most ingenious of such devices was a vein graft, devised by Conley, in which a connection between the tracheal airway and the pharynx was made by inserting a piece of vein into this region to act as a conduit for air and thus permit speech. This worked quite well, but had the disadvantage that it sometimes allowed aspiration to be associated with its presence. In some cases of advanced carcinoma of the larynx, it is possible to perform a near-total laryngectomy, using the techniques of Pearson, by which a permanent air channel is maintained so that speech may be utilized with relative ease. Although these patients must usually wear a tracheostomy tube, they are usually pleased with their ability to converse with this technique.[7,26,82,89,107,119,139]

Artificial fistulous tracts, dependent upon a prosthetic device, have been popularized by Singer, Panje, Sisson and others. These tracts are essentially fistulous connections between tracheal airway and oesophageal lumen. In all of these techniques, a small prosthetic device, tube or button, is placed in the septum separating the airway from the food passage. This permits the patients to pass vibrating air into his oesophagus or pharynx and then modify its vibrations by using his tongue, pharynx and lips so that he can produce intelligible speech.[16,119,120]

CONCLUSIONS

Although laryngeal cancer has undoubtedly been present for centuries, we do not have definite records of it. It is clear that there were occasional cases reported in early Greece and Rome, but the small population and the short life expectancy, unassociated with the use of tobacco, made it a less important cause of death than the infectious diseases, pestilence, wars and other causes of death. The social use of tobacco was introduced in the mid 1500s. Populations increased and longevity increased from the 30-year level of the medieval years until, by 1850, man, at birth, could look forward to 40 years of life. Until Billroth did the first total laryngectomy for cancer in 1873, no effective therapy for these tumours was known. Following that landmark case, further surgery was attempted and these surgical endeavours went from total laryngectomy to narrow-field laryngectomy — to be followed by wide-field laryngectomy and radical en bloc resection of larynx with associated lymphatic drainage fields. From this point, with the advent of effective antibiotics and radiotherapy, the pendulum swung back toward reconstruction of the surgical defect. Then came the effort to minimize the operative defect with conservation surgical techniques which were dependent upon a more complete understanding of the nature of the disease, the anatomy and physiology of the larynx, and the selective surgical procedures which could be utilized to remove the involved segments of the larynx with complete excision of the tumour while leaving the patient with a functioning larynx. These changes and improvements in technique have been of great benefit to the patient and have revolutionized the outlook, care and longevity of the patient with cancer of the larynx. From the time of the first laryngectomy, the serious significance of loss of voice has been well understood by physicians and many devices, artificial larynges and techniques for teaching oesophageal speech have been developed. We live in exciting times in which laryngeal cancer is considered a preventable disease; however, once it is present, effective means of care and techniques for developing speech are available. The evolution of this process makes a fascinating study.

It is of special interest to note that in all of prehistoric and historic time, until the first laryngectomy done by Billroth in 1873, 120 years ago, cancer of the larynx was a disease with 100% mortality. Since that time, and especially in the past 40 years, improvements in knowledge and understanding of the nature and natural history of the disease, coupled with new surgical techniques and advances in radiation therapy, have altered the outlook for the patient to the extent that the five-year cure rate is now over 80%, the operative mortality is a very reasonable 1% or 2%, and the outlook for the afflicted individual is much more hopeful than was previously the case. The most hopeful feature of all this is that the individual, with better understanding of the aetiological importance of tobacco smoking in laryngeal cancer, has the opportunity to prevent or avoid this disease and never has to confront the serious problems with which it is beset.

On the basis of historical perspectives, it seems safe to predict that new and increasingly effective modalities and treatments for the prevention, therapy, and rehabilitation of patients with laryngeal cancer will yet appear and make this disease one less feared in the future

ACKNOWLEDGEMENTS

The author would like to thank Gert Brieger, MD, and Edward T. Mormon, PhD, of the Institute of the History of Medicine, Johns Hopkins University, Baltimore, Maryland, for their generous help and assistance in locating materials and in loaning the materials used in the illustrations.

The author is also deeply indebted to Mrs Cora Damon, Librarian at the Mid-Maine Medical Center in Waterville, Maine, for her many hours of work in locating materials which were essential to the background for this work.

CHRONOLOGY

Laryngoscopy

	Celsus. Mentioned dentist's mouth mirror 'specillum'
1743	Leveret. Oral speculum and snare for removal of polyps
1804	Bozzini. Light conductor and oral speculum
1829	Babington. Glottisscope demonstrated to Hunterian Society
1837	Liston. Method of exploring larynx
1844	Avery. Directed illuminator for laryngoscope
1855	Garcia. Laryngeal mirror with which he first observed his own larynx
1858	Czermak. Confirmed usefulness of laryngeal mirror
1858	Turck. Confirmed usefulness of laryngeal mirror
1866	Turck. Treatise on diseases of the larynx
1850	Mackenzie. Indirect laryngoscopy and biopsy
1895	Kirstein. Proximal illuminated laryngoscope Brunnings. Killian. Jackson. Combined endotracheal anaesthesia with laryngoscope — introduced under direct vision — added distal illumination Clerf.
1913	Janeway. Open-sided laryngoscope with distal illumination — battery in handle
1941	Miller. Long straight blade, open on side distal illumination
1943	MacIntosh. Curved, open-sided blade with distal illumination
1972	Jako. Wide-mouthed scope, dual distal illumination for use with laser
1972	Ikeda. Fibre-optic laryngoscopy
1980	Yanagisawa. Videorecording of laryngeal pathology and function

Laryngectomy

100 AD	Araeteus. Referred to laryngeal cancer
200	Galen. 'Malignant ulceration of the throat'
1565	Sir John Hawkins. Took tobacco to England
1585	Sir Walter Raleigh. Introduced the use of tobacco to the court in England
1732	Morgagni. Autopsy findings in laryngeal cancer
1809	Pathology of the membrane of the larynx and bronchia
1824	Development of achromatic microscope
1826	Porter. Treatise on surgical pathology of larynx and trachea
1829	Albers. Removed larynx of an animal
1833	Brauers. Laryngofissure, tumour treated with cautery
1835	Trousseau. First documented tracheostomy for laryngeal tumour
1837	Trousseau, Belloc. Laryngeal phthisis
1844	Ehrmann. First to remove laryngeal polyp, following tracheotomy two days previously
1850	Virchow. Cellular pathology re diagnosis of cancer
1851	Green. First to describe cystic and malignant growths of larynx
1851	Laryngofissure for removal of cancer— recurrence — death one year
1851	Buck. Laryngofissure with tracheotomy for extensive intralaryngeal lesion; recurrence — death 15 months later
1854	Garcia. Use of laryngeal mirror
1854	Langenbeck. Recommended laryngectomy — unsuccessfully
1855	Buck. Excision of cancer via thyrotomy
1856	Koeberle. Suggested possibility of total laryngectomy
1858	Krakowizer. First in America to demonstrate the vocal cords
1858	Cutter. Demonstrated new two-tube laryngoscope: one tube for observation and one for light
1856–1858	Bouchut. Intubation of larynx for croup
1856	Jacobi. Had a mirror made with which he examined the larynx of one of his patients
1858	Virchow. Rise of histopathology; first accurate study of tumours

1859   Maxwell. Not only had a mirror made, with which he examined the larynx of his patients, but with which aid he carried out local treatments

1860   Stangenwald. Read a description of Garcia's laryngoscope to the New York Medico-Chirurgical College on 14 June

1861   Krackowizer. Stated that he 'was the first person in America who had seen vocal cords in a living subject'.

1861   von Bruns. Indirect laryngoscopy for removal of large polyp of vocal cord

1861   Green. Predicted: 'If that instrument can be brought into general use, I am confident that the profession will be able to cure diseases which are now too frequently overlooked.' Became one of the first in America to apply topical medications to the larynx

1861   Elsberg. Began a series of lectures on laryngology in the Medical Department of the City of New York University

1861   Lewin. First recorded removal of laryngeal tumour with the aid of a laryngoscope

1863   Sands. Laryngofissure with first long-term control of laryngeal cancer

1863   Elsberg. Promoted the importance of the laryngoscope and invented many instruments (brush, sponge carrier, porte-caustic, fumigation tube and electropole). One of the founders of the American Laryngological Association (and its first president). He utilized the laryngoscope to take biopsies of the larynx

1865   Cutter. Attempted photography of the larynx

1866   Watson. First total laryngectomy for syphilis—for constant aspiration of food and saliva. (There is some suggestion that this was a post-mortem procedure.)

1866   Cutter. Laryngofissure, without tracheotomy, for removal of laryngeal growth

1866   Solis-Cohen. Gave detailed account of the method of using the laryngoscope

1867   Voltolini. First used galvanocautery in laryngeal surgery

1867   Solis-Cohen. Laryngofussure with long-term survival (20 years)

1870   Czerny. Reported many laryngectomies on dogs, and that it was a feasible operation

1871   Lushka. Gave an accurate description of the larynx

1871   Mackenzie. Treatise on laryngeal tumours, indirect laryngeal biopsy. Advocated use of laryngoscope. Reported 100 cases of his own and 89 of other laryngologists

1873   Wagner. Organized the Laryngological Society of New York

1873   Billroth. First total laryngectomy for cancer. Precepts: 'diagnosis, excision, cure, rehabilitation'

1874   Heine. Second laryngectomy: six-month survival

1874   Maas. Third laryngectomy: two-week survival; fourth laryngectomy: four-day survival

1874   Billroth. His second laryngectomy: four-day survival

1874   Langenbeck. First wide-field laryngectomy; extended laryngectomy with neck dissection

1875   Bottini. First successful laryngectomy with long-term survival (sarcoma of larynx)

1875   Harvard Medical School, New York College of Physicians and Surgeons included laryngology in its curriculum

1876   Isambert. Classified laryngeal tumours as intrinsic and extrinsic

1877   Foulis. Total laryngectomy, Glasgow

1877   Solis-Cohen. Total extirpation of larynx for adenocarcinoma, attaching the free end of the trachea to the skin of the midline of the neck

1878   Billroth. First conservative hemilaryngectomy — recurrence of tumour after six months

1878   MacEwen. First to intubate larynx for anaesthetic purposes

1878   von Bruns. Collected 19 laryngofissures on 15 patients. Two survivors of one year or more

1878   Knapp. Joint Section on Ophthalmology and Otolaryngology formed by the American Medical Association under the chairmanship of Hermann Knapp of New York

1878   Elsberg. Founded the American Laryngological Association

1879   Krishaber. Classified cancer of the larynx as intrinsic or extrinsic and observed that the intrinsic lesions grow more slowly than do the extrinsic ones

1879   Lange. First laryngectomy in the USA

1879   Caselli. Voice prosthesis

1880   Tiersch. Laryngectomy with long-term survival

1880   Mackenzie. Stated: 'Endolaryngeal treatment . . . the radical removal of an ill-defined tumour cannot be efficiently accomplished by this method'

1880–1883 Elsberg, Solis-Cohen, Knight, Lefferts. Founded the Archives of Laryngology

1881   Foulis. Collected case reports of 32 laryngectomies from literature and reported not one alive after one year

1881   Gluck. Two-stage laryngectomy—devised to reduce aspiration of secretions and infection of the skin of the neck

1881	Foulis. Reported 27 total laryngectomies, 50% mortality within first week (pneumonia, pyaemia or collapse; 25% recurrence within 10 months of operation). No survival of one year
1882	O'Dwyer. First intubated patient with laryngeal airway
1884	French. Perfected method of photographing larynx
1885–1888	O'Dwyer. Intubation of larynx
1886	Solis-Cohen. Favoured limited surgery Semon, Butlin — England Okada — Japan Bruno — Germany
1886	Youtis, Czerny. Favoured total laryngectomy
1886	Cassanelo. First total laryngectomy in Uruguay
1886	Solis-Cohen, Cisneros. Reported 108 laryngectomies done from 1876 to 1886, 21 'cures.' This report included 60 cases reported by Zesas, with 15 'cures'; operative mortality: 45%–50%
1887	*Journal of Laryngology and Rhinology* reported 103 laryngectomies (39% died of immediate effects of operation between the time of operation and eight weeks postoperatively, over half from pneumonia). Recurrence of tumour in 20%. Total laryngectomy was not considered to be successful unless the patient lived more than 12 months, as it was felt that tracheostomy alone would accomplish this. Only 8.5% of the cases (a total of 9 patients out of 103) met this criterion
1887	Mackenzie and Crown Prince Frederick of Germany
1887	Störck. First case with pseudovoice following laryngectomy
1888	Sendziak. Reported 110 laryngectomies, perioperative mortality 45%
1889	Voltolini. First peroral laryngeal surgery with external illumination
1891	Solis-Cohen. Improved tracheal stoma by severing trachea
1892	Crile. First total laryngectomy in America
1892	Solis-Cohen. Successful total laryngectomy reported to Philadelphia County Medical Society
1893	Perez. First total laryngectomy in Argentina
1894	Gluck. Single-stage operation for laryngectomy
1895	Kirstein. Developed laryngoscope 'autoscopy of larynx'
1895	Röentgen. Discovered X-rays
1895	Rotter (Hartley). First to close pharyngeal wound with sutures
1896	First publication of *The Annals of Otology, Rhinology and Laryngology* and the *Laryngoscope*
1897	Bulhaóes. First total laryngectomy in Brazil
1898	Curies discovered radium
1900	Bisi. Reported from Argentina many laryngeal operations, from cordectomy to total laryngectomy
1900	Kuhn. Flexible metal intubation tube, long enough to protrude from mouth
1900	Delavan. First to say that surgery for laryngeal cancer should be done by trained teams of surgeons in certain hospitals
1901	Kraus. Four hundred and fifty cases: 13% alive without recurrence after one year, 1% after three years
1902	Delavan. Discussed the use of radium
1906	Crile. Suggested importance of lymphatic dissection in head and neck tumours
1909	Chiari. Surgery only treatment which produces positive cures. Stressed advantage of total over partial laryngectomy
1912	Killian. Suspension laryngoscopy
1913	Trotter. First practical method of resection of tumours of supraglottic larynx and lateral pharyngeal wall
1913	Bloodgood. Recommended en bloc dissection of nodes of neck
1913	Gluck, Sorensen. Developed technique of removing larynx from above, thereby reducing sepsis by closing pharyngeal defect first
1915–1920	Orthovoltage 200–400 kV radiotherapy
1915	Razetti. First total laryngectomy in Venezuela
1921	St Clair Thomson. Observed that carcinoma of the vocal cord usually originates on the anterior third of the cord
1922	Coutard. Demonstrated fractional radiation can control laryngeal cancer
1922	Okada. Removed regional lymph nodes, except in well-localized intrinsic cancer
1922	Delavan. Reported that Quick had treated 156 laryngeal cancers with radium
1922	MacKenty. Reported 31 laryngectomies without operative mortality
1922	Gluck, Sevenson. Reported 160 of their own procedures, the last 63 without a fatality
1925–1940	Surgery treatment of choice for intrinsic cancer of larynx; radiotherapy for extrinsic cancer
1927	Portmann. Reported roentgen therapy often used for cancer of the larynx
1927	Clerf. Reported surgical procedures so satisfactory that roentgen therapy should be condemned
1927	Jackson. Reported on 45 laryngofissure

patients, 29 three-year cures, many salvages by subsequent total laryngectomy

1927   Semken. Described and advocated radical neck dissection

1928   New. Two-stage laryngectomy

1930   Supravoltage therapy

1931   Jackson, Babcock. Wide-field laryngectomy

1932   New. Palliative roentgen therapy recommended. Some cases of severe damage were being reported

1934   New, Waugh. Seventy-three laryngectomies with one death

       Martin, Ellis. Popularized aspiration biopsy

1935   Cetra. Presented 200 laryngectomies with 5% operative deaths and 25%–32% survival with no recurrence

1936   Buckley. Roentgen therapy only for lesions of soft parts of the larynx. A fixed cord is a contraindication

1938   Crowe, Broyles. Narrow-field laryngectomy for 'operable and intrinsic growths of the larynx' (no invasion of either cartilage or lymphatics). Preservation of thyroid cartilage periosteum for repair

1938   Müller. Related lung cancer to the use of tobacco

1940   Martin. Recommended radiotherapy for extrinsic cancers. He did not feel total laryngectomy could be safely combined with radical neck dissection

1940   Clerf. Pointed out special relationship between anterior commissure lesions and pre-epiglottic space

1940   Jackson. Popularized narrow-field laryngectomy for intrinsic lesions

1940–1960 Radiation therapy for early cancer and surgery for advanced cancer of the larynx

1940   Portmann. Advocated use of temporary pharyngostome

1940   Riveros. First total laryngectomy in Paraguay

1941   Cobalt-60 available

1942   Clerf. Prophylactic neck dissection

1942   Kernan. Laryngectomy with neck dissection is preferred operation for extrinsic cancer

1944   Sylvestre-Benis. In Argentina, on the basis of 250 cases, recommended either partial or complete radical (either unilateral or bilateral) neck dissection, at time of laryngectomy

1944   Brown, McDowell. Recommended preservation of spinal accessory nerve and resection of platysma as part of specimen

1944   Vasconselos, Barretto. Laryngectomy using pharyngeal clamp which obviates need to open pharynx

1946   New. Laryngectomy with subsequent radical neck dissection in 568 cases, 78% operable, 60% 5-year cures

1947   Alonso. First practical conservation surgery — supraglottic laryngectomy with preservation of voice

1947   Martin. Extrinsic cancer of the larynx is primarily a surgical problem, to be followed by neck dissection later if necessary

1947   De Sel, Agra. Recommended bilateral cervical node resection in all cases of laryngectomy, except in those with move-able cords or lesions of the anterior commissure

1947   Cleves. First total laryngectomy in Colombia

1948   Desjardins. Reported 7–8% 5-year cures of patients treated with roentgen therapy for inoperable carcinoma of the larynx

1951   Martin. Surgical technique for laryngectomy and neck dissection standardized, opposed prophylactic neck dissection

1951   Cobalt-60 first used for teletherapy

1952   Alonso. Advocated conservation surgery, partial vertical and partial horizontal laryngectomies with nodal dissections, temporary pharyngostomy

1952   Edgerton. One-stage excisional–reconstructive laryngectomy

1953   Negus. One-stage excisional–reconstructive total laryngectomy

1953   Conley. One-stage excisional–reconstructive total laryngectomy

1960   Jessberg. Recommended radiotherapy for early intrinsic lesions and laryngectomy with radical neck dissection for extrinsic lesions

1960   Regules. In Uruguay, partial vertical and horizontal laryngectomies, 90 cases

1961   Postoperative radiation

1962   Clinical staging system for cancer of the larynx

1962   Suarez. In Argentina, 580 cases partial laryngectomy

1964   Goldman, Silverstone. Preoperative radiation

1965   Federal legislation passed requiring all cigarette packages to carry health hazard warning labels

1971   All cigarette advertising banned on television in the USA

1974   Goldman. Use of indirect laryngoscopy for biopsy of laryngeal tumours

1987–1988 The International Union Against Cancer and the American Joint Committee on Cancer publish a single global TNM classification system for staging laryngeal cancer

1988   The Laryngeal Cancer Association founded

ERAS IN LARYNGEAL CANCER

Prehistory Death by asphyxiation

Early history Tracheotomy; death permitted from cancer

1873–1900 Laryngectomy with high operative death rate and high morbidity; cures rare

1900–1925 Debate about need for biopsy, endolaryngeal, surgery, thyrotomy or laryngectomy. Laryngectomy only for favourable (intrinsic) cancers; radiation therapy gaining favour for extrinsic lesions

1925–1940 Radiation therapy; restricted use of laryngectomy. Although more knowledgeable in laryngeal problems and endolaryngeal techniques, most laryngologists lacked skill and knowledge in general surgery requisite for good laryngectomy care

1940–1960 Period of enlarging scope of laryngectomy, including laryngopharyngeal cancer with the addition of radical neck dissection; beginning of use of radiotherapy in combination with surgery

1960–present Period of combined therapy, pre- and postoperative radiotherapy. Period of reconstruction and rehabilitation and increased use of conservation techniques to preserve laryngeal function. The use of chemotherapy, both as therapy for cancer and as induction therapy prior to surgery in the effort to make otherwise inoperable lesions manageable by surgery. Cobalt-60, the linear accelerator, and the use of the laser have each, in their own way, contributed to the better control and therapy of laryngeal lesions in these years. The introduction of computerized axial tomography and magnetic resonance imaging have contributed greatly to improvement in the diagnostic capability of the physician and thus to the care of the patient.

REFERENCES

1. Absolon K B 1977 Theodore Billroth in Vienna 1867–1880. Aust N Z J Surg 47: 837–844
2. Adams F 1929 The genuine works of Hippocrates translated from the Greek with a preliminary discourse and annotations. William Wood, New York
3. Adams F 1856 Aretaeus the Cappadocian, edited and translated by London , and printed for the Sydenham Society, pp 249–255
4. Adler I 1912 Primary malignant growths of the lungs and bronchi. Longmans Green, New York
5. Alberti P W 1975 Panel discussion: the historical development of laryngectomy. II. The evolution of laryngology and laryngectomy in the mid-19th century. Laryngoscope 85: 288–298
6. Alonso J M 1947 Conservative surgery of the larynx. Trans Am Acad Ophthalmol Otolaryngol 51: 633–642
7. Asai R 1965 Asai's new voice production method: a substitution of human speech. Trans 8th Int Congr Otorhinolaryngol. Tokyo
8. Babin R W, Kahane J C, Freed R E.1990 Exercise in paleo-otolaryngology: head and neck examination of two Egyptian mummies. Ann Otol Rhinol Laryngol 99: 742–748
9. Ballenger J J 1991 Diseases of the nose, throat, ear, head and neck, 14th edn. Lea and Febiger, Philadelphia
10. Baretto P M 1975 Panel discussion: the historical development of laryngectomy. IV. The South American contribution to the surgery of laryngeal cancer. Laryngoscope 85: 299–321
11. Birkitt H S 1923 Transatlantic development of rhinolaryngology. Laryngoscope 33: 1–16
12. Blitzer A 1979 Mechanisms of spread of laryngeal carcinoma. Bull N Y Acad Med 55: 813–821
13. Bocca E 1975 Supraglottic cancer. Laryngoscope 85: 1318–1326
14. Bocca E, Pignataro O 1967 A conservation technique in radical neck dissection. Ann Otol Rhinol Laryngol 76: 975–978
15. Bocca E, Pignataro O, Mosciaro O 1968 Supraglottic surgery of the larynx. Ann Otol Rhinol Laryngol 77: 1005–1026
16. Brodnitz F S, Conley J J 1967 Vocal rehabilitation after reconstructive surgery for laryngeal cancer. Folia Phoniatr 19: 89–97
17. Brunschwig A 1943 Panlaringectomy for advanced carcinoma of the larynx. Surg Gynecol Obstet 76: 390–394
18. Bryce D P 1979 The management of laryngeal cancer. J Otolaryngol 8: 105–126
19. Bryce D P, Ireland P E, Rider W D 1963 Experience in the surgical and radiological treatment of 500 cases of carcinoma of the larynx. Ann Otol Rhinol Laryngol 72: 416–430
20. Cady B, Rippey J H, Frazell E L 1968 Non-epidemoid cancer of the larynx. Ann Surg 67: 116–120
21. Cancer facts and figures 1991 American Cancer Society
22. Carden E, Ferguson G B 1973 A new technique for microlaryngeal surgery in infants. Laryngoscope. 83: 691–699
23. Clark W D, Quinn F B 1984 Erroneous reporting of errors. Am Med Assoc 252: 207–208
24. Clerf L H 1940 Cancer of the larynx: an analysis of two hundred and fifty operative cases. Arch Otolaryngol 32: 484–498
25. Conley J J, Vonfraenkel P H 1956 Historical aspect of head and neck surgery. Ann Otol Rhinol Laryngol 65: 643–655
26. Conley J J, De Amesti F, Pierce M K 1958 A new surgical technique for the vocal rehabilitation of the laryngectomized patient. Ann Otol Rhinol Laryngol 67: 655–664
27. Crowe S J, Broyles E N 1938 Carcinoma of the larynx and total laryngectomy. Proc Am Laryngol Soc 60: 47–63
28. Cummings C W, Fredrickson J M, Harker L A, Krause CJ, Schuller D E 1986 Otolaryngology—head and neck surgery. Mosby, St Louis
29. Delavan D B 1902 The results of treatment of laryngeal cancer by means of the X-ray. Laryngoscope 12: 299–302
30. Devine K 1963 Laryngectomy. Vicissitudes in the development of a good operation. Arch Otolaryngol 78: 816–825
31. Doll R, Hill A B 1950 Smoking and carcinoma of the lung. Br Med J 30: 739–748
32. Donegan W L 1965 An early history of total laryngectomy. Surgery 57: 902–905
33. El-Najjar M, Aufderheide A C, Ortner D J 1985 Preserved human remains from the Southern region of the North American Continent: Report of autopsy findings. Hum Pathol 16: 273–276
34. Facts on cancer of the larynx 1987 American Cancer Society
35. Fenton R A 1947 A brief history of otolaryngology in the United States from 1847 to 1947. Arch Otolaryngol 46: 153–162
36. Ferlito A 1985 Diagnosis and treatment of verrucous squamous cell carcinoma of the larynx: a critical review. Ann Otol Rhinol Laryngol 94: 575–579
37. Ferlito A 1986 Diagnosis and treatment of small cell cancer of the larynx: a critical review. Ann Otol Rhinol Laryngol 95: 590–600
38. Ferlito A 1987 Malignant laryngeal epithelial tumors and lymph node involvement: therapeutic and prognostic considerations. Ann Otol Rhinol Laryngol 96: 542–548
39. Figi F A 1950 Removal of carcinoma of the larynx with immediate skin graft for repair. Ann Otol Rhinol Laryngol 59: 474–486
40. Figi F A, Havens F Z, Erich J B 1947 Carcinoma of the larynx. Methods and results of treatment. Surg Gynecol Obstet 85: 623–629

41. Finzi N S, Harmer D 1928 Radium treatment of intrinsic carcinoma of the larynx. Br Med J 2: 886–889
42. Freer OT 1922 Carcinoma of the larynx treated locally with radium emanation. A clinical report. J Am Med Assoc 79: 1602–1606
43. Freudenthal W 1906 Experiences with radium in diseases of the throat and nose. J Adv Ther 24: 279–287
44. Friedberg S A, Faber L P 1970 Surgery for unanticipated mediastinal and tracheal extension of recurrent laryngeal cancer. Surg Clin North Am 50: 1051–1058
45. Garrison F H 1939 History of medicine with medical chronology suggestions for study and bibliographic data. Saunders, Philadelphia
46. Gerlings P G 1968 Laryngeal carcinoma — some considerations with reference to the illness of Emperor Frederick III. Eye, Ear, Nose and Throat Monthly 47: 58–66
47. Giles C 1956 Suicidal laryngectomy. J Forensic Med 3: 91–93
48. Gindhart T D, Johnston W H, Chism S E, Dedo H H 1980 Carcinoma of the larynx in childhood. Cancer 45: 1683–1687
49. Goldman J L, Roffman J D 1975 Indirect laryngoscopy. Laryngoscope 85: 530–533
50. Goldman J L, Cheren R V, Silverstone S M, Zak F G 1967 Combined irradiation and surgery for cancer of the larynx and laryngopharynx. In: Conley J J (ed) Cancer of the head and neck. Butterworths, Washington
51. Gregg J B, Gregg P S 1978 Dry bones, Dakota territory reflected. Sioux Falls South Dakota
52. Gussenbauer C 1874 Ueber die erste durch Th. Billroth am Menschen ausgeführte Kelkopf-Exstirpation und die Anwendung eines künstlichen Kehlkopfes. Arch Klin Chir 17: 343–356
53. Holinger P H 1975 Panel discussion: the historical development of laryngectomy. I. Introduction of panel on historical development of the laryngectomy. Laryngoscope 85: 287
54. Holinger P H 1975 Panel discussion: the historical development of laryngectomy. V. A century of progress of laryngectomies in the northern hemisphere. Laryngoscope 85: 322–332
55. Ikeda S 1970 Flexible bronchofiberscope. Ann Otol Rhinol Laryngol 79: 916–923
56. Jesberg N 1958 Carcinoma of the larynx. Contralateral metastasis in lesions approaching the midline. Laryngoscope 68: 1251–1256
57. Jesberg N 1960 Laryngectomy: past, present and future. Ann Otol Rhinol Laryngol 69: 184–198
58. Kemler J L 1947 Bilateral thyrotomy for carcinoma of the larynx. Laryngoscope 57: 704–724
59. Kirchner J A 1986 A historical and histological view of partial laryngectomy. Bull N Y Acad Med 62: 808–817
60. Kirchner J A 1989 What have whole organ sections contributed to the treatment of laryngeal cancer? Ann Otol Rhinol Laryngol 98: 661–667
61. Kirchner J A, Carter D 1987 Intralaryngeal barriers to the spread of cancer. Acta Otolaryngol 103: 503–513
62. Koltai P J, Nixon RE 1989 The story of the laryngoscope. Ear Nose Throat J 68: 494–501
63. Konrad H R, Hopla DM, Bussen J, Griswold FC 1981 Use of videotape in diagnosis and treatment of cancer of the larynx. Ann Otol Rhinol Laryngol 90: 398–400
64. Lederman M 1975 Panel discussion: the historical development of laryngectomy. V I. History of radiotherapy in the treatment of cancer of the larynx 1896–1939. Laryngoscope 85: 333–353
65. LeJeune F E 1951 The surgical treatment of early carcinoma of the larynx. Laryngoscope 61: 488–495
66. LeJeune F E, Lynch M G 1955 The value of laryngofissure operation. Ann Otol Rhinol Laryngol 64: 256–262
67. Leroux-Robert J 1956 Indications for radical surgery, partial surgery, radiotherapy and combined surgery and radiotherapy for cancer of the larynx and hypopharynx. Ann Otol Rhinol Laryngol 65: 137–153
68. Leroux-Robert J 1975 Panel discussion on glottic tumors. IV. A statistical study of 620 laryngeal carcinomas of the glottic region personally operated upon more than five years ago. Laryngoscope 85: 1440–1452
69. Lewin P K, Harwood-Nash D C 1977 X-ray computed axial

tomography of an ancient Egyptian brain. Int Reg Commun Sys Med Sci 5: 78
70. Lewin P K 1987 First stereoscopic images from CT reconstructions of mummies. Am J Radiol 151: 1249
71. Lin J I 1984 Occasional notes. Virchow's pathological reports on Frederick III's cancer. J Am Med Assoc 311: 1261–1264
72. Lin J I 1985 Death of a Kaiser. Landfall Press
73. Liston R 1837 Practical surgery. Churchill, London
74. Loré J 1988 An atlas of head and neck surgery, 3rd edn. Saunders, Philadelphia
75. Lowry W S 1975 Alcoholism in cancer of the head and neck. Laryngoscope 85: 1275–1280
76. Lucente F E 1973. The impact of otolaryngology on world history. Trans Am Acad Ophthalmol Otolaryngol 77: 424–428
77. Mackenty J R 1926 Cancer of the larynx. Arch Otolaryngol 3: 205–232, 305–337
78. Mackenzie J N 1900 A plea for early naked-eye diagnosis and removal of the entire organ, with the neighboring area of possible lymphatic infection in cancer of the larynx. Trans Am Laryngol Assoc 22: 56–65. (Cited by C Jackson and C L Jackson 1939 in Cancer of the larynx. Saunders, Philadelphia)
79. Mackenzie M 1880 Diseases of the pharynx, larynx and trachea William Wood, New York
80. Mackenzie M 1880 A manual of diseases of the nose and throat, vol 1. Churchill, London, pp 342, 518
81. Mackenzie M 1888 The fatal illness of Frederick the Noble. Sampson Low, Marston, Searle and Rivington, London
82. Majer E H, Reider W 1973 Laryngectomy with preservation of the air passages. ORL J Otorhinolaryngol Relat Spec 35: 200–204
83. Marx M, D'Auria S H 1988 Three-dimensional CT reconstructions of an ancient human Egyptian mummy. Am J Radiol 150: 147–149
84. Massey R U 1987 The ninety-nine day Kaiser. Conn Med 51:61
85. McInnis W D, Egan W, Aust J B 1976 The management of carcinoma of the larynx in a prominent patient, or did Morell Mackenzie really cause World War I? Am J Surg 132: 515–522
86. McNally W D 1932 The tar in cigarette smoke and its possible effects. Am J Cancer 16: 1502–1514
87. Meurman Y 1953 Extended cordectomy for intrinsic laryngeal cancer: application and results. Plastic covering of excision surface. In: Proc 5th Int Congr Otol Rhinol Laryngol. Amsterdam
88. Minnigerode B 1986 The disease of Emperor Frederick III. Laryngoscope 96: 200–203
88a. Montgomery W W 1989 Surgery of the upper respiratory system, 2nd edn. Lea & Febiger, Philadelphia
89. Morrison W W 1931 The production of voice and speech following total laryngectomy. Arch Otolaryngol 14: 413–431
90. Muller F H 1940 Tabakissbrauch und Lungencarcinoma. Z Krebsforshung 38–86
91. New G B 1928 A two-stage laryngectomy. Surg Gynecol Obstet 47: 826–830
92. New G B, Figi F A, Havens F Z, Erich J B 1947 Carcinoma of the larynx. Methods of treatment and results. Trans Am Acad Ophthalmol Otolaryngol 85: 623–629
93. Norris C M 1958 Technique of extended fronto-lateral partial laryngectomy. Laryngoscope 68: 1240–1250
94. Norris C M. 1979 Contributions of Philadelphia to early laryngology. Ann Otol Rhinol Laryngol 88: 128–131
95. Notman D H N, Tashijian J, Aufderheide A C, Cass OW, Shane O C III, Berquist T H, Gray J E, Gedgaugas E 1986 Modern imaging and endoscopic biopsy in Egyptian mummies. Am J Radiol 146: 93–96
96. Ober W B 1970 The case of the Kaiser's cancer. Pathol Annu 5: 207–216
97. Ogura J H 1955 Surgical pathology of cancer of the larynx. Laryngoscope 65: 867–926
98. Ogura J H 1976 Progress of otolaryngology in head and neck surgery. Ann Otol Rhinol Laryngol 85: 425–427
99. Ogura J H, Bello J A 1952 Laryngectomy and radical neck dissection for carcinoma of the larynx. Laryngoscope 62: 1–52
100. Ogura J H, Dedo H H 1965 Glottic reconstruction following subtotal glottic-supraglottic laryngectomy. Laryngoscope 75: 856–878

101. Ogura J H, Spector G J 1976 The larynx. In: Nealon T F (ed) Management of the patient with cancer. Saunders, Philadelphia, pp 206–238

102. Ogura J H, Marks J E, Freeman R B 1980 Results of conservation surgery for cancers of the supraglottis and pyriform sinus. Laryngoscope 90: 591–600

103. Ogura J H, Sessions D G, Ciralsky R H 1975 Conservation surgery for carcinoma of the supraglottic larynx. Laryngoscope 85: 180–1815

104. Orton H B 1938 Cancer of the larynx. Immediate and ultimate results of operation in one hundred and two cases. Arch Otolaryngol 28: 153–192

105. Orton H B 1956 Surgery of carcinoma of the larynx. Arch Otolaryngol 64: 205–206

106. Paparella M M, Shumrick D A 1980 Otolaryngology. Saunders, Philadelphia

107. Pearson B W 1986 Near total laryngectomy. In: Cummings C W, Fredrickson J M, Harker L A, Krause C J, Schuller D E (eds) Otolaryngology head and neck surgery, vol 3. Mosby, St Louis pp 2117–2132

108. Pratt L W 1987 Presidential remarks: Fabricius of Aquapendente. Trans Am Laryngol Assoc 108: 13–17

109. Pressman J, Dowdy A, Libby R, Fields M 1956 Further studies upon the submucosal compartments and lymphatics of the larynx by the injection of dyes and radioisotopes. Ann Otol Rhinol Laryngol 65: 963–980

110. Putney F J 1958 Preventive dissection of the neck in cancer of the larynx. Ann Otol Rhinol Laryngol 67: 136–144

111. Rosenberg P J 1971 Total laryngectomy and cancer of the larynx. Arch Otolaryngol 94: 313–316

112. Ryland F A 1837 Treatise on the diseases and injuries of the larynx and trachea. Longman, London

113. Schall L A 1938 Laryngectomy: its place in the treatment of laryngeal cancer. Penn Med J 41: 261–267

114. Schall L A 1951 Symposium: Carcinoma of the larynx. IV. Cancer of the larynx — five year results. Laryngoscope 61: 517–522

115. Schall L.A 1954 The patient after laryngectomy. In Ellis M (ed) Modern trends in diseases of the ear nose and throat. Butterworths, London

116. Schuessler W W 1944 Self inflicted excision of the larynx and thyroid and division of the trachea and esophagus with recovery. JAMA 125: 551–552

117. Silver C E 1981 Surgery for cancer of the larynx and related structures. Churchill Livingstone, New York

118. Silver C E 1991 Laryngeal cancer. Thieme, New York

119. Singer M I 1983 Tracheoesophageal speech: vocal rehabilitation after total laryngectomy. Laryngoscope 93: 1454–1465

120. Singer M I, Blair E D 1979 Tracheoesophageal puncture: a surgical prosthetic method for postlaryngectomy speech restoration. Third international symposium on plastic and reconstructive surgery of the head and neck. New Orleans, Louisiana

121. Sisson G A, Bytell D E, Becker S P 1977 Mediastinal dissection — 1976: indications and newer techniques. Laryngoscope 87: 751–759

122. Sisson G A, Bytell D E, Edison B D, Yeh S Jr 1975 Transsternal radical neck dissection for control of stomal recurrences—end results. Laryngoscope 85: 1504–1510

123. Skolnik E M, Yee K F, Wheatley M A 1975 Panel discussion on glottic tumors. V. Carcinoma of the laryngeal glottis: therapy and end results. Laryngoscope 85: 1453–1466

124. Snow J S, Norton M L, Saluja T S 1976 Fire hazard during CO_2 microsurgery of the larynx and trachea. Anesth Analg 55: 146–147

125. Som M L 1970 Conservation surgery for carcinoma of the supraglottis. J Laryngol Otol 84: 655–678

126. Stell P M 1973 The first laryngectomy for carcinoma. Arch Otolaryngol 98: 293

127. Stell P M 1975 The first laryngectomy. J Laryngol Otol 89: 353–358

128. Strong M S, Jako G J 1972 Laser surgery in the larynx. Early clinical experience with continuous CO_2 laser. Ann Otol Rhinol Laryngol 81: 791–798

129. The Encyclopedia Americana 1991 International Edition Grolier, Danbury

130. The New Encyclopedia Britannica, Macropaedia, 1973 15th edn.William Benton, Chicago

131. The New Encyclopedia Britannica, Macropaedia, 1973 vol 13. Helen Hemingway Benton, Chicago

132. St Clair Thomson 1926 Cancer of the larynx. Arch Otolaryngol 3: 37–42

133. Trendelenburg F. 1871 Arch Klin Chir 12: 112

134. Trotter W. 1920 A method of lateral pharyngotomy for the exposure of large growths in the epilaryngeal region. J Laryngol Otol 35: 289–295

135. Trotter W. 1929 Operations for malignant disease of the pharynx. Br J Surg 16: 485–487

136. Trotter W.1931 Some principles in the surgery of the pharynx. Lancet 2: 833–836

137. Trousseau A, Belloc H 1837 Traité pratique de la phthisis laryngée de la laryngite chronique et des maladies de la voix. Baillière, Paris

138. Tucker G F, Smith H R 1962 A histological demonstration of laryngeal connective tissue compartments. Trans Am Acad Ophthalmol Otolaryngol 66: 308–318

139. Tucker H M, Wood B G, Levine H, Katz R 1979 Glottic reconstruction after near total laryngectomy. Laryngoscope 89: 609–618

140. Urteaga O, Pack G T 1966 On the antiquity of melanoma. Cancer 19: 607–610

141. US Department of Health Education and Welfare 1964 Smoking and health

142. Walsh T E, Beamer P R 1930 Epidermoid cancer of the larynx occurring in two children with papilloma of the larynx. Laryngoscope 40: 1110–1124

143. Ward G E, Hendrick J W 1950 Tumors of the head and neck. Williams and Wilkins, Baltimore, pp 590–617

144. Webster N 1936 Webster's Universal Dictionary of the English Language. The World Syndicate Publishing Company, Springfield, Massachusetts

145. Weir N F 1973 Theodore Billroth. The first laryngectomy for cancer. J Laryngol Otol 87: 1161–1169

146. Wells C 1963 Ancient Egyptian pathology. J Laryngol Otol 77: 261–265

147. Wookey H 1942 Surgical treatment of carcinoma of the pharynx and upper esophagus. Surg Gynecol Obstet 75: 499–506

148. Work W P 1952 Carcinoma of the larynx; cervical metastasis: surgical treatment. Laryngoscope 62: 61–74

149. Wynder E L, Graham E A 1950 Tobacco smoking as a possible etiologic factor in bronchogenic carcinoma a study of six hundred and eighty-four proved cases. Cancer 3: 11–27

150. Wynder E L, Graham E A 1976 Environmental factors in cancer of the larynx. A second look. Cancer 38: 1591–1601

151. Wynder E L, Stellman S D 1977 Comparative epidemiology of tobacco related cancers. Cancer Res 37: 4608–4622

152. Yanagisawa E, Godley F, Mutah H 1987 Selection of video cameras for stroboscopic videolaryngoscopy. Ann Otol Rhinol Laryngol 96: 578–585

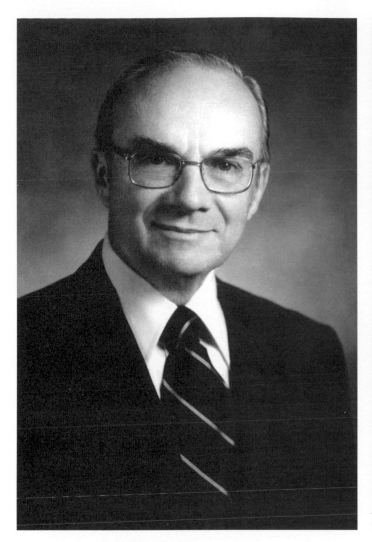 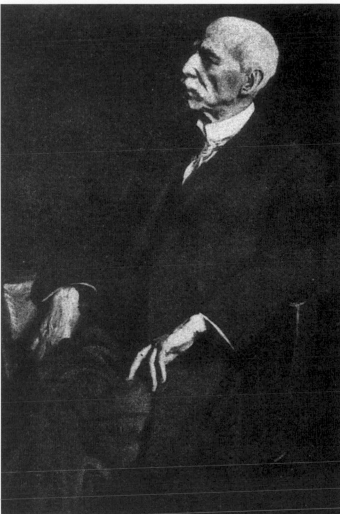

Fig. 1.1 *Left*. John A. Kirchner MD. His contributions to the understanding of laryngeal disease through the use of whole-organ sections has been significant to the development of conservation surgical techniques.

Fig. 1.2 *Right*. Manuel Garcia, Spanish singing teacher who first viewed his own vocal cords and initiated the use of indirect laryngoscopy as a diagnostic and therapeutic procedure. (*Annals of Medical History*, 1933, new series, 5: 154.)

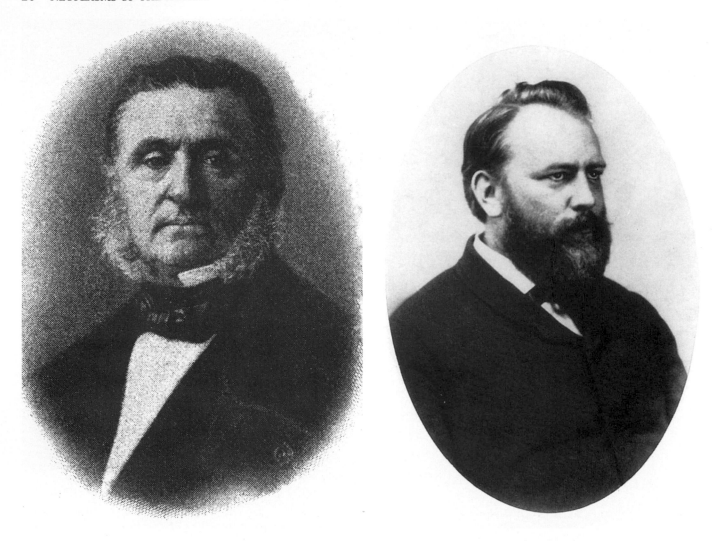

Fig. 1.3 *Left.* Armand Trousseau (1801–1867), French physician and author of an important text on Phthisie Laryngée. (*Biographisches Lexikon hervorragender Aerzte des neunzehnten Jahrhunderts*, 1901, edited by Julius Pagel. Urban & Schwartzenberg, Berlin, p 1731.)

Fig. 1.4 *Right.* Theodore Billroth (1829–1894), Viennese surgeon, known as the 'father of visceral surgery' who performed the first total laryngectomy for cancer. (Portrait file, Institute of the History of Medicine, The Johns Hopkins University, Baltimore, MD.)

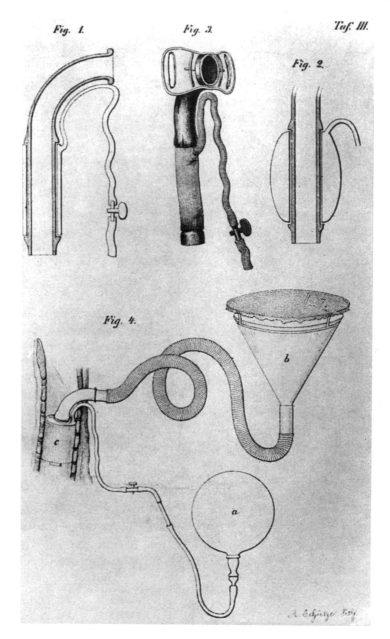

Fig. 1.5 *Above*. Langenbeck's 'tampon cannula', designed by the German surgeon Rudolf Konrad von Langenbeck (1810–1887), modified by Friedrich Trendelenburg (1844–1925), Leipzig, and used by Billroth in performing the first laryngectomy. (*Journal of Laryngology and Otology*, 1973, 87: 1166.)

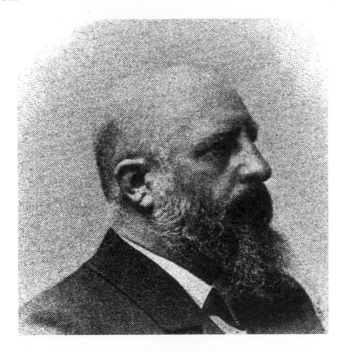

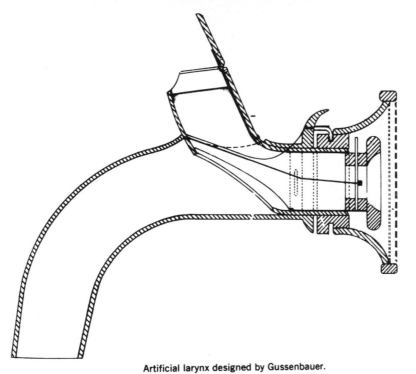

Artificial larynx designed by Gussenbauer.

Fig. 1.6 *Top.* Carl Gussenbauer, MD (1842–1903), German surgeon who assisted Billroth on his first laryngectomy and who designed and created the artificial larynx used by the patient in his period of rehabilitation. (*Biographisches Lexikon hervorragender Aerzte des neunzehnten Jahrhunderts*, 1901, edited by Julius Pagel. Urban & Schwartzenberg, Berlin; p 661.)

Fig. 1.7 *Bottom.* Diagram of Gussenbauer's artificial larynx showing vibrating reed which produced sound for alaryngeal speech. (*Archives of Otolaryngology*, 1973, 98: 293.)

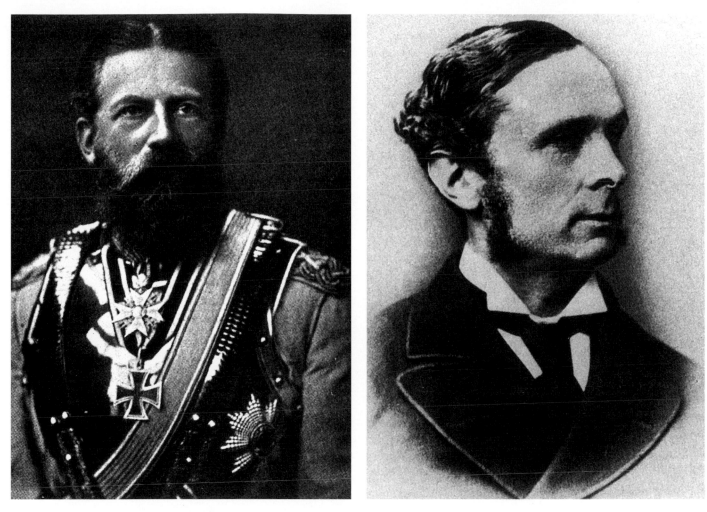

Fig. 1.8 *Left.* Prince Frederick Wilhelm III, Emperor of Germany, 1877, at the time of the Jubilee celebration for Queen Victoria. (*American Journal of Surgery*, 1976, 132: 516.)

Fig. 1.9 *Right.* Morell Mackenzie MD (1837–1892), celebrated British laryngologist who was consulted on the care of Prince Frederick Wilhelm III. (*American Journal of Surgery*, 1976, 132: 516.)

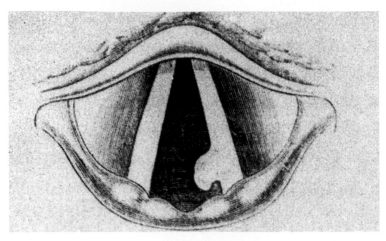

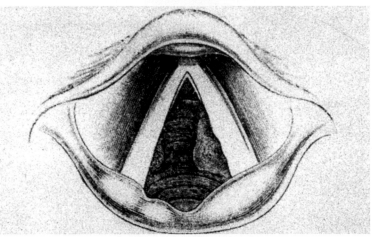

Fig. 1.10 *Top*. Drawing of the cord of Prince Frederick Whilhelm III made by Morell Mackenzie, MD, at time of his first consultation (20 May 1887). (*Pathology Annual*, 1970, p 210.)

Fig. 1.11 *Bottom*. Drawing of the vocal cord of Prince Frederick Wilhelm III ·made by Morell Mackenzie MD, on 6 November 1887, by which time the subglottic lesion could be plainly seen with the laryngeal mirror. (*Pathology Annual*, 1970, p 211.)

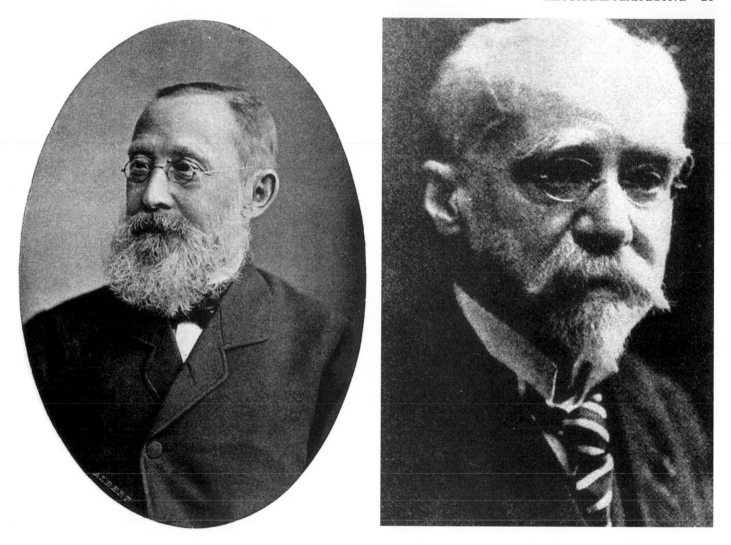

Fig. 1.12   *Left.* Rudolph Virchow MD (1821–1902), German pathologist who was known worldwide for his contributions to microscopic pathology. (Portrait file, Institute of the History of Medicine, The Johns Hopkins University, Baltimore, MD.)

Fig. 1.13   *Right.* Jacob Da Silva Solis-Cohen MD, Philadelphia laryngologist who performed the first laryngofissure which resulted in a 'permanent' cure of the cancer. (*Laryngoscope* 1975, 85: 326.)

2. Embryology and anatomy

B. K. B. Berkovitz, S. A. Hickey, B. J. Moxham

DEVELOPMENT OF THE LARYNX

The larynx is derived from the second, third, fourth and sixth branchial arches. Its development commences during the third and fourth weeks of intrauterine life.[4,9] A respiratory or laryngo-tracheal diverticulum arises ventrally from the foregut (caudal to the tuberculum impar and copula of the developing tongue) and elongates to form the tracheo-oesophageal groove. Lateral tracheo-oesophageal folds now develop to form a tracheo-oesophageal septum which separates the laryngo-tracheal diverticulum from the more dorsally situated oesophagus. Incomplete closure of the septum results in the formation of a posterior laryngeal cleft, which may persist in the neonate and cause problems with laryngeal incompetence and overspill. The oesophagus develops by way of a process of obliteration and recanalization, whilst the laryngo-tracheal diverticulum elongates and bifurcates repeatedly to form the lower respiratory tree.

The endoderm of the laryngo-tracheal diverticulum will give rise to the epithelium and glands of the larynx and trachea. These are fully differentiated by the end of the first trimester, although ciliated cells are seen initially on the vocal cords and squamous cells in the subglottis. The branchial arch mesoderm, through which the diverticulum passes, gives rise to the muscle, membranes and skeleton of the larynx. During the fifth and sixth weeks in utero, three swellings appear at the level of the future glottis: a median epiglottic swelling from the third and fourth branchial arches, and paired arytenoid swellings from the fourth branchial arch; a 'T'-shaped laryngeal introitus develops which is closed by temporary fusion of these three swellings. Patency is restored by the eighth week in utero.

During the eighth week, the thyroid cartilage starts to develop from the fourth arch, by means of two lateral chondrification centres. The level of the glottis is defined by the junction of the fourth and sixth arch mesoderm. This pattern of development is reflected by the innervation of the larynx in the adult, the supraglottic epithelium being innervated by the internal laryngeal branch of the superior laryngeal branch of the vagus (the nerve of the fourth arch), whereas the subglottis is innervated by the recurrent laryngeal branch of the vagus nerve (the nerve of the sixth arch). The level of the true vocal cords is the junctional region between the fourth and sixth branchial arches and may be innervated by both the internal and recurrent laryngeal nerves.

The arytenoid, corniculate and cricoid cartilages develop from the sixth arch. The cuneiform cartilages within the aryepiglottic folds develop from the epiglottis which itself arises from cartilage of the fourth branchial arch. The muscles of the larynx arise from the cephalad migration of epicardial mesenchyme to the region of the fourth and sixth arches. These developmental patterns are reflected in the innervation of the muscles. The persistence of the dorsal sixth arch artery on the left tethers the left recurrent laryngeal nerve in the chest, whilst its involution and disappearance on the right allows the right recurrent laryngeal nerve to ascend until it meets (and thus hooks around) the right subclavian artery.

During the development of the thyroid cartilage, the ventral displacement of its median portion results in the creation of the false and true vocal cords. Within the latter, a condensation of mesenchyme results in the formation of the vocal ligament along the cephalad margin of the crico-vocal membrane. Above the vocal cord, the epithelium evaginates to form the ventricles and saccules of the larynx.

The hyoid bone is associated with the larynx and develops from the mesenchyme of the second and third branchial arches. The second arch gives rise to the styloid processes, stylohyoid ligaments, lesser horns and upper body of the hyoid bone; the third arch gives rise to the lower part of the body of the hyoid and the greater horns.

THE ADULT LARYNX

The adult larynx is situated in the midline of the neck at the level of the third to sixth cervical vertebrae. It extends from the laryngeal inlet, near the base of the tongue, to the trachea. At its inlet, the larynx communicates with the oropharynx and laryngopharynx (hypopharynx).

Few features of the larynx are visible externally. It is essentially a tube-like structure whose rigidity and form depend upon an underlying cartilaginous skeleton. Anteriorly, the larynx is almost completely covered by the infrahyoid strap muscles and by the thyroid gland. The only feature visible is the laryngeal prominence of the thyroid cartilage (the Adam's apple). This is markedly more prominent in the male larynx.

The posterior aspect of the larynx forms the anterior wall of the laryngopharynx. The laryngeal inlet (aditus) is bounded anteriorly and superiorly by the epiglottis, posteriorly and inferiorly by the mucosa of the arytenoid cartilages and the interarytenoid region, and laterally by the aryepiglottic folds. The pharynx extends along the sides of the laryngeal inlet to form the pyriform fossae. From above, the epiglottis and tongue are separated by depressions called the valleculae. The valleculae are bounded by the median and lateral glosso-epiglottic folds.

The internal anatomy of the adult larynx

The interior of the larynx (Figs 2.1 and 2.2) is divided into compartments by two paired folds (the false or vestibular cords and the true or vocal cords), and the membranes of the larynx (the quadrangular and cricovocal membranes — see Fig. 2.4). Between the laryngeal inlet and the vocal cords lies the supraglottis. The glottis lies between the vocal cords. The vestibule lies between the inlet of the larynx and the level of the vestibular folds.[9] Between the glottis and the level of the inferior margin of the cricoid cartilage lies the subglottis.[1] Between the false cords and the vocal cords are two slit-like spaces, the laryngeal ventricles or sinuses. A small pouch of mucosa (the saccule) extends upwards from the anterior end of each ventricle to lie between the supraglottis and the inner surface of the alae of the thyroid cartilage (see Fig. 2.9).

The vestibular or false cord

The false cord is a thick ridge of mucosa which covers a thin layer of connective tissue, the inferior free edge of the quadrangular membrane. It is located above the vocal cord.

The (true) vocal cord

The anterior three-fifths of the vocal cord is formed by the vocal ligament, the thickened free edge of the cricovocal membrane. Because the mucosa overlying the vocal ligament is thin and lies directly on the ligament, the cord appears pearly white in vivo. The mucosa is loosely attached to the ligaments and a potential space

exists which readily collects oedema fluid in disease. Known as Reinke's space, it extends along the length of the free margin of the vocal ligament and somewhat onto the superior surface of the cord. The posterior two-fifths of the vocal cord is formed by the vocal process of the arytenoid cartilage. The cords meet anteriorly to form the anterior commissure. Fibres of the vocal ligament pass through the thyroid cartilage to blend with the overlying perichondrium, forming Broyles' ligament. Broyles' ligament contains blood vessels and lymphatics and therefore is a potential route for the escape of malignant tumours from the larynx.

The skeleton of the larynx

The skeleton of the larynx (Figs 2.3–2.5) consists of cartilages and membranes. Because the hyoid bone is associated with the movements of the larynx, it will be considered briefly here. The function of the skeleton of the larynx is to prevent collapse of the air passages and to give attachment to a series of muscles.

The hyoid bone. The hyoid bone is U-shaped, being deficient posteriorly, and lies at the base of the tongue, thus forming the superior limit of the laryngeal skeleton. It has a multi-faceted superior surface which gives attachment to the muscles of the tongue and to the infrahyoid strap muscles. From this superior surface arise a pair of short spines (the lesser horns) which project superiorly about one-third of the way from the midline anteriorly to the posterior limits of the bone (the tips of the greater horns). The stylohyoid ligaments have their inferior attachments to the lesser horns.

The laryngeal cartilages

The major cartilages of the larynx are the thyroid, cricoid and arytenoid cartilages. The minor cartilages are the cuneiform and corniculate cartilages. The arytenoid, cuneiform and corniculate cartilages are paired. Associated with the larynx is the epiglottic cartilage.

The epiglottic cartilage, the cuneiform cartilage and the corniculate cartilages are composed of elastic cartilage. The thyroid, cricoid and arytenoid cartilages are hyaline cartilages and may ossify in old age.

The thyroid cartilage. This is the largest and most prominent cartilage, forming most of the anterior and lateral walls of the larynx.

The overall shape of the thyroid cartilage takes the form of a shield. It consists of two flattened, quadrilateral laminae which are joined anteriorly to form the laryngeal prominence (Adam's apple). Above the prominence, the laminae are separated by a deep V-shaped notch called the thyroid notch. Posteriorly, the laminae project upwards and downwards as the superior and inferior horns. On the external surface of each lamina lies an

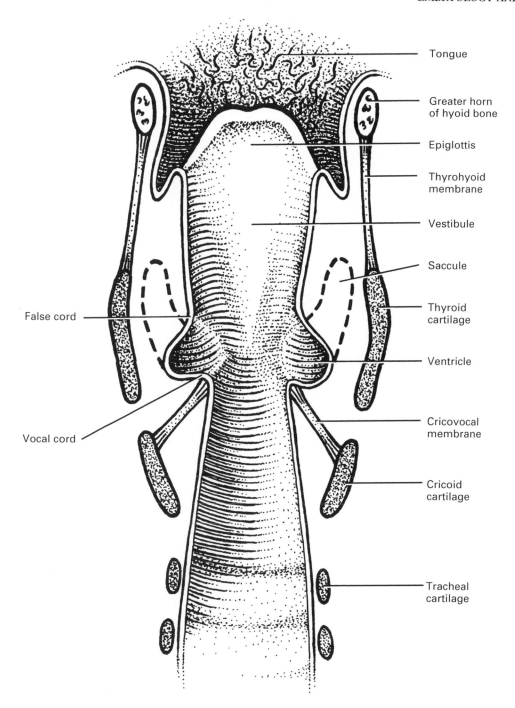

Tongue

Greater horn
of hyoid bone

Epiglottis

Thyrohyoid
membrane

Vestibule

Saccule

Thyroid
cartilage

False cord

Ventricle

Vocal cord

Cricovocal
membrane

Cricoid
cartilage

Tracheal
cartilage

Fig. 2.1   Diagram showing the internal anatomy of the larynx as displayed in a coronal section viewed from behind.

oblique line which is the site for muscle attachments. The line runs downwards and forwards from the superior horn towards the lower border of the cartilage. It is bounded above and below by a tubercle. The thyroid cartilage shows sexual dimorphism: in the male, it increases markedly in size at puberty and the thyroid prominence becomes very distinct.[1]

The cricoid cartilage. Unlike the thyroid cartilage, the cricoid cartilage forms a complete ring. Indeed, it is the only complete cartilaginous ring in the air passages. It comprises the most inferior and posterior part of the larynx and supports the entrance to the trachea. The shape of the cricoid cartilage resembles that of a signet ring, showing a narrow arch anteriorly and a flat,

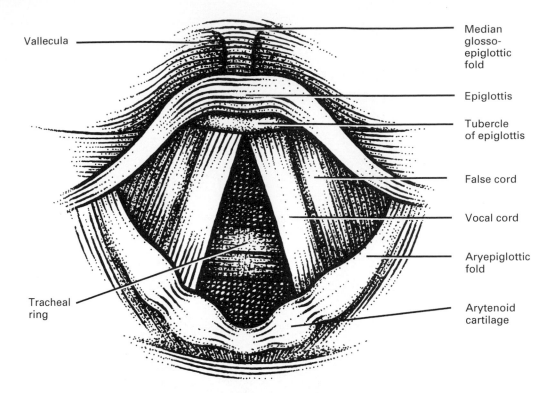

Vallecula

Median glosso-epiglottic fold

Epiglottis

Tubercle of epiglottis

False cord

Vocal cord

Aryepiglottic fold

Tracheal ring

Arytenoid cartilage

Fig. 2.2 Diagram of a laryngoscopic view of the larynx.

quadrangular lamina posteriorly. Where the arch meets the lamina are small articular facets for the inferior horns of the thyroid cartilage. The superior edge of the lamina has sloping shoulders and articular facets for the arytenoid cartilages. The cricoid cartilage may appear more prominent in the female.

The arytenoid cartilages. The arytenoid cartilages lie in the postero-inferior part of the larynx, on the superior edge of the lamina of the cricoid cartilage. They contribute to the margin of the inlet of the larynx. Each cartilage is pyramidal in shape, although the superior process (or apex) is the corniculate cartilage. The base of the arytenoid cartilage presents the articulating surface with the cricoid cartilage. The arytenoid cartilage has a process anteriorly, the vocal process (for attachment of the vocal ligament), and a process laterally, the muscular process (for the attachment of some of the muscles of the larynx).

The minor cartilages of the larynx. The corniculate cartilages surmount the arytenoid cartilages, thus completing their pyramidal shapes.

The cuneiform cartilages lie within the aryepiglottic folds at the inlet of the larynx.

Small triticeal cartilages are found in the ligaments joining the tips of the superior horns of thyroid cartilage to the tips of the greater cornua of the hyoid bone.

Articulations of the laryngeal cartilages. The inferior horn of the thyroid cartilage articulates with the cricoid cartilage at a synovial joint. This joint has a well-

developed capsule which is strengthened posteriorly by fibrous bands. The joint permits a rotary movement with activity of the cricothyroid muscle, such that the thyroid cartilage tilts forwards and downwards, with upward movement of the arch of the cricoid cartilage (see Fig. 2.15D).

The joint between the base of the arytenoid cartilage and the lamina of the cricoid cartilage is also synovial. The capsule of the joint is strengthened by the posterior crico-arytenoid ligament which is said to limit forward movement of the arytenoid cartilage. Rotation and gliding movements of the arytenoid occurs at this joint, both types of movement being responsible for opening and closing the glottis.

A synovial or cartilaginous joint links the corniculate cartilage to the arytenoid.

The epiglottis. The epiglottis consists of a thin lamina of elastic cartilage covered on all sides with mucous membrane. It is leaf-shaped, the 'stalk' or petiole providing the means of attachment to the larynx via a thyro-epiglottic ligament. A depression for this ligament lies just below the thyroid notch on the inner surface of the thyroid cartilage. The epiglottis is also anchored to the posterior surface of the body of the hyoid bone by a hyo-epiglottic ligament. The sides of the epiglottis are attached to the arytenoid cartilages by the aryepiglottic folds. Median and lateral glosso-epiglottic folds pass from the root of the tongue to the anterior surface of the epiglottis. The epiglottis projects upwards and backwards

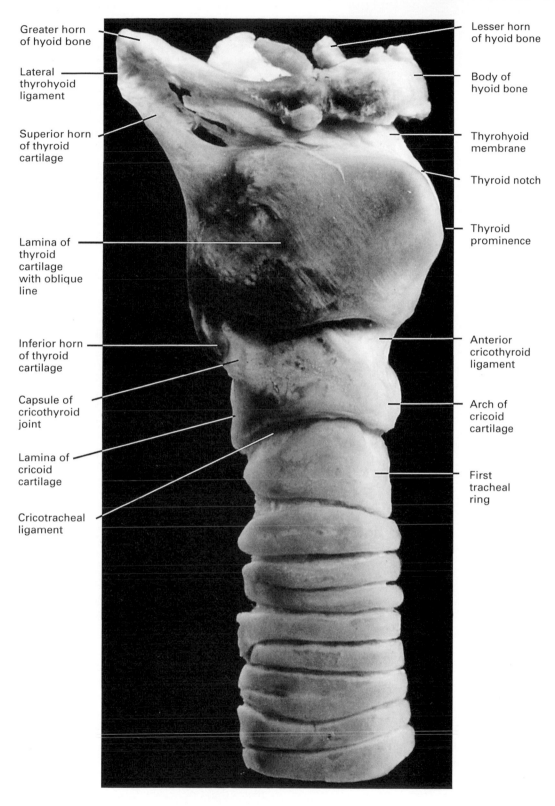

Greater horn
of hyoid bone

Lateral
thyrohyoid
ligament

Superior horn
of thyroid
cartilage

Lamina of
thyroid
cartilage
with oblique
line

Inferior horn
of thyroid
cartilage

Capsule of
cricothyroid
joint

Lamina of
cricoid
cartilage

Cricotracheal
ligament

Lesser horn
of hyoid bone

Body of
hyoid bone

Thyrohyoid
membrane

Thyroid notch

Thyroid
prominence

Anterior
cricothyroid
ligament

Arch of
cricoid
cartilage

First
tracheal
ring

Fig. 2.3 Dissection of the larynx viewed laterally.

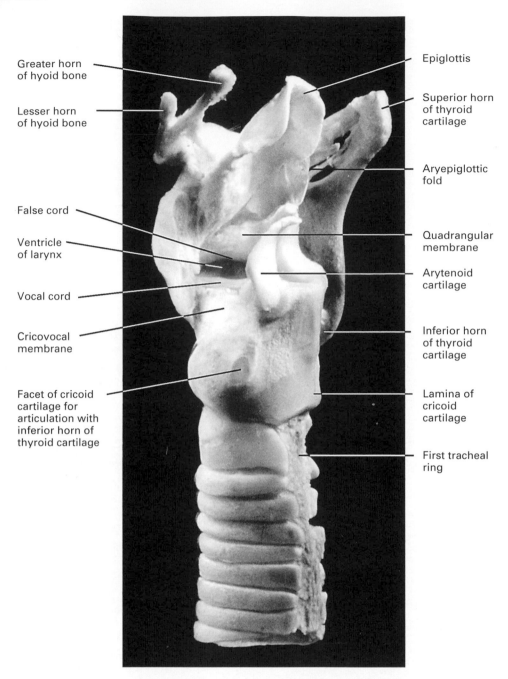

Greater horn
of hyoid bone

Lesser horn
of hyoid bone

False cord

Ventricle
of larynx

Vocal cord

Cricovocal
membrane

Facet of cricoid
cartilage for
articulation with
inferior horn of
thyroid cartilage

Epiglottis

Superior horn
of thyroid
cartilage

Aryepiglottic
fold

Quadrangular
membrane

Arytenoid
cartilage

Inferior horn
of thyroid
cartilage

Lamina of
cricoid
cartilage

First tracheal
ring

Fig. 2.4 Dissection of the larynx with the left ala of the thyroid cartilage removed, showing the internal anatomy.

over the vestibule of the larynx and gives the appearance of a 'lid'. The posterior surface of the cartilage of the epiglottis shows numerous small indentations and perforations in which lie mucous glands (see Fig. 2.10).

The laryngeal membranes

The larynx has thyrohyoid, quadrangular and cricovocal membranes. The thyrohyoid membrane is external to the larynx, whereas the paired quadrangular and cricovocal membranes are internal. All the membranes are composed of fibro-elastic tissue. There are also two ligaments, the anterior cricothyroid ligament and the cricotracheal ligament.[1]

The thyrohyoid membrane. This membrane extends from the upper border of the thyroid cartilage to the upper border of the inner surface of the hyoid bone (both body and greater horns). Between the membrane and the hyoid bone lies a bursa.

The thyrohyoid membrane is thickened in three places to form ligament-like structures. In the midline is found the median thyrohyoid ligament. At the lateral margins

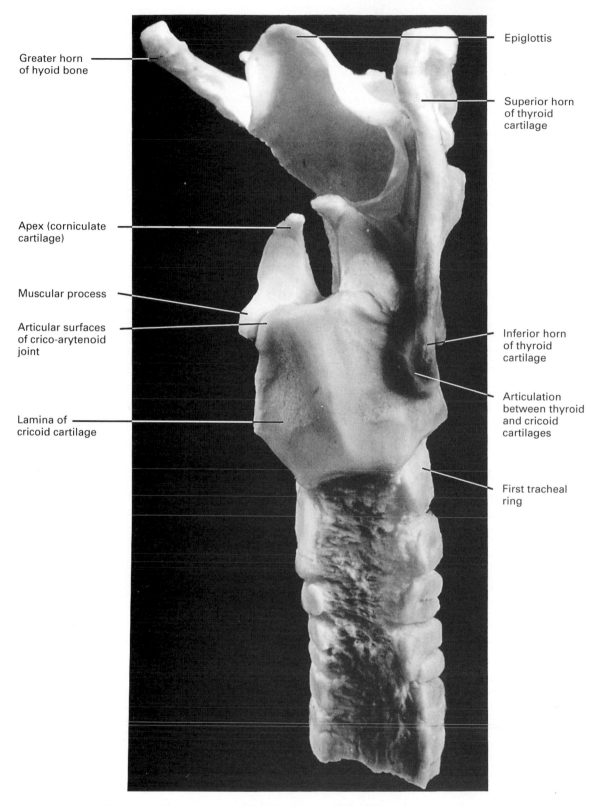

Greater horn
of hyoid bone

Epiglottis

Superior horn
of thyroid
cartilage

Apex (corniculate
cartilage)

Muscular process

Articular surfaces
of crico-arytenoid
joint

Inferior horn
of thyroid
cartilage

Articulation
between thyroid
and cricoid
cartilages

Lamina of
cricoid cartilage

First tracheal
ring

Fig. 2.5 Dissection of the larynx with the left ala of the thyroid cartilage removed, viewed posteriorly.

are found the lateral thyrohyoid ligaments, connecting the tips of the superior horns of the thyroid cartilage to those of the greater horns of the hyoid bone. The lateral ligaments may contain triticeal cartilages.

The thyrohyoid membrane is pierced by the superior laryngeal vessels and the internal laryngeal nerves as they pass into the larynx (see Fig. 2.16).

The quadrangular membrane. Each quadrangular membrane passes from the lateral margin of the epiglottis to the arytenoid cartilage on its own side. It is often poorly defined. The membrane shows two free borders. The upper and posterior border forms the aryepiglottic fold. The lower border forms the false cord. Within the aryepiglottic folds lie the cuneiform cartilages.

The cricovocal membrane. This membrane is more pronounced than the quadrangular membrane, and arises from the side of the larynx at the upper border of the arch of the cricoid cartilage. It passes internally, deep to the lamina of the thyroid cartilage, to become attached anteriorly to the inner surface of the thyroid cartilage close to the midline, and posteriorly to the vocal process of the arytenoid cartilage. The attachment of the cricovocal membrane lies half-way between the thyroid notch and inferior border of the thyroid cartilage in the female, whilst in the male it lies one-third of the way.

The cricovocal membrane has an upper free margin which passes across the larynx. This is thickened to form the vocal ligament.

The anterior (median) cricothyroid ligament. This ligament (Fig. 2.3) is considered by some anatomists to be a superficial part of the cricovocal membrane. It is situated anteriorly in the midline, passing from the upper border of the cricoid cartilage to the lower border of the thyroid cartilage.

The cricotracheal ligament. This ligament (Fig. 2.3) joins the lower border of the cricoid cartilage to the first cartilaginous tracheal ring.

The para-lumenal spaces and other relationships of the larynx

The pre-epiglottic space (Fig. 2.8) lies anterior to the epiglottis and is bounded superiorly by the hyo-epiglottic ligament, anteriorly by the thyro-hyoid membrane and the thyroid cartilage, and inferiorly by the thyro-epiglottic ligament. Inferolaterally, the pre-epiglottic space is in continuity with the paraglottic space (see below) and is often invaded from the latter by the laryngeal saccule. It is also in continuity with the mucosa of the laryngeal surface of the epiglottis via multiple perforations in the cartilage of the epiglottis. It is through these perforations that malignancies of the laryngeal surface of the epiglottis may invade the fat and areolar tissue of the pre-epiglottic space.

The paraglottic space (Fig. 2.10) lies lateral to the quadrangular and cricovocal membranes, and is bounded posteriorly by the mucosa of the pyriform fossa. Inferiorly, the space is bounded by the upper margin of the cricoid cartilage, and laterally by the thyroid ala, and cricothyroid and thyrohyoid membranes. The paraglottic space contains the laryngeal ventricle and part, or all, of the laryngeal saccule. It also contains the thyro-arytenoid muscles.

The anatomy of the paraglottic space is important in determining paths of spread to the thyro-arytenoid muscles and then to the limits of the space to become 'transglottic', before extending out of the larynx or into the subglottis.[5] Supraglottic tumours may also spread into the paraglottic space and reach the subglottis, or extend beyond the limits of the larynx. Ventricular tumours may obstruct mucous outflow from the saccule and cause its expansion within the paraglottic space to form a secondary laryngocoele; the tumour itself may also spread transglottically, and thereby fix the vocal cord. Fixation of the vocal cord is a good indicator of a tumour within the paraglottic space. The proximity of the mucosa at the pyriform fossa makes its removal in surgery mandatory for such disease.

The relationships of the larynx illustrated in Figs 2.6–2.8. See also Figs 2.9–2.12.

The histology of the larynx

The larynx is lined both internally and on its outer, posterior surface by pseudostratified, ciliated, columnar epithelium interspersed with goblet cells (Figs 2.9–2.12). The exceptions in the normal larynx are the surface of the vocal cords and the anterior surface of the epiglottis, which are covered by stratified squamous epithelium. Scattered islets of metaplastic squamous epithelium are found throughout the larynx in approximately 50% of normal larynges. In many people, the false cords are covered by squamous epithelium. Thus, the transition from respiratory to squamous epithelium is not a reliable indicator of the limits of the glottis.[6,7]

Mucous glands are scattered throughout the larynx, but are particularly numerous on the epiglottis and in the saccule (Figs 2.9 and 2.10). Taste buds are also found in the larynx, principally on the epiglottis. Melanocytes, argyrophilic and paraganglionic cells are also found in normal larynges.[2]

The muscles of the larynx

The muscles can be categorized as extrinsic or intrinsic.

The extrinsic muscles of the larynx

These muscles have an attachment outside the larynx and include the infrahyoid (strap) muscles of the neck, and the stylopharyngeus, salpingopharyngeus palatopharyngeus and inferior constrictor muscles of the pharynx.

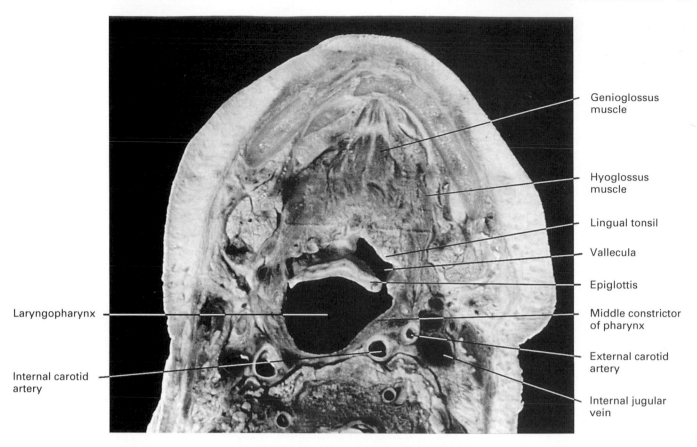

Fig. 2.6 Horizontal section of the neck at the level of the valleculae.

The extrinsic muscles are responsible for movements of the whole larynx, i.e., elevation and depression during swallowing, respiration and phonation. The thyrohyoid, stylopharyngeus, salpingopharyngeus and palatopharyngeus muscles elevate the larynx. The omohyoid, sternohyoid and sternothyroid muscles depress the larynx. Of these three latter muscles, sternothyroid is the only one that has an attachment onto the larynx and which therefore depresses the larynx by direct action. The omohyoid and sternohyoid muscles can cause depression only indirectly by way of their action on the hyoid bone.

Because the larynx and the hyoid bone are connected by the thyrohyoid membrane and muscles, elevation of the larynx occurs by the actions of the suprahyoid musculature (mylohyoid, digastric, stylohyoid and geniohyoid muscles).

The intrinsic muscles of the larynx

These muscles are confined to the larynx (Figs 2.13–2.15). Within this group are the posterior crico-arytenoid, lateral crico-arytenoid, interarytenoid, thyro-arytenoid and cricothyroid muscles. With the exception of the interarytenoid muscle, the muscles are paired.

The intrinsic muscles of the larynx are concerned mainly with the activities of the vocal cords. Extensions of the interarytenoid and thyro-arytenoid muscles (the aryepiglottic and thyro-epiglottic muscles) modify the inlet of the larynx.

Whereas most of the intrinsic muscles lie internally (under cover of the thyroid cartilage or the mucosa), the cricothyroid muscles appear on the outer aspect of the larynx.

The posterior crico-arytenoid muscle.

Attachments. This muscle arises from a broad depression on the posterior surface of the lamina of the cricoid cartilage. Passing upwards and laterally, it is inserted into the muscular process of the arytenoid cartilage.

Innervation. The recurrent laryngeal branch of the vagus nerve provides the motor supply.

Vasculature. The posterior crico-arytenoid muscle receives its blood supply from the laryngeal branches of the superior and inferior thyroid arteries.

Actions. This is the only muscle that opens the glottis and it does so in two ways (Fig. 2.15). First, the upper fibres, being almost horizontal, rotate the arytenoid cartilage. Second, the lower fibres, being more vertical, cause sliding of the arytenoid cartilage down the sloping superior margin of the cricoid cartilage.

The lateral crico-arytenoid muscle.

Attachments. This muscle originates from the lateral

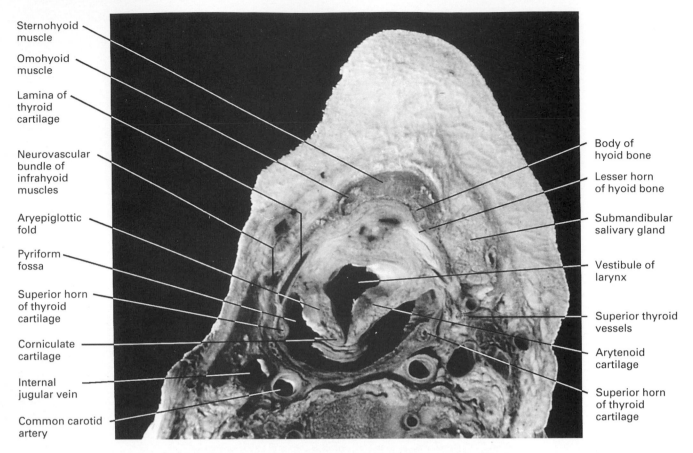

Sternohyoid muscle
Omohyoid muscle
Lamina of thyroid cartilage
Neurovascular bundle of infrahyoid muscles
Aryepiglottic fold
Pyriform fossa
Superior horn of thyroid cartilage
Corniculate cartilage
Internal jugular vein
Common carotid artery

Body of hyoid bone
Lesser horn of hyoid bone
Submandibular salivary gland
Vestibule of larynx
Superior thyroid vessels
Arytenoid cartilage
Superior horn of thyroid cartilage

Fig. 2.7 Horizontal section of the neck at the level of the ventricle of the larynx.

side of the upper border of the arch of the cricoid cartilage. It extends upwards and backwards beneath the thyroid cartilage to insert on to the muscular process of the arytenoid cartilage.

Innervation. The recurrent laryngeal nerve supplies the lateral crico-arytenoid muscle.

Vasculature. It receives its blood supply from the laryngeal branches of the superior and inferior thyroid arteries.

Actions. The lateral crico-arytenoid muscle rotates the arytenoid cartilage in a direction opposite to that of the posterior crico-arytenoid muscle, thereby closing the glottis (Fig 2.15B).

The interarytenoid muscle.

Attachments. This is a single muscle in two parts, which runs posteriorly between the muscular processes of the arytenoid cartilages (Fig. 2.14). Many of its fibres run transversely across the posterior surfaces of the arytenoids (the transverse arytenoid part), but some run obliquely from the muscular process of one arytenoid to the apex of the opposite cartilage (the oblique arytenoid part). The oblique fibres form two bands which cross to produce a distinctive X-shape. Some of the oblique fibres continue into the aryepiglottic folds as the aryepiglottic muscles.

Innervation. The muscle is innervated by the recurrent laryngeal nerve.

Vasculature. The blood supply is derived from the laryngeal branches of the superior and inferior thyroid arteries.

Actions. The interarytenoid muscle closes the glottis by approximating the arytenoid cartilages. This is accomplished by drawing the arytenoids upwards along the sloping shoulders of the cricoid lamina, without rotation (Fig. 2.15C). The aryepiglottic muscles modify the inlet of the larynx. However, their poor development limits their action as sphincters of the inlet.

The thyro-arytenoid muscle.

Attachments. This muscle lies lateral to the vocal cord. It arises on the inner surface of the thyroid cartilage in the midline. It also arises from the cricovocal membrane. The thyro-arytenoid muscle passes backwards, upwards and outwards to be inserted into the base and anterior surface of the arytenoid cartilage. The lower and deeper fibres form a distinct bundle that runs parallel with, and lateral to, the vocal ligament. This bundle is sometimes referred to as the vocalis muscle and is attached to the vocal process of the arytenoid cartilage. There is doubt as to whether the fibres of vocalis are also attached to the vocal ligament. The upper

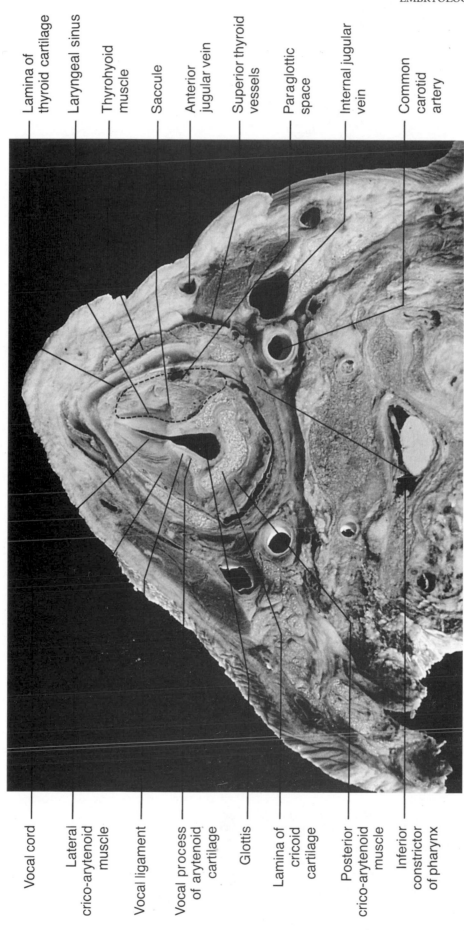

Lamina of thyroid cartilage

Laryngeal sinus

Thyrohyoid muscle

Saccule

Anterior jugular vein

Superior thyroid vessels

Paraglottic space

Internal jugular vein

Common carotid artery

Vocal cord

Lateral crico-arytenoid muscle

Vocal ligament

Vocal process of arytenoid cartilage

Glottis

Lamina of cricoid cartilage

Posterior crico-arytenoid muscle

Inferior constrictor of pharynx

Fig. 2.8 Horizontal section of the neck at the level of the vocal cords.

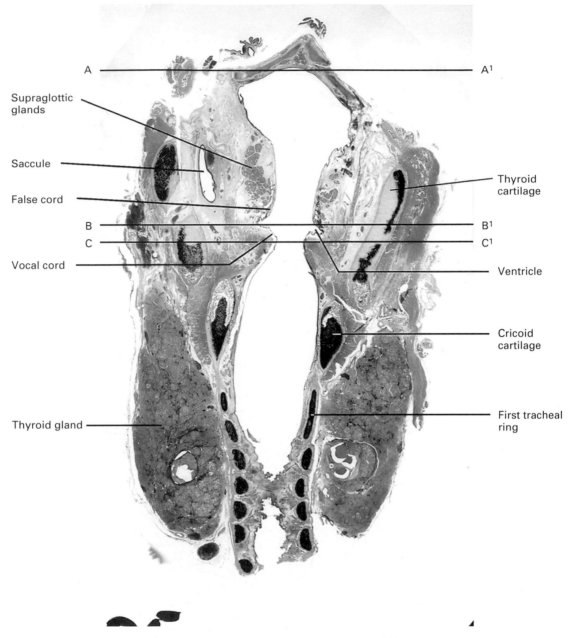

Fig. 2.9   Longitudinal section of the larynx. H&E.

fibres of the thyro-arytenoid muscle may extend into the aryepiglottic fold to form the thyro-epiglottic muscle.

Innervation. All parts of the thyro-arytenoid muscle are supplied by the recurrent laryngeal nerve.

Vasculature. The arterial blood supply is derived from the laryngeal branches of the superior and inferior thyroid arteries.

Actions. The primary function of the thyro-arytenoid muscle is to shorten the vocal ligament and adjust the tension within it during phonation. In addition, it can rotate the arytenoid cartilage medially and so aid closure of the glottis. Increased tension of the muscle increases pitch, while decreased tension decreases pitch. Contrac-

tion of vocalis will alter the profile of the vocal cord and change the timbre of the voice. The thyro-epiglottic muscles widen the inlet of the larynx.

The cricothyroid muscle.

Attachments. The cricothyroid muscle arises from the anterior and anterolateral parts of the external surface of the arch of the cricoid cartilage. Its fibres pass upwards and backwards to insert into the thyroid cartilage. Two distinct parts can be recognized. The anterior and superior fibres constitute the straight part of the cricothyroid muscle. This inserts into the lower border of the thyroid lamina. The posterior and inferior fibres constitute the oblique part of the cricothyroid

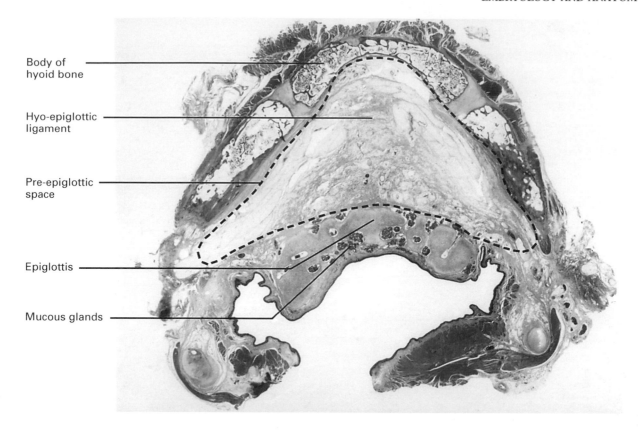

Body of
hyoid bone

Hyo-epiglottic
ligament

Pre-epiglottic
space

Epiglottis

Mucous glands

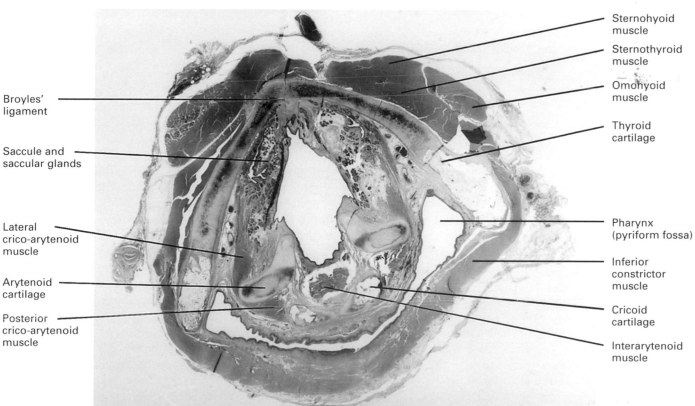

Broyles'
ligament

Saccule and
saccular glands

Lateral
crico-arytenoid
muscle

Arytenoid
cartilage

Posterior
crico-arytenoid
muscle

Sternohyoid
muscle

Sternothyroid
muscle

Omohyoid
muscle

Thyroid
cartilage

Pharynx
(pyriform fossa)

Inferior
constrictor
muscle

Cricoid
cartilage

Interarytenoid
muscle

Fig. 2.10 (*top*) Horizontal section of the larynx at the level of the hyoid bone (level A, Fig. 2.9). H&E.

Fig. 2.11 (*bottom*) Horizontal section of the larynx at the level of the ventricle (level B, Fig. 2.9). H&E.

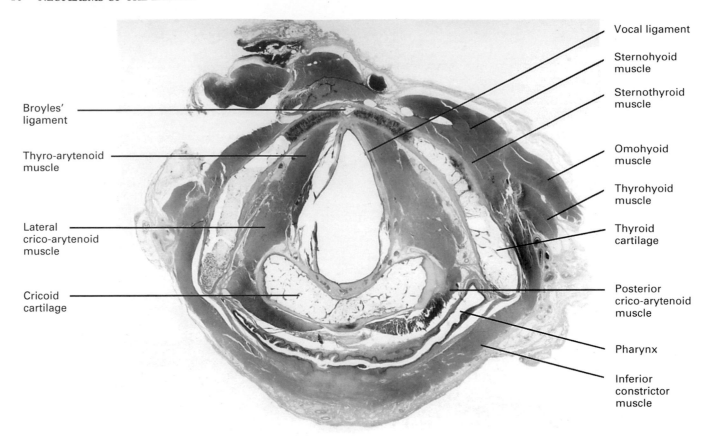

Broyles'
ligament

Thyro-arytenoid
muscle

Lateral
crico-arytenoid
muscle

Cricoid
cartilage

Vocal ligament

Sternohyoid
muscle

Sternothyroid
muscle

Omohyoid
muscle

Thyrohyoid
muscle

Thyroid
cartilage

Posterior
crico-arytenoid
muscle

Pharynx

Inferior
constrictor
muscle

Fig. 2.12   Horizontal section of the larynx at the level of the vocal cords (level C, Fig. 2.9). H&E.

muscle. This inserts into the inferior horn of the thyroid cartilage.

Innervation. Unlike the other intrinsic muscles of the larynx, the cricothyroid muscle is innervated not by the recurrent laryngeal nerve, but by the external branch of the superior laryngeal nerve.

Vasculature. The muscle is supplied by the cricothyroid branch of the superior thyroid artery and by the inferior laryngeal branch of the inferior thyroid artery.

Actions. The cricothyroid muscle elongates the vocal ligaments. This is accomplished by elevating the arch of the cricoid cartilage and tilting back the upper border of its lamina (Fig. 2.15D). As a result, the distance between the angle of the thyroid cartilage and the vocal processes of the arytenoids is increased. A similar activity results if the muscles pull the thyroid cartilage forward. Indeed, this is thought to be the principal activity during phonation, as the lamina of the cricoid cartilage is held in position against the vertebral column.

The blood supply of the larynx

The blood supply of the larynx (Fig. 2.16) is derived

mainly from two pairs of arteries: the superior and inferior laryngeal arteries. The superior laryngeal artery supplies the larynx above the vocal cords. It is derived from the superior thyroid artery, a branch of the external carotid artery. The superior laryngeal artery runs down towards the larynx with the internal branch of the superior laryngeal nerve. It enters the larynx by penetrating the thyrohyoid membrane. The inferior laryngeal artery supplies the larynx below the vocal cords. It is a branch of the inferior thyroid artery which itself is derived from the thyrocervical trunk of the subclavian artery. The inferior laryngeal artery runs up and into the larynx, deep to the lower border of the inferior constrictor muscle. It is accompanied in its course by the recurrent laryngeal nerve. The cricothyroid branch of the superior thyroid artery may also supply the larynx.

Venous return from the larynx occurs via superior and inferior laryngeal veins. These run parallel to the laryngeal arteries. They drain into the superior and inferior thyroid veins respectively (Fig. 2.17).

The lymph vessels draining the larynx above the vocal cords accompany the superior laryngeal artery, pierce the thyrohyoid membrane, and end in the upper deep cervical lymph nodes. Below the vocal cords, some of the

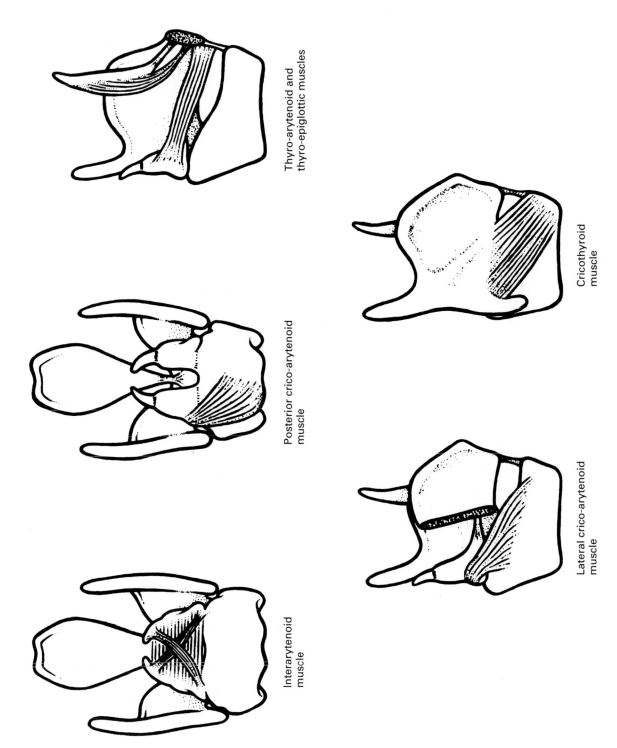

Thyro-arytenoid and thyro-epiglottic muscles

Cricothyroid muscle

Posterior crico-arytenoid muscle

Lateral crico-arytenoid muscle

Interarytenoid muscle

Fig. 2.13 Diagram illustrating the intrinsic muscles of the larynx.

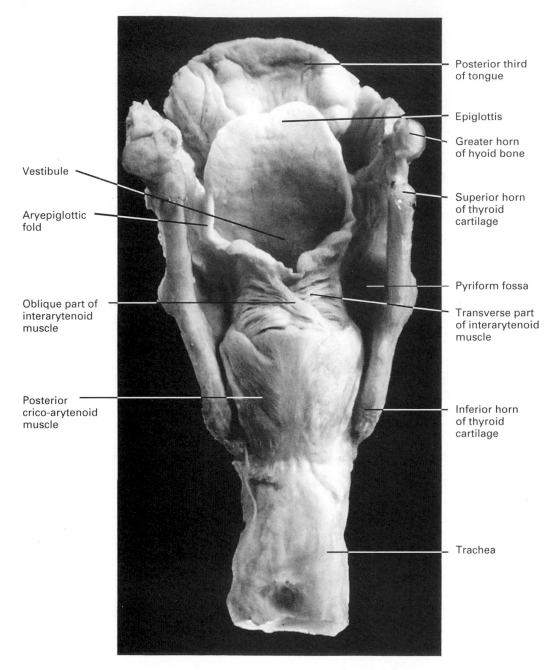

Fig. 2.14 Dissection of the posterior surface of the larynx.

lymph vessels pass through the cricovocal membrane to reach the prelaryngeal (Delphian) and/or pretracheal lymph nodes. Others run with the inferior laryngeal artery to join the lower deep cervical nodes. Figure 2.17 summarizes the lymphatic drainage of the larynx.

The innervation of the larynx

The vocal cords form a dividing line for both the sensory and the secretomotor innervation of the mucosa within the larynx. Above the vocal cords, the mucosa is innervated by the internal laryngeal branch of the superior laryngeal nerve. Below the vocal cords, the mucosa is supplied by the recurrent laryngeal nerve. The vocal cords themselves are innervated by both nerves.

The motor supply to the intrinsic muscles of the larynx is derived mainly from the recurrent laryngeal nerve. The cricothyroid muscle, however, is supplied by the external branch of the superior laryngeal nerve (Fig. 2.16).

Thus, the chief nerves supplying the larynx are the superior laryngeal and recurrent laryngeal branches of the vagus, both of which contain sensory and motor fibres.

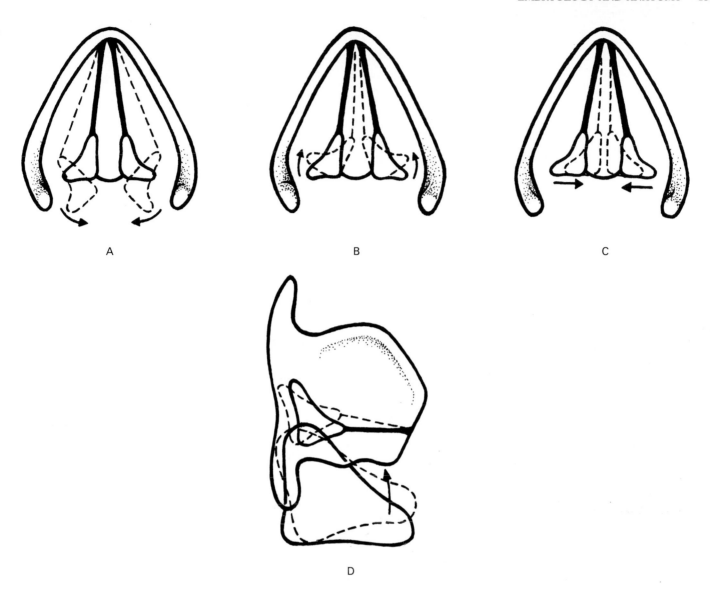

A   B   C

D

Fig. 2.15   Diagram illustrating movements of the laryngeal joints. A, B, C: crico-arytenoid joints; D: cricothyroid joints.

The superior laryngeal nerve leaves the trunk of the vagus at its inferior ganglion. It curves downwards and forwards by the side of the pharynx, medial to the internal carotid artery. It divides into external and internal branches. The external branch continues downwards and forwards on the lateral surface of the inferior constrictor muscle to end in the cricothyroid muscle. The internal branch is larger and enters the larynx after piercing the thyrohyoid membrane. On entering the larynx, the nerve divides into an ascending branch (which supplies the mucosa of the pyriform fossa), and a descending branch (which supplies the supraglottic mucosa). On the medial wall of the pyriform fossa, descending branches give twigs to the transverse inter-arytenoid muscle and continue behind the cricoid cartilage as fine filaments which communicate with the

recurrent laryngeal nerve (the ansa Galeni).

The origins of the recurrent laryngeal nerves differ according to side. The right recurrent laryngeal nerve issues from the vagus nerve in front of the subclavian artery. It then passes below and behind the artery. The left recurrent laryngeal nerve arises in the thorax (on the arch of the aorta). Both nerves run up the neck towards the larynx in 'grooves' between the oesophagus and trachea, giving branches to each. The upper part of the recurrent laryngeal nerve then passes between, or in close relation to, the branches of the inferior thyroid artery and in intimate proximity to the posteromedial aspect of the thyroid gland. It enters the larynx by passing deep to, or between, the fibres of the cricopharyngeus muscle at its attachment to the lateral aspect of the cricoid cartilage, supplying the muscle as it passes. The recurrent laryngeal

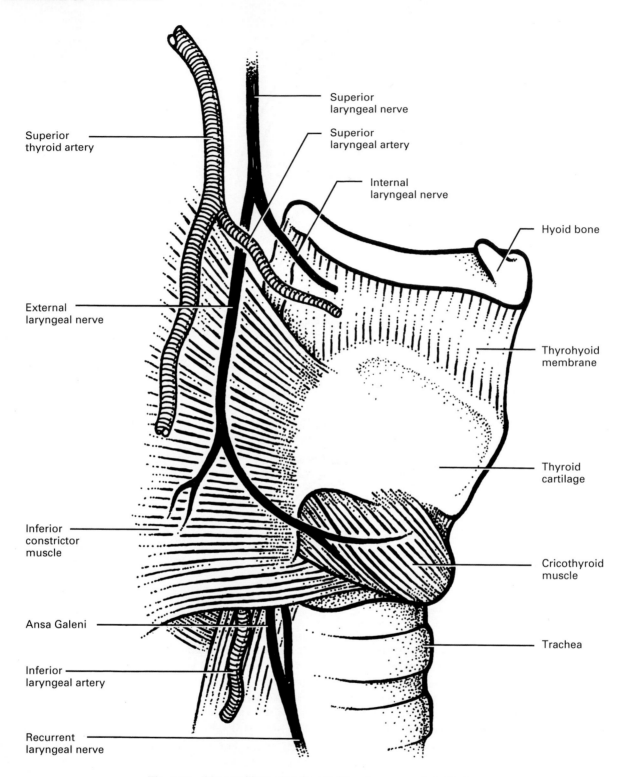

Fig. 2.16 Diagram illustrating the arterial and nerve supply to the larynx.

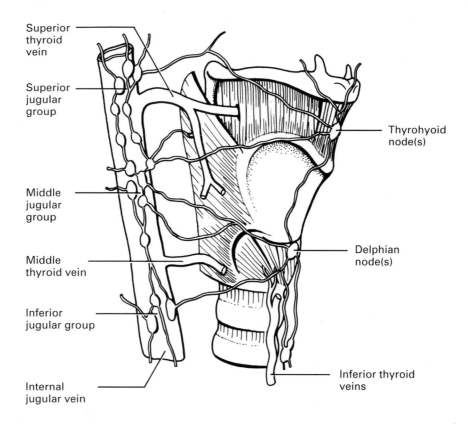

Fig. 2.17   Diagram illustrating the venous and lymphatic drainage of the larynx (after Tucker[8]).

nerve passes posterior to the crico-thyroid joint (although in 15–20% of cases it passes anterior to it or around it). It then usually divides into two branches, an anterior motor branch and a posterior sensory branch. A communicating branch reaches the superior laryngeal nerve via the ansa Galeni. Once inside the larynx, the recurrent laryngeal nerve supplies all the intrinsic muscles of the larynx (save for the cricothyroid muscle) and the mucosa of the subglottis and glottis.

Parasympathetic, secretomotor fibres run with both the superior and recurrent laryngeal nerves to glands throughout the larynx. Sympathetic fibres run to the larynx with its blood supply, having their origin in the superior and middle cervical ganglia.

THE INFANT LARYNX

The infant larynx differs markedly from the adult larynx.[8] It is relatively smaller and this has two main consequences. First, it s lumen is disproportionately narrower than the adult, and second, it lies higher in the neck than the adult larynx. The tip of the epiglottis is located at the level of the intervertebral disc between the first and second cervical vertebrae. This high position is associated with the ability of the infant to use its nasal airway to

breathe while suckling. The epiglottis is Ω-shaped, with a furled petiole, and the laryngeal cartilages are soft and more pliable than those of the adult larynx (a fact which may predispose to airway collapse in inspiration, leading to the clinical picture of laryngomalacia). The thyrohyoid ligament is relatively short, making emergency cricothyrotomy extremely difficult. The mucosa of the supraglottis is more loosely attached than it is in the adult larynx, and it exhibits multiple submucosal glands. Inflammation of the supraglottis will therefore rapidly result in gross oedema due to the laxity of the supraglottic soft tissues. The mucosa is also lax in the subglottis, the narrowest part of the infant larynx measuring 3.5 mm in diameter in neonates. Swelling at this point rapidly results in severe respiratory obstruction.

THE FUNCTIONAL ANATOMY OF THE LARYNX

Not only is the larynx the organ of phonation, it is also important in airway maintenance. Temporary closure of the larynx occurs physiologically in three situations: speech, swallowing, and just before sneezing and coughing. During swallowing, the airway is protected by the sphincteric action of the interarytenoid muscle and by the adductors of the glottis. The larynx is elevated and anteriorly displaced below the base of the tongue by the contraction of the suprahyoid muscles. A combination of these two actions produces a rotational displacement of the epiglottis which comes to lie, to a greater or lesser extent, over the laryngeal inlet. Respiration is also momentarily inhibited.

Prior to sneezing and coughing, the vocal cords are apposed and the respiratory muscles contract, producing a build up of intrathoracic pressure prior to explosive, expulsive expiration.

Phonation, the production of sounds by the larynx for articulation by the palate, tongue, teeth and lips, depends on the co-ordinated movements of the abdominal and thoracic muscles of respiration and the intrinsic musculature of the larynx. During phonation, the vocal cords, which are held in abduction during quiet respiration, are approximated and vibrate. The intensity of the sound produced is dependent on the velocity of the expired air and the disposition of the vocal cords with respect to each other. The deeper pitch of the adult male voice depends on the greater length of the vocal cords (15 mm in males compared with 11 mm in females). In individual subjects, the length of the vocal cord varies as a result of the change in the disposition of the cricoid cartilage with respect to the thyroid cartilage, which in turn is dependent on the degree of contraction of the cricothyroid muscles.

Both pitch and quality (or timbre) of the voice depend upon the tension in the vocal cords. Such tension is dependent on the degree of contraction of the cricothyroid and thyro-arytenoid muscles. The shape of the vocal cord is variable and depends on the degree of contraction of the vocalis portion of the thyro-arytenoid muscles.

Whilst variation in cord shape has a direct effect on the quality of the voice produced, the timbre of the voice is directly dependent on the state of the cordal mucosa and the relative laxity of the submucosal Reinke's space. The expiratory airflow induces a rippling of the mucosa of the cord overlying Reinke's space and it is the integrity of this 'mucosal wave' which determines the 'normality' of the timbre of the voice (Fig. 2.18). Its integrity may be disrupted by inflammation or neoplasia, resulting in a change of timbre and the production of a hoarse, abnormal voice, characteristic of diseases affecting the vocal cords. The mucosal wave may be 'frozen' with stroboscopic light during endoscopic examination (Fig. 2.19). Using such instruments, the detection of lesions affecting the mucosal wave is possible at an earlier stage in their development than when using conventional illumination.[3]

ACKNOWLEDGEMENTS

We are grateful to Mr F. Sambrook for photographic assistance, and to the President and Council of the Royal College of Surgeons of England for permission to use the dissected material illustrated. We thank Professor Sir Donald Harrison for providing Figs 2.9–2.12.

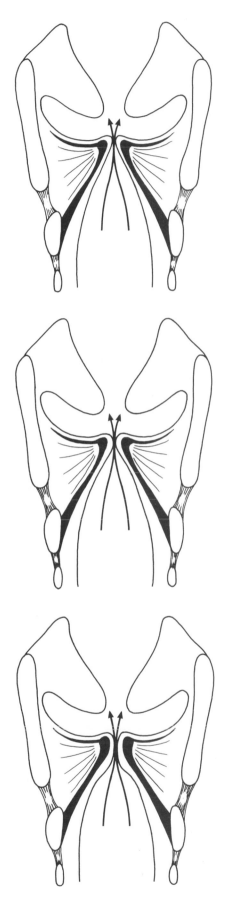

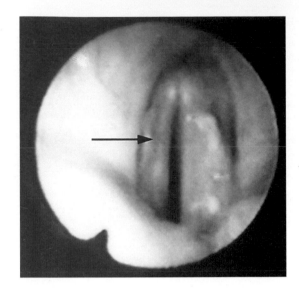

Fig. 2.18 (*left*) Diagram of a longitudinal section through the larynx illustrating the glottic mucosal wave associated with the vocal cords.

Fig. 2.19 (*above*) Glottic mucosal wave (arrow) as visualized with a stroboscopic laryngoscope.

REFERENCES

1. Berkovitz BB, Moxham BJ 1988 A textbook of head and neck anatomy. Wolfe Medical Publications Ltd, London
2. Friedmann I, Ferlito A 1988 Granulomas and neoplasms of the larynx. Churchill Livingstone, Edinburgh
3. Kitzing P 1985 Stroboscopy — a pertinent laryngological examination. J Otolaryngol 14: 151–157
4. Langman J 1989 Medical embryology, 6th edn. Williams and Wilkins, Baltimore
5. Silver CE 1981 Surgery for cancer of the larynx and related structures. Churchill Livingstone, London
6. Stell PM, Gregory I, Watt J 1978 Morphometry of the epithelial lining of the human larynx. I. The glottis. Clin Otolaryngol 3: 13–20
7. Stell PM, Gregory I, Watt J 1980 Morphology of the human larynx. II. The subglottis. Clin Otolaryngol 5: 389–395
8. Tucker HM 1987 The larynx. Thieme Medical Publishers Inc, New York
9. Weir N 1987 Anatomy of the larynx and tracheobronchial tree. In: Scott-Brown's Otolaryngology, vol 1, 5th edn. Butterworth, London

3. Epidemiology

J. A. H. Waterhouse

INTRODUCTION

Epidemiology provides a general picture of a disease, mainly through its quantitative aspects. It summarizes the interplay between the features of the disease and those of the population in which it occurs. Its impact on that population can be measured in terms which can be compared, legitimately and properly, with its impact on populations otherwise constituted in terms of their make-up by sex, age, climate, ethnicity, occupation, etc. or with the impact of different diseases. Correspondingly it can be used to measure changes in relation to time, or to geographical situation, or to environmental circumstances. Essentially, it represents an extension of experience, the experience of an individual clinician being inadequate, in itself, to furnish a sufficient range and variety of cases, and generally being incapable of providing detailed characteristics of the source population. By suitably linking together the data available from all clinical sources in an identifiable and defined area whose population details are known, appropriate measures can be obtained and used for comparison and evaluation in relation to others.

Most epidemiological measures are presented in the form of rates, where the numbers of those who have succumbed to the disease are set against the totality of those who might have succumbed — or, more properly, were, or are, at risk of the disease — together with those who did contract it. Thus, out of the whole population under review, the proportion affected by the disease provides a useful measure of its impact. Those 'affected by the disease' may refer to cases diagnosed, or to deaths from the disease, or it may include both, within a period of time which is usually a calendar year. Rates based on deaths as certificated, and collected centrally, provided the first measures, and these have been available for many countries for well over a century. In addition to the crude rate, which sets all deaths from the disease against the total population, mortality rates are usually available by sex and age group, and often also by other population subdivisions, such as geographic localities.

More recently, and mostly within the last thirty years, cancer registries have been set up in order to collect together the records of newly diagnosed cases of the disease occurring within a defined geographical area. If the population of that area is known in sufficient detail, the registry can supply rates of incidence of the disease by age group and sex, and possibly in relation to other features, such as ethnic group. In contrast to mortality rates, these incidence (or morbidity) rates can be much more useful in describing the impact of the disease, especially if survival is good and eventual death may be attributable to causes other than the cancer. Tables of incidence by site, sex and age group, have been collected from cancer registries and published at quinquennial intervals by the International Agency for Research on Cancer (IARC) at Lyon in a series of volumes (*Cancer Incidence in Five Continents*[1,2,6,10,11]) of which the sixth is almost completed. In the period of a quarter-century, these volumes have increased very considerably in their range of source data, especially in their coverage of the world, though there are still many important lacunae where it would be very desirable to be able to obtain good epidemiological information to aid in the classification of possible aetiological and environmental factors.

AGE AND SEX

Rather more men than women suffer from laryngeal cancer; the ratio varies between different countries from 20 or above down to about 4, though the majority fall into the range 6 to 10. The majority will fall into the age range from 50 to 75 when first presenting. Naturally, there will be some differences between countries, and over time periods, but they are relatively small. Figure 3.1 shows the distribution by age of new male patients in each of three decades for the Birmingham Cancer Registry covering a population of just over five million people in the Midlands of England. The shapes of the distributions are very similar, and although the numbers of cases in the last decade were 43% greater than in the

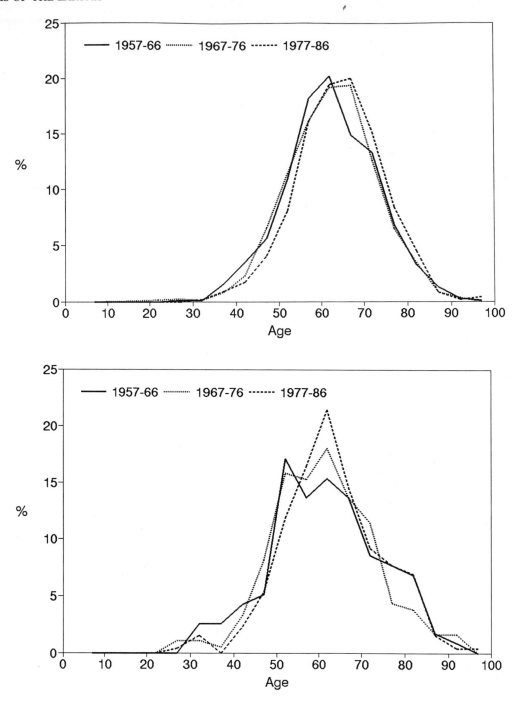

Fig. 3.1 (*top*) Distribution (%) of cases by age (5-year age groups) for each of three decades: males.

Fig. 3.2 (*bottom*) Distribution (%) of cases by age (5-year age groups) for each of three decades: females.

first (which were just over 1000), the mean ages for each decade were 62.7, 62.8 and 62.9 years. Figure 3.2 shows a similar set of graphs for females from the same population. It is very much more irregular since the numbers are smaller (just over 100 in the first decade) but they increase by 123% in the twenty years between the first and third decades. Again, in terms of their mean ages, the changes are small, being successively 61.8, 61.6 and 63.4. However, the large increase in numbers is typical of the experience of many countries in a similar period, and is generally ascribed to the increase of smoking among women.

Figure 3.3 shows that the increase in numbers of cases by year has been reasonably steady, though subject to irregular fluctuations. For two reasons the vertical scale of Figure 3.3 has been chosen to be a logarithmic one: first, in order to display simultaneously the numbers for two sexes without too wide a separation between them (since their ratio is nearly ten to one), and secondly, to permit legitimately the comparison of their slopes, or rates of increase. For this latter purpose it is clear that the number of females is increasing more rapidly than the number of males, since the upward trend in females is steeper, though the actual number of new female cases each year is less than the number of new male cases.

The numbers of new cases of either sex presenting each year will of course depend essentially on the size of the population under review and on the severity of the disease in that population. In order to characterize the impact of the disease on the population, and to facilitate comparison with other situations, the numbers of cases need to be classified by sex and age group and set against the corresponding classes in the description of the population, thus obtaining the incidence rates by sex and age group. These rates are shown in Figure 3.4, again using a logarithmic vertical scale for the same reasons as above. Figure 3.4 clearly shows that the general shape of the curve is the same for each sex, despite the ratio of around 10:1 of the absolute rates in the latter age groups. The small peak in the female rate around the age of 30 is almost certainly fortuitous rather than indicative of any real factor influencing the disease at that age in women. The general pattern of the incidence curves by sex is very similar to those of many other countries, as may be found from their data provided in *Cancer Incidence in Five Continents*,[1,2,6,10,11] or in *Patterns of Cancer in Five Continents*.[12] The shape at the upper end is unlikely to show any marked divergence from a broadly smooth curve, any apparent departure being the result of the small numbers of cases found in the extreme age groups, where diagnosis may be difficult.

The data from the Birmingham Cancer Registry have been collected in a uniform manner over a period of more than thirty years, and have always included very full descriptions of the primary tumour, its extent, histology and treatment. Moreover, the regularity and quality of follow-up have also been consistently good. For these reasons, a series of clinical cancer monographs has been based on the data, of which the second volume is entitled *Cancer of the Larynx*.[7] Data from a period of twenty-five years were available at the time of preparation of that book, and this period was divided into five quinquennial

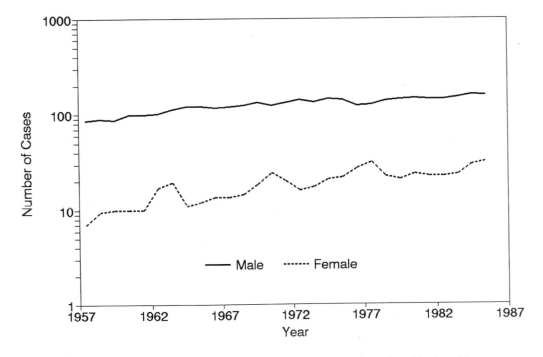

Fig. 3.3   Numbers of cases (2-point moving average) by year and sex (logarithmic scale).

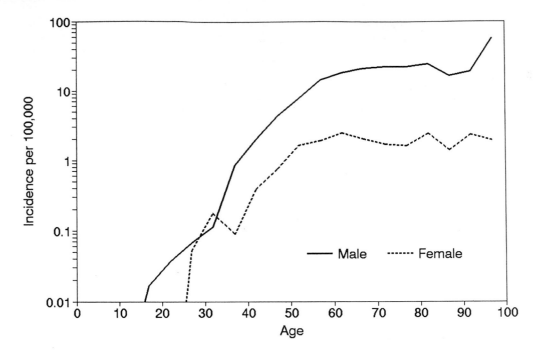

Fig. 3.4 Incidence (per 100 000) by age (5-year groups) and sex (logarithmic scale).

periods. To these data a further quinquennial period can now be added so that secular changes over the spell of thirty years can be examined in detail. The numbers of cases amount to 3778 males and 561 females; these numbers are more usefully examined in three decennial periods to avoid the irregularities inevitable in finer subdivisions, due to small numbers in certain categories.

Figure 3.5 shows the incidence by age for males in each of the three decades 1957–66, 1967–76 and 1977–86. Clearly, they are very similar, both in shape and position; furthermore, the rates for the first decade are consistently lower than for both the others, while the rates for the last decade fall below the middle one only at the rate for age 50. The age groups used for this graph, and for the next, encompass ten years in order to match the spacing of the decades. One result of this aggregation of the age groups is to reduce the fluctuations seen in earlier graphs, since the numbers in each group are increased. A similar effect is found in Figure 3.6, for female incidence rates. In presenting these graphs, the overall range of age has been restricted for purposes of clarification. The greater degree of separation between the three curves in Figure 3.6 emphasizes the more rapid rise in the incidence of the disease in females.

This clear separation facilitates the demonstration of 'cohort' incidence rates. The term 'cohort' is used for convenience in epidemiology to describe a group defined in a particular manner, which, in this application, is a group of people (women, since Figure 3.6 refers to female rates) of a similar age, and thus born within a few years of each other. Take for instance the group of women of

mean age 50 in the first decade, whose risk of developing laryngeal cancer is represented by the first point on the lowest curve in Fig. 3.6. This age group refers to those aged between 45 and 54 in the first decade (1957–66): their central year of birth will be 1912, though their years of birth can range from 1903 to 1921 – very few being in the extreme years of the range. After the expiry of ten years, they will be ten years older (mean age 60), and the time period is now that of the second decade (1967–76) so that their risk of laryngeal cancer is now represented by the second point (age 60) on the second curve. Finally, after the lapse of a further ten years their mean age will have become 70 and the period is now that of the third decade. Their risk is represented by the third point on the third curve. Linking together the three points discussed here provides the incidence rates curve for the 1912 cohort, shown in Figure 3.7, together with three other cohort curves constructed in a similar way from Figure 3.6. In the sense that such cohort curves describe the pattern of incidence by age in relation to birth-year, they represent more realistically lifetime risks for all those of a 'generation' defined by the central birth-year. They may also be interpreted to show the results of secular changes: the fact that the curves for successively more recently born cohorts in Figure 3.7 show consistently higher rates of incidence suggests that younger women may be exposed increasingly to some aetiological factors, such as smoking. Smoking among women is known to have been increasing in the past few decades, and it is also known as an aetiological factor in cancer of the larynx (see, for instance, Tuyns[9]). However, the connection is not proved

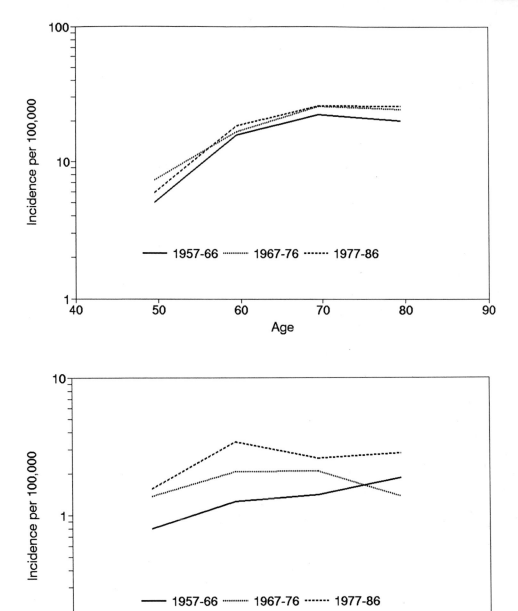

Fig. 3.5 (*top*) Incidence (per 100 000) by age (10-year groups) for each of three decades (logarithmic scale): males.

Fig. 3.6 (*bottom*) Incidence (per 100 000) by age (10-year groups) for each of three decades (logarithmic scale): females.

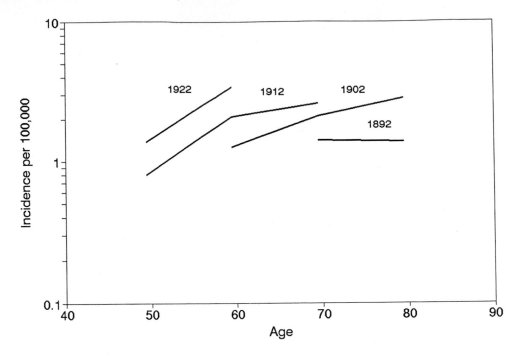

Fig. 3.7 Sections of cohort age incidence curves by central birth year: females.

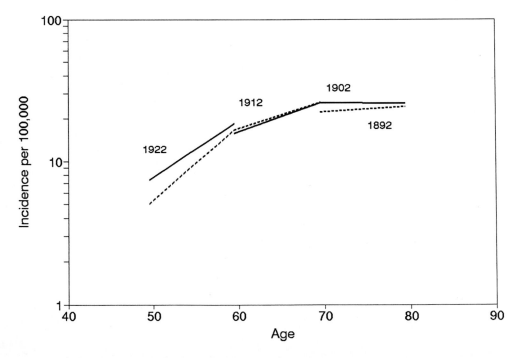

Fig. 3.8 Sections of cohort age incidence curves by central birth year: males.

by such statements; it can be established only by specific studies set up for that purpose.

Figure 3.8 shows in the same way the birth–cohort curves for males. Here, the separation between successive curves is not so striking as among the females, but it is of the same pattern in that successively more recently-born cohorts have higher incidence rates.

STANDARDIZATION OF RATES TO LEGITIMIZE COMPARISONS

Not only do the incidence rates change with time, sex and age, but they are also influenced by changes in the characteristics of the population base which form the denominators of the rates. Populations naturally change over time, but their structures, in terms of sex, age, ethnicity etc., can also differ markedly between countries. Is it possible to make legitimate comparisons of rates under such circumstances?

A full comparison of two sources of data can be made by comparing the shapes of the incidence rate curves by age, for each sex separately, on the same graph. If both the incidence rates by age group (usually five-year) and the population in the same groups are available for each source, then a single ratio may be found to express their relationship by setting the crude incidence rate (total of cases regardless of age — but for one sex — divided by the total of the population for that sex) of one against a computed crude rate; this rate is obtained by applying each age-specific rate from the second source to the population of that age-group in the first population, thus providing a set of 'expected' cases which would have occurred if the first population had experienced the age-specific rates of the second. Clearly, the situation could be reversed and the same procedure followed. The resultant ratio will be slightly – but usually not very – different.

If one population can be taken as a standard, the method described above can be used to obtain a single incidence rate for any other population, and thereby avoid the major distorting effect of differences in age structure. The Japanese epidemiologist Segi[8] was the first to construct a standard population which he designed to be intermediate between the preponderantly young pattern of developing countries and the rather older pattern of the developed countries. With relatively minor amendments of his original work, the *World Standard Population* is now generally accepted as a basis for comparison of morbidity or mortality rates worldwide. Such rates are described as world standardized rates (WSR).

WORLD VARIATIONS IN INCIDENCE OF LARYNGEAL CANCER

Figure 3.9, taken from *Patterns of Cancer in Five Continents*,[12] in a form of presentation very characteristic of Segi, gives an indication of the wide difference in incidence over the world, from Sao Paulo in Brazil to the Japanese in Los Angeles for men, and from Blacks in Connecticut to the Japanese in Miyagi, Japan, for women. These figures had been taken from the fifth volume of *Cancer Incidence in Five Continents*[6] and they refer of course to morbidity rates from cancer registries, all of which must satisfy minimum standards of quality of data to qualify for admission. Five of the male populations in Figure 3.9 have rates above 10. However, the countries (registries) included in Figure 3.9 number forty, and have been chosen to give the widest possible geographical representation. Of the total of 137 (excluding rural/urban subdivisions) in the whole of the fifth volume, there are 16 with male rates above 10. High rates are found in

Brazil, Spain, Italy, France, India and among black populations in the USA. From previous volumes, though including fewer sources of data, the same groups account for the highest rates. Figure 3.9 shows that the pattern for females differs somewhat from that for males, and, of course, covers a much smaller range.

Figure 3.10 shows — separately for males and females — the distribution of the WSRs from each of the five volumes of *Cancer Incidence in Five Continents*.[1,2,6,10,11] Again, these exclude subdivisions (rural/urban) or aggregates (all Canada, all Scotland, etc.). They are not symmetric distributions but are all positively skew, with a 'tail' to the right which increases from the first to the fifth volume. Table 3.1 shows, in the 'medians' and in the 'highest rates', the increases found in the male WSRs after successive five-year intervals.

By utilizing the WSRs in the foregoing discussion, the wide variations in population age structure between the many different registries have been virtually eliminated. However, a better appreciation of the impact of the disease on populations from various parts of the world can be obtained from the shape of the age incidence curve. Figure 3.11 shows four such graphs of incidence rates by sex and age (five-year groups). The irregularities, especially in the female rates, can be largely ignored since they are due to the small number of cases compared to those in males. Sweden shows a pattern typical of many developed countries of mainly European stock; Puerto Rico is not very dissimilar, except in that the rates in both sexes are higher than in Sweden, above the age of fifty. In comparison, the female rates in French Bas-Rhin are diminutive, but the male rates are much higher. This is typical of several other French registries. For Bombay, the curves approximate two nearly straight parallel lines, showing little evidence of flattening at the upper ages. Bombay does, in fact, possess the highest rates for each sex, at the upper extremity of the age range.

When appropriate environmental and geographical data are available, and can be correlated to sufficiently detailed incidence tabulations, they can lead to the formulation of hypotheses of aetiology, which again can be tested from subsequent data, suitably selected for the purpose. Among these may be the co-incidence of diseases, or perhaps the enhanced incidence of a cancer among the sequelae of a chronic disease. A number of such examples are already known, but there may be many yet to find, which may provide valuable indications of detailed pathogenesis.

Table 3.1 Changes of WSR over 20 years in two parameters of the world distribution

Volume number	I	II	III	IV	V
Median	3.4	4.3	5.3	5.7	5.9
Highest rate	8.6	13.8	14.1	17.6	17.8

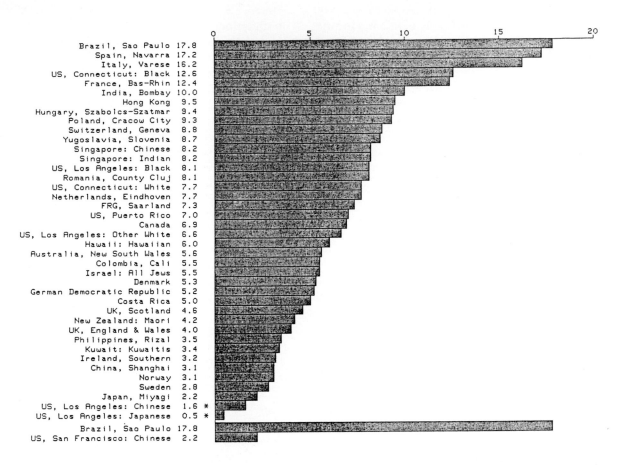

Brazil, Sao Paulo	17.8	
Spain, Navarra	17.2	
Italy, Varese	16.2	
US, Connecticut: Black	12.6	
France, Bas-Rhin	12.4	
India, Bombay	10.0	
Hong Kong	9.5	
Hungary, Szabolcs-Szatmar	9.4	
Poland, Cracow City	9.3	
Switzerland, Geneva	8.8	
Yugoslavia, Slovenia	8.7	
Singapore: Chinese	8.2	
Singapore: Indian	8.2	
US, Los Angeles: Black	8.1	
Romania, County Cluj	8.1	
US, Connecticut: White	7.7	
Netherlands, Eindhoven	7.7	
FRG, Saarland	7.3	
US, Puerto Rico	7.0	
Canada	6.9	
US, Los Angeles: Other White	6.6	
Hawaii: Hawaiian	6.0	
Australia, New South Wales	5.6	
Colombia, Cali	5.5	
Israel: All Jews	5.5	
Denmark	5.3	
German Democratic Republic	5.2	
Costa Rica	5.0	
UK, Scotland	4.6	
New Zealand: Maori	4.2	
UK, England & Wales	4.0	
Philippines, Rizal	3.5	
Kuwait: Kuwaitis	3.4	
Ireland, Southern	3.2	
China, Shanghai	3.1	
Norway	3.1	
Sweden	2.8	
Japan, Miyagi	2.2	
US, Los Angeles: Chinese	1.6	*
US, Los Angeles: Japanese	0.5	*
Brazil, Sao Paulo	17.8	
US, San Francisco: Chinese	2.2	

* Rates based on less than 10 cases

Fig. 3.9 World standardized rates (WSR) of incidence for 40 representative source in five continents. *Above*: male; *opposite page*: female.

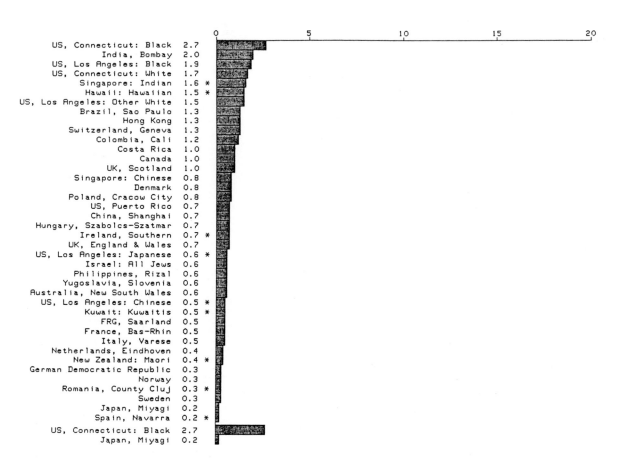

		0	5	10	15	20
US, Connecticut: Black	2.7					
India, Bombay	2.0					
US, Los Angeles: Black	1.9					
US, Connecticut: White	1.7					
Singapore: Indian	1.6 *					
Hawaii: Hawaiian	1.5 *					
US, Los Angeles: Other White	1.5					
Brazil, Sao Paulo	1.3					
Hong Kong	1.3					
Switzerland, Geneva	1.3					
Colombia, Cali	1.2					
Costa Rica	1.0					
Canada	1.0					
UK, Scotland	1.0					
Singapore: Chinese	0.8					
Denmark	0.8					
Poland, Cracow City	0.8					
US, Puerto Rico	0.7					
China, Shanghai	0.7					
Hungary, Szabolcs-Szatmar	0.7					
Ireland, Southern	0.7 *					
UK, England & Wales	0.7					
US, Los Angeles: Japanese	0.6 *					
Israel: All Jews	0.6					
Philippines, Rizal	0.6					
Yugoslavia, Slovenia	0.6					
Australia, New South Wales	0.6					
US, Los Angeles: Chinese	0.5 *					
Kuwait: Kuwaitis	0.5 *					
FRG, Saarland	0.5					
France, Bas-Rhin	0.5					
Italy, Varese	0.5					
Netherlands, Eindhoven	0.4					
New Zealand: Maori	0.4 *					
German Democratic Republic	0.3					
Norway	0.3					
Romania, County Cluj	0.3 *					
Sweden	0.3					
Japan, Miyagi	0.2					
Spain, Navarra	0.2 *					
US, Connecticut: Black	2.7					
Japan, Miyagi	0.2					

* Rates based on less than 10 cases

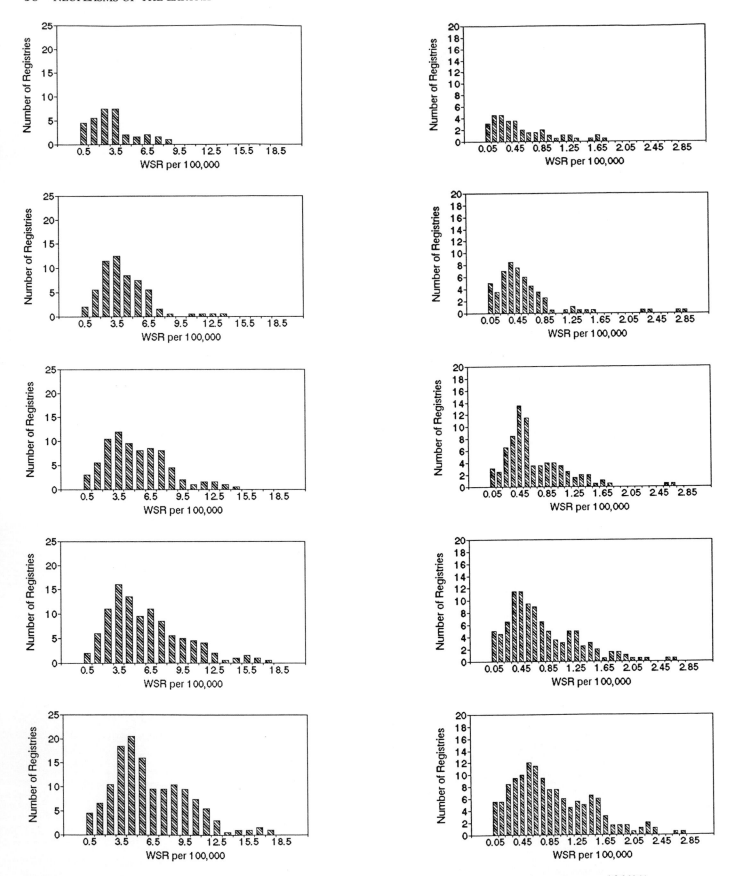

Fig. 3.10 Distribution by WSR of individual sources in each of five successive volumes of *Cancer Incidence in Five Continents*[1,2,6,10,11].
Left: male; *right*: female.

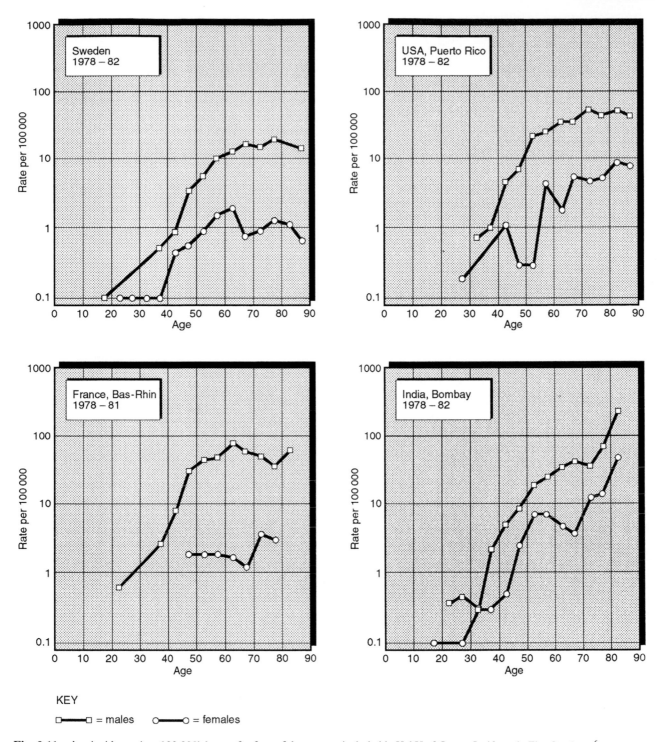

KEY

□——□ = males   ○——○ = females

Fig. 3.11 Age incidence (per 100 000) by sex for four of the sources included in Vol V of *Cancer Incidence in Five Continents*[6] (logarithmic scale).

MULTIPLE PRIMARY CANCERS

Not far removed from the preceding reference to the co-incidence of diseases is the incidence of multiple primary cancers, where it is clear, by the application of stringent and agreed rules, that one is not a metastasis of the other. It has been shown by Robin *et al* that there is an excess of second primary cancers, when the first primary is larynx, in both men and women, and that their number is statistically significantly raised above expectation.[7] The principal sites of the second primaries are: bronchus and lung; mouth and tongue in both sexes, and pharynx (but not nasopharynx); colorectum; and skin.

The same study found an association with social class, the ratio of observed to expected being highest in classes I and II when the second primary was colorectal, and high in classes III, IV and V for bronchus. These associations were for males only, partly because the smaller numbers of females were inadequate to demonstrate additional relationships, and partly also because the five social classes used here are based on occupation: I is professional and senior executive, II managerial, below I, III is for skilled workers, being sometimes subdivided into non-manual and manual, IV is semi-skilled workers, and V unskilled workers. This study found that the risk of a second primary among laryngeal cancer cases was increasing over the 25 years of the survey, and also concluded that there was no evidence of any influence of therapeutic radiation in the causation of second primaries.

SUBSITES

The standard WHO *International Classification of Diseases*[5] (ICD) in its 9th Revision (ICD-9) includes provision of a fourth digit to subdivide the principal three-figure categories into greater detail. As a site of cancer, larynx is classified 161, and the additional ('decimal') digits provided are:

161.0	Glottis, vocal cord
.1	Supraglottis
.2	Subglottis
.3	Laryngeal cartilage
.8	Other
.9	Unspecified

Site detail by fourth digit was requested for the fifth volume of *Cancer Incidence in Five Continents*,[6] and most registries provided it. In the presentation of the data from such registries the last three categories were grouped together, which, since .3 is extremely rare, amounts to a measure of the uncertainty or of the inadequacy of information available. A relatively large proportion of the whole site classified in that category therefore throws some doubt on the completeness of the first three groups.

For many registries, however, that proportion is low, and so is that in .2 (subglottis). The ratio of glottis to supraglottis in males is then near to 2:1, though for blacks in the USA it is closer to 1:1. In each of the four French registries, and in Basel and Zaragoza, the ratio is 1:2. In females, the ratio is usually 1:1, though sometimes, as for blacks in the USA, it is 1:2, or even 1:3. Further information in subsequent volumes may help to indicate how these subsites change with time.

Figures 3.12 and 3.13, from Robin *et al*,[7] show the trends of incidence by sex for each of the three principal subsites, by quinquennium. The vertical scale is logarithmic, in order to legitimize the direct comparison of the slopes. The females show a clear upward trend for all three subsites, running closely parallel and thus at the same rate of increase, with glottis and supraglottis in close proximity. The males, on the other hand, show only a slight increase for glottis and possible downturns for the other two subsites in the last quinquennium. It has not yet proved possible to obtain comparable data for the quinquennium 1982–1986; such data might help to indicate whether the downturn continues in the males for both supra- and subglottis.

Figures 3.14 and 3.15, also from Robin et al,[7] serve to demonstrate the age incidence curves in each sex for the three subsites under review. They are generally similar in shape to the overall curve (i.e., for all larynx), when allowance is made for the irregularities in the females due to smaller numbers, and their spacing follows what has already been shown in the previous pair of figures: that, for males, glottis is the commonest, followed by supraglottis and then subglottis; for females, the curves for glottis and supraglottis almost coincide, while subglottis is the least frequent.

Table 3.2 shows the distribution by subsites for males within each of the five social classes (as defined earlier). The two extreme social classes, I and V, show the greatest differences, I with 69% which were at the glottis, compared with V with 55%, and likewise for subglottis, but in the opposite direction for supraglottis. The other social classes show intermediate figures. No ready explanation is available for these differences.

Table 3.2 Distribution of subsites by Social Class

Subsite	Social Class					
	I	II	III	IV	V	NK
Glottis	69	64	65	62	55	70
Supraglottis	22	25	26	28	36	20
Subglottis	5	4	3	5	3	3
Not specified	4	7	6	5	6	7
	(100)	(100)	(100)	(100)	(100)	(100

Note. Based on 2337 cases. Percentages have been rounded up for simplicity.

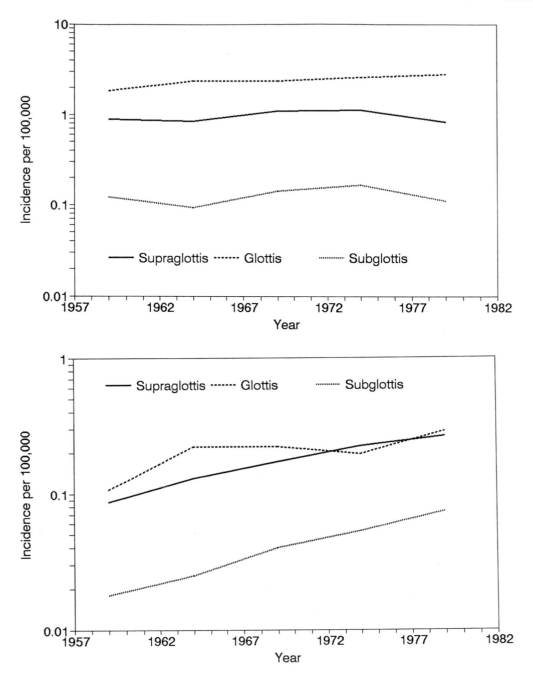

Fig. 3.12 (*top*) WSR by quinquennium and subsite (logarithmic scale): males.

Fig. 3.13 (*bottom*) WSR by quinquennium and subsite (logarithmic scale): females.

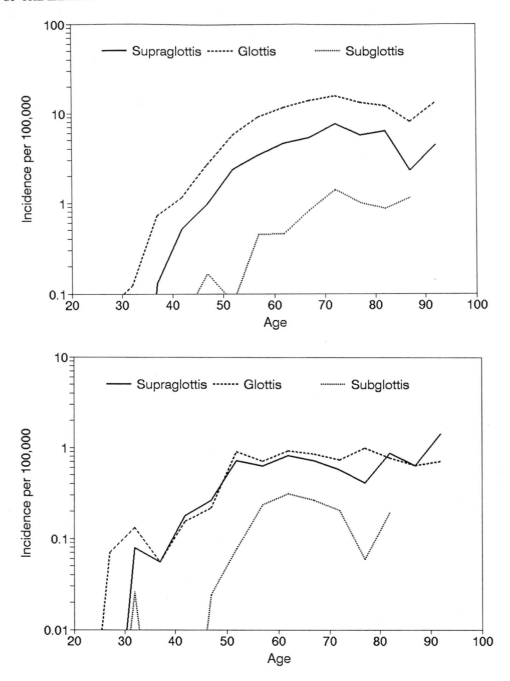

Fig. 3.14 (*top*) Age incidence (per 100 000) by subsite (logarithmic scale): males.

Fig. 3.15 (*bottom*) Age incidence (per 100 000) by subsite (logarithmic scale): females.

SURVIVAL

Figure 3.16 shows the annual age-adjusted survival rates by sex and subsite. Age-adjusted survival rates take into account (usually from life tables) the increasing mortality, from causes other than cancer, with advancing age, and thus render comparisons virtually unaffected by differences in the initial age structure of the laryngeal patients. Survival rates for glottis tumours are remarkably similar in both sexes, and are clearly very much better than they are for either of the other two subsites. Survival rates for both supraglottis and subglottis in men are almost identical, while in women they differ markedly after two years – subglottis cases experiencing a sudden drop in survival. This result could be an artefact of the particular group of cases of subglottis cancer in females, which numbered only forty-one.

ENVOI

Study of the variations of behaviour in relation to histology, to TNM[3] or other staging system, or to treatment, both initial and subsequent, can provide a fuller picture of laryngeal cancer from an epidemiological viewpoint. Much of the detailed analysis has been undertaken extensively in the monograph *Cancer of the Larynx* by Robin et al,[7] and it is unnecessary to repeat it here. The reader seeking further detail of this kind should therefore consult this volume for information.

The potential quantitative information to be gained from collecting together a full description of each case, at presentation and examination, of treatments given, and with follow-up listing subsequent development or extensions of the growth and treatment, to ultimate death with immediate cause and condition of tumour if still present, is very great, especially if the data are collected in a strictly consistent way. Fortunately there are several standard systems of description now available to promote uniformity and comparability; these include ICD-O (*International Classification of Diseases — Oncology*),[4] which includes a detailed histological classification, and the TNM[3] for size of tumour, node involvement and metastases. These, together with others not yet so widespread in use, will help in providing broader epidemiological contributions for the clinical management of the disease.

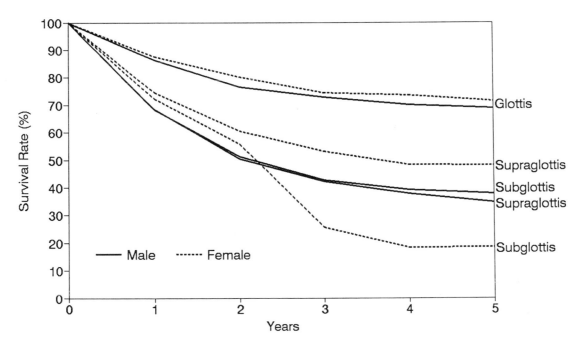

Fig. 3.16   Survival rate (%) by subsite and sex.

REFERENCES

1. Doll R, Payne P, Waterhouse J 1966 Cancer incidence in five continents, Vol I. UICC, Geneva
2. Doll R, Muir C, Waterhouse J 1970 Cancer incidence in five continents, Vol II. UICC, Geneva
3. Harmer M H 1978 TNM classification of malignant tumours. Union Internationale Contre le Cancer (UICC), Geneva
4. ICD-O (International classification of diseases — oncology) 1976 WHO, Geneva
5. International classification of diseases (ICD), 9th revision 1977 WHO, Geneva
6. Muir C, Waterhouse J, Mack T, Powell J, Whelan S 1987 Cancer incidence in five continents, Vol V. IARC, Lyon
7. Robin P E, Powell J, Holme G M, Waterhouse J A H, McConkey C C, Robertson J E, 1989 Cancer of the larynx. MacMillan, London
8. Segi M 1977 Graphic presentation of cancer incidence by site and by area and population. Segi Institute of Cancer Epidemiology, Nagoya (Japan)
9. Tuyns A J 1982 Incidence trends of laryngeal cancer in relation to national alcohol and tobacco consumption. In: Magnus K (ed) Trends in cancer incidence. Hemisphere Publishing Corporation, Washington
10. Waterhouse J, Muir C S, Correa P, Powell J 1976 Cancer incidence in five continents, Vol III. IARC, Lyon
11. Waterhouse J, Muir C, Shanmugaratnam K, Powell J 1982 Cancer incidence in five continents, Vol IV. IARC, Lyon
12. Whelan S, Parkin D M, Masuyer E 1990 Patterns of cancer in five continents, IARC, Lyon

4. Laryngeal cancer: a preventable disease

D. F. N. Harrison

Despite the ineffectiveness of much cancer research, which hitherto has been related primarily to animal experimentation rather than to molecular biology, there is good evidence that the causes of many human cancers are now recognizable. All can be partly, if not entirely, eliminated or avoided, yet there is little evidence that this is happening or likely to happen. Epidemiologists have shown that the risk of developing most of the commoner cancers varies greatly in relation to where you live, your ethnic group, or your age — often in relation to all three. Some of the variation between population groups is possibly due to genetic differences in susceptibility but cannot explain changes in risk over time, or differences in national populations after migration, such as in nasopharyngeal carcinoma. The activation of polycyclic aromatic hydrocarbons by aryl hydrocarbon hydroxylase (AHH) to epoxides, which, in turn, form covalent bonds with RNA and DNA, is a prominent feature in carcinogenesis.[7] AHH inducibility has been determined in lymphocytes in 90 patients with laryngeal cancer, and a significantly high percentage (21%) had high levels compared with controls (11%).[10] Mitogen-stimulated human lymphocytic studies of AHH activity show individual variations which have a single autosomal locus of genetic control. It may be that there is a genetic difference in susceptibility to smoke carcinogens, for not everybody who smokes heavily develops lung or laryngeal cancer.[9]

There is, however, a recognizable correlation between the incidence of some cancers and environmental factors — particularly in relation to socioeconomic structure and personal habits. In Norway, the incidence of laryngeal cancer amongst nickel refinery workers has been reported to be 3.9 times the expected rate.[11] Asbestos exposure appears to double the risk of laryngeal cancer[1] but, when these data are adjusted for smoking and alcohol, this relationship becomes tenuous.[2] Indeed, most longitudinal studies which include latency period and incidence, show no excess deaths from laryngeal cancer in asbestos workers. Similar studies relating to the possible role of industrial carcinogens (such as mustard gas) in laryngeal cancer, and studies on textile workers and those involved in the production of irritant materials such as sulphuric acid, have failed to consider adequately the significance of associated smoking or use of alcohol. This is not to say, however, that exposure to sulphuric acid fumes, or those of isopropyl oils, plays no part in the production of this tumour.

Risk factors are those contributing to the cause of a cancer, most of which are considered to be environmental. The epidemiologist recognizes three types of risk, all of which are of importance to the oncologist.

Absolute risk

This is a measure of the occurrence of cancer as shown by incidence or mortality rates. The various factors which are responsible for the risk may not be evenly spread throughout a population, neither may they affect all individuals who are exposed to the same degree.

Relative risk

This is the measure of risk, and is the term most commonly used in cancer statistics. A large relative risk suggests strong association of a risk factor with a specific cancer and is recognized when evidence suggests that this factor forms part of the complex process that increases the probability of the cancer developing. Freedom from this factor will then decrease the likelihood of the cancer forming, i.e., non-smokers are less likely to develop laryngeal cancer.

Attributable risk

This is defined as a measure of the amount of disease in a specific population that would be prevented by alteration in the risk factor, and is probably the most important estimate of risk for practical cancer control. Estimates give a figure of 25% for cancer deaths but 50% for cardiovascular disease. However, it is obvious that such figures must relate to a wide variety of factors such as expectation of life, socioeconomic state and, perhaps of greatest statistical importance, the reliability of recorded data. However, reduction of the recognizable risks for cancer, e.g., smoking and alcohol, together with effective control of hypertension, would prevent over 70% of all premature deaths — and result in a dramatic increase in the world's geriatric population!

How then does laryngeal cancer fit into this epidemiological pattern, and is it really preventable? It is relatively uncommon, so that the accuracy of available statistics depends upon the inclusion of every individual patient. Incidence statistics must always be considered against the background of relevant populations, and especially their age structure. An 'age pyramid' deformed by war, emigration, falling birth-rate or excessive females, will inevitably lead to changes in cancer incidence, irrespective of risk factors. Despite this, within the head and neck, cancer of the larynx and hypopharynx remains the commonest cancer, although in recent years the incidence of oral cancer has been increasing in many countries.

Between 1940 and 1950, a real increase in the incidence of laryngeal cancer was reported from many countries, and there is anecdotal evidence that the mortality from this disease rose by a factor of nine in Italy over the previous two decades. Scandinavian countries, Uruguay, Puerto Rico and parts of the United States all noted an increase which ranged from 5.5 to 7.8 per 100 000 population. However, low figures were recorded in Singapore, Syria and Australia. The world record was held by the Chiang Mai Province in Northern Thailand, with figures of 18.4 per 100 000 male population and 3.4 per 100 000 females. All blamed the smoking of a particularly strong tobacco.

Every race appears to be susceptible, except possibly the indigenous Indians of North and South America. However, those whose religion forbids smoking and the drinking of alcohol — such as the Mormons of Utah and the Seventh Day Adventists — have a particularly low risk of laryngeal and lung cancer. It is also less common amongst the Jews, who tend to smoke and drink less than many other races, an excellent example of the effect social mores have upon an avoidable disease. The site of the neoplasm with the larynx is also influenced by geographical and racial factors, although, as yet, there is no rational explanation for this variation.

Laryngeal cancer at all sites — glottic, supraglottic or subglottic — occurs most frequently between the ages of 55 and 65 years although, when set against the background of the age pyramid in individual populations, the age-corrected incidence continues to rise up to 75 years, and with an ageing population the total number of patients can be expected to increase. 'You have to live long enough to develop any cancer.' This is well illustrated by consideration of the changes now taking place in China.

At the death rate of the 1940s, about half the children born in China could expect to die before middle age. Current death rates, however, suggest that 90% will survive through middle age due to control of malnutrition and infectious diseases. The prime cause of premature death is now tobacco-related disease, particularly laryngeal and lung cancer. In the 1950s, a popular Chinese slogan was 'Food, shelter and a cigarette for everybody' and in 1989, the Chinese consumed one third of the world's cigarettes — 1600 billion. Current trends suggest that by 2025 the incidence of lung and laryngeal cancer will be 900 000 cases per year. This could mean that 50 million Chinese now aged under 20 years will eventually die from tobacco-related disease. In Beijing, smoking is already popular among young women, and, as in the United Kingdom, this will inevitably lead to a higher risk of neoplasia early in their lives.[17]

Below the age of 35 years, men and women appear to run similar risks of developing this neoplasm, and this continues until the incidence curves separate around 40 to 50 years. Younger women may therefore be more susceptible, and with an increasing number of young women smokers there may well be a dramatic increase in the number of women with laryngeal cancer. Indeed, within the United Kingdom this is already seen in the incidence of lung cancer.

Despite clear evidence that the majority of patients with laryngeal cancer are smokers, a small number of cases occur in non-smokers, suggesting the importance of indigenous factors or unusual sensitivity to passive smoking. Non-smokers who live with smokers are at double the risk of death from lung cancer, and there is some evidence that this may also be true for laryngeal cancer.

Although the incidence of laryngeal cancer shows a close correlation with tobacco consumption, neither the geographical nor the ethnic distribution of the cancer mirrors that of lung cancer. The possibility of a synergistic interaction between alcohol and tobacco may explain some differences, and the increase in the United Kingdom of female laryngeal cancer correlates well with change in social habits over the last two decades. Cigarette smoking is largely a 20th-century phenomenon for, until the 1880s when the manufacture was mechanized, snuff and chewing were more popular — although no safer. In World War 1, cigarette rations were largely responsible for the initiation of large numbers of young men and women and, by World War 2, female emancipation had ensured that over 25% of women in Europe and the USA smoked. This habit still retains, however, an inverse relationship with educational attainment, and is now rare amongst doctors in many countries. However, advertising has influenced the young of every country in all social strata, although there is some evidence that the proportion of smokers decreases as the years of education increase!

Most commentators agree that reduction in cigarette smoking should be the prime aim of all health programmes. With this aim in mind, it may appear overambitious to rely heavily on the effects of education. Although partially effective in reducing smoking in the young, over-emphasis may suffer from the law of diminishing returns — merely reinforcing the present level of consumption. In many poor countries it is the least of the health problems, and may be the only source of comfort for its population. Health education must always be viewed in perspective if it is to achieve support and success.

Epidemiological evidence supports a definitive but casual relationship between smoking and laryngeal cancer and, essentially, smoking remains the leading known preventable cause of cancer. It accounts for at least 75% of all cases of laryngeal cancer and, even more significant, perhaps, is the increased likelihood of those patients cured of their laryngeal cancer going on to develop a lung neoplasm. A figure of between 7 and 15% may increase to over 40% if the patient continues to smoke, and the original figure is itself related to the amount of tobacco used prior to the development of the original neoplasm. Some tobaccos appear to be more lethal than others, although 20 cigarettes per day appears to be the minimal risk figure. Absolute correlation is not possible, and it is a curious facet of human habit reporting that individuals appear to think in multiples of 5 or 10. Few report smoking, say, 4 or 18 cigarettes, but over 40 per day may increase the risk of a neoplasm by over 13 times by comparison with a non-smoker.

All cancers within the oral cavity, oropharynx and larynx have also been associated with alcohol consumption, although this is a less important factor in laryngeal cancer where there is minimal direct contact. Most clinical trials show an increased incidence of cancer amongst smokers who drink heavily, and this increase in relative risk is found at all levels of tobacco consumption — although there is doubt as to whether the effects are additional or synergistic.[1] Applying maximum-likelihood techniques to facilitate the estimated index or interaction, Flanders and Rothman[6] found that exposure to alcohol and tobacco increased the risk of laryngeal cancer 50% more than might be expected from a purely additive effect. Others have found them to be independent, with no evidence of synergism.[8]

Although it is generally, if erroneously, accepted that a majority of habitual smokers would like to stop (for health or financial reasons), governments give little incentive for them to do so! In 1610, King James I of England, who succinctly summarized his personal position on tobacco by saying 'A custom loathsome to the eye, hateful to the nose, harmful to the brain, dangerous to the lungs, and in the black stinking fume thereof, nearest resembling the horrible, stingian smoke of the pot that is bottomless,'[5] raised tobacco duty by 4000%, which certainly had an effect on consumption. Less effective was Hong Kong's Financial Secretary who, in 1991, announced a 200% increase in tobacco duty — eventually reduced by half following pressure from the media, trade unions and political lobbying.[12] This is not surprising, for all governments receive considerable revenue from tobacco duty, and it is depressing that the Treaty of Rome (which effectively established the European Community) — and later the Single European Act (which removed most trade barriers in 1992) — say nothing about Community health. It might be thought that it is in the interest of most governments to encourage smoking since it brings in much-needed finance and, after a respectable interval, reduces the older, non-earning population by killing them with tobacco-related diseases — of which lung cancer is the quickest and most profitable! Unfortunately, laryngeal cancer is not only less common but is much less lethal — although this is not true for any secondary lung cancer. As the incidence of both neoplasms increases in the female population, we can expect to see a dramatic increase in both tumours which, in the case of laryngeal cancer, will cost health budgets more in achieving expected cure rates. Only more surgery will prove cost-effective, for few laryngectomized patients continue to smoke.

In addition to the health consequences of tobacco consumption, there are also the often forgotten but important economic and environmental costs. The land occupied for cultivation, most of which is in the under-developed countries, has been estimated as being capable of feeding 20 million people. Perhaps of even more significance is the focusing of the multinational tobacco combines on third world markets. Hardly surprisingly, the Governments of such countries are eager to receive these revenues, and sales potential is assisted by the limited awareness of the health risks. It might even be argued that expectation of long life is so limited in many of these countries that this 'tobacco money' may indirectly assist survival by improving health facilities.[13] However, evidence suggests that local tobacco producers, let alone the indigenous population, see little of these 'tobacco profits'.[16]

Within the more affluent countries the problem is little different, with total world consumption now almost 7 million tons each year and projected to grow by 2% per year, although hopefully less in the now more resistant developed countries. The World Health Organization has estimated that three million people die each year from tobacco usage; extrapolation means that 10% of the world's population could ultimately die from tobacco-related diseases.[3]

Some mention must be made of the risks associated with marijuana smoking, as reports from Australia and the United States describe laryngeal cancer in young chronic marijuana smokers. Marijuana smoke appears to have a greater carcinogenic effect on the larynx than does tobacco smoke, and respiratory function studies have demonstrated abnormalities in the proximal rather than the peripheral airways.[4,15] This is probably due to the rapid, deep inhalation techniques used in this form of smoking, leading to the deposition of particulate matter from turbulence and inertial impaction.[14]

Health care programmes rarely reach the section of the community that most needs help, and it is unlikely that health warnings and similar devices will have any great effect upon tobacco consumption without determined governmental action. A recent study in Finland has confirmed that smokers tend to weigh less than non-smokers of similar age, possibly due to the metabolic effects of tobacco smoke. That in itself is enough to encourage young females to smoke, particularly at an age when adolescent 'obesity' is a matter of great anxiety.

The lack of success in reducing the incidence of lung cancer throughout the world, and the obvious need for large numbers of the world's population to smoke, suggest that, although laryngeal cancer could be largely eliminated, this will not happen. The philosopher, and probably the psychologist, will argue that we have no moral right to interfere with an individual's right to personal autonomy, although discussions over the emotional topic of personal euthanasia suggest that such arguments are in fact conditional on local mores. If tobacco production were stopped completely, there can be little doubt that laryngeal cancer would largely disappear — but at what cost? Most national revenue is partially or even totally dependent upon tobacco, and many countries rely on its growth for their existence. In many parts of the world, expectation of life is far short of the 70+ years confidently expected in more affluent societies, and deaths from other causes far exceed those from tobacco. Indeed, smoking may be the only solace available to these populations, and have we the right to deny them their only pleasure?

Although of prime importance to the laryngologist, laryngeal cancer is probably one of the least serious sequelae of smoking for, in general, it carries a good prognosis and, if treated early, minimal morbidity. Indeed, if people are unwise enough to indulge in a habit which is clearly recognized as dangerous, which indirectly provides their fellows with revenue, should they not be allowed — even encouraged to do so? This ignores the risk to others of passive smoking, and is clearly not an acceptable argument for the caring physician, yet it appears to be one followed by most health agencies. Certainly, the means are available to prevent cancer of this organ, but there is little evidence that anybody wishes to do so!

> 'Tobacco surely was designed
> to poison and destroy mankind'
>
> Philip Freneau (1752–1832)

REFERENCES

1. Cann C I, Fried M P, Rothman K S 1985 Epidemiology of squamous carcinoma of the head and neck. Otolaryngol Clin North Am 18: 367–388
2. Chan C K, Gee J B L 1988 Asbestos exposure and laryngeal cancer. J Occup Med 30: 23–27
3. Davis R M, Smith R 1991 Addressing the most important preventable cause of death. Br Med J 303: 732–733
4. Donald P S 1986 Marijuana smoking, possible cause of head and neck cancer. Otolaryngol Head Neck Surg 94: 517–521
5. Eckholm E 1987 Cutting tobacco. Worldwide Institute, USA, paper 18 pp 6–7
6. Flanders W D, Rothman K S 1982 Interaction of alcohol and tobacco in laryngeal cancer. Am J Epidemiol 115: 371–379
7. Grover P L, Slims J B L 1973 K-region epoxides of polycyclic hydrocarbons. Biochem Pharmacol 22: 661–666
8. Hinds M W, Kolonel L N, Lee J, Hirohata T 1980 Association between cancer incidence and alcohol and cigarettes. Br J Cancer 41: 929–940
9. Kellerman G, Layten-Kellerman M, Shaw C R 1973 Genetic variation of aryl hydrocarbon hydroxylase in human lymphocytes. Am J Human Genet 25: 327–331
10. Korsgaard R, Trell E, Kitzing P 1984 Aryehydrocarbonhydroylase inducibility and smoking habits in patients with laryngeal cancer. Acta Otolaryngol 98: 368–373
11. Pederson E A, Hogetuit A C, Anderson A 1973 Cancer of the respiratory tract amongst workers at a nickel refinery in Norway. Int J Cancer 12: 32–41
12. Raw M 1991 Hong Kong tobacco tax doubled. Br Med J 302: 1422
13. Seely D R 1991 Third world targetted by tobacco firms. Arch Otolaryngol Head Neck Surg 117: 451
14. Taskin D P 1980 Respiratory status of 74 habitual marijuana smokers. Chest 78: 699–706
15. Taylor F M 1988 Marijuana as a potential respiratory tract carcinogen. South Med J 81:1213–1216
16. Tobacco use and world health — a situation analysis. 1986 PAHO Bull 20: 409–417
17. Vines G 1982 Interaction of alcohol and tobacco in laryngeal cancer. 1982 Am J Epidemiol 115: 380–388

5. Experimental carcinogenesis

U. Saffiotti

INTRODUCTION

The larynx is a target site for carcinogenesis induced by a variety of different agents. Experimental evidence shows that laryngeal carcinogenesis can be induced not only by topical exposure to carcinogens, but also by carcinogens acting through a systemic route. Experimental animal model studies have shown that different types of carcinogens and cofactors can combine their effects on the laryngeal epithelium and play a critical role in the induction of laryngeal tumours by multifactorial and synergistic mechanisms.

Most experimental findings on laryngeal carcinogenesis have resulted from studies designed to investigate tumour induction in the entire respiratory tract. In the course of such studies, only a systematic observation of induced laryngeal pathology will reveal the extent of preneoplastic and neoplastic changes in this organ.

The columnar, mucus-secretory epithelium extending from the larynx, through the trachea, to the segmental bronchi shares a common embryological origin and a basic biological homology,[71] but anatomical and functional properties give the larynx a distinct identity as a target site for carcinogenesis. Thus, while progress in the investigation of the cellular and molecular mechanisms involved in carcinogenesis in the tracheal and bronchial epithelia provides a basis for understanding the corresponding mechanisms in the larynx, a proper investigation of the basic mechanisms in laryngeal carcinogenesis will require specific studies on the reactions of the laryngeal epithelia as such, including consideration of their differences in anatomically distinct parts of the larynx.

The use of animal models, selected for their susceptibility to specific types of carcinogenesis and for their adequacy in reproducing the histogenesis and histopathology of their human counterpart, continues to provide a necessary basis for the experimental investigation of carcinogenesis.

In recent years, the remarkable progress of methods for cell biology and molecular biology has opened up a broad range of investigative opportunities in the search for the critical steps that control the induction of neoplasia in specific cell types, at the level of gene lesions and gene expression, cell growth control mechanisms and cell–cell interactions. Methods have been established for the growth and neoplastic transformation of respiratory epithelia, derived both from experimental animals and from humans. The underlying mechanisms of growth control and carcinogenesis are currently under intensive study and are beginning to be elucidated at the molecular level for several specific epithelial cell types. Extension of this effort to the laryngeal epithelium is needed in order to elucidate the mechanisms of carcinogenesis, the markers of individual susceptibility and the opportunities for prevention.

LARYNGEAL CARCINOGENESIS IN EXPERIMENTAL ANIMAL MODELS

The animal models for the experimental induction of laryngeal carcinogenesis were described in previous reviews in 1975[65] and 1985.[80] They are based on the use of the Syrian golden hamster as a species of choice, both because it reproduces the respiratory tract tumour pathology observed in human subjects, and because this species is particularly resistant to intercurrent respiratory inflammatory processes. The laryngeal carcinogens that have so far been effectively used are limited to the classes of polynuclear aromatic hydrocarbons, *N*-nitroso compounds and tobacco smoke (which contains compounds from both the above classes). The role of cofactors has also been demonstrated, especially by studies of carcinogenesis by polynuclear aromatic hydrocarbons adsorbed onto inorganic particulates and by a series of studies on multifactorial combined treatments.

For the present review, a search was made for laryngeal carcinogenic effects in the pathology database of the National Toxicology Program*, which includes the

---

*Personal communication from Drs G. A. Boorman and J. R. Hailey, National Institute of Environmental Health Sciences, National Institutes of Health, Research Triangle Park, North Carolina 27709, USA.

results on over 400 compounds that were thoroughly tested for carcinogenicity in two-year studies in rats and mice of both sexes. None of the tested compounds has revealed any carcinogenic effect on the larynx under the test conditions, and only a few laryngeal tumours were found, unrelated to experimental treatments.

The two most effective methods for the induction of laryngeal carcinomas are: (i) the repeated intratracheal instillation in hamsters of benzo[a]pyrene adsorbed onto inorganic particulates of respirable size (<5µm in diameter) suspended in saline,[57,58,62] and (ii) the intralaryngeal instillation of a direct-acting alkylating agent, such as N-methylnitrosourea.[21,78,79] The multifactorial aspects of these induction methods are discussed below.

The instillation of suspensions of benzo[a]pyrene adsorbed onto particulates has been found effective for the induction of laryngeal carcinogenesis in the hamster model, using many different inorganic particulates which are not carcinogenic when administered by themselves. They include: ferric oxide (Fe_2O_3), magnesium oxide (MgO), titanium dioxide (TiO_2), talc, crystalline silica (samples of quartz and silica sand), aluminium silicate and zirconium silicate; a lower yield of laryngeal tumours, always when combined with benzo[a]pyrene, has been reported for: aluminium oxide (A_2O_3), ferric chloride (FeC_3), carbon and iodine.[50,62,69,80]

Some of these particulate materials exert specific toxic activities because of their physicochemical surface properties. Current studies in our laboratory are investigating the pathogenetic mechanisms of inorganic particulates in respiratory carcinogenesis, especially crystalline silica. The carcinogenic activity of silica has been recognized only in the last decade by numerous epidemiological studies showing increased lung cancer risks in silicotic human subjects,[12,26,70] and in numerous experimental studies showing a marked carcinogenic activity of silica for rat lungs.[8,15,23,60,67,68] No laryngeal tumour induction was reported in any of these studies. Some aspects of cellular and molecular mechanisms involved in silica toxicity and carcinogenesis, however, may be relevant to the role played by particle deposition and cellular uptake in the respiratory epithelium, including the larynx, which is a site of impact of inhaled particles.

An important mechanism of cell injury by particulates is represented by the activation of oxygen radicals, especially when catalysed by the presence of divalent (ferrous) or trivalent (ferric) iron cations. Iron can be present as impurity, bound to negatively charged sites on the crystalline surface, e.g., on silica particles. Endogenous iron sources in cells and tissues can contribute to this reaction. Phagocytosis of insoluble particulates leads to production of oxygen radicals by macrophages and polymorphonuclear monocytes, and may thus stimulate proliferation of adjacent epithelial cells. Other proliferative stimuli may derive from cell

mediators (growth factors, cytokines) elicited by the reaction to particulates and/or other inflammatory reactions. We are investigating the hypothesis that these mechanisms play a critical role in respiratory tract carcinogenesis, including the larynx.[61,63,67]

The carcinogenic activity of several N-nitroso compounds on the laryngeal epithelium was demonstrated in the Syrian golden hamster and/or the European hamster.[2,65,80] They include di-N-ethylnitrosamine, N-nitroso-di-ethanolamine, di-N-propylnitrosamine, 2,2'-dimethyl-di-N-propylnitrosamine, 2,2'-dihydroxy-di-N-propylnitrosamine, methyl-N-propylnitrosamine, N-nitroso-hexamethylenei-mine, and N-nitroso-2,6-dimethylmorpholine. Most of the induced laryngeal tumours were benign polyps and papillomas. These nitrosamines are effective by systemic routes of administration, but the localization of target tumours varies with the route and conditions of administration.[80] Very high frequencies of laryngeal tumours were induced by N-ethyl-N-nitrosovinylamine, following weekly subcutaneous injections in hamsters.[14]

Squamous cell carcinomas of the larynx, as well as trachea and bronchi, were induced by topical application (instillation) of N-methylnitrosourea, a direct-acting alkylating nitrosamide.[21,78,79] The combined activity of this agent in multifactorial protocols will be discussed below.

Tobacco smoke, a major causative factor in human laryngeal cancer, has been shown experimentally to induce laryngeal cancer following inhalation exposure and the histopathology of laryngeal precursor lesions and invasive cancers, induced by exposure to cigarette smoke in hamsters, has been found to resemble closely the human counterpart.[4-6,9,24,25]

Inhalation exposure to a mixture of vapour-phase components of cigarette smoke (isoprene, methyl chloride, methyl nitrite and acetaldehyde) in hamsters resulted in hyperplastic and metaplastic lesions and in a significant incidence (19%) of squamous cell carcinomas of the larynx.[10]

MULTIFACTORIAL AND SYNERGISTIC INDUCTION MODELS

Combined exposures to specific carcinogens and tobacco smoke in the experimental animal models indicate that they can interact synergistically.[80] The carcinogens that have shown such activity include the polynuclear aromatic hydrocarbons 7,12-dimethylbenz[a]anthracene and benzo[a]pyrene.[22] Tests of combined exposures to diethylnitrosamine and cigarette smoke for laryngeal carcinogenesis in hamsters gave marginal[88] or negative[9] results for synergism.

Combined experimental exposures of hamsters to diethylnitrosamine given subcutaneously and to benzo[a]pyrene/ferric oxide suspensions instilled intratracheally gave enhanced carcinogenic effects in other segments of the respiratory tract, but not in the larynx.[43,44,47,77] These interactions require cautious interpretation in view of the complex tissue reactions elicited by the treatments.[69,80]

The mechanisms of the tissue reactions, involved in respiratory carcinogenesis, when mucosal damage and repair, particulate deposition and toxic effects were intrinsic components of the experimental model, were recently analysed in an experimental investigation of multifactorial carcinogenesis in the larynx, in an appropriate animal model.[34,35] These studies will be discussed here in some detail because they illustrate the importance of multiple interacting factors in the process of laryngeal carcinogenesis.*

In the animal species of choice for this study, the Syrian golden hamster, two treatment protocols were selected to identify specific topical segmental responses in the respiratory tract epithelium: intralaryngeal or intratracheal cannulations, with or without instillations of some carcinogens, particulates or vehicles. The study was designed to examine not only the effects of two different chemical carcinogens, but also the role played by the tissue damage induced by cannulation with a blunt 19-gauge stainless steel cannula on the respiratory epithelium and the underlying stroma. A plastic stop was fitted on the cannula and prevented its insertion, respectively, beyond the cricoid cartilage for intralaryngeal cannulation (ILC) or beyond the tracheal carina for intratracheal cannulation (ITC). When the cannula was gently introduced into anaesthetized hamsters, it scraped against the laryngeal and tracheal epithelium and produced focal areas of abrasion of the surface epithelium and of the underlying submucosa (mucosal wounds), respectively, only in the larynx for ILC, and in both the larynx and trachea for ITC.

The tissue reactions to mucosal wounding, evaluated by morphological and cytokinetic analysis, have been described previously.[31–36,42] They consisted of a rapid migration of epithelial secretory cells to cover the denuded wound surface, followed by marked epithelial cell proliferation (hyperplasia) and accompanied by a moderate underlying inflammatory reaction.

Two types of carcinogen were used in the multifactorial experiment.[35] One consisted of a single instillation of N-methyl-N-nitrosourea (MNU) (0.2 ml of a 1% solution in sodium citrate) given by ILC at 5 weeks of age, when the mitotic rate in the respiratory epithelium is about 25 times that of adult hamsters. The other treatment started two weeks later and consisted of 15 repeated cannulations

(once weekly) either by ILC or by ITC, with or without instillation of saline alone, or a saline suspension of ferric oxide (Fe_2O_3) particles, or a saline suspension of Fe_2O_3 particles on which the carcinogen benzo[a]pyrene (BP) had been previously adsorbed by nucleation.[35] Permutation of these variables resulted in a protocol with 14 groups, each consisting of 40 male hamsters, as shown in Table 5.1.

The animals were observed for a period extending to 78 weeks of age, at which time the surviving animals were sacrificed. All animals were examined histologically, each with multiple sections through the respiratory tract, including three cross-sections of the larynx.

The results of this study[35] provided experimental evidence of the interplay of multiple causative factors in the induction of respiratory cancers, and specifically in laryngeal carcinogenesis. Several factors were found to act as major determinants of the carcinogenic response in various segments of the respiratory tract. The two known carcinogens (single pretreatment with MNU and repeated instillations of BP-Fe_2O_3) were found not only to be critical determinants, but also to act synergistically. In addition, a major determining role was found to be played by mucosal wounding with its sequence of injury, epithelial regeneration, hyperplasia and mesenchymal reaction. Instillations of Fe_2O_3 suspensions, or even of saline alone, were found to contribute to the epithelial proliferative response.[34]

The specific effects obtained at the level of the larynx are discussed hereupon. The laryngeal tumours were diagnosed in the following categories: (a) papilloma: histologically benign epithelial tumours; (b) carcinoma in situ: epithelial lesions composed entirely of histologically malignant cells that had not invaded the surrounding stroma (most in situ lesions had the cellular features of epidermoid carcinomas); (c) carcinoma, invasive: carcinomas showing invasion of the surrounding stroma, diagnosed as epidermoid carcinomas, except for one case of combined epidermoid-adenocarcinoma and one case of small cell carcinoma.

Laryngeal inflammatory lesions, as well as epithelial hyperplasia and/or metaplasia, were found with significantly increased frequency in all groups that had received the course of ILC treatments (with or without MNU pretreatment), especially in those groups that had also received instillation of particulates and/or tracheal wounding. These findings indicate that these laryngeal tissue reactions persisted well beyond the period of treatment.

Effects of mucosal wounding

Induction of any laryngeal tumour (papillomas, carcinomas in situ or invasive carcinomas) occurred only in groups treated with one of the two carcinogens (MNU or BP) or both. No laryngeal tumours were found in any of the 101 larynges examined from groups that received no

*This study was conducted in collaboration by Drs Kevin P. Keenan and Elizabeth M. McDowell of the Department of Pathology, University of Maryland School of Medicine, Baltimore, MD and by Drs Umberto Saffiotti and Sherman F. Stinson of the Laboratory of Experimental Pathology, Division of Cancer Etiology, National Cancer Institute, Bethesda, MD, USA. I wish to thank my colleagues for their permission to discuss the results acquired jointly.

Table 5.1 Laryngeal lesions and tumours in multifactorial hamster study[1]

	Untreated control	Anaesthetized control	Treatments[2]											
			MNU	MNU, Lx wd	MNU, Lx wd, T wd	MNU, Lx wd, T wd, Sal	MNU, Lx wd, T wd, Sal, Fe_2O_3	MNU, Lx wd, T wd, Sal, Fe_2O_3, BP	MNU, Lx wd, Sal	MNU, Lx wd, Sal, Fe_2O_3	MNU, Lx wd, Sal, Fe_2O_3, BP	MNU, Lx wd, T wd, Sal, Fe_2O_3, BP	Lx wd, Sal, Fe_2O_3, BP	Lx wd, T wd, Sal
Group number	1	2	3	4	5	6	7	8	9	10	11	12	13	14
Number of larynges	37	33	34	34	35	32	35	21	33	33	27	34	31	31
Laryngitis[3]	0	1	3	9	21	22	11	7	4	15	12	27	10	10
(%)		3	9	26	60	69	31	33	12	45	44	79	32	32
Hyper/meta[4]	0	0	1	14	18	9	13	16	4	14	16	19	12	6
(%)			3	41	51	28	37	76	12	42	59	56	39	19
Papilloma	0	0	1[a]	0	4[f]	1[g]	0	2[l]	0	2[p]	1[s]	5[w]	2[bb]	0
(%)			3		11	3		10		6	4	15	6	
Ca in situ[5]	0	0	0	1[d]	0	3[h]	1[j]	5[m]	0	4[q]	2[t]	9[x]	1[cc]	0
(%)				3		9	3	24		12	7	26	3	
Ca (EC)[6]	0	0	1[b]	0	0	0	0	4[n]	0	0	1[u]	2[y]	0	0
(%)			3					19			4	6		
Ca (SCC)[7]	0	0	0	0	0	0	0	0	0	0	0	1[z]	0	0
(%)												3		
All Ca[8]	0	0	1[c]	1[e]	0	3[i]	1[k]	11[o]*	0	4[r]	3[v]	12[aa]	1[dd]	0
(%)[9]			3	3		9	3	33		12	11	26	3	

[1] = Lesions and tumours at 22–78 weeks of age. Modified from reference (35).

[2] = MNU: N-methylnitrosourea, single dose by ILC. Other treatments, once weekly for 15 weeks: Lx wd = larynx wound; T wd = tracheal wound; Sal = saline; Fe_2O_3 = ferric oxide; BP = benzo[a]pyrene.

[3] = Number of lesions and percentage (%) of larynges examined with lesion (percentage rounded to the nearest whole number).

[4] = Epithelial hyperplasia and/or metaplasia.

[5] = Carcinoma in situ.

[6] = Epidermoid carcinoma.

[7] = Small cell carcinoma.

[8] = Total number of carcinomas of hamsters (22–78 weeks of age) with carcinoma (in situ, invasive or both).

[9] = Percentage.

[a–dd] = Mean time to tumour (age in weeks). a = 78, b = 78, c = 78, d = 56, e = 56, f = 66, g = 48, h = 45, i = 45, j = 56, k = 56, l = 27, m = 48, n = 54, o = 45, p = 52, q = 51, r = 51, s = 78, t = 52, u = 39, v = 47, w = 66, x = 73, y = 71, z = 78, aa = 73, bb = 63, cc = 78, dd = 78.

* = Includes one carcinoma in situ and one combined epidermoid-adenocarcinoma, both at 21 weeks.

carcinogens, including the 31 larynges of group 14 that received 15 instillations of saline by ITC and were therefore subjected to repeated laryngeal and tracheal wounding. Wounding alone thus failed to induce any tumours.

The effect of wounding on carcinogenesis became apparent in the groups that received one or both carcinogens, indicating that wounding was a significant factor in determining the frequency of tumour induction. Tracheal wounding, involving larger tissue areas than was the case with laryngeal wounding, was found to extend its effects to the entire respiratory tract, including the larynx. Group 8 and 11 received the single MNU instillation by ILC followed by repeated instillations of BP-Fe_2O_3 in saline, respectively, by ITC in group 8 and by ILC in group 11. Both groups therefore had the same doses of carcinogens and both had laryngeal wounding, but only group 8 had additional tracheal wounding. Group 8 had 2 papillomas and 11 carcinomas of the larynx (two of which as early as 21 weeks) in 23 larynges examined, whereas group 11 (no tracheal wounding) only had 1 papilloma and 3 carcinomas in 27 larynges examined. In the absence of MNU pre-

treatment, groups 12 and 13 both received repeated doses of BP-Fe_2O_3 in saline and laryngeal wounding, but only group 12 also had tracheal wounding: group 12 developed 5 papillomas, 9 carcinomas in situ and 3 invasive carcinomas in 34 larynges examined, and group 13 (no tracheal wounding) only two papillomas and one carcinoma in situ in 31 larynges examined. In the absence of BP, both groups 6 and 9 had a single dose of MNU by ILC, followed by repeated saline instillations, respectively, by ITC for group 6 and by ILC for group 9: tracheal wounding resulted in a higher incidence of inflammatory and epithelial hyperplastic/metaplastic lesions in the larynx, and in the occurrence of one papilloma and 3 carcinomas in situ in the 32 larynges of group 6 examined, versus no tumours in 33 larynges for group 9.

Instillations of saline or of Fe_2O_3 in saline did not induce clear and consistent effects in the larynx.

Effects of repeated instillations of benzo[a]pyrene

The carcinogenic effect of BP was the strongest one among those tested in this multifactorial protocol. In the presence of all other factors (MNU pretreatment, laryngeal and tracheal wounding and instillation of saline and Fe_2O_3) BP instillations were a determinant factor for the highest tumour induction in the larynx. Group 8 (BP and all other factors) in 23 larynges examined had a total of 13 laryngeal tumours: 2 papillomas, 6 carcinomas in situ and 5 invasive carcinomas (4 epidermoid and one combined epidermoid-adenocarcinoma). For comparison, the groups that received MNU pretreatment and both laryngeal and tracheal wounding, with or without saline or Fe_2O_3 (groups 5, 6 and 7), in a combined total of 102 larynges, had 5 papillomas, 4 carcinomas in situ and no invasive carcinomas. In the absence of MNU pretreatment, repeated instillations of BP-Fe_2O_3 by ITC (group 12, 34 larynges) induced 5 papillomas, 9 carcinomas in situ, and 3 invasive carcinomas (2 epidermoid and one small cell carcinoma), whereas the corresponding group 14 (without BP-Fe_2O_3, 31 larynges) had no tumours at all.

Effects of a single intralaryngeal instillation of N-methyl-N-nitrosourea

A single dose of MNU, delivered in the larynx in 5-week-old hamsters, had a remarkable effect, not only as a determining cofactor in respiratory tract carcinogenesis, but also as a complete carcinogen for the induction of benign and malignant tumours in several distant organs and tissues, including oral/pharyngeal mucosa, oesophagus, forestomach, pancreas, biliary tract and large intestine, as well as vascular tumours and sarcomas.[35] These findings indicate the powerful systemic carcinogenic activity of this alkylating agent in young hamsters. The MNU dose was selected because it gave a minimal direct carcinogenic response in the respiratory tract in the absence of cofactors (1 papilloma and 1 epidermoid carcinoma in 34 examined larynges of group 3). In the larynx, pretreatment with MNU, followed by repeated instillations of saline by ITC (group 6, 32 larynges) gave rise to 1 papilloma and 3 carcinomas in situ and to significantly increased incidences of inflammatory lesions and epithelial hyperplasia/metaplasia, compared with group 14 (no MNU pretreatment, 31 larynges) which had no laryngeal tumours. The respiratory tumour response in hamsters receiving repeated instillations of BP-Fe_2O_3 by ILC (groups 11 and 13), or by ITC (groups 8 and 12), was significantly influenced by MNU pretreatment for the induction of tracheal and lung tumours, but not for laryngeal tumours.

CONSIDERATIONS ON THE ROLE OF MULTIFACTORIAL MECHANISMS

Cancer of the larynx can be experimentally induced not only by exposure to a number of individual carcinogens, but by combined exposures to interacting carcinogens, and also by interaction of carcinogens with other factors that influence the expression of carcinogenic effects. A special kind of interaction is that with chemopreventive agents that are capable of inhibiting the process of carcinogenesis.

The comparisons discussed above for a multifactorial model of laryngeal carcinogenesis show that tracheal wounding had a marked effect on the response not only in the trachea itself, but also in the larynx and in the bronchopulmonary airways. These effects resulted in the increased occurrence and severity of inflammatory and epithelial proliferative lesions as well as in enhanced carcinogenic responses. The role of mucosal damage, repair and reaction strongly suggests the participation of mechanisms involving cell–cell mediators in determining the carcinogenic response in the respiratory tract, including the larynx.

The reaction to toxic and carcinogenic agents, to insoluble particulates and to mucosal injury involves not only the airway lining epithelium, but also the adjacent mesenchymal tissue. In the experimental model discussed above,[34, 35] the epithelial and stromal reactions following mechanical mucosal abrasion represent a likely source of cellular mediators providing prolonged stimulation of cell proliferation. Following neoplastic transformation of target epithelial cells by the carcinogens, such persistent stimulation is likely to lead to clonal growth of the transformed cells with the establishment of a neoplasm.

The role of growth factors, cytokines and oxygen radicals as cell–cell mediators in the control of cell proliferation and neoplastic transformation of the respiratory epithelium has recently become a subject of investigation and represents a possible basis for the interpretation of the effects of cell injury and repair and of inflammatory reactions on the adjacent development of neoplastic growth.[61]

It is tempting therefore to formulate the hypothesis that human laryngeal cancer may derive from the interaction of multiple different causative factors and mechanisms. Among them, the following factors are to be considered: direct deposition of different chemical carcinogens; deposition and penetration of particulate materials; indirect effects of carcinogens adsorbed through the entire respiratory tract; topical or systemic effects of toxic agents on epithelial cells and on adjacent mesenchymal cells; consequent hyperplastic epithelial response and underlying inflammatory response; DNA damage and growth stimulation of epithelial cells, not only by carcinogens, but also by reactive oxygen species released by the chronic inflammatory process; growth and/or differentiation control by growth factors and cytokines released by the inflammatory cells and/or by the stimulated epithelial cells, e.g., transforming growth factor beta, tumour necrosis factor, platelet-derived growth factor, interleukins and other cytokines.

The well documented aetiological role of cigarette smoke can be interpreted as representing, by itself, a complex combination of the above mentioned factors. The role of alcohol consumption, especially in combination with smoking, also can be interpreted as contributing to these mechanisms of chronic cell injury and repair reactions.

Research on the chemoprevention of respiratory carcinogenesis was begun in the 1960s, following the demonstration that vitamin A not only inhibited squamous differentiation of the respiratory epithelium, but also prevented the induction of bronchogenic carcinoma in the hamster model.[66] Initial research on these mechanisms[7,11,19,29,73] developed into a wide program of studies that has now reached the stage of clinical trials for human cancer chemoprevention.[72,74]

OPPORTUNITIES FOR INVESTIGATING CELLULAR AND MOLECULAR MECHANISMS OF LARYNGEAL CARCINOGENESIS

Systematic studies need to be devoted specifically to the investigation of cellular and molecular characteristics of the laryngeal epithelium in the process of carcinogenesis. Several approaches have been developed for such studies on other segments of the respiratory tract, including the trachea, bronchi and peripheral lung airways. Our laboratory has contributed to several of these developments.

After animal models had been established for respiratory carcinogenesis at a given site, methods were developed for in vitro culture of target tissue segments from the animal model. Organ culture methods were first used to characterize the target epithelia morphologically, cytokinetically and biochemically.[7,11,17,18,29,30] Subsequently, methods were established for culture of tracheal epithelial cells, for combined in vivo/in vitro cultures, and for re-epithelization by cultured epithelial cells of denuded tracheal segments implanted subcutaneously in syngeneic animals.[13,30,39,40,45,46,48,49,55,59,64,82] Neoplastic transformation was induced experimentally in rat tracheal epithelial cells in culture.[51,76,83–86] Culture in serum-free media with defined growth factors was used to identify specific cellular requirements for added growth factors and for neoplastic transformation of rat tracheal cells.[13, 83, 85, 86] A fetal rat pulmonary alveolar type II epithelial cell line was established[38] and its responses to toxic and carcinogenic agents are currently under study (Saffiotti et al, unpublished observations).

Specific efforts were addressed to the development of appropriate methods for the culture and characterization of human respiratory epithelia, obtained in viable form from surgical or immediate autopsy specimens.[16,81,87] These methods made it possible to evaluate the specific reactions of target human respiratory epithelia to differentiation control factors, growth factors, toxic agents and carcinogens. Unfortunately, no specific work has been done to characterize laryngeal epithelia by these methods, in comparison with other segments of the respiratory tract.

Methods were subsequently developed for cell culture of human bronchial epithelia, especially in serum-free media,[20,37,41] and continuously growing ('immortalized') cell lines of human bronchial epithelium were obtained by means of infection or transfection with SV40 genes and, most effectively, by infection with an adenovirus 12/SV40 hybrid virus.[56] It is interesting that immortalization of normal human bronchial epithelial cells was obtained also by transfection with human papillomaviruses 16 and 18, since human papillomaviruses are associated with human laryngeal papillomatosis.[89] The transformation of the SV40-immortalized cells to fully malignant phenotypes (growing as carcinomas in nude mice) was obtained by further transfection with the oncogenes v-Ha-*ras* or v-Ki-*ras*, or with a combination of the oncogenes c-*raf*-1 and c-*myc*.[3,52–54] It is of interest that activation of c-*raf*-1, the cellular homologue of the viral oncogene v-*raf*, has been implicated in some types of human tumours, including laryngeal carcinoma.[28]

Studies on the structural and functional properties of differentiated cell types, including specific respiratory epithelial cell types from different segments of the airways, have been greatly assisted by critical advances in the methods for cell biology and molecular biology, applied to specific target epithelial cells from both experimental animals and human subjects, making it possible to correlate human and animal pathology and cell biology with specific mechanisms of carcinogenesis and with specific molecular pathways. New fields of investigation have been opened by advances in molecular biology. Research on cellular growth factors and cytokines, and on their receptors, has shown their increasingly important role in carcinogenesis, and their localization in tissues and cells can be studied by immunohistochemical and molecular markers.[1,75]

Detection and characterization of altered gene expression, especially of mutated oncogenes and tumour-suppressor genes, in experimental and human respiratory tumours, has provided initial data on the genetic mechanisms involved in the process of respiratory tract carcinogenesis.[27,59]

A complex but critical network of gene changes, cellular and molecular mediators and control factors is presently under intense investigation in order to elucidate the molecular mechanisms that determine neoplastic transformation in specific respiratory target cells, both in culture and in vivo.

In conclusion, current rapid progress in the methods of cellular and molecular biology, coupled with the availability of previously established animal models, offers unprecedented opportunities for an in-depth analysis of the causative mechanisms and the cellular control factors that determine laryngeal carcinogenesis. Elucidation of cellular control factors is likely to yield critical clues to the identification of individual host susceptibility factors, and these in turn will become a potential basis for the selective prevention of laryngeal cancer in high-risk subjects.

Direct study of laryngeal cell biology and carcinogenesis mechanisms has lagged behind corresponding studies of other segments of the respiratory tract. It is both a challenge and a timely opportunity for laryngologists to attack and elucidate the basic mechanisms of carcinogenesis in the larynx.

REFERENCES

1. Aaronson S A 1991 Growth factors and cancer. Science 1991 254: 1146–1153

2. Althoff J, Mohr U, Lijinsky W 1985 Comparative study on the carcinogenicity of N-nitroso-2,6-dimethylmorpholine in the European hamster. J Cancer Res Clin Oncol 109: 183–187

3. Amstad P, Reddel R R, Pfeifer A, Malan-Shibley L, Mark G E, Harris C C 1988 Neoplastic transformation of a human bronchial epithelial cell line by a recombinant retrovirus encoding viral Harvey ras. Mol Carcinog 1: 151–160

4. Bernfeld P, Homburger F, Russfield AB 1974 Strain differences in the response of inbred Syrian hamsters to cigarette smoke inhalation. J Natl Cancer Inst 53: 1141–1157

5. Bernfeld P, Homburger F, Russfield A B 1979 Cigarette smoke-induced cancer of the larynx in hamsters (CINCH): a method to assay the carcinogenicity of cigarette smoke. Prog Exp Tumor Res 24: 315–319

6. Bernfeld P, Homburger F, Soto E, Pai K J 1979 Cigarette smoke inhalation studies on inbred Syrian golden hamsters. J Natl Cancer Inst 63: 675–689

7. Clamon G H, Sporn M B, Smith J M, Saffiotti U 1974 α- and β-Retinyl acetate reverse metaplasias of vitamin A deficiency in hamster trachea organ culture. Nature 250: 64–66

8. Dagle G E, Wehner A P, Clark M L, Buschbom R L 1986 Chronic inhalation exposure of rats to quartz. In: Goldsmith D F, Winn D M, Shy C M (eds) Silica, silicosis and cancer. Preager, New York, pp 255–266

9. Dontenwill W, Chevalier H-J, Harke H-P, Lafrenz U, Reckzeh G, Schneider B 1973 Investigations on the effects of chronic cigarette smoke inhalation in Syrian golden hamsters. J Natl Cancer Inst 51: 1781–1832

10. Feron V J, Kuper C F, Spit B J, Reuzel P G J, Woutersen R A 1985 Glass fibers and vapor phase components of cigarette smoke as cofactors in experimental respiratory tract carcinogenesis. In: Mass M J, Kaufman D G, Siegfried J M, Steele V E, Nesnow S (eds). Carcinogenesis — a comprehensive survey, vol 8. Cancer of the respiratory tract. Predisposing factors. Raven Press, New York, pp 93–118

11. Genta V M, Kaufman D G, Harris C C, Smith J M, Sporn M B, Saffiotti U 1974 Vitamin A deficiency enhances binding of benzo[a]pyrene to tracheal epithelial DNA. Nature 247: 48–49

12. Goldsmith D F, Winn D M, Shy C M 1986 Silica, silicosis, and cancer. Praeger, New York, pp 1–536

13. Gray T, Rundhaug J, Nettesheim P 1991 Critical variables controlling cell proliferation in primary cultures of rat tracheal epithelial cells. In Vitro Cell Dev Biol 27A: 805–814

14. Green U, Althoff J 1982 Carcinogenicity of vinylnitrosamine in Syrian golden hamsters. J Cancer Res Clin Oncol 102: 227–233

15. Groth D H, Stettler L E, Platek S F, Lal J B, Burg J R 1986 Lung tumors in rats treated with quartz by intratracheal instillation. In: Goldsmith D F, Winn D M, Shy C M (eds) Silica, silicosis, and cancer. Praeger, New York, pp 243–253

16. Harris C C, Autrup H, Stoner G D, Trump B F 1978 Carcinogenesis studies in human respiratory epithelium. An experimental model system. In: Harris C C (ed) Pathogenesis and therapy of lung cancer. Marcel Dekker, New York, pp 559–607

17. Harris C C, Kaufman D G, Sporn M B, Boren H, Jackson F, Smith J M, Pauley J, Dedick P, Saffiotti U 1973 Localization of benzo[a]pyrene-3$_H$ and alterations in nuclear chromatin caused by benzo[a]pyrene–ferric oxide in the hamster respiratory epithelium. Cancer Res 33: 2842–2848

18. Harris C C, Kaufman D G, Sporn M B, Smith J M, Jackson F, Saffiotti U 1973 Ultrastructural effects of N-methylnitrosourea on the tracheobronchial epithelium of the Syrian golden hamster. Int J Cancer 12: 259–269

19. Harris C C, Sporn M B, Kaufman D G, Smith J M, Jackson F E, Saffiotti U 1972 Histogenesis of squamous metaplasia in the hamster tracheal epithelium caused by vitamin A deficiency or benzo[a]pyrene–ferric oxide. J Natl Cancer Inst 48: 743–761

20. Harris C C, Yoakum G H, Lechner J F, Willey J C, Gerwin B I, Banks-Schlegel S, Masui T, Mark G 1986 Growth, differentiation, and neoplastic transformation of human bronchial epithelial cells. In: Harris C C (ed) Biochemical and molecular epidemiology of human cancer. Alan R. Liss, New York, pp 213–226

21. Herrold K M 1970 Upper respiratory tract tumors induced in Syrian hamsters by N-methyl-N-nitrosourea. Int J Cancer 6: 217–222

22. Hoffmann D, Rivenson A, Hecht S S, Hilfrich J, Kobayashi N, Wynder E L 1979 Model studies in tobacco carcinogenesis with the Syrian golden hamster. Prog Exp Tumor Res 24: 370–390

23. Holland L M, Wilson J S, Tillery M I, Smith D M 1986 Lung cancer in rats exposed to fibrogenic dusts. In: Goldsmith D F, Winn D M, Shy C M (eds) Silica, silicosis and cancer. Praeger, New York, pp 267–279

24. Homburger F 1975 "Smokers' larynx" and carcinoma of the larynx in Syrian hamsters exposed to cigarette smoke. Laryngoscope 85: 1874–1881

25. Homburger F, Soto E 1979 Animal model of human disease: carcinoma of the larynx in hamsters exposed to cigarette smoke. Am J Pathol 95: 845–848

26. International Agency for Research on Cancer. Silica. 1987 In: IARC Monographs on the evaluation of carcinogenic risk of chemicals to humans, vol 42. Silica and some silicates. International Agency for Research on Cancer, Lyon, pp 39–143

27. Kaighn M E, Gabrielson E W, Iman D S, Pauls E A, Harris C C 1990 Suppression of tumorigenicity of a human lung carcinoma line by nontumorigenic bronchial epithelial cells in somatic line hybrids. Cancer Res 50: 1890–1896

28. Kasid U, Pfeifer A, Weichselbaum R R, Dritschilo A, Mark G E 1987 The raf oncogene is associated with a radiation-resistant human laryngeal cancer. Science 237: 1039–1040

29. Kaufman D G, Baker M S, Harris C C, Smith J M, Boren H, Sporn M B, Saffiotti U 1972 Coordinated biochemical and morphologic examination of hamster tracheal epithelium. J Natl Cancer Inst 49: 783–792

30. Kaufman D G, Baker M S, Smith J M, Henderson W R, Harris C C, Sporn M B, Saffiotti U 1972 RNA metabolism in tracheal epithelium: alteration in hamsters deficient in vitamin A. Science 177: 1105–1108

31. Keenan K P, Combs J W, McDowell E M 1982 Regeneration of hamster tracheal epithelium after mechanical injury. I. Focal lesions: quantitative morphologic study of cell proliferation. Virchows Arch (Cell Pathol) 41: 193–214

32. Keenan K P, Combs J W, McDowell E M 1982 Regeneration of hamster tracheal epithelium after mechanical injury. II. Multifocal lesions: stathmokinetic and autoradiographic studies of cell proliferation. Virchows Arch (Cell Pathol) 41: 215–229

33. Keenan K P, Combs J W, McDowell E M 1982 Regeneration of hamster tracheal epithelium after mechanical injury. III. Large and small lesions: comparative stathmokinetic and single pulse and continuous thymidine labeling autoradiographic studies. Virchows Arch (Cell Pathol) 41: 231–252

34. Keenan K P, Saffiotti U, Stinson S F, Riggs C W, McDowell E M 1989 Morphological and cytokynetic responses of hamster airways to intralaryngeal or intratracheal cannulation with instillation of saline or ferric oxide particles in saline. Cancer Res 49: 1521–1527

35. Keenan K P, Saffiotti U, Stinson S F, Riggs C W, McDowell E M 1989 Multifactorial hamster respiratory carcinogenesis with interdependent effects of cannula-induced mucosal wounding, saline, ferric oxide, benzo[a]pyrene and N-methyl-N-nitrosourea. Cancer Res 49: 1528–1540

36. Keenan K P, Wilson T S, McDowell E M 1983 Regeneration of hamster tracheal epithelium after mechanical injury. IV. Histochemical, immunological, and ultrastructural studies. Virchows Arch (Cell Pathol) 43: 213–240

37. Lechner J F, Haugen A, McClendon I A, Pettis E W 1982 Clonal growth of normal adult human bronchial epithelial cells in a serum free medium. In Vitro 18: 633–642

38. Leheup B P, Federspiel S L, Guerry-Force M L, Wetherall N T, Commers P A, DiMari S J, Haralson M A 1989 Extracellular matrix biosynthesis by cultures fetal rat lung epithelial cells. I. Characterization of the clone and the major genetic types of collagen produced. Lab Invest 60: 791–807

39. Marchok A C, Cone V, Nettesheim P 1975 Induction of squamous metaplasia (vitamin A deficiency) and hypersecretory activity in tracheal organ cultures. Lab Invest 33: 451–460

40. Mass J M, Kaufman D G, Siegfried J M, Steele V E, Nesnow S 1985 Carcinogenesis — a comprehensive survey, vol 8. Cancer of the respiratory tract. Predisposing factors. Raven Press, New York, pp 1–468

41. Masui T, Wakefield L M, Lechner J F, La Veck M A, Sporn M B, Harris C C 1986 Type β transforming growth factor is the primary differentiation-inducing serum factor for normal human bronchial epithelial cells. Proc Natl Acad Sci USA 83: 2438–2442

42. McDowell E M, Keenan K P, Huang M 1984 Effects of vitamin A-deprivation on hamster tracheal epithelium: a quantitative morphologic study. Virchows Arch (Cell Pathol) 45: 197–219

43. Montesano R, Saffiotti U, Ferrero A, Kaufman D G 1974 Synergistic effects of benzo[a]pyrene and diethylnitrosamine on respiratory carcinogenesis in hamsters. J Natl Cancer Inst 53: 1395–1397

44. Montesano R, Saffiotti U, Shubik P 1970 The role of topical and systemic factors in experimental respiratory carcinogenesis. In: Hanna M G, Nettesheim P, Gilbert J R (eds) Inhalation carcinogenesis. Atomic Energy Commission Symposium Series No. 18, Oak Ridge, TN, pp 353–371

45. Mossman B T, Craighead J E 1978 Induction of neoplasms in hamster tracheal grafts with 3-methylcholanthrene-coated Lycra fibers. Cancer Res 38: 3717–3722

46. Mossman B T, Ezerman E B, Adler K B, Craighead J E 1980 Isolation and spontaneous transformation of cloned lines of hamster tracheal epithelial cells. Cancer Res 40: 4403–4409

47. Nettesheim P, Creasia D A, Mitchell T J 1975 Carcinogenic and cocarcinogenic effects of inhaled synthetic smog and ferric oxide particles. J Natl Cancer Inst 55: 159–169

48. Nettesheim P, Griesemer R A 1978 Experimental models for studies of respiratory tract carcinogenesis. In: Harris C C (ed) Pathogenesis and therapy of lung cancer. Marcel Dekker, New York, pp 75–188

49. Nettesheim P, Marchok A C 1983 Neoplastic development in airways epithelium. In: Klein G, Weinhouse S (eds) Advances in cancer research, vol 39. Academic Press, New York, pp 1–70

50. Niemeier R W, Mulligan L T, Rowland J 1986 Cocarcinogenicity of foundry silica sand in hamsters. In: Goldsmith D F, Winn D M, Shy C M (eds) Silica, silicosis and cancer. Praeger, New York, pp 215–227

51. Pai S B, Steele V E, Nettesheim P 1983 Neoplastic transformation of primary tracheal epithelial cell cultures. Carcinogenesis 4: 369–374

52. Pfeifer A M A, Jones R T, Bowden P E, Mann D, Spillare E, Klein-Szanto A J P, Trump B F, Harris C C 1991 Human bronchial epithelial cells transformed by the c-raf-1 and c-myc protooncogenes induce multidifferentiated carcinomas in nude mice: a model for lung carcinogenesis. Cancer Res 51: 3793–3801

53. Pfeifer A M A, Lechner J F, Masui T, Reddel R R, Mark G E,

Harris C C 1991 Control of growth and squamous differentiation in normal human bronchial epithelial cells by chemical and biological modifiers and transferred genes. Environ Health Perspect 80: 209–220

54. Pfeifer A M A, Mark G E III, Malan-Shibley L, Graziano S, Amstad P, Harris C C 1989 Cooperation of c-raf-1 and c-myc protooncogenes in the neoplastic transformation of simian virus 40 large tumor antigen-immortalized human bronchial epithelial cells. Proc Natl Acad Sci USA 86: 10 075–10 079

55. Randell S H, Comment C E, Ramaekers C S, Nettesheim P 1991 Properties of rat tracheal epithelial cells separated based on expression of cell surface α-galactosyl end groups. Am J Respir Cell Mol Biol 4: 544–554

56. Reddel R R, Ke Y, Gerwin B I, McMenamin M, Lechner J F, Su R T, Brash D E, Park J B, Rhim J S, Harris C C 1988 Transformation of human bronchial epithelial cells by infection with SV40 or adenovirus-12/SV40 hybrid virus, or transfection via strontium phosphate coprecipitation with a plasmid containing SV40 early region genes. Cancer Res 48: 1904–1909

57. Saffiotti U 1969 Experimental respiratory tract carcinogenesis. Progr Exp Tumor Res 11: 302–333

58. Saffiotti U 1970 Experimental respiratory tract carcinogenesis and its relation to inhalation exposure. In: Hanna M G, Nettesheim P, Gilbert J R (eds) Inhalation carcinogenesis. Atomic Energy Commission Symposium Series No. 18, Oak Ridge, TN, pp 27–54

59. Saffiotti U 1987 Human lung cancer and experimental pathogenic models: an increasingly close connection. In: McDowell E M (ed) Lung carcinomas. Churchill Livingstone, Edinburgh, pp 370–393

60. Saffiotti U 1990 Lung cancer induction by silica in rats, but not in mice and hamsters: species differences in epithelial and granulomatous reactions. In: Seemayer N H, Hadnagy W (eds) Environmental hygiene II. Springer-Verlag, New York, pp 235–238

61. Saffiotti U 1991 Lung cancer induction by crystalline silica. In: D'Amato R, Slaga T J, Farland W H, Henry C (eds) Relevance of animal studies to the evaluation of human cancer risk. John Wiley, New York, pp 51–69

62. Saffiotti U, Cefis F, Kolb L H 1968 A method for the experimental induction of bronchogenic carcinoma. Cancer Res 28: 104–124

63. Saffiotti U, Daniel L N, Mao Y, Ahmed N 1991 DNA damage induced by combined exposure to crystalline silica (CS) and hydrogen peroxide. FASEB J 5: A1603

64. Saffiotti U, Harris C C 1979 Carcinogenesis studies on organ cultures of animal and human respiratory tissues. In: Griffith A C, Shaw C R (eds) Carcinogens: identification and mechanisms of action. Raven Press, New York, pp 65–82

65. Saffiotti U, Kaufman D G 1975 Carcinogenesis of laryngeal carcinoma. Laryngoscope 85: 454–467

66. Saffiotti U, Montesano R, Sellakumar A R, Borg S A 1967 Studies of experimental lung cancer: inhibition by vitamin A of the induction of tracheobronchial squamous metaplasia and squamous cell tumors. Cancer 20: 857–864

67. Saffiotti U, Stinson S F 1988 Lung cancer induction by crystalline silica: relationships to granulomatous reactions and host factors. Envir Carcino Revs (J Envir Sci Hlth) C6: 197–222

68. Saffiotti U, Stinson S F 1989 Lung cancer induced by crystalline silica in rats, but not in mice and hamsters: species differences in epithelial and granulomatous reactions to silica. Proc Amer Assoc Cancer Res 30: 113

69. Saffiotti U, Stinson S F, Keenan K P, McDowell E M 1985 Tumor enhancement factors and mechanisms in the hamster respiratory tract carcinogenesis model. In: Mass M J, Kaufman D G, Siegfried J M, Steele V E, Nesnow S (eds). Carcinogenesis — a comprehensive survey, vol 8. Cancer of the respiratory tract. Predisposing factors. Raven Press, New York, pp 63–92

70. Simonato L, Fletcher A C, Saracci R, Thomas T L (eds) 1990 Occupational exposure to silica and cancer risk. IARC scientific publication No. 97. International Agency for Research on Cancer, Lyon, pp 1–124

71. Sorokin S P 1970 The cells of the lung. In: Nettesheim P, Hanna M G, Deatherage J W Jr (eds) Morphology of experimental respiratory carcinogenesis. Atomic Energy Commission Symposium Series No. 21, Oak Ridge , T N, pp 3–43

72. Sporn M B 1991 Carcinogenesis and cancer: different perspectives

on the same disease. Cancer Res 51: 6215–6218

73. Sporn M B, Clamon G H, Dunlop N M, Newton D L, Smith J M, Saffiotti U 1975 Activity of vitamin A analogues in cell cultures of mouse epidermis and organ cultures of hamster trachea. Nature 253: 47–50

74. Sporn M B, Newton D L 1979 Chemoprevention of cancer with retinoids. Fed Proc 38: 2528–2534

75. Sporn M B, Roberts A B (eds) 1990 Peptide growth factors and their receptors (2 vols). Handbook of experimental pharmacology, vol 95. Springer-Verlag, Berlin, New York

76. Steele V E, Marchok A C, Nettesheim P 1977 Transformation of tracheal epithelium exposed in vitro to N-methyl-N'-nitro-N-nitrosoguanidine (MNNG). Int J Cancer 20: 234–238

77. Stenbäck F G, Ferrero A, Shubik P 1973 Synergistic effects of diethylnitrosamine and different dusts on respiratory carcinogenesis in hamsters. Cancer Res 33: 2209–2214

78. Stinson S F, Lilga J C 1980 Morphogenesis of neoplasms induced in the hamster trachea with N-methyl-N-nitrosourea. Cancer Res 40: 609–613

79. Stinson S F, Reznik-Schüller H M, Reznik G, Donahoe R 1983 Spindle cell carcinoma of the hamster trachea induced by N-methyl-N-nitrosourea. Am J Pathol 111: 21–26

80. Stinson S F, Saffiotti U 1985 Experimental laryngeal carcinogenesis. In: Ferlito A (ed) Cancer of the larynx. CRC Press, Boca Raton, pp 5–54

81. Stoner G D, Katoh Y, Foidart J-M, Myers G A, Harris C C 1980 Identification and culture of human bronchial epithelial cells. In: Harris C C, Trump B F, Stoner G D (eds) Methods in cell biology, vol 21. Normal human tissue and cell culture. A. Respiratory, cardiovascular, and integumentary systems. Academic Press, New York, pp 15–35

82. Terzaghi M, Nettesheim P 1963 Combined in vivo–in vitro studies of neoplastic development in rat respiratory tissues. In: Reznik-Schüller H M (ed) Comparative respiratory tract carcinogenesis, vol II. Experimental respiratory tract carcinogenesis. CRC Press, Boca Raton, pp 189–197

83. Thomassen D G 1986 Role of spontaneous transformation in carcinogenesis: development of preneoplastic rat tracheal cells at a constant rate. Cancer Res 46: 2344–2348

84. Thomassen D G, Gray T E, Mass M J, Barrett J C 1983 High frequency of carcinogen-induced early, preneoplastic changes in rat tracheal epithelial cells in culture. Cancer Res 43: 5956–5963

85. Thomassen D G, Kaighn M E, Saffiotti U, Lerman M I 1986 Effects of viral oncogenes on the neoplastic progression of rat tracheal epithelial (RTE) cells: evidence for a multistep process. Proc Amer Assoc Cancer Res 27: 135

86. Thomassen D G, Saffiotti U, Kaighn M E 1986 Clonal proliferation of rat tracheal epithelial cells in serum-free medium and their responses to hormones, growth factors and carcinogens. Carcinogenesis 7: 2033–2039

87. Trump B F, Resau J, Barrett L A 1980 Methods of organ culture for human bronchus. In: Harris C C, Trump B F, Stoner G D (eds). Methods in cell biology, vol 21. Normal human tissue and cell culture. A. Respiratory, cardiovascular and integumentary systems. Academic Press, New York, pp 1–14

88. Wehner A P, Busch R H, Olson R J 1976 Effects of diethylnitrosamine and cigarette smoke on hamsters. J Natl Cancer Inst 56: 749–756

89. Willey J C, Broussoud A, Sleemi A, Bennett W P, Cerutti P, Harris C C 1991 Immortalization of normal human bronchial epithelial cells by human papillomaviruses 16 or 18. Cancer Res 51: 5370–5377

6. Special techniques in diagnostic pathology

L. Barnes

During the last decade there have been enormous advances in the fields of immunology, molecular biology and genetics. The new technologies that have led to these advances are no longer confined to research laboratories but are now integral components of a modern-day surgical pathology laboratory. These new test procedures not only permit pathologists to make more specific and accurate diagnoses but also allow for more objective means of evaluating tumours and, in some instances, provide previously unavailable information that may be useful in the diagnosis and clinical management of patients. An overview of some of these current methods follows.

IMMUNOPEROXIDASE STAINS

Immunoperoxidase stains, perhaps more than any other procedure, have revolutionized the practice of surgical pathology. With these stains, pathologists are often able to make diagnoses with a greater degree of confidence than in the past.

These stains are antigen–antibody reactions that rely on the binding of a specific antibody to a specific cell component. A chromogen is then used to visualize and locate the immunoreaction in tissue. The stains are, however, time-consuming and expensive. On average, they take one to two days to perform, and, in order to be reliable, they must be carried out by experienced personnel under stringent quality-controlled conditions.

Currently, over one-hundred antibodies are available. Antibodies can be developed not only against tumour antigens but also against immunoglobulins, various haematopoietic cells, hormones, infectious agents, and a variety of cellular components (intermediate filaments, neurosecretory granules) (Figs 6.1–6.3).

Immunostains offer several advantages over electron microscopy. First, in contrast to electron microscopy, which requires forethought of need and special fixation, immunoperoxidase stains can be done on formalin-fixed, paraffin-embedded tissue. Second, electron microscopy requires expensive equipment while immunostains do not. Lastly, several different tissue blocks can be examined as opposed to only minute fragments of tissue with the electron microscope. Thus, sampling errors are less of a problem.

In addition to diagnosis, immunoperoxidase stains can also be used for prognostic purposes. Gallo et al[11] employed immunoperoxidase stains for S–100 protein and lysozyme to identify intratumoral and peritumoral Langerhans cells (T-zone histiocytes) in 88 patients with squamous cell carcinoma of the larynx. They observed that patients with tumours that had a high or intermediate density of Langerhans cells had a significantly better survival than did those with a low density of cells. The actuarial five-year survival rates were respectively 60%, 62% and 0%.

ELECTRON MICROSCOPY

With the availability of immunoperoxidase stains, and for reasons noted above, the use of electron microscopy in diagnostic pathology has become less popular. There are occasions, however, when antibodies are not available to perform immunoperoxidase stains or when immunoperoxidase stains are inconclusive or do not support the light microscopic evaluation. In these instances, electron microscopy may be of use.

FLOW CYTOMETRY

In surgical pathology, flow cytometry is used primarily to determine tumour ploidy. The principle is simple, and either fresh or formalin-fixed, paraffin-embedded tissue can be used for analysis. The tissue is first disaggregated and a suspension of nuclei is obtained and stained with propidium iodide. The nuclei are then passed singly through a flow cytometer where the DNA content is analysed and ultimately recorded on a histogram.

Flow cytometric studies on squamous cell carcinoma of the larynx indicate that 45 to 90% of all tumours are aneuploid.[7,8,12,25,30] The clinical significance of ploidy

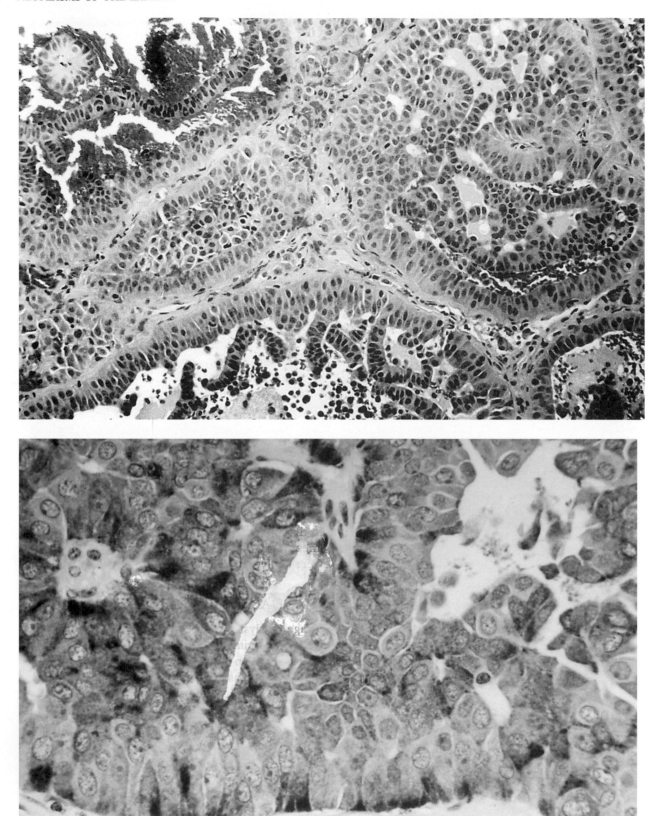

Fig. 6.1 (*top*) Biopsy of a laryngeal tumour that might be mistaken for a non-specific adenocarcinoma. H&E, ×100. See Fig. 6.2.

Fig. 6.2 (*bottom*) The tumour in Fig. 6.1 was immunostained for chromogranin. The results indicate a neuroendocrine neoplasm, specifically an atypical carcinoid (large cell neuroendocrine carcinoma, moderately differentiated neuroendocrine carcinoma). ×250.

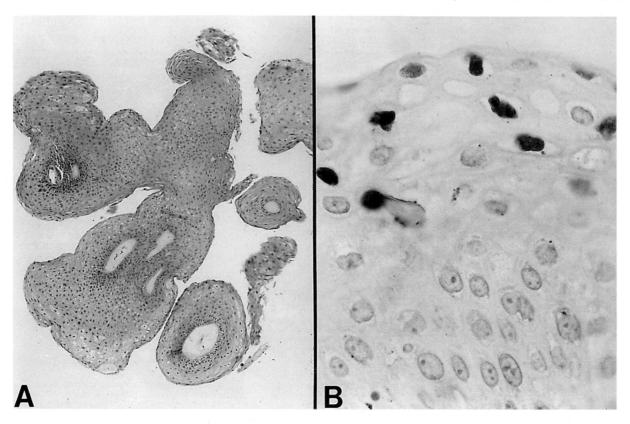

Fig. 6.3   A. Non-keratinized squamous papilloma of the larynx occurring in a 10-year-old boy. H&E, ×20. B. Same papilloma immunostained for human papillomavirus. Note the positive intranuclear staining. ×315.

patterns in the larynx, however, is both confusing and controversial. Some indicate that there is no correlation between tumour ploidy and survival while others indicate that patients with aneuploid tumours have a more favourable outcome.[8,12,30] Still others, conversely, have found that diploid tumours are associated with a better prognosis[14] (Fig. 6.4). Although Rua et al[25] have noted that the overall survival rates of patients with diploid and aneuploid tumours are comparable, they did observe that aneuploid tumours with a well-differentiated pattern are associated with a poor prognosis.

Laryngeal ploidy patterns have also been used to predict response to irradiation and chemotherapy. The results again are confusing. Some investigators have observed that non-diploid tumours respond better to both irradiation and chemotherapy while others have found no relationship between tumour ploidy and subsequent response to either of these therapeutic modalities.[1,14,26,30] Walter et al,[35] on the other hand, indicate that TINOMO glottic tumours that are aneuploid are more radioresistant than are diploid lesions and should be treated primarily with surgery.

Part of the above controversy may be related to tumour heterogeneity. El-Naggar et al[7] studied 21 squamous cell

carcinomas of the larynx by flow cytometry and observed that 76% were heterogeneous in DNA content. According to these investigators, the calculated probability of missing aneuploidy if only one, two, three or four tissue samples was analysed was 33%, 17%, 8% and 3%, respectively.

IMAGE ANALYSIS

Image analysis, like flow cytometry, is used in surgical pathology primarily to determine tumour ploidy. It, too, can be done on fresh or formalin-fixed, paraffin-embedded tissue as well as on tumour imprints. In contrast to flow cytometry which uses nuclear suspensions, image analysis requires that the nuclei be on microscope slides. The slides are then stained with the Feulgen reaction and examined under a microscope with an attached computerized digital imaging system. With this procedure, only 100 to 300 cells are usually examined, and since the cells are viewed through a microscope before the DNA is quantified by the computer, the examiner has the advantage of selecting only tumour cells for analysis. This is in contrast to flow cytometry where literally thousands of cells are examined but the examiner has no absolute control over whether normal or abnormal cells are examined.

Counts
full scale

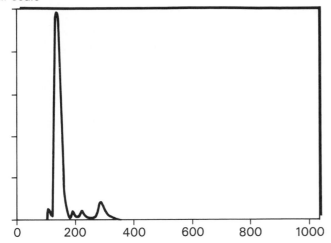

Fig. 6.4 Squamous cell carcinoma of the larynx that was diploid by flow cytometry.

Image analysis is therefore ideally suited for small specimens such as vocal cord biopsies. It is well known that the histological evaluation of mucosal biopsies of the larynx is very subjective and varies not only between different pathologists but also with the same pathologist viewing the same material over different time intervals. It is also well known that not all dysplasias or carcinomas-in-situ of the vocal cords progress to invasive carcinomas.

Image analysis of vocal cord biopsies in conjunction with routine histopathological evaluation offers a more objective means of evaluating these biopsies. Recent studies employing imaging analysis of vocal cord biopsies indicate that aneuploidy can be seen not only in biopsies that show severe dysplasia or carcinoma-in-situ but also in some biopsies that show histologically only mild or moderate dysplasia[4,22] (Fig. 6.5). As Munick-Wikland et al[22] have stated, 'Aneuploidy cannot (always) be equated with cancer, but it is a reflection of a genomic instability which, if unchecked, may culminate in carcinoma.' Initial results certainly indicate that those patients with vocal cord biopsies that show aneuploidy should be followed (? even treated) very closely.

MORPHOMETRY

Morphometry is the study of disease through precise morphological measurements.[15,24] It is more objective than ordinary descriptive morphology and deals with finite figures, such as number of mitoses per unit area, nuclear size, cell volume, tumour thickness, etc. Such measurements, in some instances, may allow pathologists to distinguish between benign, malignant, or borderline malignant neoplasms with greater confidence, or may even have prognostic value. Future developments in mor-

phometry may ultimately lead to automated screening and diagnosis of cytological and histological specimens on a routine basis.

IN-SITU HYBRIDIZATION AND POLYMERASE CHAIN REACTION

In-situ hybridization (ISH) and polymerase chain reaction (PCR) are powerful, highly specific and sensitive procedures for detecting targeted DNA.[6,36] Both can be applied to fresh as well as formalin-fixed, paraffin-embedded tissue. The methodologies involved are complex and beyond the scope of this chapter.

Both procedures have many applications. They are of particular value in identifying infectious agents and genetic abnormalities and in detecting oncogene expression.

ISH is of immense value to pathologists, since the microscopic tissue sample used in analysis remains intact and therefore allows the pathologist to localize the targeted DNA to a specific cell or cell component.

In the larynx, ISH and PCR have been used to detect and genotype human papillomaviruses (HPV). It is now known that juvenile papillomatosis of the larynx is related primarily to HPV 6 and 11. Human papillomaviruses, particularly HPV 16, have also been detected in some squamous cell carcinomas of the larynx, raising speculation that HPV may also be involved in carcinogenesis.[16]

HORMONE RECEPTORS

Since the larynx is a secondary sex organ and the majority of laryngeal carcinomas occur in men, speculation exists on whether these tumours are hormonally dependent and, if so, whether antihormonal therapy may be of therapeutic value.

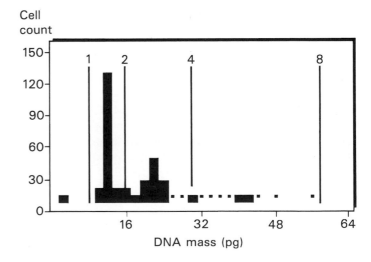

Fig. 6.5 Squamous cell carcinoma of the larynx that was aneuploid by image analysis.

Androgen receptors have been found in normal laryngeal mucosa and laryngeal squamous carcinoma in both sexes.[31,34] The incidence of finding these receptors in laryngeal carcinomas, however, has varied from 28 to 91%.[31-34]

Mattox et al[18] studied 11 patients with advanced or metastatic squamous cell carcinoma (10 laryngeal, 1 floor of mouth) who were treated with antiandrogen therapy, and observed only three short-lived responses (1, 2 and 2.5 months) in nine patients whose tumours could be evaluated. They concluded that future clinical trials of treating patients with antiandrogen therapy did not appear warranted.

Oestrogen and progesterone receptors (OR, PR) have also been evaluated in patients with squamous cell carcinoma of the larynx.[9,29,34] Virolainen et al[34] studied cytosol preparations of 26 squamous cell carcinomas of the larynx (21 primary, 4 recurrent, and 1 neck metastasis) and observed detectable OR in 69%. Only three tumours, however, contained greater than 10 fmol/mg of receptor. They also found detectable levels of PR in 53%, none of which were greater than 10 fmol/mg. Schuller et al[29] studied OR and PR in 65 patients with head and neck cancer from various sites. They found only two patients who had OR in excess of 10 fmol/mg, and none with PR that exceeded this limit. They concluded that head and neck cancers do not contain sufficient concentrations of OR and PR to be worthy of any optimistic response to antihormonal therapy.

Using an immunoperoxidase method, Ferguson et al[9] examined the distribution of OR and PR in normal and non-neoplastic larynges. They noted in all instances that the receptors were localized to the nuclei of the vocalis muscle, perivocalis mesenchymal tissue, or lamina propria. None was found in normal or neoplastic epithelium. To explain the discrepancy between their study in which no OR or PR was found in laryngeal carcinoma and those in which these receptors have been found, they postulated that the difference was probably related to the procedure. Most assays of OR and PR in laryngeal carcinomas employ a tissue homogenate (cytosol) and the positive results may therefore represent contamination of the cytosol with OR and PR containing vocalis muscle and/or mesenchymal tissue.

ONCOGENES

Oncogenes are normal genes that are involved in the control of normal cell growth and differentiation.[3,5,10,17,19-21,28] When abnormally activated, they may play an important part in neoplastic transformation. There are many oncogenes, some of which can be correlated with clinical prognosis. This is particularly true of the N-*myc* oncogene and neuroblastoma and *erb*-B2 and breast cancer.

In laryngeal carcinoma, epidermal growth factor receptor (EGFR) is receiving increasing attention. Its significance, however, is controversial. Scambia et al[28] observed that EGFR was significantly higher in moderate to poorly differentiated squamous cell carcinomas of the larynx and, therefore, serves as a marker for more biologically aggressive tumours. Miyaguchi et al,[20,21] on the other hand, found no association between EGFR and the degree of differentiation. They also noted that EGFR was in general not expressed in either normal or dysplastic laryngeal epithelium. Miyaguchi et al[21] did observe, however, that laryngeal carcinomas associated with an increased expression of EGFR were more likely to recur following irradiation. Kearsley et al,[17] in contrast, concluded that quantification of EGFR does not yield any important prognostic information. Obviously, more work is needed to assess the impact of EGFR and other oncogenes upon prognosis in laryngeal carcinoma.

CYTOGENETICS

Although cytogenetics is a valuable adjunct in haematology, its role in the assessment of solid tumours has been limited.[23,27] This, in part, is due to the fact that often only large or advanced neoplasms have been studied, which characteristically demonstrate multiple and complex karyotypic alterations. Consequently, it has been difficult to distinguish primary from secondary chromosomal changes. Only by studying precursor lesions or smaller tumours can this issue be resolved.

By recognizing early and consistent karyotypes, investigators may better understand the complex process of clonal selection and tumour progression and, accordingly, develop more effective treatment strategies. Unique genetic alterations, if they can be identified, may assist pathologists in diagnosis or might even provide an additional prognostic parameter, e.g., the Philadelphia chromosome and chronic myelogenous leukemia.

Chromosomal analysis of squamous cell carcinoma of the head and neck have also revealed complex abnormalities.[2] The most consistent finding to date, according to Gollin et al,[13] is the 1 p21–p22 breakpoint.

ACKNOWLEDGEMENTS

This work was supported in part by the Pathology Education and Research Foundation, University of Pittsburgh School of Medicine, Pittsburgh, PA, USA. The author also wishes to express his appreciation to Ms Donna Bowen for secretarial assistance, and to Ms Linda Shab and Mr Jeffrey Levis for illustrations.

REFERENCES

1. Campbell B H, Schemmel J C, Hopwood L E, Hoffman R G 1990 Flow cytometric evaluation of chemosensitive and chemoresistant head and neck tumors. Am J Surg 160: 424–426
2. Carey T E, van Dyke D L, Worsham M J, Bradford C R, Babu V R, Schwartz D R, Hsu S, Baker S R 1989 Characterization of human laryngeal primary and metastatic squamous cell carcinoma cell lines UM-SCC-17A and UM-SCC-17B. Cancer Res 49: 6098–6107
3. Cline M J 1989 Biology of disease. Molecular diagnosis of human cancer. Lab Invest 61: 368–380
4. Crissman J D, Zarbo R J 1991 Quantitation of DNA ploidy in squamous intraepithelial neoplasia of the laryngeal glottis. Arch Otolaryngol Head Neck Surg 117: 182–188
5. Dolcetti R, Pelucchi S, Maestro R, Rizzo S, Pastore A, Boiocchi M 1991 Proto-oncogene allelic variations in human squamous cell carcinomas of the larynx. Eur Arch Otorhinolaryngol 248: 279–285
6. Eisenstein B I 1990 The polymerase chain reaction. A new method of using molecular genetics for medical diagnosis. N Engl J Med 322: 178–182
7. El-Naggar A, Lopez V, Luna M, Garsney L, Batsakis J G 1991 Intratumoral heterogeneity of DNA content in laryngeal squamous carcinoma. Lab Invest 64: 64A, abstract 372
8. Feinmasser R, Freeman J L, Noyek A 1990 Flow cytometric analysis of DNA content in laryngeal cancer. J Laryngol Otol 104: 485–487
9. Ferguson B J, Hudson W R, McCarty K S Jr 1987 Sex steroid receptor distribution in the human larynx and laryngeal carcinoma. Arch Otolaryngol Head Neck Surg 113: 1311–1315
10. Friend S H, Dryja T P, Weinberg R A 1988 Oncogenes and tumor–suppressing genes. N Engl J Med 318: 618–622
11. Gallo O, Libonati G A, Gallina E, Fini-Storchi O, Giannini A, Urso C, Bondi R 1991 Langerhans cells related to prognosis in patients with laryngeal carcinoma. Arch Otolaryngol Head Neck Surg 117: 1007–1010
12. Goldsmith M M, Cresson D S, Postma D S, Askin F B, Pillsbury H C 1986 Significance of ploidy in laryngeal cancer. Am J Surg 152: 396–402
13. Gollin S M, Whiteside T, Johnson J, Sheer M E 1991 Consistent cytogenetic alterations in six squamous cell carcinomas of the head and neck. Am J Hum Genet 49: 241, abstract 1319
14. Guo Y–C, DeSanto L, Osetinsky G V 1989 Prognostic implications of nuclear DNA content in head and neck cancer. Otolaryngol Head Neck Surg 100: 95–98
15. Hall T L, Fu Y S 1985 Biology of disease. Applications of quantitative microscopy in human pathology. Lab Invest 53: 5–21
16. Hoshikawa T, Nakajima T, Uhara H, Gotoh M, Shimosato Y, Tsutsumi K, Ono I, Ebihara S 1990 Detection of human papillomavirus DNA in laryngeal squamous cell carcinomas by polymerase chain reaction. Laryngoscope 100: 647–650
17. Kearsley J H, Leonard J H, Walsh M D, Wright G R 1991 A comparison of epidermal growth factor receptor (EGFR) and c-erb B-2 oncogene expression in head and neck squamous cell carcinomas. Pathology 23: 189–194
18. Mattox D E, von Hoff D D, McGuire W L 1984 Androgen receptors and antiandrogen therapy for laryngeal carcinoma. Arch Otolaryngol 110: 721–724
19. Merritt W D, Weissler M C, Turk B F, Gilmer T M 1990 Oncogene amplification squamous cell carcinoma of the head and neck. Arch Otolaryngol Head Neck Surg 116: 1394–1398
20. Miyaguchi M, Olofsson J, Hellquist H B 1990 Expression of growth factor receptor in laryngeal dysplasia and carcinoma. Acta Otolaryngol 110: 309–313
21. Miyaguchi M, Olofsson J, Hellquist H B 1991 Expression of epidermal growth factor receptor in glottic carcinoma and its relation to recurrence after radiotherapy. Clin Otolaryngol 16: 466–469
22. Munick-Wikland E, Kuylenstierna R, Lindholm J, Auer G 1991 Image cytometry DNA analysis of dysplastic squamous epithelial lesions in the larynx. Anticancer Res 11: 597–600
23. Nowell P C 1990 Cytogenetics of tumor progression. Cancer 65: 2172–2177
24. Pesce C M 1987 Biology of disease. Defining and interpreting diseases through morphometry. Lab Invest 56: 568–575
25. Rua S, Comino A, Fruttero A, Cera R, Semeria C, Lanzillotta L, Boffetta P 1991 Relationship between histologic features, DNA flow cytometry, and clinical behavior of squamous cell carcinomas of the larynx. Cancer 67: 141–149
26. Sakr W, Hussan M, Zarbo R J, Ensley J, Crissman J D 1989 DNA quantitation and histologic characteristics of squamous cell carcinoma of the upper aerodigestive tract. Arch Pathol Lab Med 113: 1009–1014
27. Sandberg A A 1988 Chromosomal lesions and solid tumors. Hosp Practice 23: 93–106
28. Scambia G, Panici P B, Battaglia F, Ferrandina G, Almadori G, Paludetti G, Maurizi M, Mancuso S 1991 Receptors for epidermal growth factor and steroid hormones in primary laryngeal tumors. Cancer 67: 1347–1351
29 Schuller D E, Abou-Issa H, Parrish R 1984 Estrogen and progesterone receptors in head and neck cancer. Arch Otolaryngol 110: 725–727
30. Stell P M 1991 Ploidy in head and neck cancer. A review and meta-analysis. Clin Otolaryngol 16: 510–516
31. Toral I, Ciliv G, Gursel B, Ozdem C 1990 Androgen receptors in laryngeal carcinoma. Eur Arch Otorhinolaryngol 247: 244–246
32. Tuohimaa P T, Kallio S, Heinijoki J, Aitasalo K, Virolainen E, Karma P, Tuohimaa P J 1981 Androgen receptors in laryngeal carcinoma. Acta Otolaryngol 91: 149–154
33. Vecerina-Volic S, Romic-Stojkovic R, Krajina Z, Gamulin S 1987 Androgen receptors in normal and neoplastic laryngeal tissue. Arch Otolaryngol Head Neck Surg 113: 411–413
34. Virolainen E, Tuohimaa P, Aitasalo K, Kytta J, Vanharanta-Hiltunen R 1986 Steroid hormone receptors in laryngeal carcinoma. Otolaryngol Head Neck Surg 94: 512–517
35. Walter M A, Peters G E, Peiper S C 1991 Predicting radioresistance in early glottic squamous cell carcinoma by DNA content. Ann Otol Rhinol Laryngol 100: 523–526
36. Wolfe H J 1988 DNA probes in diagnostic pathology. Am J Clin Pathol 90: 340–344

7. Histological classification of laryngeal neoplasms

A. Ferlito, I. Friedmann

The classification of tumours is of considerable importance, and many attempts have been made to correlate the type of a neoplasm with its biological behaviour. There are clinical, topographical and staging classifications and those based on the microscopical features of the neoplasms. The internationally applied TNM classification is based on staging and anatomical extent of the neoplasm, but the histological features have been omitted. A histological classification of laryngeal neoplasms is of essential relevance to prognosis and treatment but the frequently changing terminology may lead to mistakes and misunderstandings. Early classifications were incomplete and too simple, having included only a few types of malignant tumour, such as squamous cell carcinoma, undifferentiated carcinoma, adenocarcinoma and sarcomas.

In 1976, Ferlito[4] proposed the classification for laryngeal carcinomas shown in Table 7.1.

To standardize the nomenclature of laryngeal tumours, the World Health Organization (WHO) published its *Histological Typing of Upper Respiratory Tract Tumours* (which included the larynx) in 1978.[24] This classification was the result of a team effort by Drs Shanmugaratnam and Sobin and several pathologists from eight countries. Table 7.2 summarizes the first version of this WHO classification.

Table 7.1 Malignant epithelial neoplasms of the larynx[4]

Carcinoma in situ
Squamous cell carcinoma
Verrucous squamous cell carcinoma
Spindle cell carcinoma
Lymphoepithelial carcinoma
Undifferentiated carcinoma
Oat cell carcinoma
Carcinoid
Adenocarcinoma in situ
Adenocarcinoma (NOS)
Giant cell carcinoma
Clear cell carcinoma
Adenosquamous carcinoma
Malignant mixed carcinoma
Mucoepidermoid carcinoma
Adenoid cystic carcinoma
Acinic cell carcinoma
Carcinosarcoma
Unclassified carcinoma

Table 7.2 Histological typing of laryngeal tumours[24]

Epithelial tumours

Benign	Squamous cell papilloma/papillomatosis
	Oxyphilic adenoma (oncocytoma)
	Others
Malignant	Carcinoma in situ (intraepithelial carcinoma)
	Squamous cell carcinoma
	Verrucous (squamous) carcinoma
	Spindle cell (squamous) carcinoma
	Adenocarcinoma
	Adenoid cystic carcinoma
	Carcinoid tumour
	Others
	Undifferentiated carcinoma

Soft tissue tumours

Benign	Lipoma
	Haemangioma
	Leiomyoma
	Rhabdomyoma
	Granular cell tumour
	Neurofibroma
	Neurilemmoma (schwannoma)
	Paraganglioma (chemodectoma)
	Others
Malignant	Fibrosarcoma
	Rhabdomyosarcoma
	Angiosarcoma
	Kaposi's sarcoma
	Others

Tumours of bone and cartilage

Benign	Chondroma
	Others
Malignant	Chondrosarcoma
	Others

Tumours of lymphoid and haematopoietic tissues
Miscellaneous tumours
Secondary tumours
Unclassified tumours

In 1987, Hyams and Heffner[12] proposed a classification of primary neoplasms of the larynx which is an adaptation of the WHO classification (Table 7.3).

Table 7.3   Classification of neoplasms of the larynx[12]

Benign
  Epithelial
    Squamous cell papilloma
    Cyst, epithelial
    Oncocytoma
    Adenoma
      Pleomorphic adenoma (benign mixed tumour)
  Mesodermal, neuroectodermal
    Benign granular cell tumour
    Chondroma
      Osteochondroma
    Haemangioma
      Lymphangioma
    Fibroma
    Fibrohistiocytoma
    Leiomyoma
    Rhabdomyoma
    Lipoma
    Giant cell tumour (? of soft tissue)
    Neurilemmoma (schwannoma, neurinoma)
    Neurofibroma
    Paraganglioma (extra-adrenal)
  Premalignant epithelial abnormalities
  Benign squamous hyperplasia (keratosis) with or without epithelial atypia

Malignant
  Epithelial
    Squamous cell carcinoma
    Verrucous carcinoma
    Spindle cell carcinoma
    Undifferentiated small cell (? oat- cell) carcinoma
    Adenocarcinoma (carcinoid tumour)
    Adenoid cystic carcinoma
    Mucoepidermoid carcinoma
  Mesodermal, neuroectodermal
    Fibrosarcoma
    Malignant fibrohistiocytoma
    Synovial sarcoma
    Rhabdomyosarcoma
    Angiosarcoma
    Kaposi's sarcoma
    Liposarcoma
    Chondrosarcoma
    Lymphoma
    Plasmacytoma
    Neurofibrosarcoma
    Malignant melanoma
  Teratoid neoplasms (benign and malignant)
    Dermoid cyst
    Teratoma
    Hamartoma
    Choristoma
    Teratocarcinoma
  Metastatic neoplasms involving the larynx

Table 7.4   Primary and metastatic malignancies of the larynx[15]

Primary malignancies
  Epithelial cancers
    Squamous cell carcinoma
      Carcinoma in situ
      Superficially invasive
      Verrucous carcinoma
      Pseudosarcoma
      Anaplastic
      Transitional cell
      Lymphoepithelial
    Small cell or oat cell carcinoma
    Adenocarcinoma
      Mucoepidermoid carcinoma
      Adenocarcinoma
      Adenoid cystic carcinoma
      Non-specific adenocarcinoma
    Paraganglioma
    Carcinoid
    Oncocytoid carcinoma
    Melanoma
  Non-epithelial cancers
    Sarcomas
      Fibrosarcoma
      Chondrosarcoma
      Rhabdomyosarcoma
      Leiomyosarcoma
      Hemangiomyosarcoma
      Giant cell sarcoma
      Lymphosarcoma

Metastatic malignancies
  Renal cell carcinoma
  Thyroid carcinoma
  Breast
  Lung
  Prostate
  Gastrointestinal tract

In 1989, Lawson et al[15] proposed the classification illustrated in Table 7.4.

The WHO classification of upper respiratory tract tumours was recently reviewed by the following experts: K. Shanmugaratnam (Singapore), L. H. Sobin (USA), L. Barnes (USA), A. Cardesa (Spain), A. Ferlito (Italy), I. Friedmann (England), D. K. Heffner (USA), H. B. Hellquist (Sweden), V. J. Hyams (USA), G. R. F. Krueger (Germany), C. Micheau (France), A. Nascimento (Brazil). The classification, published in 1991,[25] is outlined in Table 7.5.

CONSIDERATIONS

Many new laryngeal neoplasms have been recognized in recent years (Table 7.6), demanding an applicable and acceptable histopathological classification of benign and malignant neoplasms of the larynx. The new histological classification of tumours of the upper respiratory tract and ear, compiled by the above-mentioned WHO team, has been based — like the earlier version — on the microscopical features of the neoplasm. Although appreciative of the important diagnostic role of modern immunohistochemical methods, especially in the differential diagnosis of poorly differentiated and round cell neoplasms, the definition of each neoplasm has been essentially based on evidence supplied by routine histological staining methods.[26]

The neoplasms added to the new version of the WHO classification are marked with an asterisk in Table 7.5.

The vague category 'others' has been discarded, and so too have some doubtful entities such as oxyphilic adenoma (oncocytoma) and 'undifferentiated' carcinoma: the former because it is not a true neoplasm, the latter because it has been attributed to a heterogeneous group of laryngeal neoplasms notoriously difficult to distinguish.

Ferlito and Friedmann believe that the application of electron microscopy and of immunohistochemical methods, with an ever-increasing arsenal of antibodies and recently-developed molecular biology techniques, will enable a more accurate identification and therefore a more reliable classification of neoplasms of the larynx.[5] The new WHO classification is more comprehensive than before, but some neoplasms described in the literature have not been included, e.g., sebaceous carcinoma, mucoid adenocarcinoma, malignant granular cell tumour, malignant myoepithelioma, malignant mesenchymoma, laryngeal blastoma.[2,3,13,14,16,27]

Of the important group of neuroendocrine neoplasms of the larynx, only carcinoid tumour and paraganglioma were listed in the earlier WHO classification; atypical carcinoid tumour and small cell neuroendocrine carcinoma have now been added. It is important to note that some cases of atypical carcinoid and/or metastatic neoplasms may have been diagnosed as 'adenocarcinoma' in the past.

The terminology used in this book coincides largely with that of the second edition of the WHO's histological typing of laryngeal tumours.

Table 7.5 Histological typing of laryngeal tumours[25]

Epithelial tumours and precancerous lesions
Benign
    Papilloma
    Papillomatosis
    Pleomorphic adenoma★
    Basal cell (basaloid) adenoma★

    Dysplasia and carcinoma in situ
      Squamous cell dysplasia
        Mild dysplasia
        Moderate dysplasia
        Severe dysplasia
      Carcinoma in situ

Malignant
    Squamous cell carcinoma
    Verrucous squamous cell carcinoma
    Spindle cell carcinoma
    Adenoid squamous cell carcinoma★
    Basaloid squamous cell carcinoma★
    Adenocarcinoma
    Acinic cell carcinoma★
    Mucoepidermoid carcinoma★
    Adenoid cystic carcinoma
    Carcinoma in pleomorphic adenoma★
    Epithelial–myoepithelial carcinoma★
    Clear cell carcinoma★
    Adenosquamous carcinoma★
    Giant cell carcinoma★
    Salivary duct carcinoma★
    Carcinoid tumour
    Atypical carcinoid tumour★
    Small cell carcinoma★
    Lymphoepithelial carcinoma★

Soft tissue tumours
Benign
    Aggressive fibromatosis★
    Myxoma★
    Fibrous histiocytoma★
    Lipoma
    Leiomyoma
    Rhabdomyoma
    Haemangioma
    Haemangiopericytoma★
    Lymphangioma★
    Neurilemmoma
    Neurofibroma
    Granular cell tumour
    Paraganglioma

Malignant
    Fibrosarcoma
    Malignant fibrous histiocytoma★
    Liposarcoma★
    Leiomyosarcoma★
    Rhabdomyosarcoma
    Angiosarcoma
    Kaposi sarcoma
    Malignant haemangiopericytoma★
    Malignant nerve sheath tumour★
    Alveolar soft part sarcoma★
    Synovial sarcoma★
    Ewing sarcoma★

Tumours of bone and cartilage
Benign
    Chondroma

Malignant
    Chondrosarcoma
    Osteosarcoma★

Malignant lymphomas

Miscellaneous tumours
Benign
    Mature teratoma★

Malignant
    Malignant melanoma★
    Malignant germ cell tumours★

Secondary tumours
Unclassified tumours

★Oncotypes new to the second edition.

Table 7.6   New neoplastic entities diagnosed in the larynx

Histological type	Author (s)	Year
Squamous cell carcinoma with osteoclast-like cells	Ferlito et al[6]	1987
Basaloid squamous cell carcinoma	Wain et al[28]	1986
Typical carcinoid	Gehanno et al[8]	1980
Atypical carcinoid	Goldman et al[9]	1969
Small cell neuroendocrine carcinoma	Olofsson and van Nostrand[21]	1972
Acinic cell carcinoma	Montes Noriega[20]	1974
Clear cell carcinoma	Ferlito[4]	1976
Giant cell carcinoma	Ferlito[4]	1976
Salivary duct carcinoma	Ferlito et al[7]	1981
Epithelial–myoepithelial carcinoma	Mikaelian et al[18]	1986
Sebaceous carcinoma	Martinez-Madrigal et al[16]	1991
Mucoid adenocarcinoma	Tsang et al[27]	1991
Malignant myoepithelioma	Ibrahim et al[13]	1991
Laryngeal blastoma	Eble et al[3]	1985
Junctional naevus	Seals et al[23]	1986
Fibrous histiocytoma	Rolander et al[22]	1972
Leiomyoblastoma	Mori et al[20a]	1992
Synovial sarcoma	Miller et al[19]	1975
Alveolar soft part sarcoma	Michaels[17]	1984
Ewing sarcoma	Abramowsky and Witt[1]	1983
Malignant mesenchymoma	Kawashima et al[14]	1990
Mycosis fungoides[*]	Hood et al [10]	1979
Burkitt's lymphoma[*]	Michaels[17]	1984
Mast cell sarcoma[*]	Horny et al[11]	1986

[*] Primary lesion in the larynx.

REFERENCES

1. Abramowsky C R, Witt W J 1983 Sarcoma of the larynx in a newborn. Cancer 51: 1726–1730
2. Busanni-Caspari von W, Hammar C H 1958 Zur Malignität der sogenannten Myoblastenmyome. Zentralbl Allg Pathol 98: 401–406
3. Eble J N, Hull M T, Bojrab D 1985 Laryngeal blastoma. A light and electron microscopic study of a novel entity analogous to pulmonary blastoma. Am J Clin Pathol 84: 378–385
4. Ferlito A 1976 Histological classification of larynx and hypopharynx cancers and their clinical implications. Pathologic aspects of 2052 malignant neoplasms diagnosed at the ORL Department of Padua University from 1966 to 1976. Acta Otolaryngol 342 (suppl): 1–88
5. Ferlito A, Friedmann I 1990 Poorly-differentiated laryngeal malignancies. ORL J Otorhinolaryngol Relat Spec 52: 63–64
6. Ferlito A, Friedmann I, Recher G 1987 Squamous cell carcinoma of the larynx with osteoclast-like giant cells. J Laryngol Otol 101: 393–398
7. Ferlito A, Gale N, Hvala A 1981 Laryngeal salivary duct carcinoma. A light and electron microscopic study. J Laryngol Otol 95: 731–738
8. Gehanno P, Lallemant Y, Groussard O, Blanchet F, Veber F, Guedon C, Rame J A 1980 Apudomes en O.R.L à propos de 6 observations (dont 1 chémodectome et 1 carcinoïde du larynx); critique du concept d'apudome. J Fr Otorhinolaryngol 29: 7–18
9. Goldman N G, Hood C I, Singleton G T 1969 Carcinoid of the larynx. Arch Otolaryngol 90: 91–93
10. Hood A F, Mark G J, Hunt J V 1979 Laryngeal mycosis fungoides. Cancer 43: 1527–1532
11. Horny H P, Parwaresch M R, Kaiserling E, Muller K, Olbermann M, Mainzer K, Lennert K 1986 Mast cell sarcoma of the larynx. J Clin Pathol 39: 262
12. Hyams V J, Heffner D K 1987 Laryngeal pathology. In: Tucker HM (ed) The larynx. Thieme, New York
13. Ibrahim R, Bird J, Sieler M W 1991 Malignant myoepithelioma of the larynx with massive metastatic spread to the liver: an ultrastructural and immunocytochemical study. Ultrastruct Pathol 15: 69–76
14. Kawashima O, Kamei T, Shimizu Y, Shizuka T, Nakayama M 1990 Malignant mesenchymoma of the larynx. J Laryngol Otol 104: 440–444

15. Lawson W, Biller H F, Suen J Y 1989 Cancer of the larynx. In: Myers E N, Suen J Y (eds) Cancer of the head and neck, 2nd edn. Churchill Livingstone, New York
16. Martinez-Madrigal, Casiraghi O, Khattech A, Nasr-Khattech R B, Richard J-M, Micheau C 1991 Hypopharyngeal sebaceous carcinoma: a case report. Hum Pathol 22: 929–931
17. Michaels L 1984 Pathology of the larynx. Springer-Verlag, Berlin
18. Mikaelian D O, Contrucci R B, Batsakis J G 1986 Epithelial–myoepithelial carcinoma of the subglottic region: a case presentation and review of the literature. Otolaryngol Head Neck Surg 95: 104–106
19. Miller L H, Santaella-Latimer L, Miller T 1975 Synovial sarcoma of the larynx. Trans Am Acad Ophthalmol Otolaryngol 80: 448–451
20. Montes Noriega B 1974 Adenomas de laringe. An Otorrinolaringol Ibero Am 1: 98–105
20a. Mori H, Kumoi T, Hashimoto M, Uematsu K 1992 Leiomyoblastoma of the larynx: report of a case. Head Neck 14: 148–152
21. Olofsson J, van Nostrand AWP 1972 Anaplastic small cell carcinoma of larynx. Ann Otol Rhinol Laryngol 81: 284–287
22. Rolander T, Kim O J, Shumrick D A 1972 Fibrous xanthoma of the larynx. Arch Otolaryngol 96: 168–170
23. Seals J L, Shenefelt R E, Babin R W 1986 Intralaryngeal nevus in a child. A case report. Int J Pediatr Otorhinolaryngol 12: 55–58
24. Shanmugaratnam K, Sobin L H 1978 Histological typing of upper respiratory tract tumours. International histological classification of tumours. World Health Organization, Geneva
25. Shanmugaratnam K 1991 Histological typing of tumours of the upper respiratory tract and ear. World Health Organization. International histological classification of tumours, 2nd edn. Springer-Verlag, Berlin
26. Sobin L H 1989 International histological classification of tumours, 2nd edn. Cancer 63: 907
27. Tsang Y W, Ngan K C, Chan J K C 1991 Primary mucoid adenocarcinoma of the larynx. J Laryngol Otol 105: 315–317
28. Wain S L, Kier R, Vollmer R T, Bossen E H 1986 Basaloid–squamous carcinoma of the tongue, hypopharynx, and larynx: report of 10 cases. Human Pathol 17: 1158–1166

8. Recurrent respiratory papillomatosis

H. K. Kashima, B. G. Leventhal

INTRODUCTION

The essential clinical and histological features of laryngeal papillomata were described by Sir Morell Mackenzie in the late 19th century. Recognition of 'warts in the throat' has been ascribed to Marcellus Donatus in the 17th century. Victor Egon Ullman demonstrated a transmitting agent when he injected a cell-free filtrate from laryngeal papilloma and successfully produced papillomas on his own arm as well as on the arm of an associate.[35]

The first successful peroral excision of laryngeal papilloma was described by Koderik in 1750, and surgical excision by thyrotomy was performed by Brauers in 1883. Improved illumination and magnification of the operating microscope established endoscopic excision as a reliable and preferred method for papilloma ablation.[6] The operating microscope and the surgical laser are recent refinements that enhance precise surgical excision. A wide variety of agents have had unsuccessful trials as topical adjuvants to surgical excision; of these, podophyllum has had the longest-standing use.[13] Interstitial and teletherapy have been used in the treatment of papillomatosis, but growth disturbance in pediatric laryngeal cartilages and increased risk for malignant transformation of previously benign laryngeal papillomata has been recognized and these modalities are no longer used.[36] In recent years anti-neoplastic agents have been utilized with limited success.[18] Biological modifiers, notably interferon, were found effective in numerous pilot studies during the 1980s and led to several randomized trials. The results of these multi-institutional interferon trials are reviewed in the section discussing treatment.

TERMINOLOGY AND DEFINITIONS

Recurrent respiratory papillomatosis (RRP) denotes benign regrowths of papillomata with particular predilection for the larynx (Fig. 8.1) and trachea. The nasal vestibule, nasopharyngeal surface of the soft palate, lower tracheobronchial mucosa and peripheral lung field are less often involved. The lesions are histologically benign (Figs 8.2, 8.3) but typically exhibit regrowth after total surgical excision — hence the designation 'recurrent'.

Recurrent respiratory papillomatosis is conventionally classified according to age at disease onset. Approximately half the cases are designated *juvenile-onset* (JO); initial symptoms appear during infancy or childhood up to age 12 years. *Adult-onset (AO) RRP* initially presents after 20 years of age and has peak incidence during the third and fourth decades but may appear as late as 60–70 years of age. Initial presentation of papilloma between the ages 12 and 20 years is virtually unknown.

Juvenile-onset (JO) RRP characteristically presents with multiple lesions predominantly affecting the true and false cords. Hoarseness is the cardinal symptom and, due to the small size of the larynx and rapid regrowth of papilloma, airway compromise necessitates frequent and repeated surgical excisions. Males and females are afflicted in equal numbers, and the disease has been regarded as entering spontaneous remission at puberty — although there are no data to support this view.

Adult-onset (AO) RRP, histologically indistinguishable from JO-RRP, occurs more frequently in males; the papillomatous lesions are often solitary, and upper airway obstruction is less frequently observed than in JO-RRP due, in part, to the larger laryngotracheal dimension. Although papilloma recurrence after surgical excision occurs, severe upper airway obstruction is rare.

INCIDENCE

Laryngeal papilloma is the commonest benign laryngeal neoplasm and has world-wide distribution. On the basis of a mail survey of American otolaryngologists, an estimate of 1500 new cases per year in the United States was made.[34] The estimate of 7.1 new cases per 1 million population agrees closely with the prevalence rate of 0.8 cases of juvenile-onset papillomatosis per 100 000 population reported in a study from Denmark.[5] The term juvenile laryngeal papillomatosis (JLP) was coined to

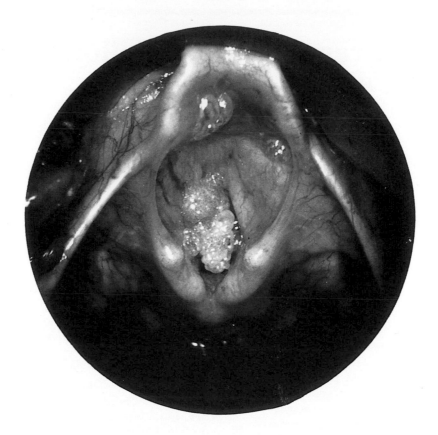

Fig. 8.1 Large mass of papillomata causing severe obstruction of the glottis. Others scattered on the posterior surface of the epiglottis. (Courtesy of Dr B. Benjamin, Sidney, and the editor of *Journal of Laryngology and Otology*.)

designate papillomatous growths which have a predilection for the larynges of paediatric patients, in whom hoarseness dramatically catapults into life-threatening airway obstruction — even after meticulous surgical excision. The alternative designation of recurrent respiratory papillomatosis (RRP) recognizes the persistent regrowth with predilection for the entire respiratory tract.

The precise numbers of AO- and JO-RRP are not known, but it is likely that the total case numbers are approximately equal. The male-to-female ratio is equal in JO-RRP, but in AO-RRP males predominate over females by at least two-to-one — and as much as four-to-one. The numbers of AO and JO-RRP are influenced by the size of the human papillomavirus (HPV) reservoir, and current evidence is that the prevalence of genital HPV infection is increasing steadily.

EPIDEMIOLOGY

Clinical observations suggest that transmission of HPV infection from mother to child occurs during passage through an infected birth canal. In a review of 109 case records of juvenile-onset respiratory papillomatosis, there was only a single case born by caesarean section.[30] On the basis of a questionnaire survey, the clinical triad of a *first born delivered vaginally* to a *young* (teenaged) *mother* was present in partial or complete form in 72% of juvenile onset RRP patients, 36% of AO-RRP patients, 29% of juvenile controls and 38% of adult controls. This feature distinguishing JO-RRP patients was significant at the 0.05 level for birth rank and method of delivery, and at 0.01 level for maternal age.[17]

The prevalence of genital condyloma in women of child-bearing age far exceeds the number of new cases of respiratory papillomatosis; the risk of transmission from a mother with HPV infection to her newborn has been estimated to be in the range of 1:80 to 1:1500.[30] More precise definition of risk factors associating respiratory papillomatosis with maternal condyloma is needed before caesarean section can be advocated in order to reduce the risk of respiratory papillomatosis developing in newborns.

Adult-onset recurrent respiratory papillomatosis has been presumed to occur on the basis of sexual contact, namely, orogenital exposure. AO-RRP subjects reported more life-time sex partners (P<0.01) and a higher frequency of oral sex (P<0.05) than reported by adult controls.[17]

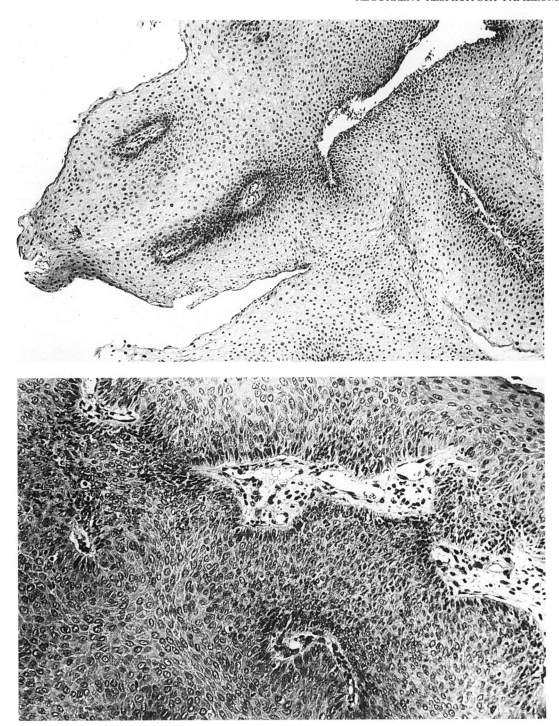

Fig. 8.2 (*top*) Juvenile-type squamous papilloma of the larynx from a 2-year-old child. Cross-cut papillae showing the fibrovascular central stalks covered by well-differentiated squamous epithelium. H&E, ×16 OM. (Courtesy of Professor A. Ferlito, Padua.)

Fig. 8.3 (*bottom*) Same case as in Fig. 8.2. There are slight dysplastic changes in this area. H&E, ×40 OM. (Courtesy of Professor A. Ferlito, Padua.)

Some cases of 'adult-onset' papillomatosis have a life-long history of hoarseness — suggesting the alternative possibility that initial viral transmission may have occurred at childbirth but remained dormant until diagnosed in adulthood.

Transmission of viral infection through oropharyngeal secretions is rare. There are no documented cases of papillomatosis occurring among siblings or family members who are constantly exposed to oral secretions from papilloma patients.

AETIOLOGY — HISTOGENESIS

The histopathological similarity of respiratory papilloma and cutaneous warts has been recognized for many years. Light-microscopic and electron-micrographic evidence of virus-like particles in papillomatous lesions had been reported, but precise identification of human papilloma virus (HPV) in respiratory papilloma was not achieved until the early 1980s, when molecular biological techniques identified HPV types 6 and 11 as the causative agents.[27] Specific subtypes of HPV 6 have been correlated with extent of spread and clinical severity of papilloma; HPV 6-C (HPV 11) is associated with a subset of patients with extensive anatomical disease, including spread of papillomatous growths into the trachea and lungs.[27]

HPV types 6 and 11 are also implicated as causative agents in genital condyloma. The relevance of maternal condyloma to laryngeal papilloma was recognized by Hajek in his case report of 1956 describing the occurrence of maternal condyloma in association with a newborn subsequently diagnosed as having respiratory papillomatosis.[10] A history of maternal condyloma is recognized in 30–50% of juvenile-onset recurrent respiratory papillomatosis.[29]

CLINICAL MANIFESTATIONS

Juvenile-onset papillomatosis is suspected and detected on the basis of hoarseness, often present from the time of birth. Hoarseness is also the common initial symptom in patients with adult-onset (AO) RRP. Upper airway obstructive symptoms of varying severity can worsen during intercurrent upper respiratory tract infection, and initial presentation may occur as an airway emergency — particularly among pediatric patients. Endoscopic excision effectively restores a safe airway, but rapid regrowth of papilloma necessitates repeated excisions in a subset of patients so that 100 or more endoscopic operations may be necessary to maintain a safe and adequate airway. The intervals between operations usually lengthen as the JO-RRP patient approaches puberty. This diminished clinical severity is attributable to increased laryngeal size and possible reduced papilloma growth rate. A proportion of patients may experience spontaneous remission from papilloma regrowth. An undetermined proportion of patients continue to experience regrowth of papilloma, some with papilloma extension from the larynx to the trachea, bronchi and lungs.

Pulmonary papilloma is initially manifested as an asymptomatic non-calcified nodule in the lung parenchyma; these nodules slowly enlarge and central cavitation occurs. In spite of alarming radiographic features, the clinical manifestations are surprisingly mild and the clinical course unexpectedly long. The ultimate outcome is progressive respiratory failure and death. At present there is no satisfactory treatment for pulmonary papilloma; a proportion of pulmonary papilloma have foci of squamous metaplasia and some of squamous cell carcinoma, often unsuspected and undetected until postmortem examination. HPV-6 and 11 have been identified in pulmonary papilloma.[37]

PATHOLOGY

Papilloma lesions occur exclusively in squamous epithelium, and sites at which squamous and ciliary epithelium are juxtaposed appear particularly susceptible. Hence the limen vestibuli in the anterior nose, the nasopharyngeal surface of the soft palate, the mid-zone of the laryngeal surface of the epiglottis, the upper and lower surfaces of the vocal folds, the carina and bronchial spurs, and the peripheral lung — all exhibiting squamo-ciliary junctions — have been specified as sites of predilection.[15]

The tracheostoma and the healed stoma, where squamous metaplasia in the stomal tract joins with ciliated tracheal epithelium, is an iatrogenic squamo-ciliary junction, and papilloma commonly develops at this site. The distal tip of the tracheotomy tube in the lower thoracic trachea induces a circumferential zone of squamous metaplasia and a cuff of papilloma invariably occurs at this site. Risk of papilloma extension into the lower respiratory tract is increased in patients who have had tracheotomy; for this reason meticulous and repeated endoscopic excision is strongly advocated in preference to tracheotomy.[37]

The characteristic clinical appearance of papilloma is that of a multi-nodular growth, each with a subepithelial vascular tuft. Clinically, the lesions may be sessile and broad-based or exophytic and arising from a narrow stalk. Varying degrees of epithelial atypia can occur and these cases require careful follow-up and repeated biopsies. The occurrence of epithelial atypia, particularly when severe, has been alleged to have association with rapid papilloma regrowth and increased risk of progression to carcinoma.[28] Atypia has been associated with DNA hyperploidy, a factor associated with increased risk for malignant transformation. Some 3–5% of patients with recurrent growths undergo malignant transformation.[32] Irradiation therapy and tobacco usage have been implicated as cofactors predisposing to this change.[16] Inasmuch as malignant transformation has been noted in the larynx, trachea and lungs, specimens obtained at each operation should be carefully labelled to identify their source so that any histological change of concern can be related precisely to the tissue of origin.

TREATMENT

The clinical course of recurrent respiratory papillomatosis is predictably unpredictable. There is consensus opinion that AO-RRP is less severe than JO-RRP, whether assessed on the basis of disease extent, clinical symptoms or the frequency and total number of operations. The cornerstone of papilloma management is endoscopic excision under optimal magnified visualization. CO_2 laser excision of exophytic and airway obstructive lesions seeks to achieve lesion ablation and maximum preservation of normal respiratory epithelium. Atraumatic instrumentation to minimize unintentional mucosal injury is important in avoiding creation of new lesion sites.

Tracheotomy and/or irradiation therapy are treatment modalities usually invoked under desperate clinical circumstances — both adversely affect the clinical course: tracheotomy by promoting mucosal spread of disease,[37] and irradiation by enhancing the risk of malignant degeneration.[16]

Treatment: non-surgical adjuvants

Podophyllin and colchicine have been employed in the local control of genital papillomata.[18] Dedo has used local application of podophyllin in laryngeal papillomatosis as an adjunct to surgery, and reports that disease control is better than with surgery alone.[7] Abramson et al[1] have used photodynamic activation of a haematoporphyrin derivative (HPD) with an argon pump dye laser with a red light output of 630 nm. Two to three days prior to surgery the patients receive a haematoporphyrin product which selectively accumulates in the papilloma and increases efficacy of the argon laser effect. In one patient, a complete clinical response was achieved, and the latent HPV 11 genome, previously present in morphologically normal laryngeal tissues, was eliminated.[1]

Smith and coworkers[31] observed inhibition of papilloma regrowth in 6 of 8 patients receiving 5-fluorouracil as a 0.5–5% aerosol into the larynx and tracheobronchial tree. Frequent administration (twice daily) of the agent was required; bronchospasm, coughing and tracheal bleeding occurred. Intravenous bleomycin at 7 U/m^2 twice weekly to a total of 240 U/m^2 produced a complete response in at least one patient with severe endotracheal disease. Bleomycin has pulmonary toxicity which may occur after a cumulative dose of 400 U.[26]

Isotretinoin at 1–2 mg/kg per day was used in six patients and achieved one partial and three complete responses.[23] In a limited randomized study, six patients received 13-*cis*-retinoic acid (CRA) at 100 mg/m^2 for one year; three received placebo. The intraoperative intervals were lengthened from 7.4 months to 15.8 months in patients receiving CRA; the placebo group also had longer intraoperative intervals, improving from 5 months (preCRA) to 19.4 months post-CRA. This trial was terminated when two of six patients receiving CRA experienced toxicity sufficiently severe to cause withdrawal from therapy; dose reduction was necessary in three patients. Toxicity was predominantly mucocutaneous and characterized by dryness, peeling and cracking of skin, particularly of the face and lips; in one subject these changes caused bleeding.[2]

α-Interferon has been an agent of major interest in slowing the growth of RRP.[25] In 1976 a group of Scandinavian investigators noted clinical response in all seven RRP patients treated with natural leukocyte interferon.[9] A trial with poly IC:LC, an artificial interferon inducer, likewise produced a clinical response, albeit accompanied by systemic toxicity.[19] These and other uncontrolled observations[8,33] led to several randomized studies including a 12-month controlled cross-over study with six months treatment with lymphoblastoid interferon α-n–1 (Wellferon, Beckenham, Kent) in 1988. Sixty-six patients with clinically severe JO-RRP were randomized to receive α-n–1 interferon 5 mU/m^2 daily for 28 days and 5 mU/m^2 three times weekly for 5 months or to observation for the initial 6 months and then crossed-over for the second six months of the study. A scoring system to quantify the amount of papilloma present at each operation (see above) was used[14] and demonstrated significant differences between the lesion scores during the interferon treatment and the observation periods. Eight of 57 patients achieved a complete remission — defined as two consecutive papilloma-free operative laryngoscopies — and 19 patients achieved a partial remission, defined as a 50% reduction in the lesion (composite) score.[21] At about the same time Benjamin reported that, in a 10-patient cross-over study using Wellferon, complete remission occurred in two of nine assessable patients and partial remission occurred in four.[3]

Sixty of the original 66 patients who entered the α-n–1 interferon cross-over study continued or restarted the agent after completion of the one-year trial; some patients used interferon continually for five years at dose rates of 2 mU daily or 4 mU three times per week. Late follow-up of these 60 patients reveals that there were 22 complete remissions with average duration greater than 550 days, and 15 patients remained in complete remission at the time of last analysis. There were 25 partial remissions with median duration of 400 days; seven patients remained in partial remission at the time of last analysis. Fourteen of 28 patients, who had tracheotomy[14] at the time of entry into the study, were safely decannulated. Sustained complete and partial remission occurred irrespective of papilloma severity, sex or age; two dose rates produced similar results. The presence of anti-interferon antibody did not appear to affect the degree or course of this response.[20]

Healy et al[11] evaluate human leukocyte (blood-bank) interferon efficacy in a multi-institutional study of 123 patients randomly assigned either to receive interferon, 2 mU/m² for seven days then 2 mU/m² three times weekly for one year, or not to receive interferon. The growth rate of papillomas in the interferon group was significantly lower than in the control group during the first six months, but the degree of difference diminished during the second six months and, despite continued interferon administration, was not significantly less at the end of a year. It was concluded that the interferon effect was not durable.

Zenner et al[38] administered α-2C interferon at a rate estimated to be 4.5 mU/m² daily for six weeks and three times per week thereafter; of 20 patients, 11 achieved complete remission and 7 achieved partial remission. The foregoing trials are in agreement that interferon can alter the clinical course of RRP. The comparative merits of each of several interferons is not established. These agents should be administered at an adequate dose and for a sufficient duration. The long-term toxicity of interferon, particularly following extended use, is uncertain.

On the basis of the above, our current management of RRP is as follows:

1. Microendoscopic excision at fixed intervals tailored to individualized need (2-, 4- or 6-monthly) with documentation of anatomic extent, nature and rate of papilloma regrowth. Surgical objectives are first: maximum preservation of laryngeal anatomy and function; second: airway preservation and restoration; third: voice; and fourth: achievement of a papilloma-free status.
2. Consider IFN adjuvant in patients with moderately severe disease (composite score 6 or above), and/or accelerated growth rate or expanding extent of papilloma.
3. Administer IFN dose of 2 mU/m² per day or 4 mU/m² every other day for 6 months. Discontinue IFN if no response; continue IFN for additional 6 months if partial response; continue IFN for 3 months after complete response.

CLINICAL COURSE AND PROGNOSIS

The natural history of respiratory papilloma varies from that of an isolated lesion, permanently eradicated after a single or limited number of endoscopic excisions, to those lesions demonstrating a pattern of progressive and widespread mucosal extension, with the development of multifocal disease sites and a requirement for a hundred or more endoscopic excisions. An undetermined proportion of cases may undergo spontaneous regression.

Multi-focal papillomata with widespread mucosal extension involving the larynx, tracheobronchial tree, lung, nose and nasopharynx are rarely encountered as an initial presentation. Tracheobronchial and pulmonary extension of a papilloma rarely occurs in the absence of a preceding tracheotomy.[37]

The question of spontaneous remission in respiratory papillomatosis is unanswered. In a review of 77 patients observed at the Mayo Clinic, Majoros et al[24] reported that 85% became 'free of disease' without specifying age at remission or duration of remission. Holinger,[12] and Bjork and Weber,[4] in separate clinical reviews, noted that patients with adult-onset recurrent respiratory papillomatosis were more likely to attain remission than were juvenile-onset patients. These reports support the view that most cases of RRP are self-limited and achieve clinical remission. Papilloma relapse during pregnancy may occur in a subset of patients who have been clinically disease-free for many years.

Dedo and Jackler[7] reported on 10 patients with normal and indirect laryngoscopic examination in whom papilloma was found at suspension microlaryngoscopy performed on the following day; their report attests that mirror laryngoscopy, even when performed by experts, may overlook small and isolated papilloma persistence. Steinberg et al[33] have demonstrated the presence of HPV-DNA in histologically normal laryngeal epithelial biopsies from papilloma patients with disease elsewhere in the respiratory tract. These observations lead to recognition that 'complete remission' from papillomatosis can be defined on clinical, histological or viral bases. An asymptomatic patient cannot be presumed to be in papilloma remission. The once widely held view that spontaneous remission of papilloma occurs at puberty is open to question inasmuch as JO-RRP recurrences into early and late adulthood are often encountered. Some patients, alleged to have achieved complete remission at puberty, have had papilloma recurrence as late as 30 and 40 years later.[22] Administration of exogenous hormones (testosterone and/or progesterone) have not altered the clinical course of papilloma recurrences.

A practical and reliable method of staging clinical severity of papilloma is required to assess the course of disease and the efficacy of alternative treatments. In the past, clinical assessment of disease severity has been based on either the frequency of operations, the interval between operations, or the total number of endoscopic excisions performed within a specified time. The criteria or indication for each operation have not been strictly defined, some operations are performed for the relief of hoarseness, others for the relief of airway impairment, and still others, for 'prophylaxis'. A numerically scored papilloma severity rating — based on the anatomical extent of disease, the nature of the individual growth (whether sessile or exophytic), and the degree of airway encroachment — was used in a multicentre clinical trial evaluating interferon efficacy. A composite score was derived to describe overall severity (1–6 mild, 7–12 moderate, 13 or more severe) and to monitor the trend of disease.[14]

The relationship of the severity of disease to HPV subtypes has been analysed; HPV 6C(11) was associated with cases having widespread mucosal disease,[27] and was also identified in squamous cell carcinomas arising from previously benign recurrent respiratory papilloma.[16] The influence of host immune factors in determining the severity of disease is not known.

REFERENCES

1. Abramson A L, Waner M, Brandsma J 1988 The clinical treatment of laryngeal papillomas with hematoporphyrin therapy. Arch Otolaryngol Head Neck Surg 114: 795–800
2. Bell R, Hong W K, Itri L M, McDonald G, Strong M S 1988 The use of cis-retinoic acid in recurrent respiratory papillomatosis of the larynx: a randomized pilot study. Am J Otolaryngol 9: 161–164
3. Benjamin B N, Gatenby P A, Kitchen R, Harrison H, Cameron K, Basten A 1988 Alpha-interferon (Wellferon) as an adjunct to standard surgical therapy in the management of recurrent respiratory papillomatosis. Ann Otol Rhinol Laryngol 97: 376–380
4. Bjork H, Weber C 1956 Papilloma of the larynx. Acta Otolaryngol 46: 499–516
5. Bomholt A 1988 Juvenile laryngeal papillomatosis. An epidemiological study from the Copenhagen Region. Acta Otolaryngol 105: 367–371
6. Cohen S R, Geller K A, Seltzer S, Thompson J W 1980 Papilloma of the larynx and tracheobronchial tree in children. Ann Otol Rhinol Laryngol 89: 497–503
7. Dedo H, Jackler R K 1982 Laryngeal papilloma: results of treatment with the CO_2 laser and podophyllum. Ann Otol Rhinol Laryngol 91: 425–430
8. Goepfert H, Sessions R B, Gutterman J U, Cangir A, Dichtel W J, Sulek M 1982 Leukocyte interferon in patients with juvenile laryngeal papillomatosis. Ann Otol Rhinol Laryngol 91: 431–436
9. Haglund S, Lundquist P-G, Cantell K, Strander H 1981 Interferon therapy in juvenile laryngeal papillomatosis. Arch Otolaryngol 107: 327–332
10. Hajek E F 1956 Contribution to the etiology of laryngeal papilloma in children. J Laryngol Otol 70: 166–168
11. Healy G B, Gelber R D, Trowbridge A L, et al 1988 Treatment of recurrent respiratory papillomatosis with human leukocyte interferon: results of a multi-center randomized clinical trial. N Engl J Med 319: 401–407
12. Holinger P 1950 Papilloma of the larynx: a review of 109 cases with a preliminary report of aureomycin therapy. Ann Otol Rhinol Laryngol 59: 547–564
13. Holinger P H 1968 Laryngeal papilloma, a review of etiology and therapy. Laryngoscope 78: 1462–1474
14. Kashima H, Leventhal B, Mounts P, and the Papilloma Study Group 1985 Scoring system to assess severity in recurrent respiratory papillomatosis. Papillomaviruses: molecular and clinical aspects. In: Howley P M, Broker T R (eds) UCLA symposia on molecular and cellular biology, new series, vol 32. Alan R Liss, New York, pp 125–136
15. Kashima H, Mounts P, Kuhajda F, Goodstein M, Leventhal B 1992 Sites of predilection in recurrent respiratory papillomatosis. Laryngoscope (in press)
16. Kashima H, Wu T C, Mounts P, Heffner D, Cachay A, Hyams V 1988 Carcinoma ex-papilloma: histologic and virologic studies in whole-organ sections of the larynx. Laryngoscope 98: 619–624
17. Kashima H K, Shah F, Lyles A, Glackin R, Muhammad N, Turner L, Van Zandt S, Whitt S, Shah K 1992 A comparison of risk factors in juvenile-onset and adult-onset recurrent respiratory papillomatosis. Laryngoscope 102: 9–13
18. Leventhal B G, Kashima H K 1985 Chemotherapy of papillomavirus infection. In: Howley P M, Broker T R (eds) UCLA symposia on molecular and cellular biology, new series. Alan R

Liss, New York, pp 235–247
19. Leventhal B G, Whisnant J, Kashima H K, Levy H, Biggers W P 1985 Recurrent respiratory papillomatosis. J Biol Response Mod 4: 525–530
20. Leventhal B G, Kashima H K, Mounts P, Thurmond L, Chapman S, Buckley S 1991 A long-term study of lymphoblastoid interferon in recurrent respiratory papillomatosis. N Engl J Med 325: 613–617
21. Leventhal B G, Kashima H K, Weck P W et al 1988 Randomized surgical adjuvant trial of interferon alpha-nl in recurrent papillomatosis. Arch Otolaryngol Head Neck Surg 114: 1163–1169
22. Linderg H, Elbrond O 1989 Laryngeal papilloma: clinical aspects in a series of 231 patients. Clin Otolaryngol 14: 333–342
23. Lippman S M, Garewal H S, Myeskens F L Jr 1989 Retinoids as potential chemopreventive agents in squamous cell carcinoma of the head and neck. Preventive Med 18: 740–748
24. Majoros M, Parkhill E, Devine K D Papilloma of the larynx in children. Am J Surg 108: 470–475
25. McCabe B F, Clark K F 1983 Interferon and papillomatosis. The Iowa experience. Ann Otol Rhinol Laryngol 92: 2–7
26. Mehta P, Heold N 1980 Regression of juvenile laryngobronchial papillomatosis with systemic bleomycin therapy. J Pediatr 97: 479–480
27. Mounts P, Kashima H K 1984 Association of human papillomavirus subtype and clinical course in respiratory papillomatosis. Laryngoscope 94: 28–44
28. Quick C A, Foucar E, Dehner L P 1979 Frequency and significance of epithelial atypia in laryngeal papillomatosis. Laryngoscope 89: 550–560
29. Quick C A, Kryzyzek R A, Watts S L, Foras A J 1980 Relationship between condylomata and laryngeal papilloma. Ann Otol Rhinol Laryngol 89: 467–471
30. Shah K, Kashima H K et al 1986 Rarity of caesarean delivery in cases of juvenile onset respiratory papillomatosis. Obstet Gynecol 68: 795–799
31. Smith H G, Healy G B, Vaughn C W, Strong M S 1985 Topical chemotherapy of recurrent respiratory papillomatosis. Laryngoscope 95: 900–904
32. Solomon D, Smith R, Kashima H 1985 Malignant transformation in non-irradiated recurrent respiratory papillomatosis: report of a case and review of the literature. Laryngoscope 95: 900–904
33. Steinberg B, Topp W C, Schneider P S, Abramson A L 1983 Laryngeal papillomavirus infection during clinical remission. New Engl J Med 388: 1261–1264
34. Strong M S et al 1979 Recurrent respiratory papillomatosis. In: Healy G B et al (eds) Laryngotracheal problems in the pediatric patient. Charles C. Thomas, Springfield
35. Ullman E V 1923 On the etiology of the laryngeal papilloma. Acta Otolaryngol 5: 317–334
36. Walsh T E, Beamer, P R 1950 Epidermoid carcinoma of the larynx occurring in two children with papilloma of the larynx. Laryngoscope 60: 1110–1124
37. Weiss M D, Kashima H K 1983 Tracheal involvement in laryngeal papillomatosis. Laryngoscope 93: 45–48
38. Zenner H P, Kley W, Claros P et al 1985 Recombinant interferon alpha-2c in laryngeal papillomatosis: preliminary results of a prospective multi-center trial. Oncology 42 (suppl 1): 15–18

9. Precursors of squamous cell carcinoma

I. Friedmann, A. Ferlito

A pessimistic pathologist is the best guarantee of surgical success (from 'Gallery of Mirrors' by J. R. Wilson)

INTRODUCTION

The squamous epithelium of the vocal cord is prone to undergo moderate to severe morphological changes, which may be difficult to interpret. Comparative studies have been hampered both by the inherent difficulties and also by the terminological inexactitudes. Gynaecological pathologists have paved the way to a better understanding of the problem of dysplasia and carcinoma in situ that figure prominently in the early diagnosis and treatment of squamous carcinoma.[12,15,32]

The term 'precancerous' was coined nearly a hundred years ago by Dubreuilh, cf. Grundmann.[33] The concept of 'pre-cancer' assumes that the development of invasive cancer is preceded by a slow process during which the normal epithelium passes through various stages of hyperplasia followed, perhaps after several years, by malignant change limited to the surface epithelium and lasting many years.[15]

The clinical terms 'keratosis', 'hyperkeratosis', 'leukoplakia' and 'pachydermia' have been applied to a form of hyperplasia of the laryngeal epithelium (Fig. 9.1). These conditions have their counterparts in the mucosa of the mouth and pharynx and of the vulva, vagina and cervix. In fact, such changes are common to all mucous membranes with epithelium that is normally of the non-keratinized, stratified squamous type. Although much effort has been expended in seeking to define the supposed differences between keratosis, hyperkeratosis, leukoplakia and pachydermia, it now seems apparent that they are merely variants of a single type of reactive keratotic change that the term 'keratosis' would most appropriately denote.

Clinicians generally use the term 'leukoplakia' to indicate any white plaque or patch, 'erythroplakia' for reddish patches of raised epithelium, and 'erythroleukoplakia' for mixed forms of white and red mucosal changes, but such clinical terms are descriptive and unsuitable as a diagnosis. 'Pachydermia' is another descriptive clinical term used to indicate large areas involved by leukoplakia, but there is naturally no place for it in the histological diagnosis.

The precursory lesions of squamous cell carcinoma of the larynx present a major challenge to pathologists and clinicians as assessment of dysplastic lesions of the vocal cord is a subjective approach.

The natural history of neoplastic development in experimental models, and presumably in humans too, may be separated into three distinct stages: initiation, promotion and progression.[49] The last is divided into two different substages: one including epithelial abnormalities potentially capable of progression into an invasive neoplasm (such as dysplasia and carcinoma in situ), the second being characterized by the development of an invasive cancer. Since most of the early neoplastic development occurs subclinically, accurate clinical diagnosis is fraught with difficulty, even with direct microscopic laryngoscopy. Accurate identification of epithelial abnormalities of the laryngeal mucosa requires biopsy and microscopic evaluation[22] (Fig. 9.2).

Some of the histopathological terms used include:
Squamous metaplasia. This denotes the replacement of respiratory epithelium by stratified squamous epithelium, a change common even in the subglottic region of the non-smoking, non-bronchitic urban adult[55] and human fetal larynx.[54] The process involves the superficial epithelium in particular but may affect the seromucous glands (Figs 9.3, 9.4). Squamous metaplasia is usually the result of persistent trauma or chronic irritation. Experimental studies have shown that it is capable of reverting to normal surface epithelium.
Squamous cell hyperplasia. This is a benign change in which the epithelium becomes thicker without cellular atypia. Such thickening is due to an increase in prickle cell and/or basal cell layers. Squamous cellular differentiation is well preserved and this epithelial anomaly is reversible. Squamous cellular hyperplasia is not a precancerous lesion.

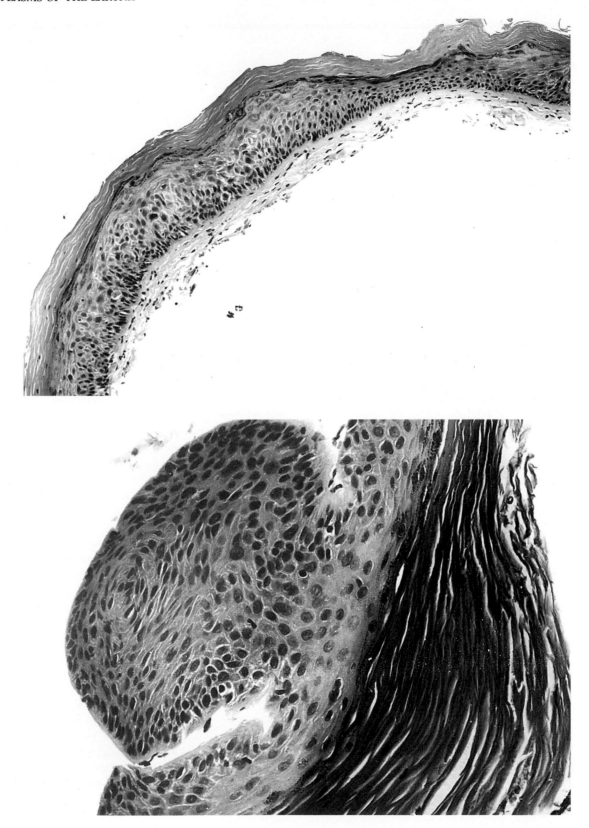

Fig. 9.1   Biopsy of the vocal cord showing keratotic squamous epithelium with some enlargement and irregularity of the nuclei and stratification of the surface layers bordering on LIN I. H&E, ×160.

Fig. 9.2   Hyperkeratotic squamous epithelium with an unusual, large cellular structure bulging through a wide gap of the basal lamina; probably an artefact in a biased section. H&E, ×400.

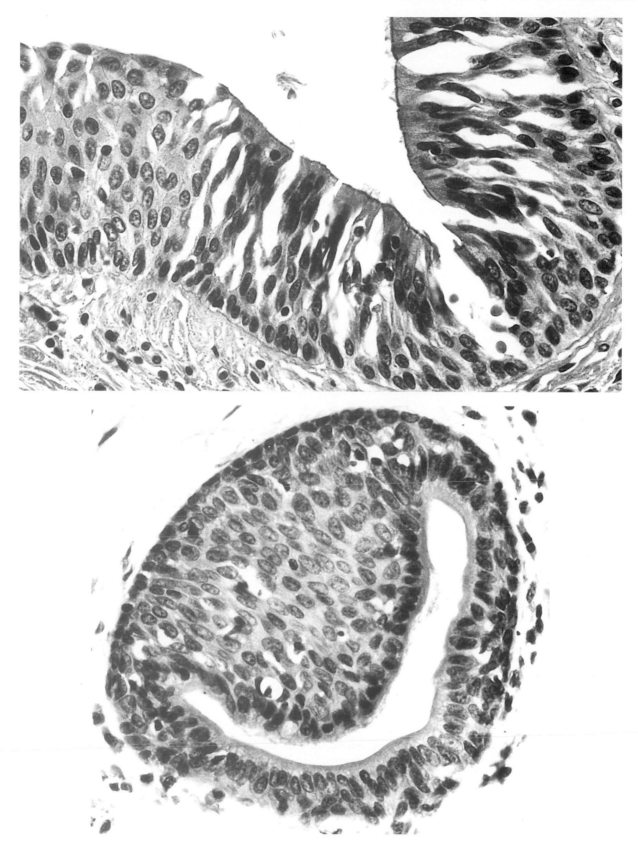

Fig. 9.3 (*top*) Vestibular fold mucosa. Note squamous metaplasia extending (on the left) and replacing the ciliated, respiratory-type epithelium (on the right). H&E, ×400.

Fig. 9.4 (*bottom*) Squamous metaplasia of a gland. H&E, ×400.

Pseudo-epitheliomatous hyperplasia. This lesion shows an irregular overgrowth of squamous epithelium with epithelial extension into the stroma. The hyperplastic epithelium may simulate well-differentiated squamous cell carcinoma, especially when it appears detached from the surface; however, the absence of atypical epithelial cells and the presence of an inflammatory infiltrate are helpful in arriving at the correct diagnosis. The pseudo-epitheliomatous reaction is a frequent feature of granular cell tumours, of various specific chronic inflammatory conditions (tuberculosis in particular), of mycotic diseases, of certain repair processes and of primary eosinophilic granuloma of the larynx.[25] There is no evidence that pseudo-epitheliomatous hyperplasia is a potentially malignant lesion, and treatment depends on the nature of the sub-epithelial disease.[22]

CLASSIFICATION AND HISTOLOGY

Although none of the classifications, whether on clinical or histological grounds, is entirely satisfactory or reliable, changes in the squamous epithelium of the larynx can be considered under these headings:

> Keratosis–Hyperplasia
> Dysplasia: low grade (LIN I)
> Dysplasia: moderate (LIN II)
> Dysplasia: high grade and carcinoma in situ (LIN III)
> Microinvasive carcinoma

In North America the classification proposed at the Centennial Conference on Laryngeal Cancer[45] is usually used: keratosis, keratosis with atypia, carcinoma in situ, carcinoma in situ with microinvasion. Others have based their classification on the degree of cellular atypia.

In Europe, a classification defined by Kleinsasser[43] has been widely applied, consisting of three classes: class I = simple squamous cell hyperplasia; class II = squamous cell hyperplasia with atypia; class III = carcinoma in situ. Although the classifications use a different terminology, they distinguish three categories which more or less coincide.

Keratosis

This is a pathological feature due to the production of keratin on the surface of the epithelium. Squamous differentiation is well preserved and a granular layer is often apparent. Keratinization without nuclei is called orthokeratosis; with retained nuclei it is called parakeratosis. Hyperplasia of the stratum spinosum or prickle cell layer (acanthosis) occurs with keratinization, and the proportions of acanthosis and keratinization can vary considerably. The basal membrane remains intact. Papillary keratosis of the larynx may be confused with verrucous carcinoma of the larynx.[6]

Dyskeratosis represents a faulty or premature keratinization of individual squamous cells (Fig. 9.5).

Crissman[16,17] uses the term 'keratosis' both because excess keratin formation is a common feature of the changes observed and because the term has historical precedent. This author recognizes three groups or grades, according to the severity of keratosis: grade I, mild keratosis characterized by hyperkeratosis, acanthosis, slight pseudo-epitheliomatous hyperplasia and no individual cell atypia; grade II, moderate keratosis characterized by grade I changes with parakeratosis with or without hyperkeratosis, pronounced pseudo-epitheliomatous hyperplasia and slight individual cell atypia; and grade III, severe keratosis characterized by grade I and grade II changes with marked dyskeratosis, keratin–pearl formation, numerous mitoses, prominent cellular atypia, loss of orderly epithelial maturation.

According to the classification of 'hyperplastic aberrations of the laryngeal mucosa' introduced by Kambic and Lenart in 1971[41] and reviewed in 1986,[42] the lesions are described as simple, abnormal and atypical hyperplasias and cancers (intraepithelial and invasive), and atypical hyperplasia is further characterized as 'risky epithelium'. The presence of dyskeratotic cells and the stromal reaction are considered significant features indicative of the malignant tendency of such a lesion.

The present authors agree that the degree of keratinization is of little or no assistance in determining the malignant change of a dysplastic lesion.[22,26–28] Kambic and Gale[42] found that the degree of keratinization differed little in these lesions whether they were described as 'hyperplasias' or as 'dysplasias'.

Mestwerdt's original definition of microinvasive cancer of the cervix was based on the depth of invasion.[44] It has since been recognized in various organs, including the larynx. The concept of microinvasive cancer and the correlation between the size of the tumour and the incidence of lymphatic spread and recurrence has been confirmed.[13]

Dysplasia: laryngeal intraepithelial neoplasia

We have benefited greatly from the extensive studies on the development of invasive squamous cell carcinoma in the uterine cervix. Lesions of the uterine cervix, traditionally categorized as dysplasia and carcinoma in situ have been encompassed in a single diagnostic category of intraepithelial neoplasia, e.g., cervical intraepithelial neoplasia: CIN of varying degrees. Although there is no agreement that the laryngeal carcinoma 'in situ' is biologically identical to the same lesion in the cervix, three similar grades of morphological (histological) abnormalities of the laryngeal mucosa have been recognized:

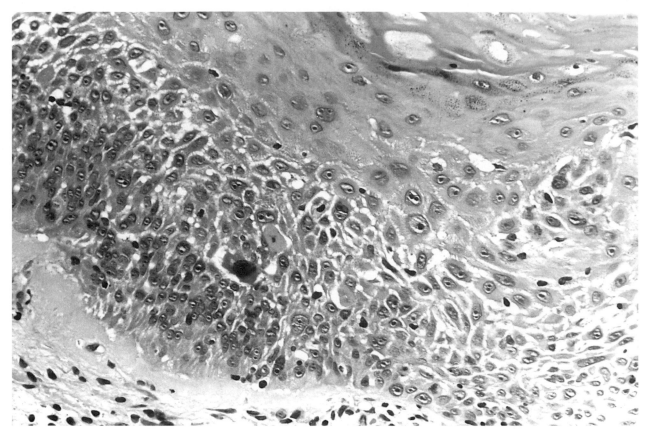

Fig. 9.5   There are scattered dyskeratotic cells in the hyperplastic and moderately dysplastic epithelium (LIN II) of the vocal cord. H&E, ×400.

laryngeal intraepithelial neoplasia grade I (LIN I) which morphologically corresponds to mild epithelial dysplasia; laryngeal intraepithelial neoplasia grade II (LIN II), morphologically equivalent to moderate epithelial dysplasia; laryngeal intraepithelial neoplasia grade III (LIN III), which includes both severe dysplasia and carcinoma 'in situ'.

Crissman and Zarbo[19] and Crissman et al[20] prefer the term 'squamous intraepithelial neoplasia' (SIN).

This classification is similar to the one proposed by Kleinsasser[43] in which severe dysplasia and carcinoma 'in situ' are also put together and form the stage III group. The time-honoured designation of dysplasia has been largely replaced by the term 'intraepithelial neoplasia' because the epithelial changes are considered to be a morphological manifestation of a neoplastic process.[19]

Histological appearances of LIN

The initial microscopical change is believed to be in the basal layer of the epithelium, and the neoplastic change gradually extends until it reaches the surface; as it extends towards the surface, it also spreads laterally in all directions within the epithelial layers. The lesion is always contained on its deep aspect by the basal lamina.

LIN I (mild dysplasia). The general tendency of the squamous epithelium to show stratification is preserved, and the superficial layers show cytoplasmic differentiation (maturation) with easily-seen intracellular bridges and keratinization (Figs 9.6, 9.7). The orientation of the cells in the lower layers is not maintained, and 'nuclear crowding' is conspicuous, with some pleomorphism and an increased nuclear–cytoplasmic ratio. Nucleoli are prominent, but mitotic figures are not common.

LIN II (moderate dysplasia). The histological changes are similar to those of grade I, but the undifferentiated (immature) cells extend to two-thirds of the thickness of the epithelium; differentiation and stratification are still seen in the superficial third of the epithelium. Mitotic figures are more numerous (Figs 9.8–9.12).

LIN III (severe dysplasia and carcinoma in situ). The non-stratified, undifferentiated cells occupy more than two-thirds of the epithelium up to its full thickness;

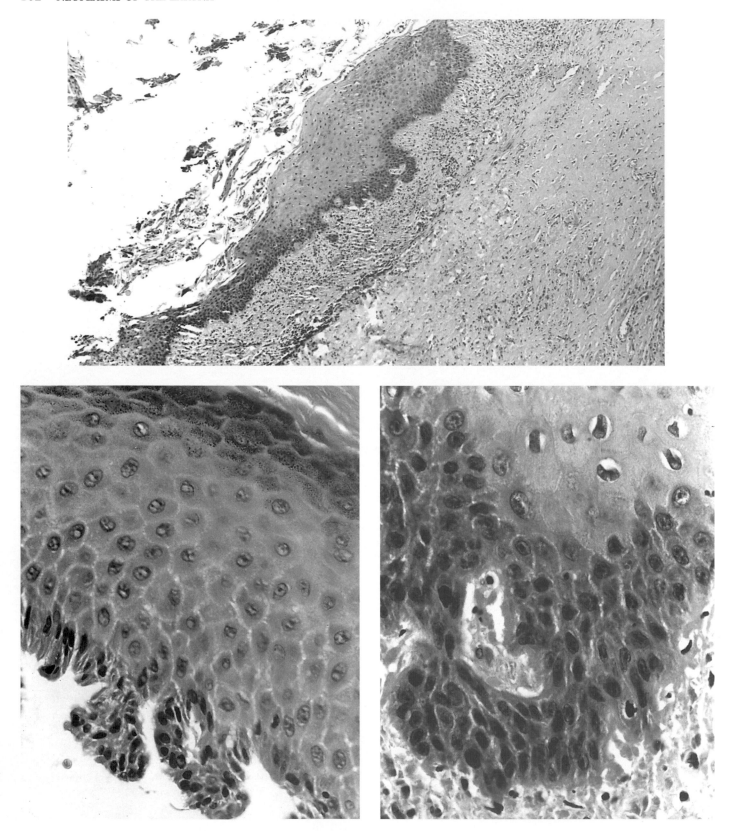

Fig. 9.6 A. (*top*) LIN I: vocal cord mucosa showing a plaque formed by hyperplastic squamous epithelium. H&E, ×160. B, C. (*bottom left, right*) Note darkly stained basal layer not extending into the prickle cell layers but showing some down-growth. H&E, ×400 and ×650.

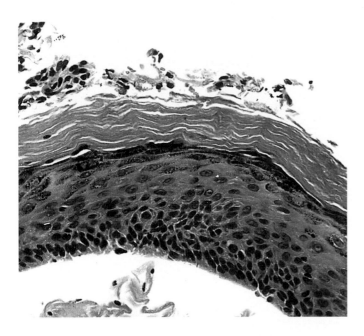

Fig. 9.7 LIN I: hyperkeratotic squamous epithelium from the vocal cord. There is marked enlargement and hyperchromasia of the nuclei crowding in the lower third of the epithelium. H&E, ×400.

this is usually accompanied by a more obvious degree of nuclear pleomorphism which may include the presence of bizarre large nuclei. Mitotic figures are seen with increasing frequency — and in all layers; not uncommonly they are of abnormal appearance. There is no keratinization in the great majority of cases, but occasionally a thin layer of keratin is seen at the surface with a complete lack of orientation of the cells below (Figs 9.13, 9.14).

The term 'carcinoma in situ' was introduced by Broders in 1932[11] who also described the first case in the larynx. It can be defined as a proliferative disorder of the epithelium displaying all the cytological and structural changes seen in overt malignant tumours but with no evidence of invasion below the basement membrane.

Carcinoma in situ may be formed by large cells with pale-staining nuclei or smaller darkly-stained cells.

Microinvasive carcinoma

This term is used to describe cases in which the neoplastic changes are confined to the basement membrane — apart from a few scattered tongues or small discrete foci of invasion. There is some controversy over the definition of the depth of invasion, in millimetres, for a cancer to be defined as microinvasive.

METHODS OF CELL CYCLE MEASUREMENT

There is a great deal of observer-difference because our approach is partly subjective and/or empirical. Self-limiting abnormalities may also be encountered in the larynx, caused by various injurious agents in common with cervical lesions where CIN I lesions can include certain self-limiting reactive or viral lesions requiring no further treatment. LIN I-type lesions of the vocal cord may be as 'overdiagnosed' as CIN I.[1,36–38] Mild intra-epithelial hyperplasia has to be distinguished from LIN I, but this can be difficult.

In a wide-ranging review, Quinn and Wright[50] have discussed the various methods which have been employed in measuring the different phases of the cell cycle and their value and/or reliability in assessing the cell's biological behaviour, ceteris paribus of a neoplasm.

The *mitotic count* is a widely used method, defined as the number of mitoses per 10 high-power fields. This may be modified to appear more accurate, as recommended by Collan and Haapasalo.[14]

Quinn and Wright[51] have pointed to various weaknesses in the mitotic count and have advocated the use of the *mitotic index*. This is based on the number of mitoses as a fraction of the interphase nuclear population.

Mitotic counts, however careful and systematic, are considered unreliable,[50,51] though they are defended by some as a helpful method.[14]

The mitotic index is preferable but it is a more laborious, painstaking and time-consuming method, difficult to adapt to prevailing laboratory conditions.

Other methods include measuring the 'labelling index' by thymidine labelling, which measures the percentage of neoplastic cells in the DNA synthetic (S) phase of the cell cycle, or by incorporating bromodeoxyuridine, which has been used in the development of the CHART method of radiotherapy.[21,53,60]

Some markers of cell activation can also be detected by nucleolar organizer regions (AgNOR), which are loops of DNA transcribing ribosomal DNA.[2] Sampling is a major handicap of this method.

Flow cytometry has been gaining in importance as an automated technique which analyses the DNA content of the cell and the cell cycle distribution. It is rapid, accurate and reproducible and can be applied on fresh, frozen and paraffin-embedded tissue.

Flow cytometry offers the best objective test method. AgNOR methods have been tested, but without convincing results.

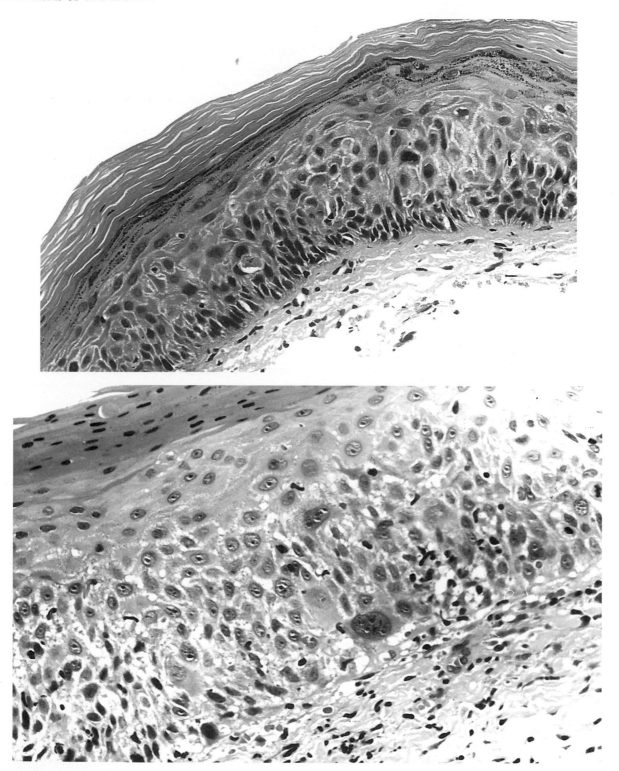

Fig. 9.8 (*top*) Same case as in Fig. 9.7. LIN II: another part of the vocal cord mucosa showing loss of polarity and marked irregularity of nuclear shape and size. There is stratification of the upper layers and a great deal of keratinization present. H&E, ×400.

Fig. 9.9 (*bottom*) LIN II: vocal cord epithelium showing good maturation; there is stratification of the surface layers showing parakeratosis. Note enlarged hyperchromatic nuclei coupled with some pleomorphism in different areas of the epithelium. There is considerable reaction in the stroma. H&E, ×400.

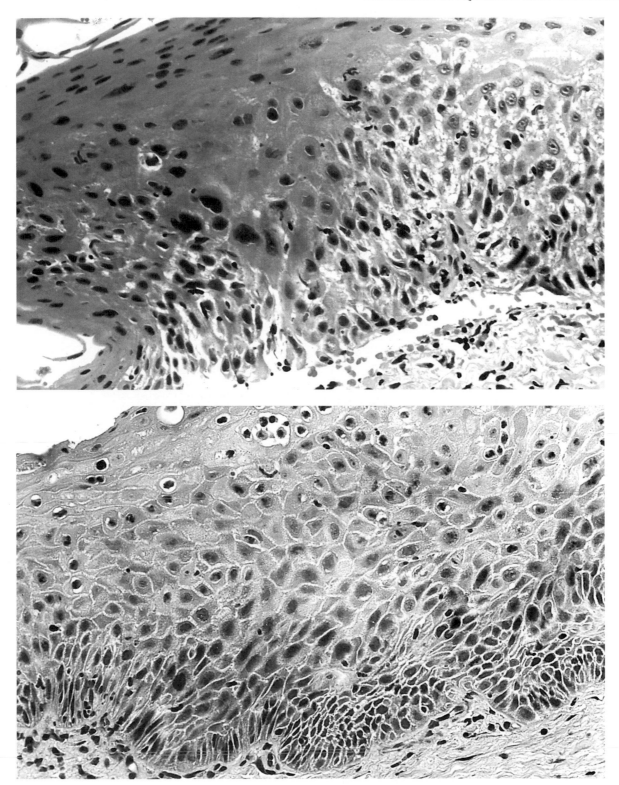

Fig. 9.10 (*top*) Same case as in Fig. 9.9. Showing a wedge-shaped area of the squamous epithelium with a cluster of enlarged hyperchromatic nuclei of irregular size and shape. No mitotic activity is apparent. The epithelium is oedematous and is infiltrated by inflammatory cells. H&E, ×400.

Fig. 9.11 (*bottom*) Repeat biopsy (about a month later) from the patient in Figs 9.9 and 9.10 showing moderately acanthotic epithelium with mild nuclear hyperchromasia. Note regularity of the prickle cell layers. There are many inflammatory cells present within the surface layer of the epithelium but there is no evidence of neoplasia. H&E, ×400.

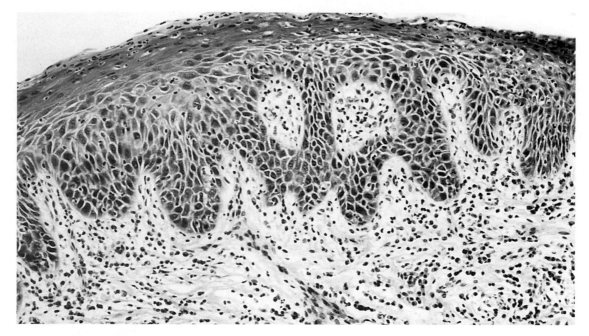

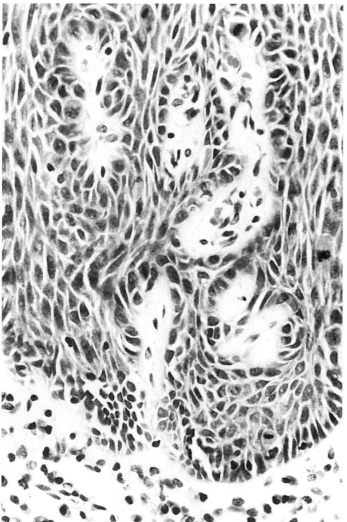

Fig. 9.12 A. (*top*) LIN II bordering on LIN III. There are crowded hyperchromatic nuclei throughout the epithelium, with marked irregularity of nuclear size and shape. There is some stratification towards the epithelial surface. H&E, ×180. B. (*bottom*) Occasional mitoses are seen. H&E, ×400.

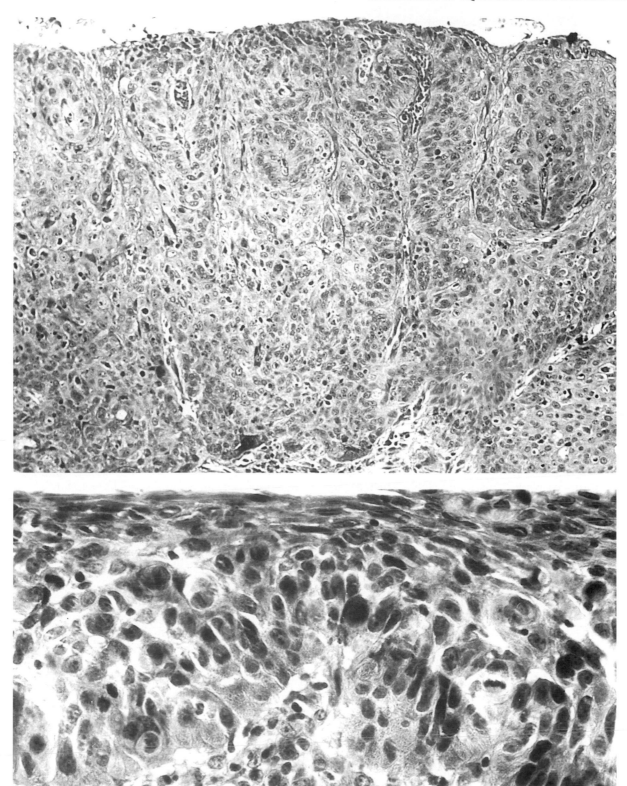

Fig. 9.13 (*top*) LIN III (carcinoma in situ). Thickened squamous epithelium showing complete loss of polarity of the cellular arrangement. Stratification is absent. There are many large darkly-stained irregular nuclei near the base and scattered in the epithelium. The basal lamina appears to be intact. H&E, ×160.

Fig. 9.14 (*bottom*) LIN III (carcinoma in situ). The epithelial surface appears to be thin but there are broad epithelial masses pushing downwards. Nuclear enlargement and hyperchromasia are noticeable and there are mitoses in the basal layer. H&E, ×400.

NEW OBJECTIVE METHODS OF GRADING

Photometry (morphometry)

Ferlito et at[23] suggested that the photometric determination of nuclear DNA content was of diagnostic assistance; DNA values above the diploid level (4n–8n) indicated malignancy, even of cells which appeared histologically benign.

Several authors[7,9,18,34,40] have found photometry of value in the assessment of nuclear atypia, sometimes masked, as in well-differentiated lesions. Increased nuclear DNA content was accompanied by the development of invasive carcinoma and a high rate of recurrence.

Morphometry was used by Kalter et al[40] in order to achieve a more objective and reproducible classification of the laryngeal lesion, especially hyperplasia with atypia (class II) and carcinoma in situ (class III) — according to Kleinsasser's classification.[43] Quantitative morphometry may be helpful in the histopathological classification of dysplastic squamous cell lesions of the laryngeal mucosa.[40]

DNA histograms

Crissman and Fu[18] have studied six patients with extensive intraepithelial alterations of the laryngeal mucosa. The nuclear DNA content was measured and DNA histograms were generated from multiple mucosal sites on Feulgen-stained sections by means of spectrophotometric microscopy. Aneuploid DNA histograms were noted in all six cases, indicative of neoplastic transformation.

Microscopically there was epithelial hyperplasia, surface keratinization and also proliferation of small, immature cells resembling basal cells in the deepest parts of the epithelium and signs of abnormal epithelial maturation presenting as 'focal areas of cytoplasmic keratinization in the lower portions of the mucosa'.[18] The DNA contents in 56 laryngeal glottic biopsy specimens with a spectrum of squamous intraepithelial neoplastic changes (SIN) were recently evaluated by image analysis.[19] Aneuploidy was observed in all SIN II and SIN III graded biopsy specimens with prominent keratinization. This, it is suggested, is a more common presentation of intraepithelial neoplasia in the laryngeal mucosa than in the 'classical' type of carcinoma in situ where the squamous epithelium is completely replaced by immature proliferating basal-like cells. The presence of keratin is irrelevant and does not affect the diagnosis of intraepithelial neoplasia LIN.

Bocking et al[9] have studied the DNA distribution pattern in squamous epithelial lesions of the larynx. The Feulgen DNA content was determined in at least 100 individual cells from dysplastic lesions. Normal euploid and atypical DNA patterns have been encountered. Cells displaying an atypical DNA distribution pattern are believed to have undergone malignant transformation. It is concluded that atypical DNA distribution recognizes malignant transformation earlier than morphological criteria.

Franzen et al[29] have examined 33 small glottic carcinomas (T1 and small T2) by malignancy grading using the 8-factor system proposed by Jakobsson et al[39] and the 4-factor system by Glanz and Eichhorn[31] together with DNA measurement. There was no significant difference in malignancy score or DNA values between tumours that recurred after a full course of radiotherapy and those that did not. These investigations indicate that neither malignancy grading nor DNA measurements can predict the clinical course in small glottic carcinomas. A recent meta-analysis on ploidy research shows that the outcome of laryngeal cancer is unaffected by ploidy.[56]

Bobrow et al[8] described a change in the expression of low-molecular-weight cytokeratin associated with the development of in situ and invasive neoplasms of the cervix as studied by means of immunohistochemical staining using monoclonal antibodies NCL-5DE, CAM 5.2 and PKK1 by Angus et al.[4] Positive staining with these monoclonal antibodies may indicate that a neoplastic lesion belongs to a CIN III type of dysplasia and that the LMW-CK positive cases (low-molecular-weight cytokeratins) would most likely progress to invasive neoplasms.[4] This may not apply to LIN III and squamous cell carcinoma of the larynx.[18]

Radio-labelled antigens

The detection of squamous cell tumours of the head and neck using radio-labelled antibodies might prove of some clinical value.[58]

HPV in precancerous lesions

Sterret et al[57] confirmed that a strong association exists between HPV infections and precancerous lesions of the uterine cervix. Their results obtained by HPV-PAP staining showed that koilocytosis was a reliable histological indicator of HPV infection of the cervix. Changes attributable to the effect of HPV occur in various grades of dysplasia, more often in lower grades.

Human papilloma virus (HPV) infection is an aetiological factor in laryngeal papilloma, and recent evidence implicates HPV in squamous neoplasms.[47] The presence of sequences related to human papilloma virus type 16 has been reported in verrucous carcinoma of the larynx.[10]

In cervical condylomas studied by in situ hybridization, nuclear atypia was found to be a sign of infection by the human papilloma viruses.[46]

Human papilloma virus types 6 and 11 were recently detected in laryngeal papilloma.[59]

DISCUSSION

In postmortem material, carcinoma in situ was found to be present in the mucosa of vocal cords in 11.4% and in the mucosa of the vestibular folds in 4.9% of the larynges examined.[5]

Published reports of cases of carcinoma in situ indicate that there are considerable discrepancies regarding its incidence.[24] In a series of 193 patients with epithelial abnormalities (hyperplasia, keratosis, dysplasia and carcinoma in situ), seen during a period of 14 years, 39 had severe dysplasia or carcinoma in situ.[35] The rates range from nil to 15% of the total number of carcinomas of the larynx collected from the literature. Two possible factors explain the discrepancies: (i) carcinoma in situ may accompany an undiagnosed invasive lesion; and (ii) carcinoma in situ may be incorrectly diagnosed by pathologists. This may be due largely to the necessarily subjective application of such criteria (known to vary even when one pathologist assesses the same case on different occasions) and to the inability of morphological features to indicate when — or even whether — the lesion will invade. In addition, the often reported observation that many invasive tumours do not pass the stage of carcinoma 'in situ', and are invasive from the start (see diagram) gives rise to questions as to the validity of this concept.[26]

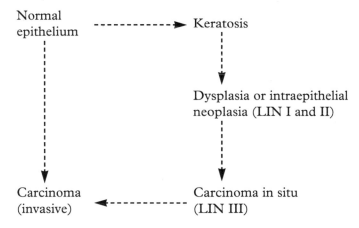

The association of carcinoma in situ and invasive cancer of the larynx is much closer than it is in the skin, cornea, or conjunctiva, and the process carries a greater threat to life.[3]

It could be argued that the relatively minor histological abnormality — under both the light- and electron-microscope — associated with grade I intraepithelial neoplasia does not warrant the 'alarming' connotation of potential malignancy which may lead to excessive treatment. These objections cannot be seriously entertained. This system of nomenclature encourages the pathologist to be precise and unequivocally to separate unrelated (reactive) changes (such as basal cell hyperplasia or simple keratinization of the epithelium) from truly neo-plastic lesions; it also spares the pathologist the sometimes impossible and always fruitless task of differentiating between severe dysplasia and carcinoma in situ.

The implications of such an approach are significant; the changes of laryngeal intraepithelial neoplasia are considered to be a morphological manifestation of a neoplastic process, not a precancerous lesion. Laryngeal intraepithelial neoplasia presents a continuous spectrum of histological abnormalities.

The above observations lead to a number of important considerations: (i) finding the abnormal morphological features of the laryngeal epithelium classified here as intraepithelial neoplasia (keratosis with atypia, epithelial dysplasia, carcinoma in situ) should alert the clinician to search for an invasive lesion nearby; (ii) this should be treated initially by local excision; and (iii) there should be a long-term follow-up, and recurrences should be dealt with appropriately to minimize the chances of invasion.

Carcinoma in situ may arise in any part of the larynx as a separate entity, but it is more common in the vocal cords — especially their anterior part. It is doubtful whether the lesion always starts in areas normally covered by stratified squamous epithelium; when the condition develops in areas ordinarily covered by transitional epithelium or by pseudostratified columnar epithelium of the respiratory-tract type, it seems likely that metaplasia to squamous epithelium has preceded the neoplastic change.

Carcinoma in situ may be multicentric in origin. If specimens are examined thoroughly, appearances typical of the condition are often found in isolated fields of otherwise apparently normal epithelium, or in a number of separate glands or their ducts. Examination of serial sections confirms that these lesions may be completely isolated from one another by areas of apparently healthy epithelium. The extent of the disease may range from small foci of microscopic size, some or all of which may eventually fuse, to involvement of almost the whole mucosa of the larynx.

Carcinoma in situ is often present in the neighbourhood of an invasive tumour. This has to be taken into account when correlating the clinical and microscopic findings. Many difficulties stand in the way of the correct microscopical diagnosis of the lesion which cannot always be arrived at on the basis of a single biopsy. Repeated and even multiple biopsies may be required, and ancillary diagnostic procedures have to be employed. Since all classifications are essentially subjective in nature, new objective methods of grading have been employed with more or less success or reliability.

In a survey of 52 international otolaryngologists, Ferlito et al[24] noted a great variety in the choice of primary therapy for laryngeal intraepithelial carcinoma in situ. Excisional biopsy (i.e., the removal of the entire lesion together with a rim of healthy tissue) is adequate for both the diagnosis and the treatment of this lesion; if the margins are not clear, re-excision or radiotherapy remain alternative options[30] together with the elimination of all potential carcinogenic factors (e.g., smoking, alcohol, occupational factors). Retinoid administration may be useful. Radiotherapy has a definite but secondary role in the treatment of all LIN cases. Frequent follow-up investigation is essential, to the degree that Rothfield et al[52] propose that the technique of tissue removal is not the critical determinant of successful outcome, but rather that compulsive follow-up is most important to the ultimate success of treatment.

The difficulties with regard to the diagnosis and terminology of carcinoma 'in situ' of the larynx make assessment of its behaviour and prognosis uncertain. Park[48] rightly warns that the assessment and treatment of lesions in the larynx that may or may not be carcinoma in situ have implications much graver than in the case of comparable lesions elsewhere. In the series reported by Hellquist et al,[35] 9 out of 39 (23%) patients in their group III (severe dysplasia or carcinoma in situ) developed invasive carcinoma.

Cancer of the larynx may be a disease of extremely long duration extending over perhaps as much as 15 to 20 years, if one includes both the pre-invasive and the invasive stages of the disease. That most laryngeal cancers begin in a pre-invasive fashion seems likely; that carcinoma in situ is not inevitably followed by invasive cancer seems just as likely. A study of 942 larynges at postmortem examination showed cells with atypical nuclei somewhere within the larynx in 84% of cases.[5] With a frequency of epithelial atypia as high as this in a population effectively healthy, as far as the larynx is concerned, the histologist should be wary of overdiagnosis with biopsies from patients whose larynx is not healthy or at least has demanded biopsy.[48] While there is general agreement that morphological assessment is fairly reliable, continued attempts are being made to develop quantitative methods derived from growth-kinetic and histometric measurements.[34]

REFERENCES

1. Al-Nafussi A I, Colquhoun M K 1990 Mild cervical intraepithelial neoplasia (CIN 1): a histological overdiagnosis. Histopathology 17: 557–561
2. Alperts B, Bray D, Lewis J, Raff M, Roberts K, Watson J D 1983 Molecular biology of the cell. Garland, New York
3. Altmann F, Ginsberg I, Stout A P 1952 Intraepithelial carcinoma (cancer in situ) of the larynx. Arch Otolaryngol 56: 121–123
4. Angus B, Kiberu S, Purvis J, Wilkinson L, Horne C H W 1988 Cytokeratins in cervical dysplasia and neoplasia: a comparative study of immunohistochemical staining using monoclonal antibodies NCL-5DE, CAM 5.2, and PKKL. J Pathol 155: 71–75
5. Auerbach O, Hammond E C, Garfinkel L 1970 Histological changes in the larynx in relation to smoking habits. Cancer 25: 92–104
6. Barnes L, Peel R L 1990 Head and neck pathology. A text/atlas of differential diagnosis. Igaku-Shoin, New York
7. Bjelkenkrantz K, Lundgren J, Olofsson J 1983 Single-cell DNA measurements in hyperplastic, dysplastic and carcinomatous laryngeal epithelia, with special reference to the occurrence of the hypertetraploid cell nuclei. Anal Quant Cytol 5: 184–188
8. Bobrow L G, Makin C A, Law S, Bodmer W F 1986 Expression of low molecular weight cytokeratin proteins in cervical neoplasia. J Pathol 148: 135–140
9. Bocking A, Auffermann W, Vogel H, Schlondorff G, Goebbels R 1985 Diagnosis and grading of malignancy in squamous epithelial lesions of the larynx with DNA cytophotometry. Cancer 56: 1600–1604
10. Brandsma J L, Steinberg B M, Abramson A L, Winkler B 1986 Presence of human papillomavirus type 16 related sequences in verrucous carcinoma of the larynx. Cancer Res 46: 2185–2188
11. Broders A C 1932 Carcinoma in situ contrasted with benign penetrating epithelium. JAMA 99: 1670–1674
12. Buckley C H, Butler E G, Fox H 1982 Cervical intraepithelial neoplasia. J Clin Pathol 35: 1–13
13. Burghardt E, Girardi F, Lahousen M, Pickel H, Tamussino K 1991 Microinvasive carcinoma of the uterine cervix (International Federation of Gynecology and Obstetrics Stage IA). Cancer 67:1037–1045
14. Collan Y, Haapasalo H 1991 Letter to the editor: The value of mitotic counting in the assessment of prognosis and proliferation in human tumours. J Pathol 163: 361–364
15. Coppleson M, Reid B 1967 Preclinical carcinoma of the cervical uterus. Pergamon, Oxford
16. Crissman J D 1979 Laryngeal keratosis and subsequent carcinoma. Head Neck Surg 1: 386–391
17. Crissman J D 1982 Laryngeal keratosis preceding laryngeal carcinoma. A report of four cases. Arch Otolaryngol 108: 445–448
18. Crissman J D, Fu Y S 1986 Intraepithelial neoplasia of the larynx: a clinicopathologic study of six cases with DNA analysis. Arch Otolaryngol Head Neck Surg 112: 522–528
19. Crissman J D, Zarbo R J 1991 Quantitation of DNA ploidy in squamous intraepithelial neoplasia of the laryngeal glottis. Arch Otolaryngol Head Neck Surg 117: 182–188
20. Crissman J D, Zarbo R J, Drozdowicz S, Jacobs J, Ahmad K, Weaver A 1988 Carcinoma in situ and microinvasive squamous carcinoma of the laryngeal glottis. Arch Otolaryngol Head Neck Surg 114: 299–307
21. Dische S, Saunders M I 1990 The rationale for continuous, hyperfractionated, accelerated radiotherapy (CHART). Int J Radiat Oncol Biol Phys 19: 1317–1320
22. Ferlito A 1990 Precancerous lesions in the larynx: diagnostic and therapeutic problems. XIV World Congr Otorhinolaryngol Head Neck Surg, Kugler & Ghedini, Amsterdam
23. Ferlito A, Antonutto G, Silvestri F 1976 Histological appearances and nuclear DNA content of verrucous squamous cell carcinoma of the larynx. ORL 38: 65–85
24. Ferlito A, Polidoro F, Rossi M 1981 Pathological basis and clinical aspects of treatment policy in carcinoma in situ of the larynx. J Laryngol Otol 95: 141–154
25. Friedmann I, Ferlito A 1981 Primary eosinophilic granuloma of the larynx. J Laryngol Otol 95: 1249–1254
26. Friedmann I, Ferlito A 1988 Granulomas and neoplasms of the larynx. Churchill Livingstone, Edinburgh
27. Friedmann I, Osborn D A 1976 The larynx. In: Symmers W St C (ed) Systemic pathology, 2nd edn, vol 1. Churchill Livingstone, Edinburgh
28. Friedmann I, Piris J 1986 Nose, throat and ears. In: Symmers W St C (ed) Systemic pathology, 3rd edn, vol 1. Churchill Livingstone, Edinburgh
29. Franzen G, Olofsson J, Klintenberg C, Brunk U 1987 Prognostic value of malignancy grading and DNA measurements in small glottic carcinomas. ORL J Otorhinolaryngol Relat Spec 49: 73–80

30. Gillis T M, Incze J, Strong S M, Vaughan C W, Simpson G T 1983 Natural history and management of keratosis, atypia, carcinoma in situ, and microinvasive cancer of the larynx. Am J Surg 146: 512–516

31. Glanz H, Eichhorn Th 1985 Die prognostische Bedeutung des histologischen 'Grading' von Stimmlippenkarzinomen. HNO 33: 103–111

32. Govan ADT, Haines R M, Langley F A, Taylor C W, Woodcock A S 1969 The histology and cytology of changes in the epithelium of the cervix uteri. J Clin Pathol 22: 283–395

33. Grundmann E 1983 Classification and clinical consequences of precancerous lesions in the digestive and respiratory tracts. Acta Pathol Jpn 33: 195–217

34. Hellquist H, Olofsson J, Gróntoft O 1981 Carcinoma in situ and severe dysplasia of the vocal cords. A clinicopathological and photometric investigation. Acta Otolaryngol 92: 543–555

35. Hellquist H, Lundgren J, Oloffson J 1982 Hyperplasia, keratosis, dysplasia and carcinoma in situ of the vocal cords — a follow-up study. Clin Otolaryngol 7: 11–27

36. Ismail S M 1991 Intra-epithelial lesions of the uterine cervix (letter). Histopathology 18: 285–288

37. Ismail S M, Colclough A B, Dinnen J S, Eakins D, Evans D M D, Gradwell E, O'Sullivan J P, Summerell J M, Newcombe R G 1989 Observer variation in histopathological diagnosis and grading of cervical intraepithelial neoplasia. Br Med J 298: 707–710

38. Ismail S M, Colclough A B, Dinnen J S, Eakins D, Evans D M D, Gradwell E, O'Sullivan J P, Summerell J M, Newcombe R 1990 Reporting cervical intra-epithelial neoplasia (CIN): intra- and interpathologist variation and factors associated with disagreement. Histopathology 16: 371–376

39. Jacobsson P A, Eneroth C M, Killander D, Moberger G, Martesson B 1973 Histologic classification and grading of malignancy in carcinoma of the larynx. Acta Radiol Ther Phys Biol 12: 1–8

40. Kalter P O, Lubsen H, Delemarre J F M, Alons C L, Veldhuizen R W, Meyer C J L M, Snow G B 1985 Quantitative morphometry of squamous cell hyperplasia of the larynx. J Clin Pathol 38: 489–495

41. Kambic V, Lenart I 1971 Notre classification des hyperplasies de l'épithélium du larynx au point de vue pronostic. J Fr Otorhinolaryngol 20: 1145–1150

42. Kambic V, Gale N 1986 Significance of keratosis and dyskeratosis for classifying hyperplastic aberrations of laryngeal mucosa. Am J Otolaryngol 7: 323–333

43. Kleinsasser O 1963 Die Klassifikation und Differentialdiagnose der Epithelhyperplasien der Kehlkopfschleimhaut auf Grund histomorphologischer Merkmale. Z Laryngol Rhinol 42: 339–362

44. Mestwerdt G 1947 Die Frühdiagnose des Kollumkarzinoms. Zentralbl Gynakol 69: 198–202

45. Miller A H 1974 Premalignant laryngeal lesions, carcinoma in situ, superficial carcinoma-definition and management. Can J Otolaryngol 3: 573–575

46. Mittal K R, Chan W, Demopoulus R I 1990 Sensitivity and specificity of various morphological features of cervical condylomas. In situ hybridization study. Arch Pathol Lab Med 114: 1038–1042

47. Mounts P, Shah K V, Kashima H 1982 Viral etiology of juvenile-onset and adult-onset squamous papilloma of the larynx. Proc Natl Acad Sci USA 79: 5425–5429

48. Park W W 1980 The histology of borderline cancer, with notes on prognosis. Springer, Berlin

49. Pitot N C 1982 The natural history of neoplastic development: the relation of experimental models to human cancer. Cancer 49: 1206–1211

50. Quinn C M, Wright N A 1990 The clinical assessment of proliferation and growth in human tumours: evaluation of methods and applications as prognostic variables. J Pathol 160: 93–102

51. Quinn C M, Wright N A 1991 Author's reply. J Pathol 163: 362–364

52. Rothfield R E, Myers E N, Johnson J T 1991 Carcinoma in situ and microinvasive squamous cell carcinoma of the vocal cords. Ann Otol Rhinol Laryngol 100: 793–796

53. Saunders M I, Dische S, Hong A, Grosch E J, Fermont D C, Ashford R F U, Maher E J 1989 Continuous hyperfractionated accelerated radiotherapy in locally advanced carcinoma of the head and neck region. Int J Radiat Oncol Biol Phys 17: 1287–1293

54. Stafford N D, Davies S J 1988 Epithelial distribution in the human fetal larynx. Ann Otol Rhinol Laryngol 97: 382–387

55. Stell P M 1991 Ploidy in head and neck cancer: a review and meta-analysis. Clin Otolaryngol 16: 510–516

56. Stell P M, Gregory I, Watt J 1980 Morphology of the human larynx. II: the subglottis. Clin Otolaryngol 5: 389–395

57. Sterret G F, Alessandri L M, Pixley E, Kulski J K 1987 Assessment of precancerous lesions of the uterine cervix for evidence of human papillomavirus infection: a histological and immunohistochemical study. Pathology 19: 84–90

58. Tranter R M D, Fairweather D S, Bradwell A R, Dykes P W, Watson-James S, Chandler S 1984 The detection of squamous cell tumours of the head and neck using radio-labelled antibodies. J Laryngol Otol 98: 71–74

59. Watanabe S, Natito Y, Kawakami T, Fukushima K, Masuda Y, Saito R, Ogura H, Fujiwara T, Yabe Y 1990 Human papillomavirus type 6 and 11 in laryngeal papillomas. Larynx Jpn 2: 165–170

60. Wilson G D, McNally N J, Dische S, Saunders M I, Des Rochers C, Lewis A A 1988 Measurement of cell kinetics in human tumours in vivo using bromodeoxyuridine incorporation and flow cytometry. Brit J Cancer 58: 423–431

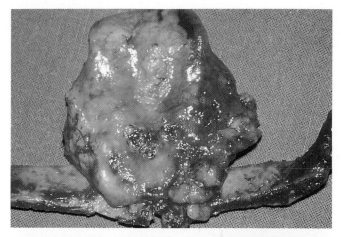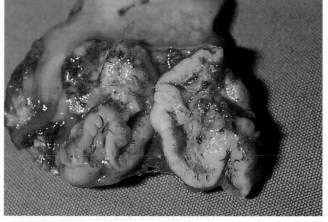

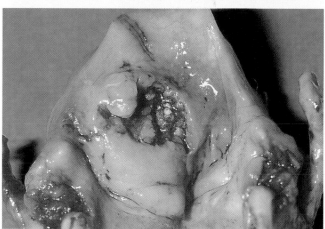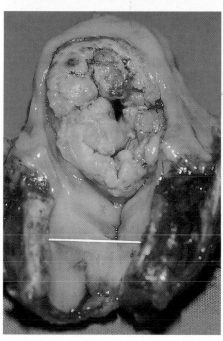

Plate 1 (*top, left*) Typical example of invasive squamous cell carcinoma at the base of the epiglottis.

Plate 2 (*top, right*) Supraglottic carcinoma of exophytic type.

Plate 3 (*bottom, left*) Exophytic carcinoma involving the base of the epiglottis.

Plate 4 (*bottom, right*) Extensive supraglottic carcinoma of ulcero-fungating type.

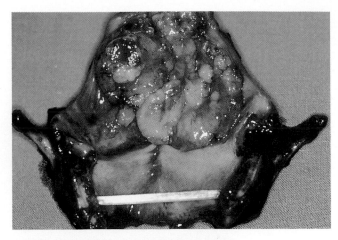

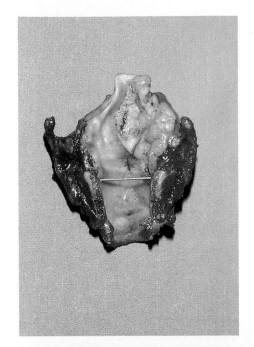

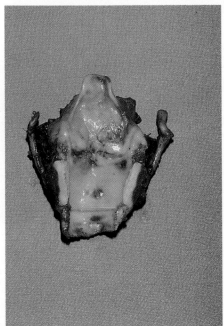

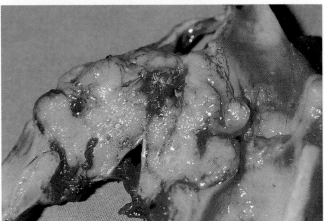

Plate 5 (*top, left*) Extensive supraglottic carcinoma of ulcero-fungating type, apparently originating in the angle between the vestibular fold and epiglottis.

Plate 6 (*top, right*) Exophytic supraglottic carcinoma spreading laterally over the edge of the epiglottis.

Plate 7 (*bottom, left*) Invasive carcinoma of the larynx.

Plate 8 (*bottom, right*) Sagittal section of Plate 7 showing massive invasion of the supraglottic, glottic and subglottic regions.

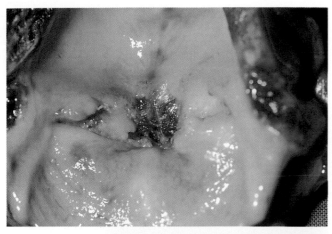

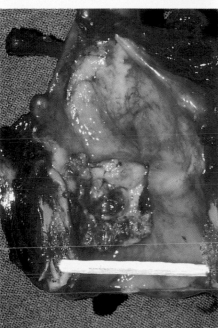

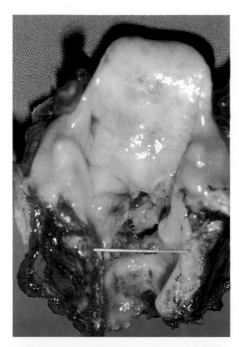

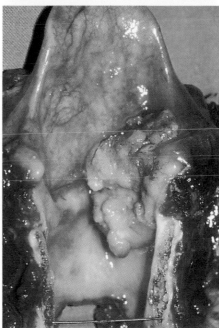

Plate 9 (*top, left*) Anterior transglottic carcinoma invading the adjacent thyroid cartilage.

Plate 10 (*top, right*) Glottic lesion extending subglottically.

Plate 11 (*bottom, left*) Glottic carcinoma with subglottic extension.

Plate 12 (*bottom, right*) Transglottic carcinoma involving the right vocal cord. It crossed the ventricle into the supraglottic region.

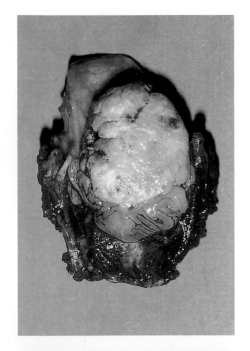

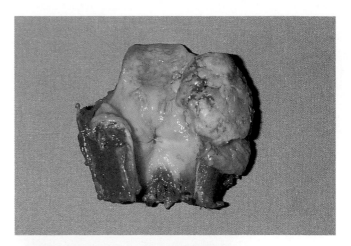

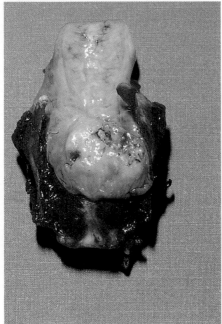

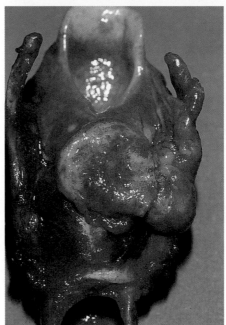

Plate 13 (*top, left*) Laryngectomy specimen showing a large tumour involving the post-cricoid region, pyriform sinus and aryepiglottic fold.

Plate 14 (*top, right*) Same case as in Plate 13. The gross specimen was opened posteriorly showing that the tumour involved the aryepiglottic fold.

Plate 15 (*bottom, left*) Very large exophytic carcinoma in the post-cricoid region.

Plate 16 (*bottom, right*) Extensive carcinoma involving the post-cricoid region and the right pyriform sinus.

10. Squamous cell carcinoma

A. Ferlito, I. Friedmann

INTRODUCTION

Araeteus appears to have been the first person to write about cancer of the larynx in the year 100 AD.[66] In 1732, Morgagni described autopsies on two deaths due to cancer of the larynx.[66] Virchow's monumental work on neoplasms contributed to the differentiation of cancer of the larynx from other common laryngeal lesions such as tuberculosis and syphilis.[89] Garcia, a Spanish singing teacher, introduced laryngoscopic investigation in 1855[32] — a technique subsequently perfected by Czermak.[15,16] The first laryngectomy was carried out by Billroth in 1873, accompanied by a high mortality of about 50%, primarily from sepsis, haemorrhage and pneumonia.[34,39,43,81] Laryngectomy was performed without previous biopsy, and pathology museums contain many examples of erroneous clinical diagnoses.

TERMINOLOGY

The most common terms are 'squamous cell carcinoma' and 'epidermoid carcinoma'.

DEFINITION

Squamous cell carcinoma is a malignant epithelial tumour which shows cellular and nuclear variability, invasion of the stroma and other definite evidence of malignancy.

INCIDENCE

The incidence of invasive squamous cell carcinoma has declined from 99% of all malignant laryngeal neoplasms in the 1970s to approximately 85–90% in recent years. In our material, the incidence is about 86% of all malignant neoplasms of the larynx. Other series show higher percentages, probably because of the inclusion of other oncotypes. Nevertheless, it has remained the most common type of laryngeal neoplasm.

In the United States, cancer of the larynx accounts for approximately 2% of all cancers and for 25% of all head and neck cancers. The American Cancer Society reported that there were 12 200 new cases in the United States during 1988.[73] Laryngeal cancer accounts for roughly 1% of all cancer mortality, amounting to about 200 000 deaths a year worldwide.[7]

HISTOGENESIS

The neoplasm arises from surface epithelium, both from stratified squamous epithelium and from columnar epithelium, which has undergone squamous metaplasia. Michaels[64] suggests that occasionally squamous cell carcinoma may arise directly from ciliated respiratory epithelium.

PATHOLOGY

Gross pathology

The gross appearance varies (see colour plate section), and the tumour may present in an exophytic, sessile, fungating or ulcerative fashion and may be papillomatous in appearance. Independent double or multiple primary cancers of the larynx may occur simultaneously or metachronously, usually displaying the same histological type.

Histopathology

Invasive squamous cell carcinoma can be graded as follows:[1]

Well differentiated (G 1)

This tumour displays polygonal prickle cells, orderly stratification, clearly visible intercellular bridges and keratinization with epithelial pearl formation (Figs 10.1 and 10.2). The nuclei are hyperchromatic and irregular in

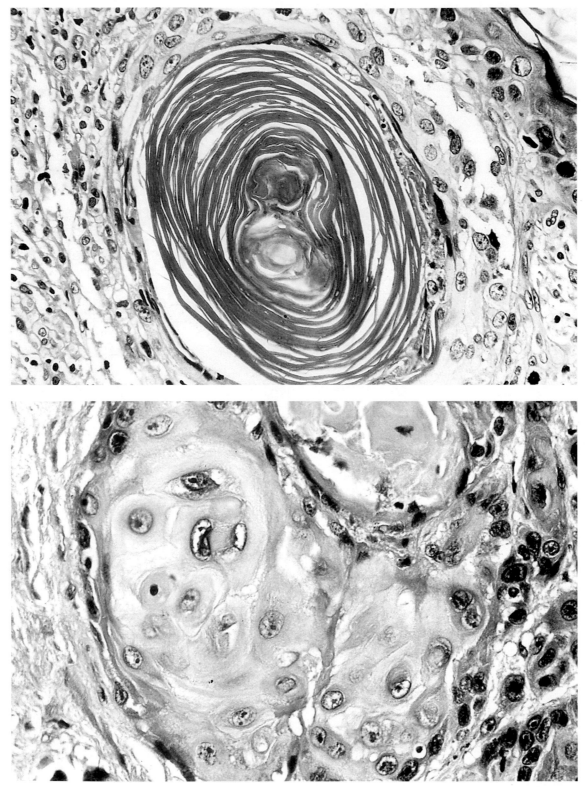

Fig. 10.1 (*top*) Well differentiated squamous cell carcinoma with keratin pearl. H&E, ×100 OM.

Fig. 10.2 (*bottom*) Well differentiated squamous cell carcinoma. H&E, ×100 OM.

size and shape, and the nuclear–cytoplasmic ratio is reduced. Atypical mitoses are rare.

Moderately differentiated (G 2)

This tumour shows polygonal prickle cells, stratification and intercellular bridge formation. Epithelial pearls are scarce or even absent (Figs 10.3, 10.4). Mitoses are frequent and atypical.

Poorly differentiated (G 3)

This tumour involves epithelial cells showing nuclear pleomorphism and hyperchromasia with scanty but distinct intercellular bridge formation. Mitoses are atypical and abundant. Keratin may be found in small amounts but it is usually missing (Figs 10.5, 10.6).

Undifferentiated (G 4)

This grading is recommended by the TNM system of classification but it is not applicable to the larynx. The concept of G4 is, in fact, a label for various oncotypes which have not been properly classified.[24]

Some squamous cell carcinomas may show areas of clear cells (Figs 10.7, 10.8) and others contain giant cells simulating a sarcoma (Figs 10.9, 10.10). In our experience, both tumours have a poor prognosis. Some irradiated neoplasms show a marked and bizarre giant cell reaction that may also occur, albeit rarely, in non-irradiated cases.

The first case of *squamous cell carcinoma with osteoclast-like giant cells* (Figs 10.11, 10.12) was described by Ferlito et al.[26] The diagnosis was supported by immunocytochemical investigation.

Other subtypes of squamous cell carcinoma include *small cell squamous carcinoma* of a tight epithelial pattern composed of relatively small cells with sharp cytoplasmic borders. A laryngeal squamous cell carcinoma in a sulphated mucopolysaccharide-rich stroma has also been described.[29] This neoplasm was called *squamous cell carcinoma with prominent myxoid stroma* and has to be distinguished from benign and malignant myxoid tissue tumours.

Immunocytochemistry

The study of intermediate filaments by immunoperoxidase methods using monoclonal antibodies has provided a new adjunct to light and electron microscopy. Intermediate filaments (also referred to as 10 nm filaments) form an important fibrous element of the cytoskeleton in almost all vertebrate cells. The cytokeratins forming tonofilament bundles are complex intermediate filaments of the cytoskeleton of epithelial cells. Several keratins have been isolated and divided into proteins of different molecular weight.

Immunohistochemically, squamous cell carcinoma of the larynx is positive for cytokeratins[11,60,79,84,85] and epithelial membrane antigen (EMA). A non-keratin protein called involucrin, which is synthesized by differentiating squamous epithelial cells, appears to be a sensitive marker of laryngeal dysplasia.[47] Involucrin has been used as a specific marker for squamous cell differentiation in lung tumours. EGF receptor (EGFR) is expressed in laryngeal neoplasms at levels significantly higher than in normal mucosa and is related to histological grading.[76]

Electron microscopy

The application of electron microscopy and indirect immunofluorescence and immunoperoxidase staining methods can assist in arriving at a more accurate histopathological diagnosis of neoplasms considered as 'undifferentiated' under the light microscope. Electron microscopy shows squamous cells with large vesicular nuclei, enlarged nucleoli, scattered intracellular tonofilament bundles attached to desmosomes and other junctional features. The Golgi apparatus is prominent in the undifferentiated cells and keratohyaline granules occur.[77,78] The basal lamina is often disrupted.[30,78]

Scanning electron microscopy

These studies of epithelial lesions of the vocal cord have yielded interesting results but the clinical value of scanning electron microscopy has remained inconclusive.[59,88] Normal squamous cell epithelium of the vocal cord at low magnification shows a uniform mosaic of polygonal cells of similar size and shape with sharp and slightly elevated cytoplasmic borders. The cell surface appears to be flat. In dysplasia, there is increased irregularity giving rise to a cobble-stone pattern. Carcinoma in situ shows a highly disorganized picture. The cells are round, swollen and protruding, with ill-defined intercellular junctions.

At higher magnification, normal squamous cell epithelium has convoluted or branching microridges. In dysplasia, carcinoma in situ and invasive carcinoma, microvilli or microvilli-like formations may be seen but regular microridges are generally missing.[48,59,88] It has been noted that not all the cells of a cytological type display identical scanning electron microscopy features. There is only an 'average' appearance for any cell type. 'Normal' and 'abnormal' surface details could be found in the same specimen, precluding any prognostic interpretation.[48]

DNA image analysis

The results of DNA-ploidy determination have remained inconclusive. Goldsmith et al[36] observed that patients with aneuploid neoplasms and a high level of DNA have

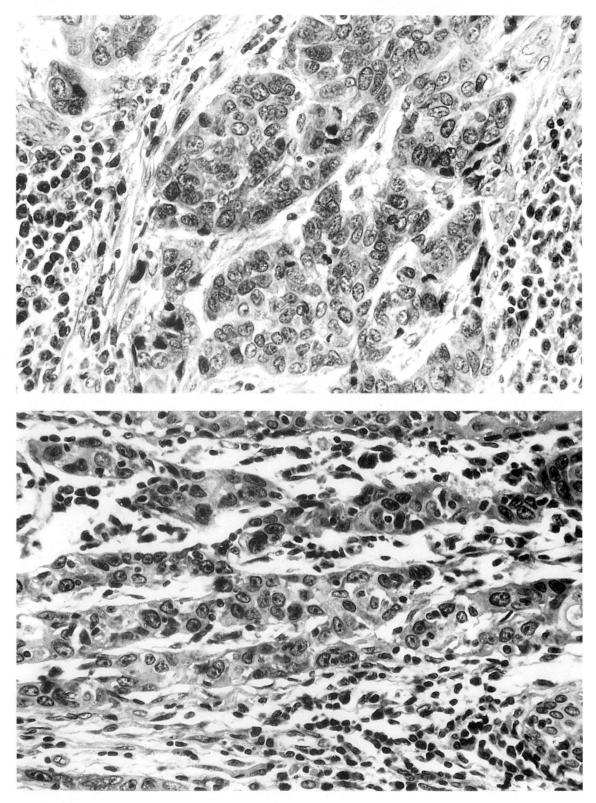

Fig. 10.3 (*top*) Moderately differentiated squamous cell carcinoma. H&E, ×100 OM.

Fig. 10.4 (*bottom*) Moderately differentiated squamous cell carcinoma. H&E, ×100 OM.

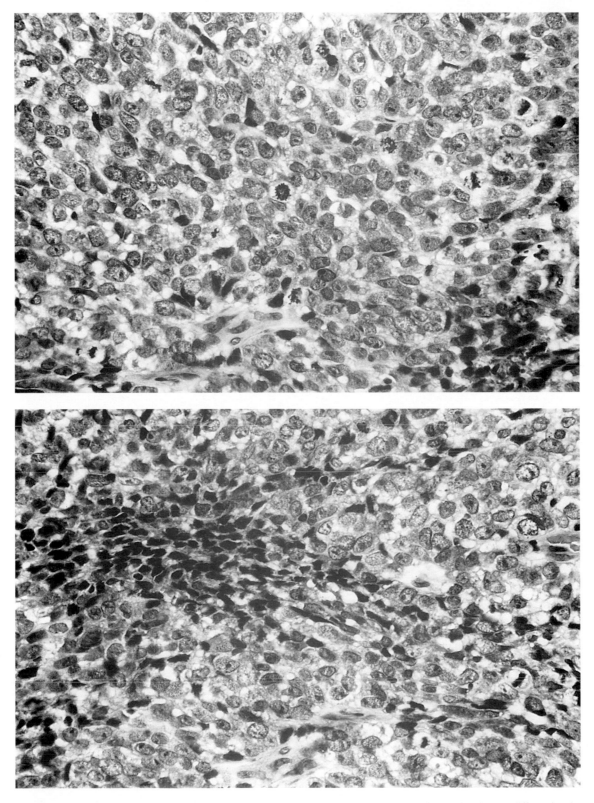

Fig. 10.5 (*top*) Poorly differentiated squamous cell carcinoma. This term replaces the earlier expression 'undifferentiated carcinoma'. The neoplasm was positive for cytokeratin and negative for CEA and leukocyte common antigen. H&E, ×100 OM.

Fig. 10.6 (*bottom*) Poorly differentiated squamous cell carcinoma. Another area of the tumour in Fig. 10.5. H&E, ×100 OM.

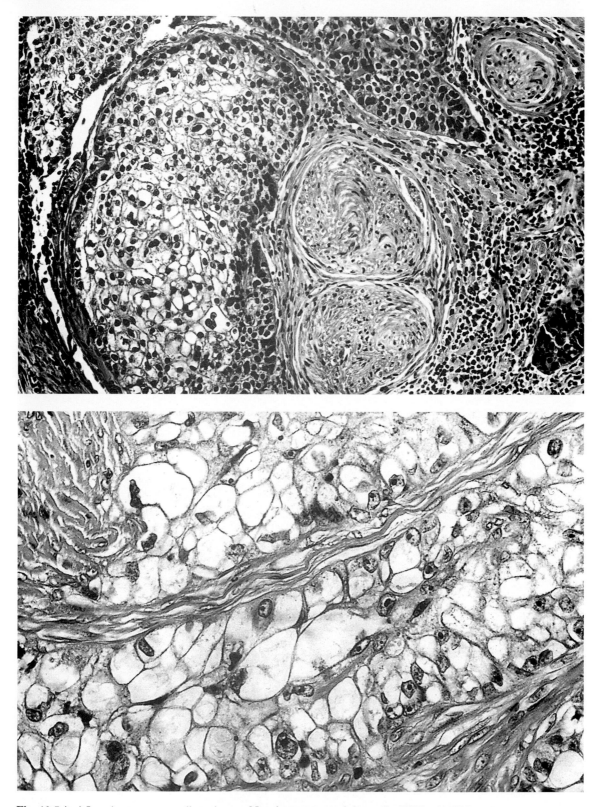

Fig. 10.7 (*top*) Invasive squamous cell carcinoma. Note large masses of clear cells. H&E, ×40 OM.

Fig. 10.8 (*bottom*) Note the cytological details of the clear cells. H&E, ×100 OM.

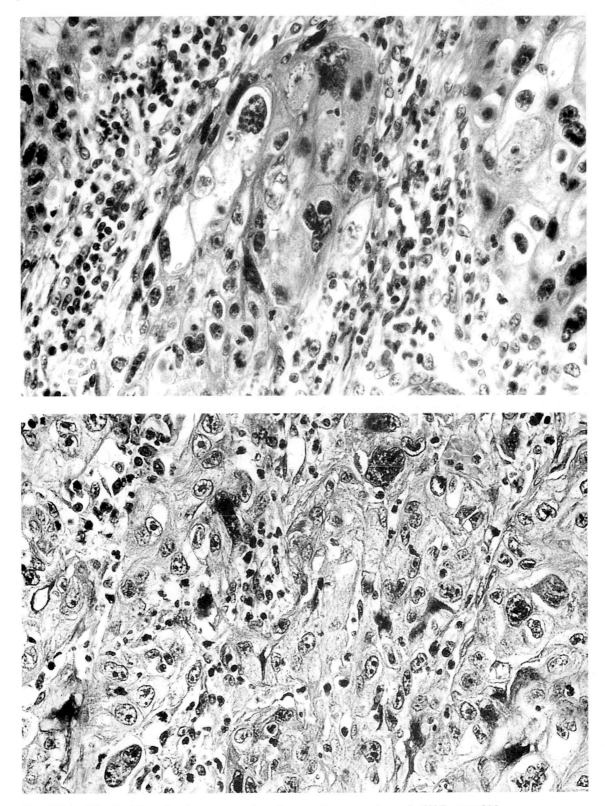

Fig. 10.9 (*top*) Poorly differentiated squamous cell carcinoma with tumour giant cells. H&E, ×100 OM.

Fig. 10.10 (*bottom*) Another area of the neoplasm with tumour giant cells. H&E, ×100 OM.

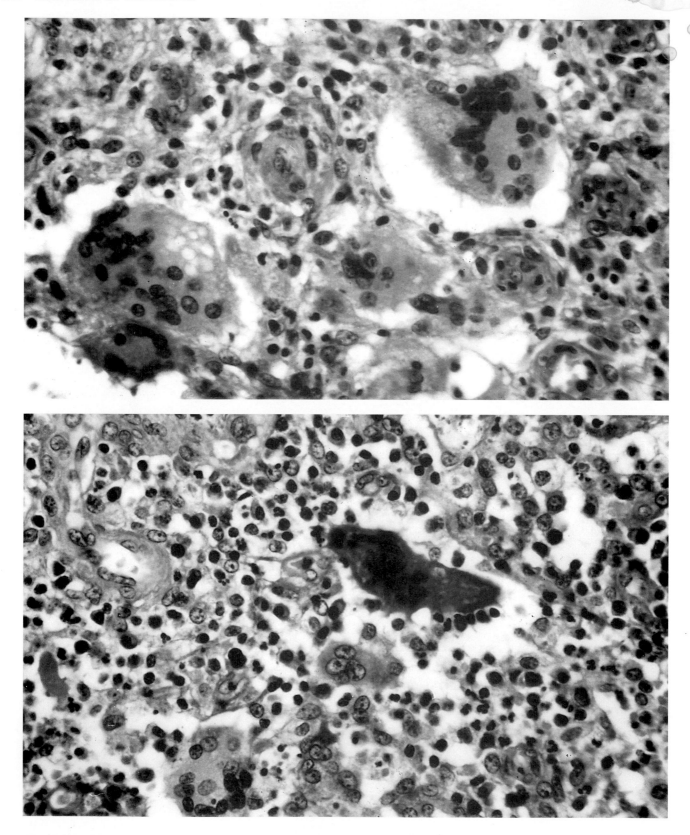

Fig. 10.11 (*top*) Squamous cell carcinoma of the larynx with osteoclast-like giant cells. H&E, ×160 OM.

Fig. 10.12 (*bottom*) Another area of the tumour in Fig. 10.11. Note the osteoclast-like giant cells and the vigorous angiogenesis. H&E, ×100 OM.

a better prognosis than patients with diploid neoplasms and low levels of DNA. Ruá et al[74] have shown that non-diploid tumours of the larynx had a poorer prognosis in the group of well-differentiated carcinomas (G1). There was some difference in the prognosis of G2 and G3 tumours. Yasuda et al[92] suggest that DNA cyto-fluorometry may be a useful prognostic parameter for glottic cancer treated by irradiation therapy. The ploidy pattern was significantly associated with the relapse-free rate, but did not correlate with the stage of the carcinoma or the cancer cell differentiation.

Tsuruta et al[87] have suggested that DNA content analysis in paraffin-embedded tissue is a helpful indicator in determining locoregional control and radiosensitivity for laryngeal cancer and in providing some biological information.

El-Naggar et al[18] have found a high intratumoral heterogeneity of DNA content in laryngeal squamous cell carcinomas with consequent variations in prognostic implications.

Stell[83] believes that ploidy has no prognostic value in cancer of the larynx.

DIAGNOSIS AND DIFFERENTIAL DIAGNOSIS

The histological diagnosis of frankly invasive squamous cell carcinoma in adequate biopsy specimens presents no difficulties. In difficult cases, immunocytochemical evaluation may be useful to distinguish squamous cell carcinoma, small cell squamous carcinoma, sarcoma, lymphoma and melanoma. Squamous cell carcinoma and small cell squamous carcinoma are negative for neuro-endocrine markers (neuron specific enolase [NSE], chromogranin, synaptophysin, protein gene product 9.5) and positive for epithelial markers (cytokeratins, EMA, carcino-embryonic antigen); sarcoma exhibits vimentin positivity and is uniformly negative for epithelial markers; lymphoma is reactive for leukocyte common antigen; melanoma is positive for NSE, S-100 and HMB-45 (a melanocyte-specific tumour marker). Electron microscopy may be a useful tool in poorly differentiated neoplasms, but its application is limited. Differential diagnosis must be made from papilloma, verrucous squamous cell carcinoma and mucoepidermoid carcinoma. The presence of cellular atypia and the absence of verrucous features indicates a classical squamous carcinoma; the presence of cells containing abundant mucus may suggest a mucoepi-dermoid carcinoma. Differential diagnosis must also be made from spindle cell squamous carcinoma, granular cell tumour and necrotizing sialometaplasia.[90]

HISTOLOGICAL GRADING OF MALIGNANCY

Various histological and cytological features have been related to prognosis and/or treatment but have not been universally accepted.[14] The histological grading of malignant neoplasms has had a chequered career since Broder's method of grading squamous cell carcinoma.[5] There are considerable limitations to the usefulness of his approach, due to the subjectivity of the criteria applied. A successful attempt to overcome such limitations has been made by Jakobsson and his colleagues at the Karolinska Institution in Stockholm, who devised a point score system for grading the malignant potential of tumours.[45] The system is based on the registration of eight micro-scopical features; four of them represent the neoplastic cell population itself (structure, differentiation, nuclear polymorphism and mitoses) whereas the remaining four criteria represent the tumour–host relationship (mode of invasion, stage of invasion, vascular invasion, cellular response).

The most important factors in the prediction of the 5-year recurrence rates were: (i) nuclear pleomorphism, (ii) mode of invasion, and (iii) total points scored; regardless of the clinical staging of the tumours, those in which the total score was between 10 and 15 showed a zero percentage of recurrence, whereas those with scores of 16 to 28 had a rate of 20–29%. The figures can be broken down further if the mode of invasion and the nuclear pleomorphism scores are taken into account. The usefulness of this work appears to be considerable — particularly because it is based on histological examin-ation of the pretreatment diagnostic biopsy specimen, which tends to produce a lower score than the final resected specimen. The results suggest that application of this method could considerably improve the value of histological examination of biopsy specimens and its contribution to the management of laryngeal carcinomas.[58] However, other workers have noted little or no correlation between the microscopical grade of laryngeal cancer and its clinical course.[42]

Glanz[33] believes that the Jakobsson system has some serious disadvantages and has developed a different grading system based on the following parameters: (i) differentiation and polymorphism of the tumour; (ii) structure and border of the tumour; (iii) vascular and perineural invasion; and (iv) cellular response of the host. The scale of each parameter has three scores.

The following histological parameters have been used by Crissman and Zarbo[13] in evaluating squamous cell carcinoma of the upper aerodigestive tract: degree and pattern of keratinization, nuclear grade, frequency of mitosis, inflammatory response, desmoplastic response, pattern of invasion and vascular invasion. The scale of each parameter has four scores. The biological malignancy of a tumour increases with the increasing pleomorphism of its cell population. Nuclear grading is a specific prognostic factor and may be evaluated as NG1 (the least favourable), NG2 (intermediate between NG1 and NG3) and NG3 (the most favourable). The increase in nuclear size and staining presumably indicates an increase in DNA content.[75] Mitotic activity should be assessed peripherally in the tumour mass, where invasion of the neighbouring healthy tissue may be adequately evaluated. A high mitotic index is an expression of high biological malignancy. All pathologists are familiar with the pitfalls inherent in the discrepancy between the morphological evidence presented by a small laryngeal biopsy specimen and the overall pattern of the same growth when examined in the laryngectomy specimen, if available. Sagittal or horizontal sectioning, stepwise or serially, gives a detailed insight into the pattern, extension and spread of an excised laryngeal neoplasm.[49–51,62] Not only may well-differentiated and poorly-differentiated areas alternate, but extensive fields of carcinoma in situ may occur in the proximity of an invasive carcinoma of the larynx or over a wide field of the mucous membrane.[31]

Expansive or infiltrative growth of a tumour has prognostic significance. Tumours of exophitic growth are less likely to metastasize than neoplasms with infiltrative margins. Moreover, pushing tumours are less likely to invade vascular structures.

The mode of invasion of a tumour (clear-cut margins or shaded margins, diffuse lesion) is not to be disregarded in establishing the degree of malignancy.

Immunocompetent cells, such as lymphocytes and plasma cells are regarded as the host's response to tumour growth, and survival rate increases with the increasing intensity of lymphocyte and plasma cell infiltration. Also the presence of eosinophilia seems to be a favourable prognostic indicator.[35] The presence of areas of necrosis is a morphological indicator of malignancy, since it means that the tumour grows quickly and has an insufficient blood supply. Necrotic foci are more frequent in poorly-differentiated than in well-differentiated squamous cell carcinomas.

SPREAD AND METASTASES

Squamous cell carcinoma of the larynx may spread by direct infiltration or by the lymphatic (Fig. 10.13), haematogenous or perineural routes. Tumour dissemination may be affected by various factors, such as the site of the primary neoplasm, the degree of cellular differentiation or the presence of any barriers to its spread, as well as by certain biological factors (largely related to tumour–host relationships). All these factors may act independently or in synergism. Invasive carcinomas lack a formed extracellular basement membrane around the invading tumour cell in the stroma. The basement membrane is also defective around tumour cells in lymph node and organ metastases. Partial basal lamina formation can be identified in certain areas of well- and moderately-differentiated carcinomas. Even in these conditions, it is usually abnormal, i.e., discontinuous, fragmented, or focally reduplicated.[2,3,57,61] Poorly differ-

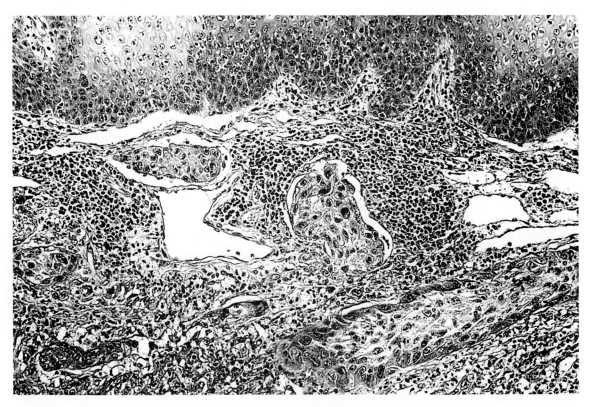

Fig. 10.13 The lymph–vascular space invaded by squamous cell carcinoma. H&E, ×40 OM.

entiated squamous cell carcinomas are less likely to have an identifiable basal lamina, suggesting active stromal invasion.[13,75]

Laryngeal cancer spreads in three dimensions, and the tumour may infiltrate beyond the anatomical boundaries of the organ in various places.[53] The pattern of direct laryngeal cancer invasion is largely determined by anatomical and mechanical features.[65] The principal structures forming a barrier to tumour spread are the hyo-epiglottic ligament, the conus elasticus and the non-ossified cartilages with their perichondrium. The fibrous sheet separating the contiguous pre-epiglottic and paraglottic spaces is not a significant barrier.[37] Less resistant to tumour invasion are the thyro-epiglottic

ligament and the cricothyroid membrane. Glandular structures may facilitate tumour spread. Muscle fibres are easily dissociated by neoplastic infiltration. The tumour may extend directly into the adjacent normal structures and it may infiltrate the glosso-epiglottic valleculae, hypopharynx, thyroid (Fig. 10.14) and trachea; it may occasionally invade the prelaryngeal muscles, sub-cutaneous tissues and overlying skin.

The growth and spread of laryngeal cancer is determined by the site of its origin. Cancer of the vocal cord originating on the free margin of the anterior half spreads initially on the surface along the length of the cord. It may circumvent the vocal ligament and occupy the space of Reinke. The lesion may extend to the

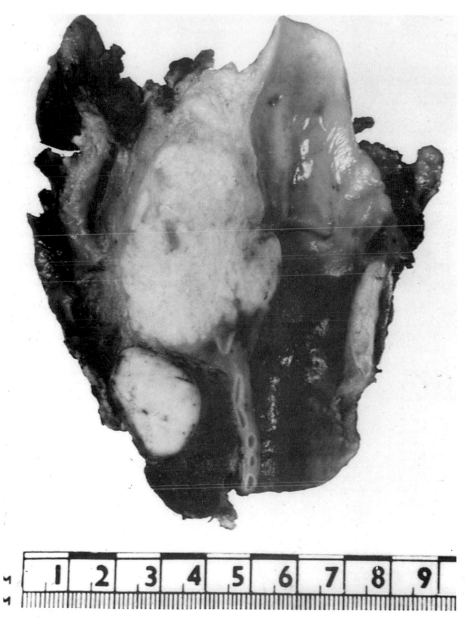

Fig. 10.14 Sagittal section through a laryngectomy specimen showing the thyroid gland infiltrated by a squamous cell carcinoma of the vocal cord.

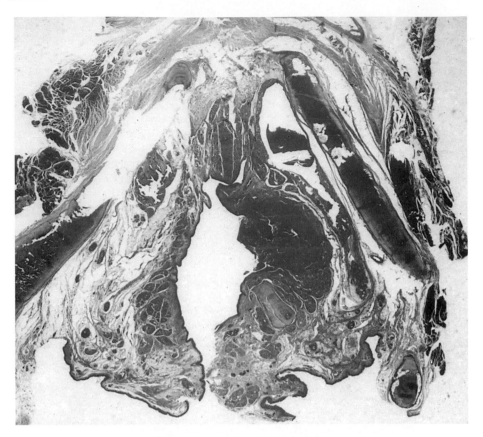

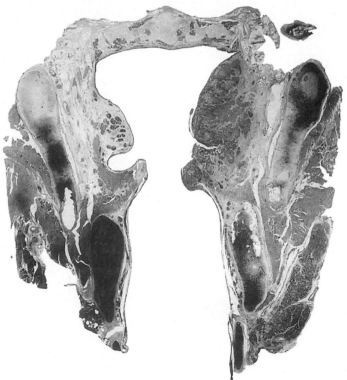

Fig. 10.15 (*top*) Transverse section showing an invasive carcinoma of the right vocal cord extending to the anterior commissure.

Fig. 10.16 (*bottom*) Coronal section of the larynx showing a squamous cell carcinoma of the right vocal cord extending upwards into the ventricle and vestibular fold.

anterior commissure (Fig. 10.15) or posteriorly to the vocal process and/or anterior surface of the arytenoid cartilage. The neoplasm may also extend upwards into the ventricle, the vestibular fold (Fig. 10.16) and the subglottic region and may thereby escape downwards through the crico-thyroid membrane.[69]

Cancer arising in the anterior commissure spreads widely, involving both vocal cords, the ventricle and ventricular fold, the base of the epiglottis and the subglottic region. Not uncommonly, it invades the lower margin of the thyroid ala and may extend through the cricothyroid membrane outside the laryngeal framework. In a set of 101 laryngectomies serially sectioned, evidence of spread through the crico-thyroid membrane was found in seven cases of glottic cancer (Fig. 10.17).[41] There may be infiltration of the Delphian lymph node.

Supraglottic cancers have been divided into *suprahyoid* laryngeal cancers (suprahyoid epiglottis, aryepiglottic fold and arytenoid) and *infrahyoid* laryngeal cancers (infrahyoid epiglottis, ventricular fold, and ventricle). Infrahyoid cancers are more common and display a clear tendency to spread into the fatty-areolar tissue of the pre-epiglottic space itself, either through the destroyed thyro-epiglottic ligament (by passing straight through the orifices of the epiglottic cartilage) or by direct destruction of the cartilage itself.[37,40,69] Suprahyoid laryngeal cancers tend to invade the tongue base and pyriform sinus rather than the pre-epiglottic space.

It has been assumed that supraglottic carcinomas do not extend to the glottic region and they have been called 'ascending cancers', but these tumours may actually infiltrate the glottic plane and subglottic region,[69] though the neoplasm may clinically appear restricted to the supraglottic region. When a supraglottic cancer invades the paraglottic space (instead of the pre-epiglottic space), inferior invasion to the glottis can easily occur. This is because the paraglottic space extends into the glottis along the medial surface of the thyroid cartilage. In a series of 100 cases, Han and Yamashita[40] recently investigated the manner of spread of supraglottic cancer by the whole-organ serial section study of surgical specimens: the glottis was involved in 48 cases and the anterior commissure in 12 cases.

Kirchner[51] believes that supraglottic cancer does not invade the laryngeal framework, a theory based on the serial sectioning of 112 surgical specimens of supraglottic cancer removed by total or partial laryngectomy: the adjacent thyroid cartilage was never invaded, regardless of the size of the tumour. However, the thyroid cartilage was invaded in 9 of the 100 cases of supraglottic cancer studied by Han and Yamashita.[40]

Subglottic carcinoma (Fig. 10.18) may go undetected at an early stage because of the lack of symptoms. In its advanced stage, it presents as a circumferential growth and may extend upwards to the vocal cords and downwards into the trachea. When the tumour grows

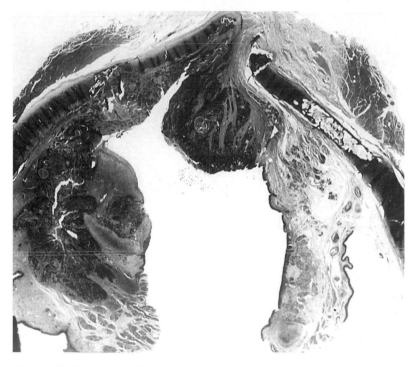

Fig. 10.17 Squamous cell carcinoma of the larynx. Transverse section at supraglottic level showing the left wall of the larynx invaded by a necrotizing papillomatous carcinoma, which at one point has broken into the thyroid cartilage. There is a large tumour occupying the anterior commissure, forming a polypoid mass protruding into the lumen.

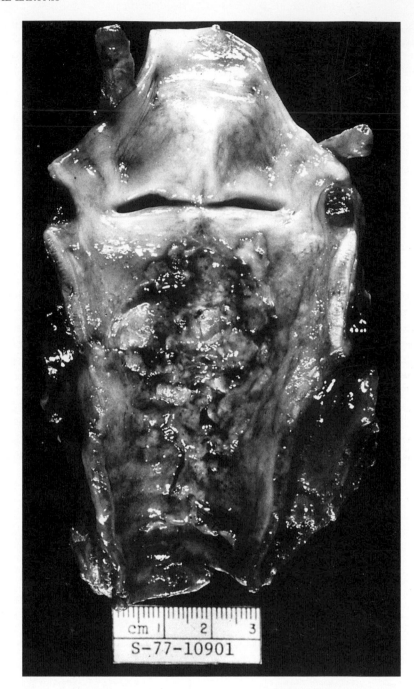

Fig. 10.18   Rare example of a primary subglottic carcinoma of the larynx. (Courtesy of Dr L. Barnes, Pittsburgh.)

anteriorly, it may perforate the cricothyroid membrane[37] and invade the thyroid gland, the anterior soft tissues and eventually the skin. If the tumour affects the posterior wall of the subglottis, it may also infiltrate the cervical oesophagus.

Invasion of the laryngeal framework is a common feature of transglottic cancers. These tumours have a prominent tendency to spread outside the larynx. Whole-organ sections suggest that transglottic cancer arises deep within the ventricle.[51]

Direct diffuse permeation of the submucosal lymphatic vessels is well known in laryngeal cancer with lymph node involvement. Direct infiltration may affect adjacent lymph nodes, particularly the prelaryngeal lymph nodes (or Delphian nodes). Direct invasion can also occur in the laryngeal cartilages and the metaplastic bone of ossified laryngeal cartilages. Patches of ossified cartilage are regularly present in the thyroid, cricoid and arytenoid cartilages. Within the thyroid cartilage, ossification invariably begins at the posterior border near the root of the inferior horn, spreading along the inferior border and reaching the midline. Ossification also extends to the upper portion of the posterior part of the laminae with the superior horn late to ossify.[41]

Non-ossified cartilage is resistant to osteoclastic erosion and direct destruction by tumour cells may go undetected. In ossified laryngeal cartilages, the tumour cells stimulate the osteoclasts to destroy the bone facing the tumour margin. Osteoclasts play an important role in the advance of the invading tumour, separated from its advancing edge by a zone of inflammatory fibrous granulation tissue. The capacity of tumour cells to erode bone in the absence of osteoclasts is probably limited and it seems that the main effect of a local infiltrating tumour is to stimulate adjacent osteoclasts by the local release of prostaglandins and other substances.[8,9,41,72] Various reasons have been suggested for the particular susceptibility of ossified cartilage to neoplastic invasion. Most important, the foci of metaplastic bone contain osteoclasts which accumulate on the bone surface in the vicinity of infiltrating carcinoma, resorbing the bone. It is only after the osteoclastic response wanes that carcinoma cells themselves impinge on the bone surface. The essentially biphasic process is the same as that of squamous carcinomas invading 'true bone'[8,71,72] and osteoclastic and osteoblastic processes are not unlike those seen in inflammatory or infectious bone-eroding processes.

It has been observed that neoplastic invasion of the thyroid cartilage occurs more frequently than may be detected by present radiological techniques.

Squamous cell carcinoma of the larynx has a high tendency to metastasize to the cervical lymph nodes. In the great majority of cases, few lymph nodes are involved. The neoplastic cells — either singly or in small emboli — are carried in afferent lymphatic vessels and become trapped in the nodal sinus system where nodal deposits may develop. The necessary local conditions for their development have remained obscure. Spreading to the lymphatic vessels is mainly by embolization, appearing first in the subcapsular sinus and subsequently spreading to the whole node parenchyma. Nodal deposits may be confined by an intact capsule, but the lesion may penetrate the capsule of the node and invade the surrounding fat and adjacent tissues. Metastases are usually ipsilateral, often bilateral and exceptionally contralateral. Localization of the cervical lymph node metastases is closely linked with the site of the primary lesion. Tumours of the supraglottic region metastasize primarily to the subdigastric and upper jugular nodes, followed closely by the midjugular nodes. The posterior cervical nodes are seldom involved and the nodes of the submandibular triangle and submental areas are rarely affected.[91] Retrograde lymph flow may produce anomalous secondary deposits.

Subglottic carcinomas metastasize at an early stage and frequently to the lower deep cervical jugular chain, prelaryngeal (Delphian) node or nodes, paratracheal nodes, lymph nodes of the recurrent nerve chain and supraclavicular nodes. The prelaryngeal lymph nodes are located above the thyroid isthmus and in front of the lower part of the thyroid cartilage.

Blood-borne metastases are uncommon in squamous cell carcinoma, but widespread dissemination to various viscera may occur in advanced stages of laryngeal cancer. The organs and structures most commonly involved are, in decreasing order: mediastinal lymph nodes, lung, liver, pleura, skeletal system, kidney, heart, spleen.[80] There have been reports of metastases to the cavernous sinus from primary squamous cell carcinoma of the larynx.[86,93] Cervical lymph nodes are always involved in cases showing distant metastases. At autopsy, visceral metastases were detected in almost 50% of supraglottic carcinoma cases (41 out of 83) versus 16.6% of glottic cancers (5 out of 30).[80] Significant distant metastases were present at autopsy in patients who died with no clinically evident squamous cell carcinoma and who might therefore have been reported as cured (Figs 10.19–10.21).[67]

The distinction between lymphatic and haematogenous spread is artificial, since dissemination of most tumours occurs through both systems.

Perineural invasion is frequent (Figs 10.22, 10.23) and often spreads along the branches of the recurrent laryngeal nerve into the thyro-arytenoid muscle, near the lower end of the thyroid ala. The longitudinal arrangement of the nerve trunks and the tendency of cancer to invade nerve sheaths enables its spread from one region to another along the perineural spaces, centrally or peripherally, sometimes traversing long distances. The nerve axons can be affected secondarily by ischaemia caused by the infiltrating neoplastic cells.

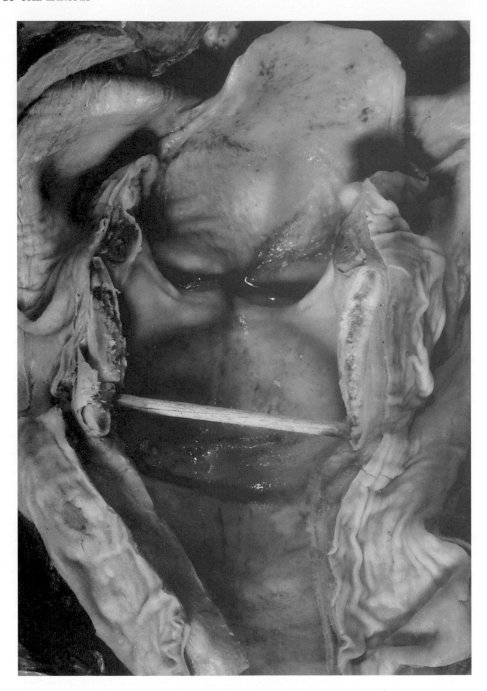

Fig. 10.19 At post mortem examination, the larynx showed no evidence of recurrent squamous cell carcinoma though distant metastases were found in the brain and heart. (Courtesy of Dr A. A. Narula, Nottingham, and the editor of *Journal of Laryngology and Otology*.)

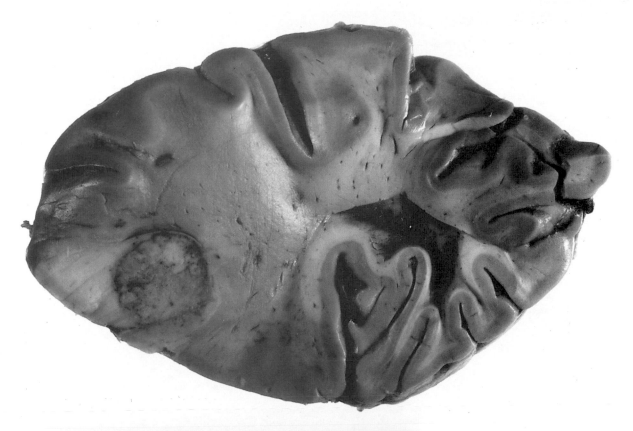

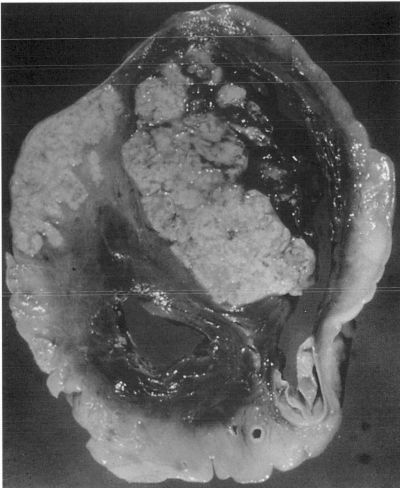

Fig. 10.20 (*top*) A tumour nodule of 1.8 cm diameter was present in the left occipital pole of the brain. (Courtesy of Dr A. A. Narula, Nottingham, and the editor of *Journal of Laryngology and Otology*.)

Fig. 10.21 (*bottom*) A 2.5 cm mass of tumour involving the anterior aspects of the heart; there was no evidence of tumour in other sites. (Courtesy of Dr A. A. Narula, Nottingham, and the editor of *Journal of Laryngology and Otology*.)

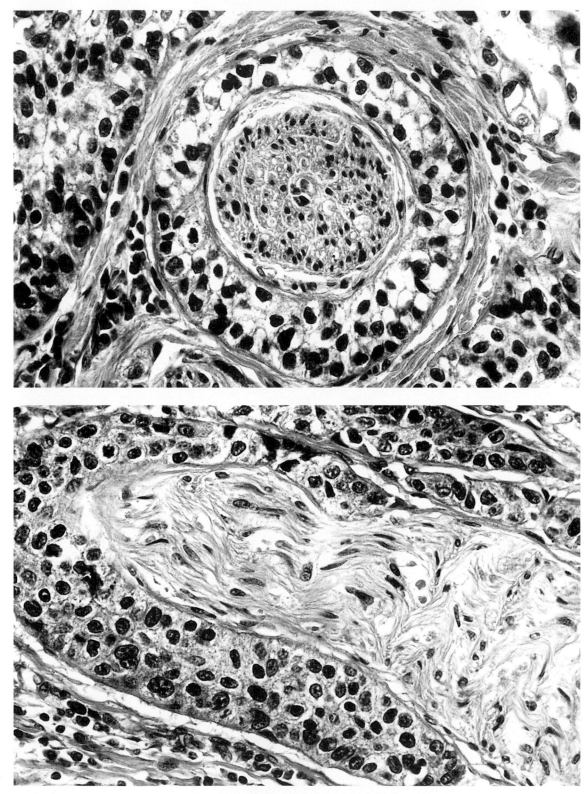

Fig. 10.22 (*top*) Squamous cell carcinoma showing perineural invasion. H&E, ×100 OM.

Fig. 10.23 (*bottom*) The same tumour as in Fig. 10.22 showing perineural invasion in another area. H&E, ×100 OM.

The metastatic process is a complex, multistep procedure. First of all the malignant cells must invade the vascular wall or lymphatic channels in order to disseminate. The tumour cells in circulation must be able to outwit body defences.

Extensive investigations have thrown light on the metastatic process and on the morphological patterns of framework invasion.[53,72]

Nevertheless, our knowledge of the mechanisms underlying the metastatic process has remained rudimentary.

IMMUNOLOGICAL PROBLEMS IN LARYNGEAL CANCER

The development of malignancy may be related to a breakdown in the body's defence mechanisms, to a defect in cell immunity and/or to the failure of its immunological surveillance.

The idea that immune response is the principle defence against neoplastic cells has had a profound influence on cancer research. Burnet[6] elaborated this concept into a theory that he termed 'immunological surveillance'.

It is important to distinguish between a surveillance mechanism and an immune response to an established tumour. The former, if it existed, eliminated any neoplastic cells as they arose. The latter, for which there is abundant evidence, may or may not prevent the spread of neoplastic cells from a primary tumour. Lymphocyte and plasma cell infiltration, a local immune response, can be regarded as an expression of the host's reactive potential against tumour cells.[22] The significance of histologically demonstrable 'host response' to carcinoma in the larynx has been studied by many researchers.[6,25] Sinus histiocytosis and germ-centre hyperplasia in nodes were found to be of limited significance. In addition to a morphological assessment of the immune reaction in the primary lesion and regional lymph nodes,[22] there are various new methods for assessing the in vivo and in vitro reactivity of immune competent cells (immunological monitoring). Blood group isoantigens A, B, and H (O), widely distributed in normal body tissues, have been employed as natural labels for the study of antigenic changes in malignant neoplasms.[12,17,38,56] Mevio et al[63] suggest the use of serum markers in the diagnosis and management of laryngeal cancer. In particular, lipid-associated sialic acid (LASA) and ferritin seem to be the most suitable markers because of their higher sensitivity at all phases of cancer disease. Several Spanish authors were able to find alterations in the expression of class I and II histocompatibility antigens in cancers of the larynx, which proved valid predictors of the behaviour and prognosis of the neoplasms.[19-21]

Stell[82] considers research for tumour markers in head and neck cancer as largely unsuccessful.

THE HETEROGENEITY OF LARYNGEAL CANCERS

Despite remarkable advances in the surgical treatment of primary neoplasms and aggressive adjuvant therapies, most cancer patients die of metastatic disease. The most formidable obstacle to the successful treatment of disseminated cancer may well be the fact that tumour cells are biologically heterogeneous.

The histological assessment of morphology has shown considerable variation between metastases and primary tumours and between one metastasis and another. Nevertheless, human cancer was considered to be clonal in nature and the clinical expression of proliferation of a single cell type. However, the application of modern methods of immunology and molecular genetics has revealed that most malignant neoplasms consist of complex subpopulations of cells.[55]

Cloning experiments have shown that, by the time of diagnosis, neoplasms may be heterogeneous, composed of cells with different biological features and metastatic potential.[28]

PARANEOPLASTIC SYNDROMES

Non-metastatic or paraneoplastic syndromes associated with squamous cell carcinoma have been reported. In general, cutaneous (acrokeratosis Bazec, acanthosis nigricans, etc.), neuromuscular (Lambert–Eaton syndrome, etc.), endocrine (ectopic adrenocorticotrophic hormone syndrome, hypercalcaemia syndrome, etc.) and haematological paraneoplastic syndromes may be distinguished.[52] Recently, Zohar et al[94] described four patients with advanced metastatic squamous cell carcinoma of the larynx and pyriform sinus with a coexisting syndrome of inappropriate antidiuretic hormone secretion. Since this syndrome is usually transient, water restriction and parenteral sodium chloride may be sufficient in overcoming the acute phase.

ASSOCIATED LESIONS

The association of squamous cell carcinoma and tuberculosis was more common before the successful application of anti-tuberculous treatment.[23] More recently, tuberculosis of various organs has been spreading among the immigrant population of Western countries.

The association of cancer of the larynx with laryngocoele,[4,10] laryngopyocoele,[44] oncocytic lesions[54] and trichinella cysts[46,80a] may also occur.

In the larynx there may be a synchronous or metachronous association of squamous carcinoma with squamous cell carcinoma in situ, verrucous squamous cell carcinoma or lymphoma.

Rarely, squamous cell carcinoma of the larynx may be associated with Hodgkin's disease[68], initially simulating cervical lymph node metastases. The finding of Hodgkin's lymphoma is often fortuitous and it follows histological examination of the neck dissection specimen. Sometimes the presence of cervical lymph node metastases is not connected with laryngeal cancer but with other malignant neoplasms arising in the thyroid gland or other structures.

In rare cases, one or more lymph nodes may simultaneously contain laryngeal and thyroid metastases.[70] A case has been reported of metastases of laryngeal cancer to cervical lymph nodes involved by chronic lymphocytic leukaemia.[27]

REFERENCES

1. American Joint Committee on Cancer 1992 Manual for staging of cancer, 4th edn. Lippincott, Philadelphia
2. Antonelli A R, Nicolai P, Cappiello J, Peretti G, Molinari Tosatti M P, Rosa D, Grigolato P G, Favret M, Maroccolo D 1991 Basement membrane components in normal, dysplastic, neoplastic laryngeal tissue and metastatic lymph nodes. Acta Otolaryngol 111: 437–443
3. Barsky S H, Siegal G, Jannotta F, Liotta L A 1983 Loss of basement membrane components by invasive tumours but not by their benign counterparts. Lab Invest 49: 140–148
4. Birt D 1987 Observations on the size of the saccule in laryngectomy specimens. Laryngoscope 97: 190–200
5. Broders A C 1926 Carcinoma grading and practical application. Arch Pathol 2: 376–381
6. Burnet F M 197 Immunological surveillance in neoplasia. Transplant Rev 7: 3–25
7. Cantrell R W 1990 The current status of laryngeal cancer. In: Inouye T, Fukuda H, Sato T, Hinohara T (eds) Recent advances in bronchoesophagology. Excerpta Medica, Amsterdam
8. Carter R L 1985 Patterns and mechanisms of bone metastases. J R Soc Med 78: 2–6
9. Carter R L, Taner N S B 1979 Local invasion by laryngeal carcinoma—the importance of focal (metaplastic) ossification within laryngeal cartilage. Clin Otolaryngol 4: 283–290
10. Celin S E, Johnson J J, Curtin H, Barnes L 1991 The association of laryngoceles with squamous cell carcinoma of the larynx. Laryngoscope 101: 529–536
11. Cortesina G, Cavallo G P, Macario M, Poggio E, Cerrato M, Prat M, Bussolati G 1988 Monoclonal antibodies against epithelial antigens in laryngeal carcinomas. An immunocytochemical and clinico-pathological investigation. J Laryngol Otol 102: 709–712
12. Cowan W K 1962 Blood group antigens on human gastrointestinal carcinoma cells. Br J Cancer 16: 535–540
13. Crissman J D, Zarbo R J 1990 Squamous cell carcinoma of the upper aerodigestive tract: histologic parameters with prognostic value. In: Fee W E Jr, Goepfert H, Johns M E, Strong E W, Ward P H (eds) Head and neck cancer, vol 2. Decker, Toronto
14. Crissman J D, Liu W Y, Gluckman J L, Cummings G 1984 Prognostic value of histopathologic parameters in squamous cell carcinoma of the oropharynx. Cancer 54: 2995–3001
15. Czermak J 1858 On the laryngeal mirror. Wien Med Wochenschr 8: 198
16. Czermak J 1859 Contributions to the examination of the larynx. Med weekly 3: 120
17. Dabelsteen E, Mygind N, Henriksen B 1974 Blood group substance A in carcinomas of the larynx. Acta Otolaryngol 77: 360–367
18. El-Naggar A K, Lopez-Varela V, Luna M A, Weber R, Batsakis J G 1992 Intratumoral DNA content heterogeneity in laryngeal squamous cell carcinoma. Arch Otolaryngol Head Neck Surg 118: 169–173
19. Esteban F, Concha A, Delgado M, Pérez-Ayala M, Ruiz-Cabello F, Garrido F 1990 Lack of MHC class I antigens and tumour aggressiveness of the squamous cell carcinoma of the larynx. Br J Cancer 62: 1047–1051
20. Esteban F, Ruiz-Cabello F, Concha A, Pérez-Ayala M, Delgado M, Garrido F 1990 Relationship of 4F2 antigen with local growth and metastatic potential of squamous cell carcinoma of the larynx. Cancer 66: 1493–1498
21. Esteban F, Ruiz-Cabello F, Concha A, Pérex-Ayala M, Sanchez-Rozas J A, Garrido F 1990 HLA-DR expression is associated with excellent prognosis in squamous cell carcinoma of the larynx. Clin Expl Metastases 8: 319–328
22. Ferlito A 1976 Histological classification of larynx and hypopharynx cancers and their clinical implications. Pathologic aspects of 2052 malignant neoplasms diagnosed at the ORL Department of Padua University from 1966 to 1976. Acta Otolaryngol 342 (suppl): 1–88
23. Ferlito A 1985 Malignant epithelial tumours of the larynx. In: Ferlito A (ed) Cancer of the larynx, vol I. CRC Press, Boca Raton
24. Ferlito A, Friedmann I 1990 Poorly-differentiated laryngeal malignancies. ORL J Otorhinolaryngol Relat Spec 52: 63–64
25. Ferlito A, Polidoro F 1979 Biological and prognostic implications of the morphologic aspects of immune reaction in lymph nodes draining head and neck cancers (a review). J Laryngol Otol 93: 153–175
26. Ferlito A, Friedmann I, Recher G 1987 Squamous cell carcinoma of the larynx with osteoclast-like giant cells. J Laryngol Otol 101: 393–398
27. Ferlito A, Recher G, Visonà A 1986 Laryngeal cancer metastatic to lymph nodes with lymphocytic leukaemia. J Laryngol Otol 100: 233–237
28. Fidler I J, Kripke M L 1977 Metastasis results from preexisting variant cells within a malignant tumor. Science 197: 893
29. Foschini M P, Fulcheri E, Baracchini P, Ceccarelli C, Betts C M, Eusebi V 1990 Squamous cell carcinoma with prominent myxoid stroma. Hum Pathol 21: 859–865
30. Friedmann I 1971 Electron microscopy in head and neck oncology. Acta Otolaryngol 71: 115–122
31. Friedmann I, Ferlito A 1988 Granulomas and neoplasms of the larynx. Churchill Livingstone, Edinburgh
32. Garcia M 1855 Observations on the human voice. Philos Magazine J Sci 10: 218
33. Glanz H K 1984 Carcinoma of the larynx. Growth, p-classification and grading of squamous cell carcinoma of the vocal cords. Adv Otorhinolaryngol 32: 1–123
34. Gluck T 1912 Die chirurgische Therapie des Kehlkopfkarzinoms Jahreskurse Artzt Fortbildung. 2: 20–41.1
35. Goldsmith M M, Cresson D H, Askin F B 1987 Part II. The prognostic significance of stromal eosinophilia in head and neck cancer. Otolaryngol Head Neck Surg 96: 319–324
36. Goldsmith M M, Cresson D H, Arnold L A, Postma DS, Askin F B, Pillsbury H C 1987 Part I. DNA flow cytometry as a prognostic indicator in head and neck cancer. Otolaryngol Head Neck Surg 96: 307–318
37. Gregor R T 1990 The preepiglottic space revisited: is it significant? Am J Otolaryngol 11: 161–164
38. Gupta Y N, Gupta S, Singh I J, Khanna N N, Agarwal M K 1985 Epithelial isoantigens A, B and H in oral carcinomas. Ear Nose Throat J 64: 51–54
39. Gussenbauer C 1874 Über die erste durch Th. Billroth am Menschen ausgeführte Kehlkopf Extirpation und die Anwendung eines künstlichen Kehlkopfes. Arch Klin Chir 17: 343–356
40. Han De-M, Yamashita K 1991 The manner of spread of supraglottic carcinoma. Larynx Jpn 2: 175–186
41. Harrison D F N 1984 Cancer of the larynx. PhD Thesis. University of London
42. Welweg-Larsen K, Graem N, Meistrup-Larsen K-I, Meistrup-Larsen U 1978 Clinical relevance of histological grading of cancer of the larynx. Acta Pathol Microbiol Immunol Scand [A] 86: 499–504
43. Holinger P H 1975 The historical development of laryngectomy. Laryngoscope 85: 322–332

44. Iversen P B, Vesterhauge S 1978 A fatal case of laryngopyocoele with cancer of the larynx. J Laryngol Otol 92: 163–167

45. Jakobsson P A, Eneroth C M, Killander D, Moberger G, Martensson B 1973 Histologic classification and grading of malignancy in carcinoma of the larynx. Acta Radiol Ther Phys Biol 12: 1–12

46. Josephson J S, Josephson G D, Dennis N N 1989 Laryngeal trichinosis with simultaneous squamous cell carcinoma. Arch Otolaryngol Head Neck Surg 115: 1384–1387

47. Kaplan M J, Mills S E, Rice R H, Johns M E 1984 Involucrin in laryngeal dysplasia. A marker for differentiation. Arch Otolaryngol 110: 713–716

48. Kenemans P, Davina J H M, de Haan R W, van der Zanden P, Vooys G P, Stolk J G, Stadhouders AM 1981 Cell surface morphology in epithelial malignancy and its precursor lesions. Scan Electron Microsc pt 3: 23–36

49. Kirchner J A 1977 Two-hundred laryngeal cancers: patterns of growth and spread as seen in serial sections. Laryngoscope 87: 474–482

50. Kirchner J A 1984 Invasion of the framework by laryngeal cancer. Surgical and radiological implications. Acta Otolaryngol 97: 392–397

51. Kirchner J A 1991 Spread and barriers to spread of cancer within the larynx. In: Silver C E (ed) Laryngeal cancer. Thieme, New York

52. Kleinsasser O 1988 Tumors of the larynx and hypopharynx. Thieme, Stuttgart

53. Lam K H, Wong J 1983 The preepiglottic and paraglottic spaces in relation to spread of carcinoma of the larynx. Am J Otolaryngol 4: 81–91

54. LeJeune F E Jr, Putman H C III, Yamase H T 1980 Multiple oncocytic papillary cystadenomas of the larynx: a case report. Laryngoscope 90: 501–504

55. Leonard R C F, Smyth J F 1985 The heterogeneity of human cancers and its influence on metastases and therapy. Eur J Cancer Clin Oncol 21: 1001–1004

56. Lin F, Liu P I, McGregor D H 1977 Isoantigens A and H in morphologically normal mucosa and in carcinoma of the larynx. Am J Clin Pathol 68: 372–376

57. Liotta L A 1984 Tumor invasion and metastases: role of the basement membrane. Am J Pathol 117: 339–348

58. Lund C, Sogaard H, Jorgensen K, Hjelm-Hansen M 1976 Epidermoid carcinoma of the larynx. V I. Histologic grading in the clinical evaluation. Acta Radiol Ther Phys Biol 15: 293–304

59. Lundgren J, Olofsson J, Hellquist H, Grontoft L 1983 Scanning electron microscopy of vocal cord hyperplasia, keratosis, papillomatosis, dysplasia and carcinoma. Acta Otolaryngol 96: 315–327

60. Malecha M J, Miettinen M 1991 Expression of keratin 13 in human epithelial neoplasms. Virchows Archiv A Pathol Anat 418: 249–254

61. Martinez-Hernandez A, Amenta P S 1983 The basement membrane in pathology. Lab Invest 48: 656–680

62. McDonald T J, DeSanto L W, Weiland L H 1976 Supraglottic larynx and its pathology as studied by whole laryngeal sections. Laryngoscope 86: 635–648

63. Mevio E, Benazzo M, Galioto P, Spriano P, Pizzala R 1991 Use of serum markers in the diagnosis and management of laryngeal cancer. Clin Otolaryngol 16: 90–92

64. Michaels L 1984 Pathology of the larynx. Springer-Verlag, Berlin

65. Micheau C, Luboinski R, Sancho H, Cachin Y 1976 Modes of invasion of cancer of the larynx. A statistical, histological, and radioclinical analysis of 120 cases. Cancer 38: 346–360

66. Myerson M C 1964 The human larynx. Thomas, Springfield

67. Narula A A, Padfield C J, Morgan D A L, MacLennan K A, Bradley P J 1988 NED survival in head and neck cancer (post-mortem correlations). J Laryngol Otol 102: 194–197

68. Nigri P T, Khasgiwala C K 1982 Unusual presentation of head and neck neoplasm. Laryngoscope 92: 1245–1246

69. Olofsson J 1985 Aspects on laryngeal cancer based on whole organ sections. Auris Nasus Larynx 12 (suppl II): 166–175

70. Pacheco-Ojeda L, Micheau C, Luboinski B, Richard J, Travagli J P, Schwaab G, Marandas P 1991 Squamous cell carcinoma of the upper aerodigestive tract associated with well-differentiated carcinoma of the thyroid gland. Laryngoscope 101: 421–424

71. Pauli B U, Kuettner K E 1985 In: Mareel M M, Calman KC (eds) Invasion. Experimental and clinical implications. Host tissue resistance to tumour invasion. Oxford University Press, Oxford

72. Pittam M R, Carter R L 1982 Framework invasion by laryngeal carcinomas. Head Neck Surg 4: 200–208

73. Rice D H, Spiro R H 1989 Current concepts in head and neck cancer. American Cancer Society, USA

74. Ruá S, Comino A, Fruttero A, Cera G, Semeria C, Lanzillotta L, Boffetta P 1991 Relationship between histologic features, DNA flow cytometry, and clinical behavior of squamous cell carcinomas of the larynx. Cancer 67: 141–149

75. Sakr W A, Hussan M K, Ensley J F, Crissman J D 1987 Correlation of DNA analysis and histologic characteristics of squamous cell carcinoma. Lab Invest 56: 67A, abstract 400

76. Scambia G, Benedetti Panici P, Battaglia F, Ferrandina G, Almadori G, Paludetti G, Maurizi M, Mancuso S 1991 Receptors for epidermal growth factor and steroid hormones in primary laryngeal tumors. Cancer 67: 1347–1351

77. Schenk P 1980 Die ultrastrukturelle Morphologie der Mitochondria im malignen Keratinozyten des Kehlkopfkarzinoms. Laryngol Rhinol Otol 59: 344–350

78. Schenk P, Konrad K 1979 Zur Ultrastruktur der Tumor-Stromagrenze des invasiven Larynxkarzinoms. Laryngol Rhinol Otol 58: 575–582

79. Shi S R, Bhan A K, Pilch B Z, Chen L B, Goodman M L 1984 Keratin antibody localization in head and neck tissues and neoplasms. J Laryngol Otol 98: 1241–1250

80. Silvestri F, Bussani R, Stanta G, Cosatti C, Ferlito A 1992 Supraglottic versus glottic laryngeal cancer: epidemiological and pathological aspects. ORL J Otorhinolaryngol Relat Spec 54: 43–48

80a. Simaskos N, Palaiologos Y, Eliopoulos P N 1992 Trichinosis and cancer of the larynx. J Laryngol Otol 106: 171–172

81. Stell P M 1981 Total laryngectomy. Clin Otolaryngol 6: 351–360

82. Stell P M 1988 Prognostic factors in laryngeal carcinoma. Clin Otolaryngol 13: 399–409

83. Stell P M 1991 Ploidy in head and neck cancer: a review and meta-analysis. Clin Otolaryngol 16: 510–516

84. Terry R M, Gray C, Bird C C 1986 Aberrant expression of low molecular weight cytokeratins in primary and secondary squamous cell carcinoma of the head and neck. J Laryngol Otol 100: 1283–1287

85. Terry R M, Gray C, Jackson P, Bird C C 1986 Expression of low molecular weight cytokeratins in the neoplastic vocal cord. J Laryngol Otol 100: 1279–1282

86. Traserra J, Comas J, Conde C, Cuchi A, Cardesa A 1990 Metastatic involvement of the cavernous sinus from primary pharyngolaryngeal tumours. Head Neck 12: 426–429

87. Tsuruta Y, Matsunaga T, Miyahara H, Tanaka O, Kanata K, Ueda K 1991 Flow cytometric analysis of DNA content in paraffin-embedded tissue in head and neck cancer (the second report) — primary lesions of the laryngeal cancer. J Otolaryngol Jpn 94: 34–40

88. Vidic B, Tucker J A, Tucker G F 1977 Surface characterization of the epithelial cells from the human plica vocalis. Ear Nose Throat J 56: 328–334

89. Virchow R 1863 Die Krankhaften Geschwülste 1863. Hirschwald, Berlin

90. Walker G K, Fechner R E, Johns M E, Teja K 1982 Necrotizing sialometaplasia of the larynx secondary to atheromatous embolization. Am J Clin Pathol 77: 221–223

91. Wenig B L, Applebaum E L 1991 The submandibular triangle in squamous cell carcinoma of the larynx and hypopharynx. Laryngoscope 101: 516–518

92. Yasuda N, Omori A, Goto T, Hisa Y, Murakami Y, Otsuki T 1990 Prognostic significance of the DNA ploidy of the early glottic cancer. J Otolaryngol Jpn 93: 1171–1190

93. Zahra M, Tewfik H H, McCabe B F 1986 Metastases to the cavernous sinus from primary carcinoma of the larynx. J Surg Oncol 31: 69–70

94. Zohar Y, Talmi Y P, Finkelstein Y, Nobel M, Gafter U 1991 Syndrome of inappropriate antidiuretic hormone secretion in cancer of the head and neck. Ann Otol Rhinol Laryngol 100: 341–344

11. Atypical forms of squamous cell carcinoma

A. Ferlito

Atypical forms of squamous cell carcinoma include verrucous squamous cell carcinoma, spindle cell carcinoma, adenoid squamous cell carcinoma, basaloid squamous cell carcinoma, lymphoepithelial carcinoma and probably giant cell carcinoma.

VERRUCOUS SQUAMOUS CELL CARCINOMA

Introduction

Friedell and Rosenthal[51] recognized this tumour in 1941 and described eight lesions of verrucoid character in the buccal mucosa and alveolar ridge of tobacco chewers. The morphologically and biologically differentiating features of this neoplasm were well defined by Ackerman,[2] who coined the term 'verrucous carcinoma' in 1948. He reported 31 cases occurring in the oral cavity, predominantly in the buccal mucosa and lower gingiva of elderly men who had a history of tobacco chewing. He stressed that verrucous carcinoma must not be confused with squamous cell carcinoma as it differs both in structural characteristics and in prognosis, which is excellent.

Terminology

The terms for designating this tumour are verrucous squamous cell carcinoma, verrucous carcinoma, verrucous cancer, verrucose squamous carcinoma[31,114] and Ackerman tumour. Other terms have been used when the tumour has involved different organs. Glanz and Kleinsasser[53,54] consider the lesion benign, and both propose the term 'verrucous acanthosis', classifying such lesions as facultative precanceroses. Conversely, the recently revised version of the WHO classification of tumours of the upper respiratory tract and ear[109] classifies the verrucous carcinoma as a distinct malignant carcinoma.

Batsakis et al[15] coined the term 'hybrid verrucous squamous carcinoma' to indicate that foci of conventional invasive squamous carcinoma also exist in a typical verrucous carcinoma.[85]

Definition

This tumour is a distinct, pathological and clinical variant of well-differentiated squamous cell carcinoma which may develop in any mucosal surface.

Incidence

The reported incidence is 1–4% of all laryngeal cancers.[43,121] Fisher[46] reported 31 cases of verrucous carcinoma of the larynx, five of which involved lymph node metastases. Some doubts have been raised concerning his diagnostic accuracy, not only because this tumour accounted for 11% of a group of 276 infiltrating carcinomas of the larynx (the highest incidence reported in the world literature to date), but also because the grade I squamous cell carcinomas found in his series amounted to only 5%. The relatively high incidence of lymph node metastases (five cases) observed by Fisher[46] might well stem from his classifying some well-differentiated squamous cell carcinomas (which have a less favourable prognosis) as verrucous carcinomas. Goethals et al[55] first mentioned that verrucous cancer can occur in the larynx in 1963. Kraus and Perez-Mesa[68] reported 105 cases in various organs, 12 of which involved the larynx. In Europe, the lesion was rarely recognized and the first reports of this tumour came from Padua University.[6,36,37,43,44] In 1975, Bak and Erdös[7] reported the first case of verrucous cancer of the larynx observed in Hungary. The tumour is primarily mentioned in English literature, but it goes unrecognized in some parts of the world.[23] Thomas et al[117] described the first case observed in India. The first report of a case of verrucous carcinoma in Africa has recently been published.[65] To date, approximately 500 cases have been reported in the literature.[1,11,19–21,27,40,48,53,57,58,60,64,70,77,80,92,93,98,103,105,111] In particular, 118 cases of verrucous carcinoma of the larynx were seen between 1976 and 1985 at the Armed Forces Institute of Pathology in Washington DC[60] and 138 were collected between 1966 and 1991 at the ENT Department of Padua University. The larynx is the most common site for this tumour within the respiratory tract and the second most common location in the body as a whole, after the oral cavity.[76] Other areas reported are the ear, rhinopharynx, nasal cavity, paranasal sinuses, oesophagus, male and female genitalia, perineum, urinary bladder and skin.

Clinical features

The tumour occurs in both sexes, but predominantly in men in their seventies and eighties. Most patients are cigarette smokers. This neoplasm has not been reported in a child's larynx. The clinical appearance of verrucous carcinoma of the larynx is a warty, pale, bulky, exophytic outgrowth usually affecting one, but sometimes both vocal cords, which initially maintain their mobility. The tumour may also occur in other parts of the larynx. The presenting symptoms may be insignificant in the early stages of this slowly-developing neoplasm. Long-standing hoarseness and dyspnoea develop due to obstruction of the laryngeal lumen by the fungating neoplasm. Occasionally the first symptom is dysphagia or haemoptysis.[71] Urgent tracheostomy may be required for the obstruction before the diagnosis has been established.[18,68] Regional lymph nodes may be enlarged due to inflammatory changes simulating a secondary tumour, but are never metastatic.

Fisher[46] and Schrader et al[106] reported some cases of verrucous cancer with lymph node metastases, but it seems that no acceptable example of a verrucous cancer of the larynx has given rise to metastases.

Aetiology and histogenesis

Human papilloma virus (HPV) has been identified in two cases of verrucous carcinoma of the vagina using Southern blot DNA hybridization under low-stringency conditions.[95] Abramson et al[1] studied tissue specimens from five patients with verrucous cancer of the larynx and analysed them for the presence of HPV by means of histological findings, immunohistochemistry and DNA hybridization. They clearly demonstrated HPV16-related DNA sequences in the tumour and in the adjacent healthy tissues in all cases. Fliss et al[48] recently conducted a retrospective clinicopathological review and tested specimens from 21 laryngeal verrucous carcinomas for the presence of HPV DNA, using the polymerase chain reaction. Their results suggested an association between this tumour and HPV types 16 and/or 18. Zachow et al[126] detected human papilloma virus DNA in anogenital verrucous carcinoma and HPV16 was found in laryngeal verrucous carcinomas too.[20,66,98] Viral infection may play an important role in verrucous carcinoma of the larynx. Fisker and Philipsen[47] reported that verrucous cancer was produced following application of the carcinogen 4-nitroquinoline-1-oxide to the oral cavity of rats three times weekly for up to 18 weeks. This tumour has also been reported in a renal transplant patient after long-term immunosuppression.[120] The tumour originates from the stratified squamous epithelium or ciliated columnar epithelium following squamous metaplasia.

Pathology

Gross pathology

The tumour appears to be a broadly implanted, non-ulcerated, exophytic, grey-white fungating mass, with papillary fronds and a locally invasive nature (Figs 11.1–11.8). The gross appearance of the tumour is quite characteristic and virtually pathognomonic. Some verrucous carcinomas can be multifocal on presentation and separated by normal skip areas of epithelium.

Histopathology

The tumour is composed of islands and solid cords of highly differentiated squamous epithelial cells. Cytological malignancy criteria are lacking or minimal (Figs 11.9–11.12). Anaplasia is absent, and this may lead to an incorrect diagnosis. Prominent koilocytotic cells with dark pyknotic nuclei have occasionally been observed (Fig. 11.13).[1] The surface is covered by a thick layer of keratinized cells (Fig. 11.14) arranged in invaginating bulbous acanthotic folds. Vertical sections of the neoplasm show epithelial spires capped by a thick parakeratotic or keratotic layer. The continuity of the irregular verrucous surface is maintained by long filiform processes of well-differentiated squamous cells. There is typically a considerable inflammatory reaction in the stroma composed of lymphocytes and plasma cells which tend to delimit the tumour mass (Figs 11.10, 11.11), the margins of which appear to be pushing and blunt (Fig. 11.11) rather than infiltrating. Epithelial pearls, keratinous cysts, micro and macro abscesses may be noted (Figs 11.15, 11.16). Foreign stromal keratin granulomas may also be seen close to epithelial pearls or around keratinized matter. Mitoses are rare and tend to be concentrated in the basal–parabasal region (Fig. 11.17); benign cellular features, coupled with the orderly maturation sequence, belie the locally destructive nature of the tumour. Invasion of the basement membrane and glandular structures (Fig. 11.18) is often seen and, if the tumour is neglected, there may be destruction of adjoining tissues, including muscle[76] and cartilage (Fig. 11.19)[50,65,69] and thyroid gland.[31] Exceptionally, perineural involvement has been reported in human[28] and experimental[47] neoplasms. Invasion of the mandible has been reported in verrucous carcinoma of the oral cavity.[2,76]

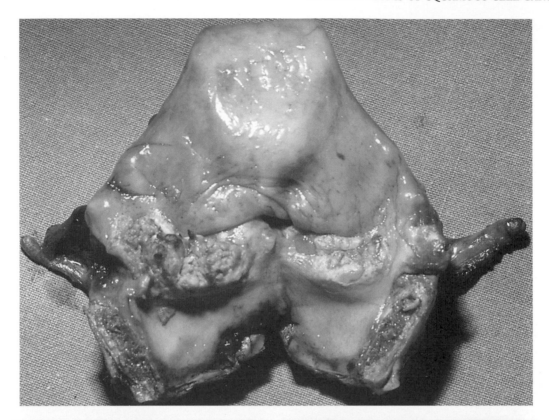

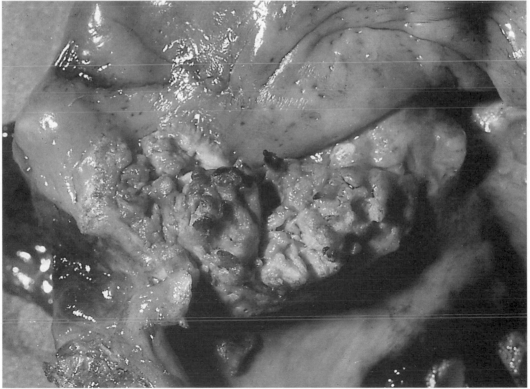

Fig. 11.1 (*top*) Laryngectomy specimen showing characteristic verrucous carcinoma involving both vocal cords, with extension into subglottis.

Fig. 11.2 (*bottom*) Detail from previous figure.

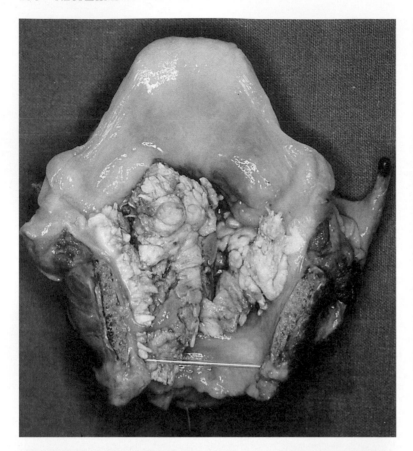

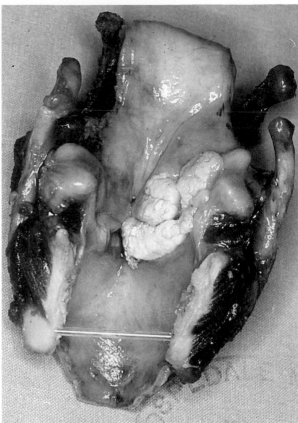

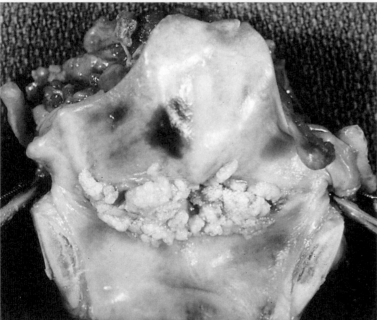

Fig. 11.3 (*top, left*) Laryngectomy specimen showing verrucous carcinoma involving three regions of the larynx.

Fig. 11.4 (*bottom*) Laryngectomy specimen showing fungating cauliflower-like tumour occupying the full length of both vocal cords, obliterating both laryngeal ventricles and extending onto the false vocal cords. (Courtesy of Professor J. Olofsson, Bergen).

Fig. 11.5 (*top, right*) Laryngectomy specimen showing a proliferating verrucous carcinoma occurring in the right glottic area and extending into the supraglottic region.

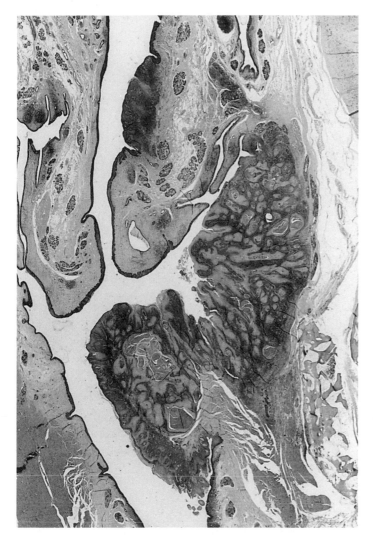

Fig. 11.6 Coronal section of the lesion in Fig. 11.5. Despite its size, the tumour is not deeply invasive.

Immunocytochemistry

This neoplasm shows positive staining for epithelial membrane antigen (EMA) and cytokeratin.[112]

Electron microscopy

The tumour is composed mainly of mature squamous epithelial cells with an overall architecture resembling normal epidermis. Desmosomes and filaments are present: numerous interdigitating membranes and well-developed desmosomes characterize the cells above the basal layer.[99] This neoplasm demonstrates a cytokinetically inactive layer of non-proliferating and non-keratinized cells between the basal germinative zones and the surface. Such a layer has not been observed in other types of squamous cell carcinoma.[99,125]

Diagnosis and differential diagnosis

Histological re-examination of laryngeal carcinomas with a verrucous macroscopic appearance has revealed that about 50% could not be accepted as verrucous carcinomas, according to conventional criteria. This fact has been observed in several series.[82,104,111] Correct diagnosis requires a close co-operation between the laryngologist and the pathologist, particularly when repeated biopsies show only a morphological pattern of diffuse keratosis, while the clinical appearance is suggestive of a malignant lesion. On examination of the larynx, the clinician often tends to overestimate the aggressiveness of this neoplasm. Conversely, the surgical pathologist tends to misinterpret the true nature of the lesion, particularly in a small biopsy specimen. Superficial biopsies may lack the characteristic histological signs, so full-thickness biopsies are a diagnostic necessity, indeed, a sine qua non.[52] It is not uncommon for multiple biopsies to be necessary to establish diagnosis when a clinically verrucous cancer contradicts a benign histological appearance.[7,18,34,65] When possible, excisional biopsy is ideal for diagnosing this lesion. Diagnosis stems from a combined clinical and histological decision, and both aspects must be properly considered.[116] Microspectrophotometric studies may be helpful in establishing the diagnosis.[45] DNA values above the diploid level (4n–8n) may prove the malignancy of cells which appear histologically benign.[44] Michaels et al[90] believe that image analysis of cells may assist in the early histological diagnosis of verrucous squamous cell carcinoma, particularly for distinguishing the tumour from benign squamous papilloma. Mean cell areas and nuclear areas are significantly larger in verrucous squamous cell carcinoma than in a squamous papilloma. The high degree of differentiation and the lack of any definite evidence of invasiveness may lead to an incorrect assumption of benignity if biopsy specimens from such a neoplasm are considered without reference to its clinical features. The tumour is thus often underdiagnosed by the pathologist.

The lesion is distinguished from a well-differentiated squamous cell carcinoma having a verrucoid or papillary pattern by its lack of cytological features of malignancy, its growth pattern and the absence of lymph node or visceral metastases. Ferlito and Recher[43] summarized the different pathological and clinical aspects of the two lesions, as shown in Table 11.1. Differential diagnosis must also be made with respect to papillary keratosis[46] and verruca vulgaris.[10,35] Papillary keratosis shows numerous, rather uniform, keratohyaline granules in the epithelial cells just beneath the keratin layer (stratum granulosum). These granules are rare or lacking in verrucous carcinoma.[9] The rete pegs are elongated, thin and pointed in papillary keratosis, whereas verrucous carcinoma is composed of bulbous rete pegs. Verruca vulgaris usually shows numerous large keratohyaline granules and

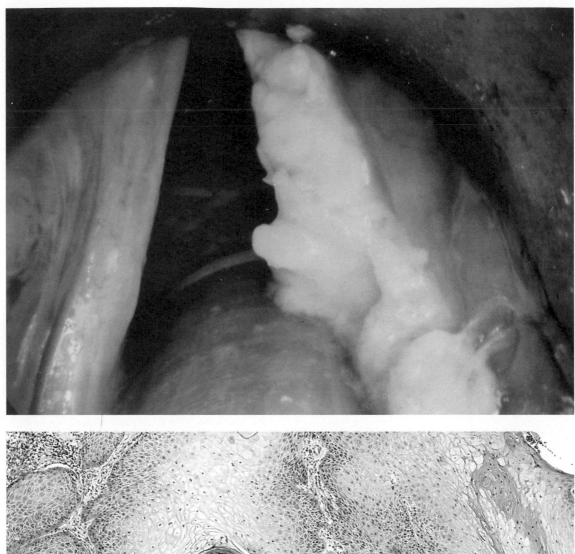

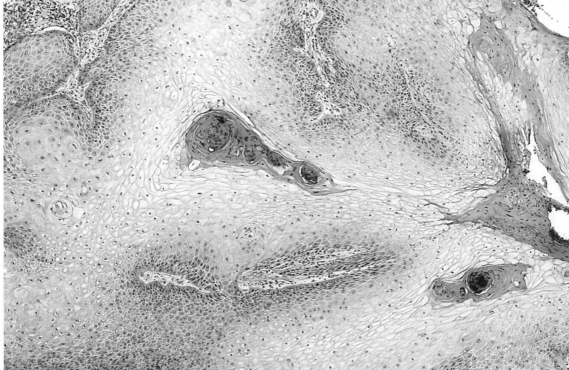

Fig. 11.7 (*top*) Verrucous carcinoma of the right vocal cord.

Fig. 11.8 (*bottom*) Microscopic pattern of verrucous carcinoma. H&E, ×16 OM.

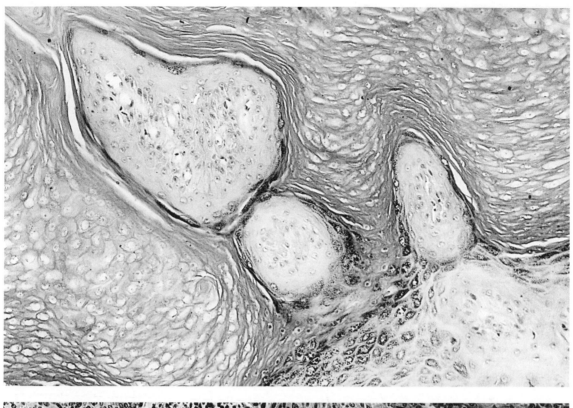

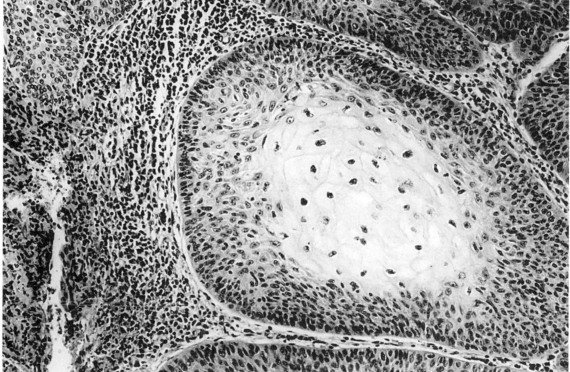

Fig. 11.9 (*top*) Marked hyperkeratosis is present. H&E, ×100 OM.

Fig. 11.10 (*bottom*) Blunt invasion of laryngeal verrucous carcinoma. A dense inflammatory reaction is present in the stroma. H&E, ×40 OM.

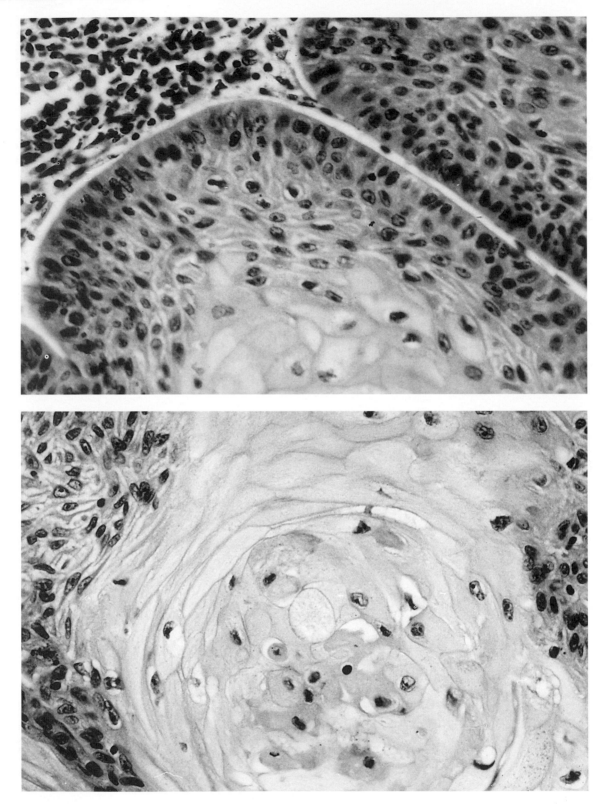

Fig. 11.11 (*top*) Detail from previous figure. H&E, ×100 OM.

Fig. 11.12 (*bottom*) Cytological criteria of malignancy are usually lacking. H&E, ×100 OM.

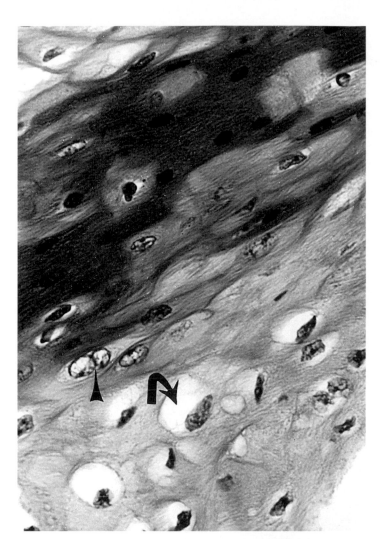

Fig. 11.13 (*top*) Koilocytotic atypia in verrucous carcinoma. Koilocyte is marked by curved arrow and surrounded by smaller koilocytotic cells with dark pyknotic nuclei. Arrowhead indicates binucleate cell. Dark area is parakeratosis. H&E, ×320. (Courtesy of Dr A. L. Abramson, New York, and the editor of *Archives of Otolaryngology*.)

Fig. 11.14 (*bottom*) The tumour is covered by prominent keratin. H&E, ×16 OM.

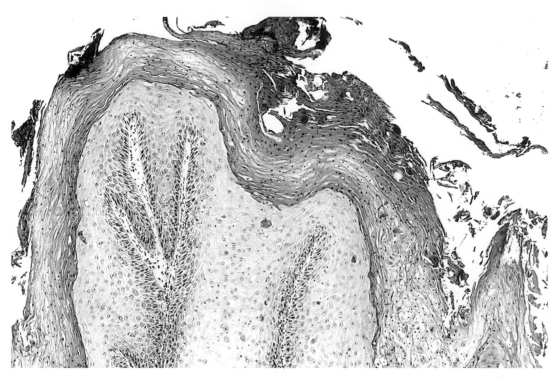

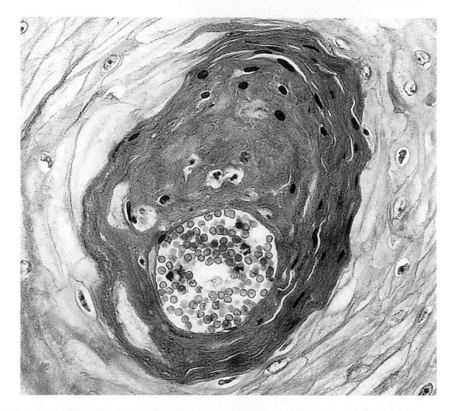

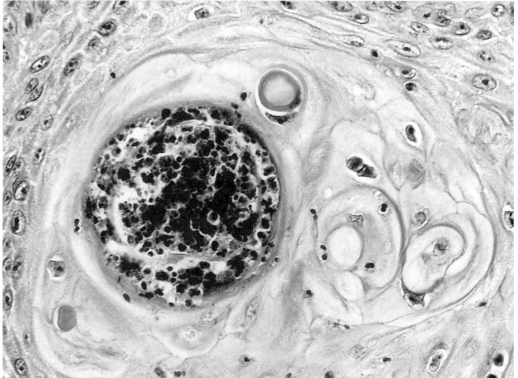

Fig. 11.15 (*top*) A keratinous cyst is observable. H&E, ×100 OM.

Fig. 11.16 (*bottom*) Micro-abscess typical of verrucous carcinoma. H&E, ×100 OM.

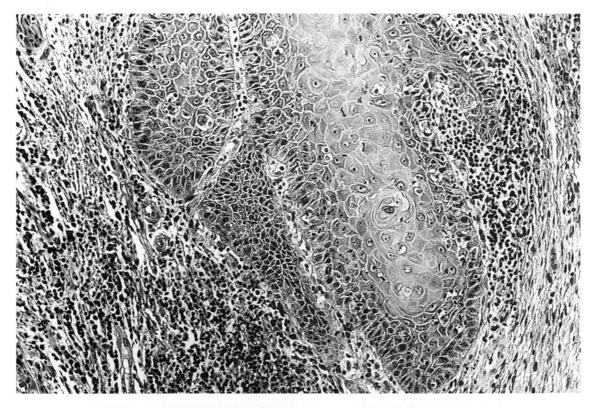

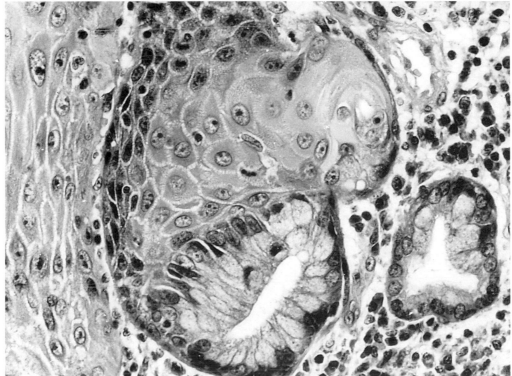

Fig. 11.17 (*top*) Dysplastic cellular changes are present in the basal–parabasal region. H&E, ×40 OM.

Fig. 11.18 (*bottom*) Glandular structure is invaded by the tumour. H&E, ×100 OM.

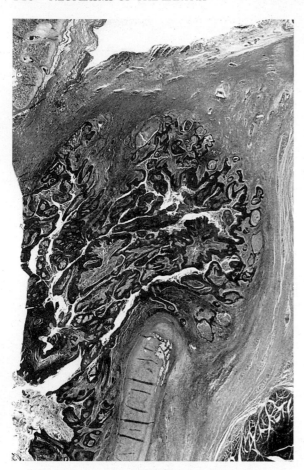

Fig. 11.19 (*top*) Lower-power view of verrucous carcinoma showing deep epithelial-lined clefts invading over the top of the thyroid cartilage. The luminal surface of the carcinoma has been artefactually lost. H&E, ×4.5 (Courtesy of Dr E. Duvall, Edinburgh, and the editor of *Journal of Laryngology and Otology*.)

Fig. 11.20 (*bottom*) A biopsy after radiotherapy illustrating anaplastic transformation of a typical verrucous carcinoma arising in the supraglottic region. The patient died of disseminated disease 10 months after radiotherapy. H&E, ×300. (Courtesy of Professor J. Olofsson, Bergen, and the editor of *Cancer*.)

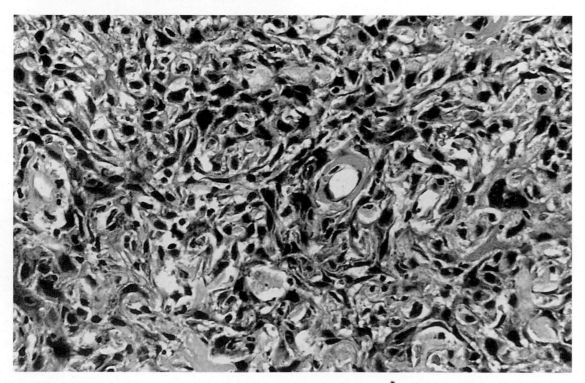

Table 11.1 Comparison of pathological and clinical findings between squamous carcinoma and verrucous squamous carcinoma

Features	Squamous cell carcinoma	Verrucous squamous cell carcinoma
Macroscopic appearance	Various appearances	Fungating, cauliflower-like tumour
Cellular differentiation	Various degrees	High
Cytological features of malignancy	Present	Absent or occasional
Margins	Infiltrating	Pushing
Cellular response	Variable	Prominent
Cleft-like spaces and small cysts	Usually absent	Present
Grade of malignancy	Moderate or high	Low
Local metastases	Usually present	Absent
Distant metastases	May be present	Absent
Prognosis	Depends on various factors, but is never as favourable as for verrucous squamous carcinoma	Excellent

koilocytotic (clear) cells.[10] These features are rare or lacking in verrucous carcinoma. Verruca vulgaris can be distinguished from papillary keratosis by the koilocytotic cells, which are present in the former but not in the latter.[9] The criteria for diagnosing verrucous squamous cell carcinoma are as follows[40]:

1. Patients are usually elderly men
2. The glottis is the most common site
3. A fungating and exophytic warty tumour formation with multiple filiform projections
4. Advancing, pushing and well-demarcated margins
5. Deeply projecting, cleft-like spaces with degenerating keratin and subsequent cystic degeneration of the central portion of the filiform projection
6. A high degree of cellular differentiation
7. The absence of cytological features of malignancy (small focal areas of cellular atypia may occasionally be present in minor components of large lesions)
8. Prominent stromal evidence of a chronic inflammatory reaction (especially the presence of lymphocytes and plasma cells)
9. Evidence of foreign-body granulomas near epithelial pearls or keratinized matter
10. Non-metastatic behaviour.

Therapy

There is considerable controversy as to the correct treatment for this tumour. At the Centennial Conference of Laryngeal Cancer held in Toronto, Hyams[63] said that it is a surgical disease since typical verrucous carcinomas do not respond to irradiation, but others hold the opposite opinion.[24,81,102,107] Lundgren et al[77] believe that verrucous carcinoma is not radio-resistant but seems less sensitive to irradiation than ordinary squamous cell carcinoma. Harwood[59] advocates irradiation with surgery in reserve. On the other hand, Ferlito and Recher[43] reviewed all reported cases of verrucous cancer of the head and neck that had been treated initially with

radiotherapy and found that the neoplasm persisted or recurred in 64 (71%) of the 90 cases treated. By contrast, only 7 (7%) of 103 patients receiving surgical treatment had recurrences.[15,18,24,28,43,104] Given the large number of irradiation-treated cases with recurrence,[43,57,77,92,97,104] this does not appear to be the treatment of choice for verrucous cancer of the larynx, quite apart from the risk of post–irradiation anaplastic or sarcomatoid changes observed (Fig. 11.20) in this or other sites.[8,17,18,24,28,49,57,68,83,87,100,112,121] The latent period for anaplastic transformation is short, usually a few months. This brief transformation time may be explained by the fact that verrucous carcinoma cells are already genetically abnormal.[1] Batsakis et al[15] and Michaels[89] suggested that anaplastic transformation is an event which is probably overestimated. The presence of cervical and distant metastases after radiation therapy has also been reported.[30,97,112] Human papilloma virus (HPV16)-related sequences were identified by DNA hybridization in five patients, which suggests that radiotherapy is contraindicated because of its potential for activating or altering HPV16-related sequences.[1] Radiation-induced DNA breaks may activate these sequences.[57] Edström et al[30] provide evidence of increased metastatic potential after irradiation for T1-2 verrucous carcinomas of the larynx as compared with the common type of squamous cell carcinoma. Radiation may have some clinical validity as a therapeutic alternative if surgical treatment is contraindicated[111] but Abramson et al[1] believe that radiotherapy should not be used unless the potential consequences and molecular mechanisms are fully explained. Hagen et al[57] recently added 12 new cases of laryngeal verrucous carcinoma and reviewed the literature concerning radiation versus surgical results. Thirty-seven patients treated with primary radiotherapy resulted in 49% cure, 51% failure and 11% deaths from anaplastic transformation. Primary surgery on 144 patients resulted in 92.4% cure, 7.6% initial failure and 3.5% deaths. Their treatment recommendations were as follows: for T1 lesions, CO_2 laser excision; for T2–T4 lesions, sound oncological extirpation. In conclusion, surgery alone seems to be the most effective form of therapy, and has been regarded historically as the treatment of choice for verrucous cancer because it has higher cure rates and lower percentages of recurrence. The lesion is usually amenable to conservative surgery (i.e., cordectomy, horizontal glottectomy, hemilaryngectomy or supraglottic laryngectomy), though total laryngectomy should be performed where necessary (e.g., evidence of cartilage invasion, extralaryngeal spread or deep infiltration of the paraglottic space). Operative treatment should not include neck dissection,[40,43,57,104,111] even though enlarged and tender lymph nodes may be palpated. In fact, histological examination of these nodes has revealed only an inflammatory reaction. Cervical and distant metastases have not been reported in non-irradiated true verrucous carcinoma. Recurrence is likely after inadequate excision of the tumour, but recurrent lesions lack any definite microscopic evidence of malignancy. Maw et al[81] claim, on the basis of only two cases, that this neoplasm can be controlled by local surgical methods such as suction diathermy, criosurgery or laser therapy. Four cases of this lesion have been successfully managed by Lee[70] using endoscopic removal. Excisional biopsy is ideal for diagnosing and treating glottic verrucous carcinoma.[19]

This tumour is highly curable when adequate surgical treatment is used without delay. The major contraindication for radiation appears to be the neoplasm's high recurrence rate, so such treatment is not recommended for this lesion.

Prognosis

The prognosis is usually excellent[33,43] when adequate treatment is adopted from the beginning. In the series of 77 cases of this tumour reported by Ferlito and Recher,[43] only three patients died for reasons directly connected with the neoplasm, one of whom had refused treatment. Of a first group of 28 cases observed at the Armed Forces Institute of Pathology between 1939 and 1976, only one patient died of this disease, following his refusal of surgical treatment.[64] This tumour shows a tendency for the development of a secondary squamous cell carcinoma in the upper respiratory tract[15,43,55,68,86,121] or in other sites. There seems to be a greater risk of second primary carcinomas developing in patients with verrucous carcinoma of the oral cavity rather than of the larynx.[24]

SPINDLE CELL CARCINOMA

Introduction

So-called carcinosarcomas and pseudosarcomas are probably a single entity, i.e., squamous cell carcinomas with spindle cell features. Most of the neoplasms classified in the past as laryngeal sarcomas were really cases of spindle cell squamous carcinoma.

Terminology

Various terms have been used to designate this tumour, such as spindle cell squamous carcinoma, spindle cell carcinoma, pseudosarcoma, pleomorphic carcinoma, carcinosarcoma, pseudosarcoma associated with squamous cell carcinoma, metaplastic carcinoma, sarcomatoid squamous cell carcinoma, pseudosarcomatous squamous cell carcinoma, collision tumour, Lane tumour, squamous cell carcinoma with sarcoma like stroma, polypoid carcinoma, monophasic spindle cell carcinoma, biphasic spindle cell carcinoma, etc. These terms reflect the controversy surrounding the origin of the 'sarcomatous' component in this lesion.[14,22,39,72,96,110]

Definition

This is a rare, controversial, biphasic variant of squamous cell carcinoma in which a pseudosarcomatous component dominates the microscopic appearance of the tumour.

Incidence

The incidence varies with different reports, mainly because of the inconsistent interpretation of microscopic features. In the series seen in Padua, the incidence is about 1% of all laryngeal malignant neoplasms. Heffner[60] mentioned 241 cases of this neoplasm seen between 1976 and 1985 at the Armed Forces Institute of Pathology. The larynx is the most common site, followed by the oral cavity and oesophagus.

Clinical features

The male sex is affected far more, and the lesion is frequently seen in patients after middle age. The symptoms are similar to those of a squamous cell carcinoma affecting the same regions of the larynx. The tumour arises predominantly from the glottic region, and the anterior commissure in particular, but also occurs elsewhere (Fig. 11.21) in the larynx as a large, grey, often ulcerated, bulky, polypoid tumour.[52] The lesion may simulate a laryngeal polyp. CT scan and MRI (Figs 11.22, 11.23) are very useful in establishing the depth of invasion for large lesions.

Histogenesis

The histogenesis of this lesion has generated considerable controversy. Basically, there are four theories: (i) a 'collision' neoplasm or a dual growth of carcinoma and sarcoma; (ii) a squamous carcinoma with an atypical, benign, non-neoplastic, pseudosarcomatous, connective-tissue reaction incapable of metastasizing; (iii) a squamous carcinoma that has developed a spindle cell component (i.e., mesenchymal metaplasia); or (iv) a sarcoma. The various histogenetic hypotheses have been reviewed by

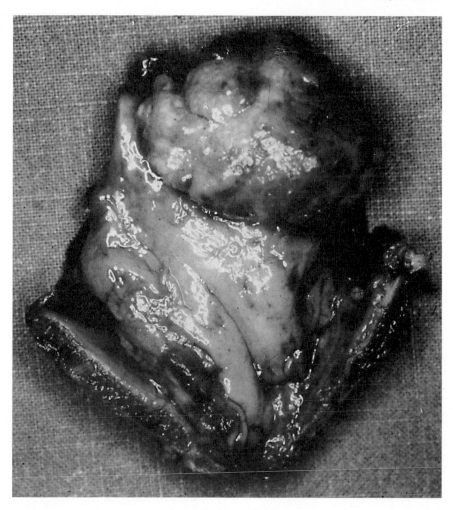

Fig. 11.21   Supraglottic laryngectomy specimen showing spindle cell carcinoma of the epiglottis.

Batsakis et al[14] and Brodsky,[22] who suggest six hypothetical histogenetic views: carcinosarcoma (collision tumour); carcinosarcoma (blastoma); spindle cell or pleomorphic carcinoma; carcinoma with pseudosarcoma; carcinosarcoma; carcinosarcoma (stromal transformation). Friedmann and Ferlito[52] suggest that the spindle-cell component is epithelial in origin, and they have provided histological evidence of transition from epithelial cells to spindle cells. The detection of keratin in fusiform tumour cells is a reliable indication that the neoplasm is a spindle cell variant of squamous cell carcinoma, and the presence of vimentin in spindle cells is suggestive of a mesenchymal phenotypic expression.[127]

Pathology

Gross pathology

Two-thirds of these tumours present a polypoid, pedunculated mass attached to the mucosa by a stalk; the others are infiltrative or sessile. The tumour surface is frequently ulcerated.

Light microscopy

The tumour is characterized by the predominance of spindle-shaped cells forming a sarcoma-like pattern and by the presence of atypical, often bizarre cells with pleomorphic nuclei (Figs 11.24, 11.25). Mitoses are typical. Osteoclast-like giant cells may occur and there may be some osteoid, chondroid or osseous metaplasia. Adequate histological examination always discloses areas of more or less differentiated squamous cell carcinoma, in situ, infiltrative or both, next to apparently sarcomatous areas (Figs 11.26–11.28). Occasionally, carcinomatous foci are found within the central area of stromal proliferation. A storiform pattern may be present. Absence of the epithelial component, which may well be lacking in small biopsy fragments, may lead to an incorrect diagnosis of sarcoma. Sometimes the lesion may simulate atypical granulation tissue. Lymph node and distant metastases usually contain squamous epithelial elements alone or both a squamous and a spindle cell element, or occasionally a spindle cell component alone.

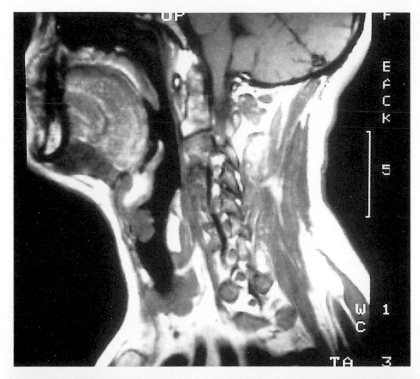

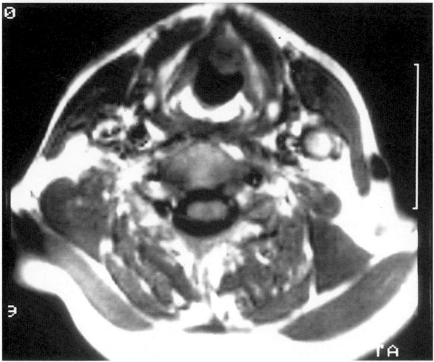

Fig. 11.22 (*top*) Spin-Echo (proton density) magnetic resonance image in sagittal projection. Polypoid mass arising in the anterior commissure.

Fig. 11.23 (*bottom*) Spin-Echo (proton density) magnetic resonance image in axial projection showing the extension of the lesion downward into the subglottic region.

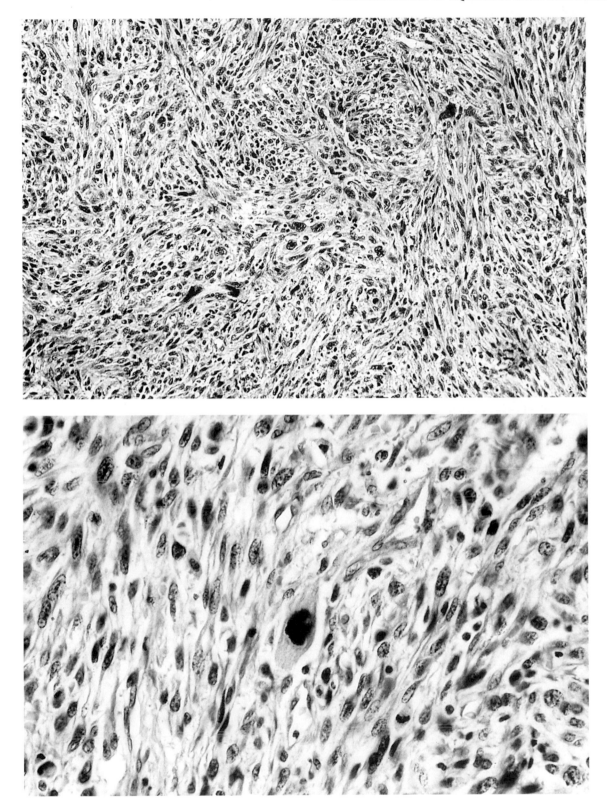

Fig. 11.24 (*top*) Sarcoma-like pattern is seen. H&E, ×40 OM.

Fig. 11.25 (*bottom*) Showing cytological details of the pleomorphic spindle cells. H&E, ×100 OM.

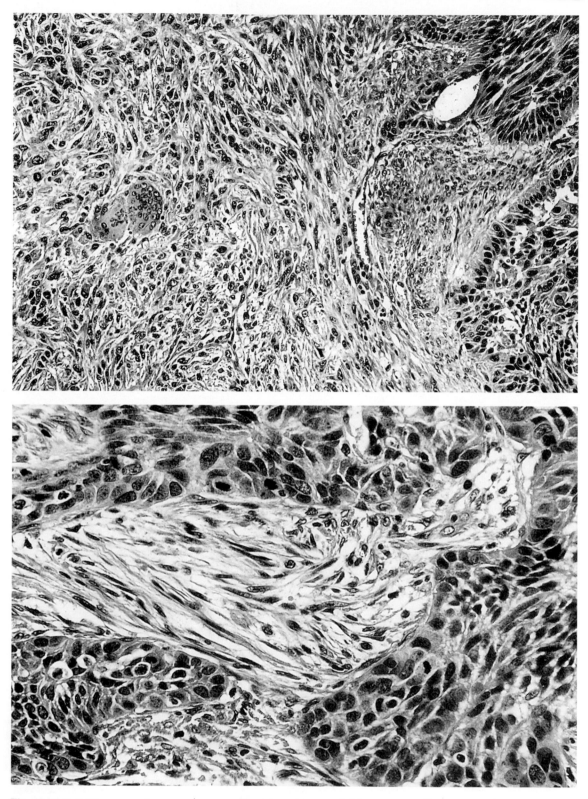

Fig. 11.26 (*top*) Microscopy shows a squamous cell carcinoma surrounded by a sarcoma-like pattern. H&E, ×40 OM.

Fig. 11.27 (*bottom*) Proliferation of squamous cell carcinoma and spindle cell component. H&E, ×100 OM.

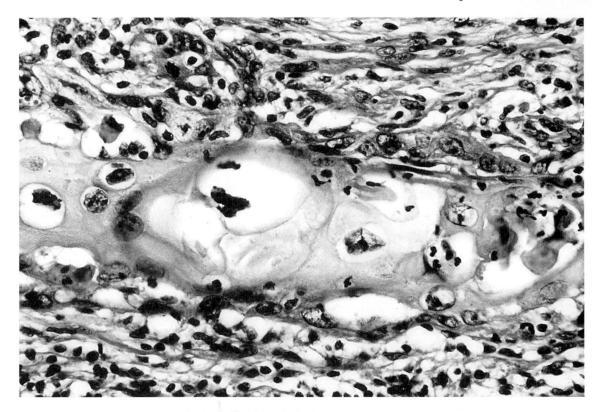

Fig. 11.28   In this biphasic neoplasm, the squamous component is well differentiated. H&E, ×100 OM.

Immunocytochemistry

This tumour may show positive staining for cytokeratin (Fig. 11.29), EMA, carcino-embryonic antigen (CEA) and vimentin; alpha-1-antitrypsin (AAT), alpha-1-antichymotrypsin (ACT) and albumin may also be positive.[86,127] In particular, individual spindle cell tumours may reveal co-expression of vimentin and keratin.[32,86,124,127]

Electron microscopy

In many tumour cells, Lichtiger et al[74] identified the presence of aggregates of keratohyaline and slender bundles of tonofilaments and occasional premelanosomes. This supports the definition of the tumour as a spindle cell squamous carcinoma. Battifora[16] carried out transmission electron microscopy studies on two cases of spindle cell squamous carcinoma and suggested that the pseudo-sarcomatous component of the tumour originates from mesenchymal metaplasia of squamous cells and that collagen is produced by these metaplastic cells. Other ultrastructural investigations support the idea that sarcoma-like elements arise through transformation of epithelial cells.[86]

In studies on spindle cell carcinoma experimentally induced in the trachea of hamsters, results were consistent with the squamous origin of the tumour.[115]

Diagnosis and differential diagnosis

The diagnosis of spindle cell carcinoma is made with relative ease if there is a squamous carcinomatous component, but becomes difficult when this is lacking. The tumour may be confused with fibrosarcoma, malignant fibrous sarcoma and spindle cell malignant melanoma. Immunocytochemical investigations to identify keratin intermediate filaments may be helpful in establishing a diagnosis of spindle cell carcinoma,[61,96,118] but a negative result does not necessarily rule out a malignant epithelial neoplasm.[32] S-100 protein is usually lacking in spindle cell carcinoma and is present in malignant melanoma. AAT and ACT may be found in spindle cell carcinoma and in malignant fibrous histiocytoma.[32] Co-expression of more than one intermediate filament type, such as keratin and vimentin, has been observed in other epithelial neoplasms, such as adenoid cystic carcinoma.[25] The presence of cervical lymph node metastases leads to the diagnosis of spindle cell carcinoma rather than sarcoma. A 'sarcomatoid' component may rarely be seen with adenocarcinoma[14] and verrucous carcinoma.[14,73] Exceptionally, a tumour may show foci of squamous carcinoma, verrucous carcinoma and spindle cell carcinoma.[78] True fibrosarcoma of the larynx is extremely rare and is a marker-negative tumour, except for vimentin.[41] The presence of numerous osteoclast-like giant cells in spindle cell

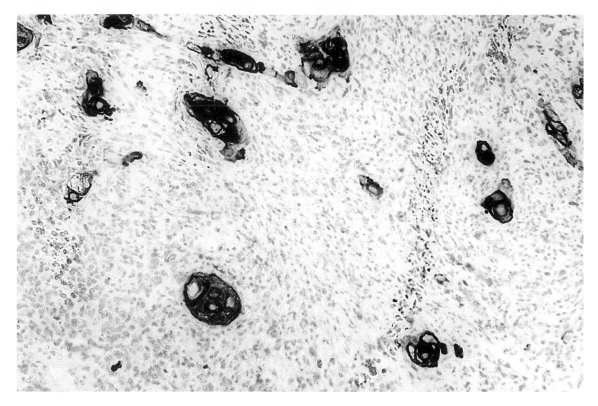

Fig. 11.29   Immunopositivity for cytokeratin in spindle cell squamous carcinoma. Anti-cytokeratin ×100 OM.

carcinoma may simulate malignant giant cell tumour of the soft parts.[5]

Therapy

The elective treatment is surgery, and neck dissection is often indicated. Radiotherapy has also been used successfully in limited lesions.

Prognosis

Patients with polypoid tumours have a better prognosis than those with ulcerative-infiltrating tumours. Survival is inversely related to depth of invasion.[73,124] Metastases to lymph nodes are frequent, and distant metastases have also occurred (Figs 11.30–11.32).[101]

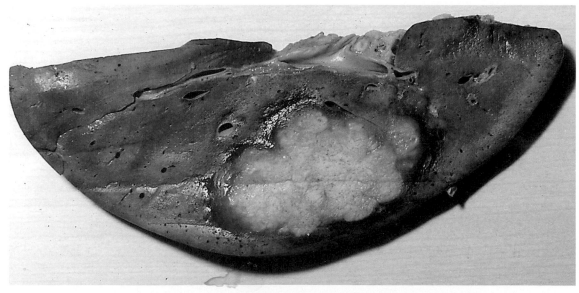

Fig. 11.30   Secondary deposit in the liver of spindle cell squamous carcinoma.

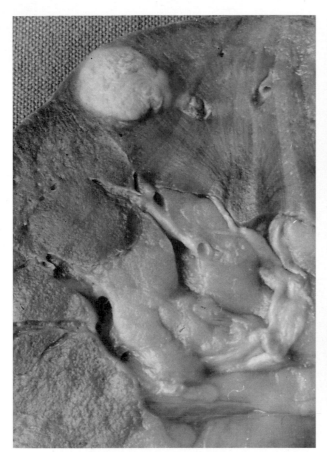 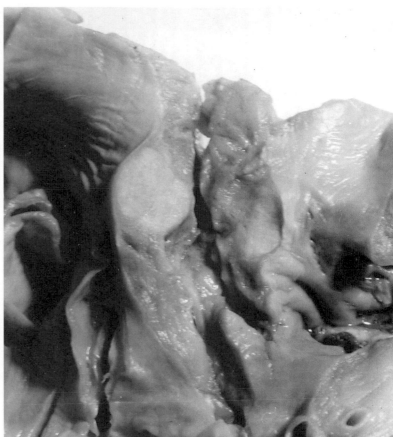

Fig. 11.31 (*left*) Isolated blood-borne deposit in the kidney of spindle cell squamous carcinoma.

Fig. 11.32 (*right*) Cardiac metastasis from spindle cell squamous carcinoma.

ADENOID SQUAMOUS CELL CARCINONA

This is an uncommon variant of squamous cell carcinoma featuring acantholysis of the malignant epidermoid cells producing pseudolumens that mimic glandular differentiation (Fig. 11.33). The neoplasm is also referred to as acantholytic squamous cell carcinoma, adenoacanthoma and pseudoglandular squamous cell carcinoma. The tumour has been observed in areas of skin exposed to the sun, in the vulva, lip, oral cavity and tongue and in the supraglottic portion of the larynx[62] and hypopharynx.[13] A differential diagnosis from adenosquamous carcinoma, adenoid cystic carcinoma and mucoepidermoid carcinoma has to be considered.[42] The neoplasm has an aggressive behaviour and a worse prognosis than conventional squamous cell carcinoma.[13]

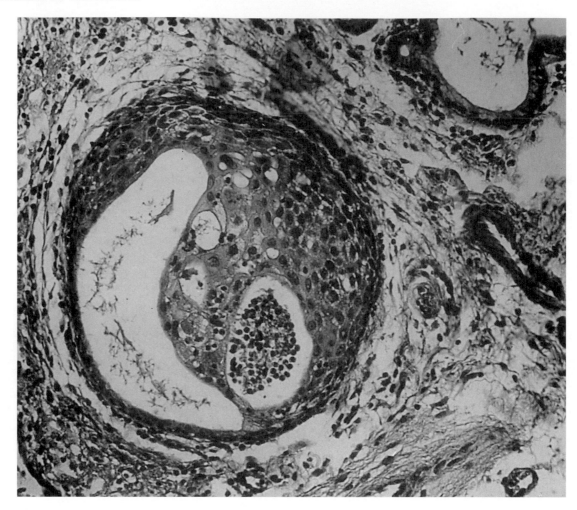

Fig. 11.33   Adenoid squamous cell carcinoma of the larynx producing pseudolumens containing cellular debris. H&E, ×100 OM.

BASALOID SQUAMOUS CELL CARCINOMA

Basaloid squamous cell carcinoma is a rare, distinct histopathological entity which was accurately described by Wain et al[123] in 1986 and recently accepted by the WHO.[109] It is a carcinoma with a mixed basaloid and squamous component and manifests a predilection for the supraglottic larynx (Fig. 11.34), hypopharynx and tongue base.[7a,b,12,75, 84,95a,108,110a,119a,123] The tumour is also called basaloid carcinoma. The basaloid pattern is associated with in situ and/or invasive squamous cell carcinoma and consists of small, crowded cells with hyperchromatic nuclei, scant cytoplasm, small cystic spaces containing material resembling mucin that stains with PAS and/or Alcian blue, foci of coagulative necrosis within the central areas of the tumour lobules (comedonecrosis) and focal areas of stromal hyalinization (Figs 11.35–11.38). The squamous carcinoma is usually well or moderately differentiated, and may be superficial or invasive. Biopsy specimens may not be representative of the whole lesion.[12] Metastases to the lymph nodes reveal both the squamous and the basaloid component.

Immunohistochemically, the tumour shows reactivity for cytokeratin, EMA, CEA, neuron-specific enolase, S-100 protein and vimentin. Ultrastructurally, the basaloid cells possess few organelles other than desmosomes, rare tonofilaments and free ribosomes.[123] The neoplasm seems to originate from a totipotent primitive cell located at the base of the pseudostratified columnar epithelium or in the proximal salivary gland ducts of the larynx.[123] The tumour may be confused with adenoid cystic carcinoma (solid or basaloid type), small cell neuroendocrine carcinoma (combined type), adenosquamous carcinoma and squamous cell carcinoma. In the case reported by McKay and Bilous,[84] and in two of our series, the initial histological diagnosis was adenoid cystic carcinoma.

The prognosis is usually worse than that of conventional squamous cell carcinoma. This tumour is regarded as a biologically high-grade malignancy with a tendency for locally aggressive behaviour and early regional and distant metastases.[75,110a] The most common sites of metastatic spread are the cervical lymph nodes, lung (Fig. 11.39), bone and skin. Surgery followed by radiation appears to be the treatment of choice, but the number of

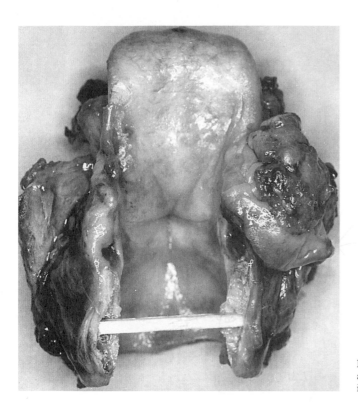

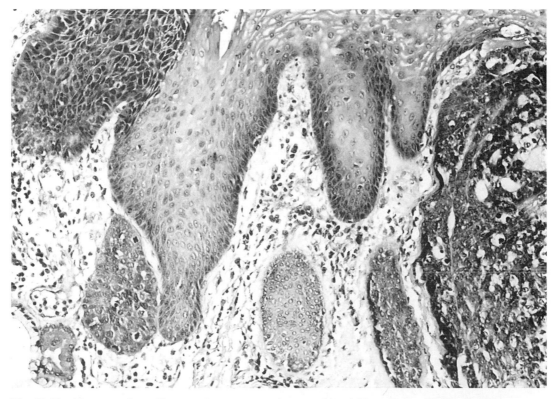

Fig. 11.34 (*left*) Basaloid squamous cell carcinoma originating from the right aryepiglottic fold and extending into the pyriform fossa. This neoplasm was initially diagnosed as a combined small cell neuroendocrine carcinoma.

Fig. 11.35   Mucosa surface with areas of squamous carcinoma and basaloid carcinoma. H&E, ×40 OM.

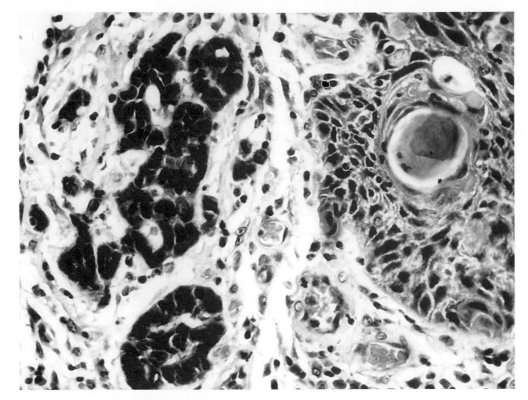

Fig. 11.36   Another area of the tumour, showing the conventional squamous component and basaloid pattern. H&E, ×100 OM.

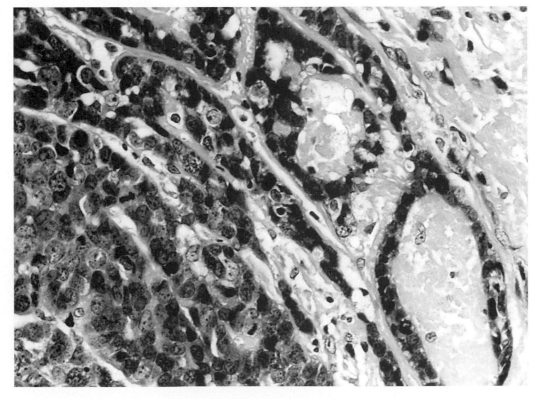

Fig. 11.37   Basaloid component with areas of stromal hyalinization. H&E, ×100 OM.

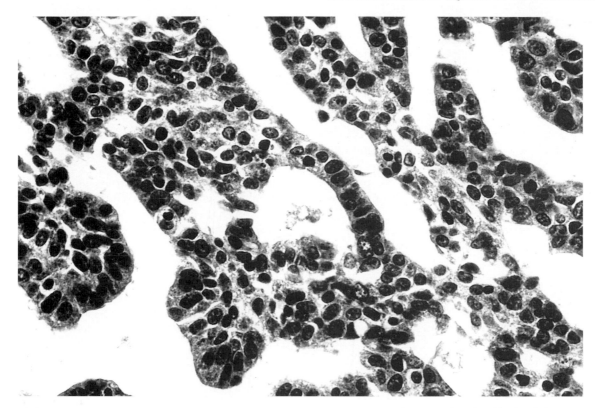

Fig. 11.38 Basaloid component showing small crowded cells with dark and hyperchromatic nuclei. Note cystic spaces. H&E, ×100 OM.

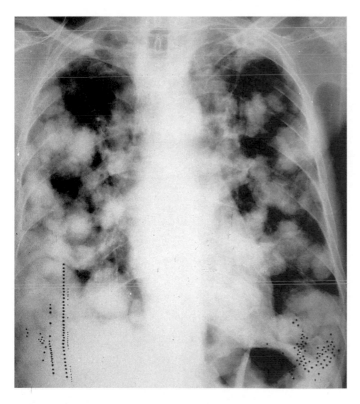

Fig. 11.39 Postero-anterior chest radiography demonstrating numerous pulmonary parenchymal metastases.

cases reported is still too limited to be conclusive.[75,84,108,123] The high incidence of distant metastases suggests that adjuvant chemotherapy may be warranted.[75,84] Three cases of basaloid squamous cell carcinoma were associated with second primary malignant tumours occurring synchronously in the upper gastrointestinal tract or larynx.[108]

LYMPHOEPITHELIAL CARCINOMA

Neoplasms histologically identical to undifferentiated carcinoma of nasopharyngeal type have been reported in the thymus, tonsil, tongue, nasal fossae, maxillary sinus, parapharyngeal area, salivary glands, lung and uterine cervix. The presence of such tumours in the larynx is not at all surprising, considering that lymphatic tissue is usually present in this organ, in the lamina propria of the mucosa in the supraglottic portion and especially in the laryngeal ventricle, which represents the 'laryngeal tonsil'. The controversial terminology for this tumour includes lymphoepithelioma, lymphoepithelial carcinoma, undifferentiated carcinoma of nasopharyngeal type and anaplastic carcinoma with lymphoid component. It is an unusual variant of squamous cell carcinoma with a conspicuous contribution of lymphocytes in its histological features. This tumour is rare but has been reported in the laryngo-hypopharyngeal regions.[4,29,38,79,88,91,113,119,122]

According to Micheau et al,[91] this neoplasm accounts for 0.2% of all laryngeal cancers. The male sex is much more affected by this neoplasm, which occurs more frequently from 50 to 70 years of age. The most common site is the supraglottic region, and the laryngeal ventricle in particular. Toker and Peterson[119] have reported a case involving the vocal cord. An early neck mass may be the presenting sign. There is an association between Epstein–Barr virus (EBV) and undifferentiated carcinoma of nasopharyngeal type but such an association has not yet been established in laryngeal neoplasms of this type. Klijanienko et al[67] reported 18 cases of undifferentiated carcinomas of the tonsillar region with a histological pattern of undifferentiated carcinoma of nasopharyngeal type, several associated with elevated EBV serum levels. In all three cases reported by Micheau et al,[91] the neoplasm was found in association with laryngocoele. A polypoid growth arising from the laryngeal ventricle may often protrude into the laryngeal lumen. The tumour is composed of large, poorly differentiated, non-keratinized cells intermingled with lymphocytes (Figs 11.40, 11.41).

The tumour cells have oval or round vesicular nuclei and prominent nucleoli. Cell margins are indistinct and the tumour often exhibits a sincytial appearance. The lymphocytes are not a neoplastic component of the tumour. As a rule, there is little fibrous tissue present. Electron microscopy of the lesion reveals that the malignant epithelial cells form tonofilaments, desmosomes and keratin fibrils. Diagnosis is not difficult if the fragment is representative. The neoplasm has to be distinguished from lymphoma. Immunocytochemical stains for epithelial membrane antigen and keratin are positive, while negative staining for leukocyte common antigen provides further documentation of epithelial differentiation. The paucity of cases reported in the literature precludes any final conclusion as to the prognosis and survival rate. The neoplasm metastasizes frequently to cervical lymph nodes and occasionally to the lungs, bone and other organs. The prognosis is usually unfavourable. Radiotherapy appears to be effective in eradicating localized disease and nodal metastases. Chemotherapy is indicated for visceral metastases.

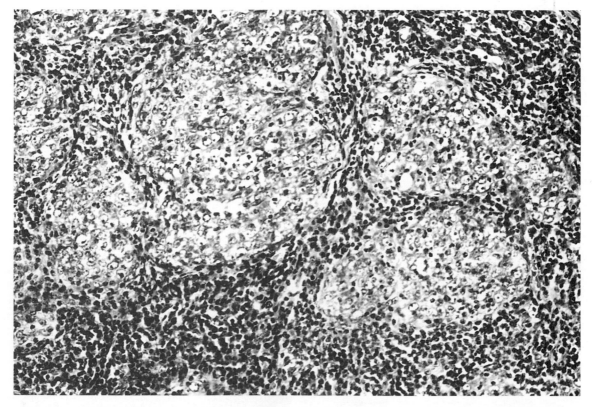

Fig. 11.40 Lymphoepithelial carcinoma. Note sheets of irregular cells with an admixture of lymphocytes. H&E, ×40 OM.

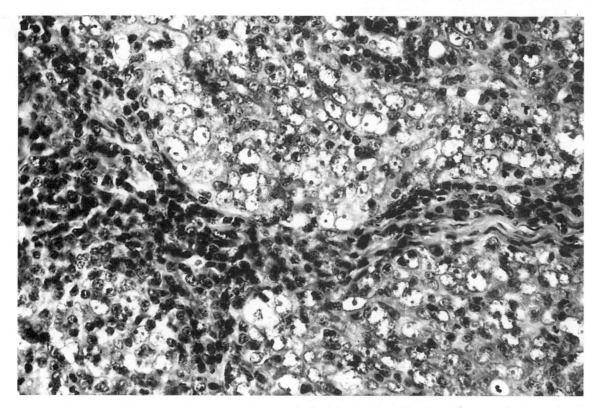

Fig. 11.41   Cohesive nest cells are surrounded by prominent stromal inflammation. The neoplastic cells have uniformly vesicular nuclei and unapparent cell borders. H&E, ×100 OM.

GIANT CELL CARCINOMA

This tumour was first described in the lung by Hadley and Bullock[56] and then by Nash and Stout.[94] The first case occurring in the larynx was reported by Ferlito[37] in 1976.

Nowadays, the WHO classification[109] of tumours of the upper respiratory tract and ear also acknowledges this tumour in the larynx, though only a few cases have been reported so far.[45]

Grossly (Fig. 11.42), the tumour is indistinguishable from a conventional squamous cell carcinoma.

Microscopically (Figs 11.43–11.45), it is composed of scattered pleomorphic, often bizarre multinucleated giant cells with intensely acidophilic vacuolated cytoplasm distributed among smaller anaplastic tumour cells and supported by a delicate fibrovascular stroma. The cells contain irregular nuclei with a coarse chromatin and prominent nucleoli. Mitoses are numerous and atypical. Leukocytes, and particularly neutrophyls and/or cell debris, are occasionally included in the cytoplasm of the tumour cells (i.e., emperipolesis). Intracytoplasmic erythrocytes may be seen. Intracellular mucin occurs in the cytoplasm of some giant cells. Syncytial formations

may be identified (Fig. 11.46). There are occasionally findings of atypical spindle cells with hyperchromatic nuclei, resembling the cells of rhabdomyosarcoma. Immunocytochemical studies have demonstrated the presence of EMA, cytokeratin and vimentin,[3,26] which is probably related to aggregates of paranuclear filaments visible ultrastructurally.[3] The cellular origin of this tumour has remained obscure. The immunohistochemical profile suggests that it displays cytokeratins characteristic of adenocarcinoma but that a subset also shows polypeptides typical of squamous carcinoma.[26] Whether this tumour is an unusual variant of squamous cell carcinoma or a poorly differentiated adenocarcinoma is still not clear, and the controversy persists. The neoplasm has to be distinguished from pleomorphic rhabdomyosarcoma and malignant fibrous histiocytoma. The presence of striations, a positive reaction to myoglobin and/or desmin and ultrastructural demonstrations of thick myofilaments, are diagnostic of rhabdomyosarcoma. The diagnosis of malignant fibrous histiocytoma is reached by exclusion.

This tumour has an extremely aggressive behaviour, and the prognosis remains unfavourable, but the lack of a sufficient number of cases does not allow conclusive considerations to be drawn. Radical surgery is indicated.

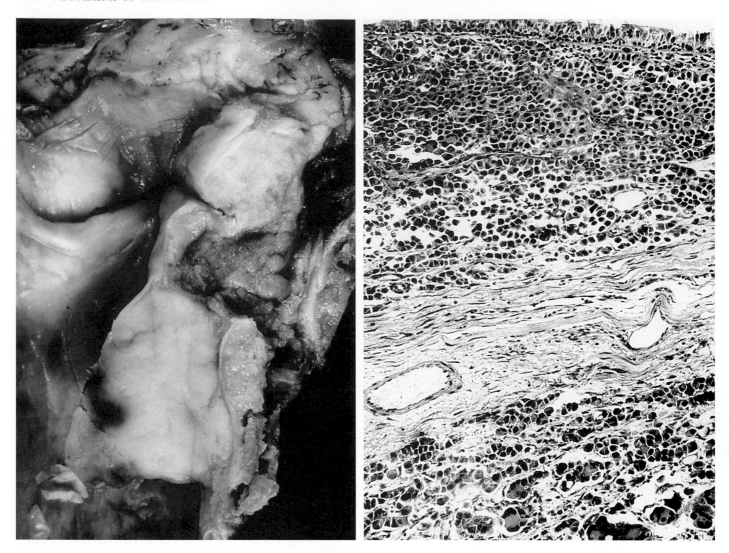

Fig. 11.42 (*left*) Giant cell carcinoma of the larynx. Sagittal section of the right half of the larynx showing the large lesion.

Fig. 11.43 (*right*) Alveolar pattern of the giant cell carcinoma. H&E, ×16 OM.

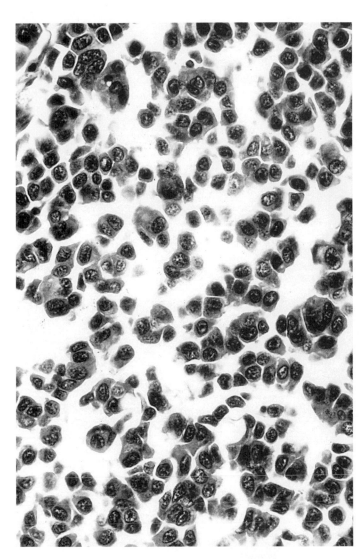

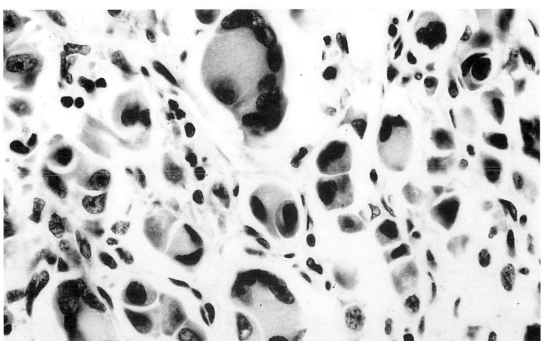

Fig. 11.44 (*top, left*) The neoplasm is composed of pleomorphic multi-nucleated giant cells. H&E, ×100 OM.

Fig. 11.45 (*bottom, left*) Note many bizarre and multinucleated giant cells. H&E, ×160 OM.

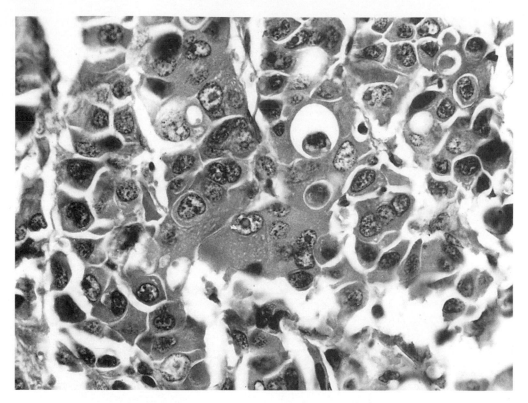

Fig. 11.46   Syncytial formations are present. H&E, ×160 OM.

REFERENCES

1. Abramson A L, Brandsma J, Steinberg B, Winkler B 1985 Verrucous carcinoma of the larynx. Arch Otolaryngol 111: 709–715
2. Ackerman L V 1948 Verrucous carcinoma of the oral cavity. Surgery 23: 670–678
3. Addis B J, Dewar A, Thurlow N P 1988 Giant cell carcinoma of the lungs. Immunohistochemical and ultrastructural evidence of dedifferentiation. J Pathol 155: 231–240
4. Alcade Navarrete J M, Perez Fernandez N, Aleman Lopez O 1991 Lymphoepithelioma of the larynx. Report of a case. In: Sacristan T, Alvarez-Vincent, Bartual J, Antoli-Candela, Rubio L (eds) Otorhinolaryngology head and neck surgery, vol II. Kugler & Ghedini, Amsterdam
5. Alguacil-Garcia A, Alonso A, Pettigrew N M 1984 Sarcomatoid carcinoma (so-called pseudosarcoma) of the larynx simulating malignant giant cell tumor of soft parts. A case report. Am J Clin Pathol 82: 340–343
6. Babighian G, Ferlito A 1974 Il carcinoma squamoso verrucoso della laringe: aspetti morfologici, istoprognosi, considerazioni terapeutiche. Atti LXI Congr Soc Ital Otorinolaringol Patol Cerv Facc vol 2, Perugia
7. Bak M Jr, Erdös M 1975 Verrucous carcinoma of the larynx. Arch Otorhinolaryngol 209: 15–22
7a. Banks E R, Frierson H F Jr, Covell J L 1992 Fine needle aspiration cytologic findings in metastatic basaloid squamous cell carcinoma of the head and neck. Acta Cytol 36: 126–131
7b. Banks E R, Frierson H F Jr, Mills S E, George E, Zarbo R J, Swanson P E 1992 Basaloid squamous cell carcinoma of the head and neck. A clinicopathologic and immunohistochemical study of 40 cases. Am J Surg Pathol 16: 939–946.
8. Bardini R, Cecchetto A, Nosadini A, Zaninotto G, Ancona E, Giordano E 1980 Il carcinoma verrucoide dell'esofago. Osservazioni su tre casi clinici. Chir Triv 20: 3–9
9. Barnes L, Peel R L 1990 Head and neck pathology. A text/atlas of differential diagnosis. Igaku-Shoin, New York

10. Barnes L, Yunis E J, Krebs F J III, Sonmez-Alpan E 1991 Verruca vulgaris of the larynx. Demonstration of human papillomavirus types 6/11 by in situ hybridization. Arch Pathol Lab Med 115: 895–899
11. Barr G S, Osborne J, Simpson J R M 1988 Late response of verrucous carcinoma of the larynx to radiotherapy. J Laryngol Otol 102: 276–279
12. Batsakis J G, El Naggar A 1989 Basaloid–squamous carcinomas of the upper aerodigestive tracts. Ann Otol Rhinol Laryngol 98: 919–920
13. Batsakis J G, Huser J 1990 Squamous carcinomas with glandlike (adenoid) features. Ann Otol Rhinol Laryngol 99: 87–88
14. Batsakis J G, Rice D H, Howard D R 1982 The pathology of head and neck tumors: spindle cell lesions (sarcomatoid carcinomas, nodular fasciitis, and fibrosarcoma) of the aerodigestive tracts, part 14. Head Neck Surg 4: 499–513
15. Batsakis J G, Hybels R, Crissman J D, Rice D H 1982 The pathology of head and neck tumours: verrucous carcinoma, part 15. Head Neck Surg 5: 29–38
16. Battifora H 1976 Spindle cell carcinoma. Ultrastructural evidence of squamous origin and collagen production by the tumor cells. Cancer 37: 2275–2282
17. Biller H F, Bergman J A 1975 Verrucous carcinoma of the larynx. Can J Otolaryngol 4: 280–283
18. Biller H F, Ogura J H, Bauer W C 1971 Verrucous cancer of the larynx. Laryngoscope 81: 1323–1329
19. Blakeslee D, Vaughan C W, Shapshay S M, Simpson G T, Strong M S 1984 Excisional biopsy in the selective management of T1 glottic cancer: a three-year follow-up study. Laryngoscope 94: 488–494
20. Brandsma J L, Steinberg B M, Abramson A L, Winkler B 1986 Presence of human papillomavirus type 16 related sequences in verrucous carcinoma of the larynx. Cancer Res 46: 2185–2188
21. Brindisi M, Cairoli G, Cappa C, Frangi R, Parmigiani F 1985 Gli istotipi non comuni dei tumori laringei. Quarantasette osser-

vazioni: inquadramento anatomo-clinico. Otorinolaringologia 35: 53–65

22. Brodsky G 1984 Carcino (pseudo) sarcoma of the larynx: the controversy continues. Otolaryngol Head Neck Surg 17: 185–197

23. Bryce D P 1979 The management of laryngeal cancer. J Otolaryngol 8: 105–126

24. Burns H F, van Nostrand A W P, Bryce D P 1976 Verrucous carcinoma of the larynx: management by radiotherapy and surgery. Ann Otol Rhinol Laryngol 85: 538–543

25. Caselitz J, Becker J, Seifert G, Weber K, Osborn M 1984 Coexpression of keratin and vimentin filaments in adenoid cystic carcinomas of salivary glands. Virchows Arch (A) 403: 337–344

26. Chejfec G, Candel A, Jansson D S, Warren W H, Koukoulis G K, Gould J E, Manderino G L, Gooch G T, Gould V E 1991 Immunohistochemical features of giant cell carcinoma of the lung: patterns of expression of cytokeratins, vimentin, and the mucinous glycoprotein recognized by monoclonal antibody A–80. Ultrastructural Pathol 15: 131–138

27. David J M, Pessy J J, Lacomme Y 1982 Carcinomes verruqueux du larynx. J Fr Otorhinolaryngol 31: 638–642

28. Demian S D E, Bushkin F L, Echevarria R A 1973 Perineural invasion and anaplastic transformation of verrucous carcinoma. Cancer 32: 395–401

29. Dockerty M B, Parkhill E M, Dahlin D C, Woolner L B, Soule E H, Harrison E G Jr 1968 Tumors of oral cavity and pharynx. In: Atlas of tumor pathology, sect IV, fasc 106. Armed Forces Institute of Pathology, Washington DC

30. Edström S, Johansson S L, Lindström J, Sandin I 1987 Verrucous squamous cell carcinoma of the larynx: evidence for increased metastatic potential after irradiation. Otolaryngol Head Neck Surg 97: 381–384

31. Elliott G B, Macdougall J A, Elliott J D A 1973 Problems of verrucose squamous carcinoma. Ann Surg 177: 21–29

32. Ellis G L, Langloss J M, Heffner D K, Hyams V J 1987 Spindle-cell carcinoma of the aerodigestive tract. An immunohistochemical analysis of 21 cases. Am J Surg Pathol 11: 335–342

33. Esteban F, Ruiz-Cabello F, Concha A, Pérez-Ayala M, Sánchez-Rozas J A, Garrido F 1990 HLA-DR expression is associated with excellent prognosis in squamous cell carcinoma of the larynx. Clin Expl Met 8: 319–328

34. Fechner R E 1981 Verrucous carcinoma. Arch Otolaryngol 107: 454–456

35. Fechner R E, Mills S E 1982 Verruca vulgaris of the larynx. A distinctive lesion of probable viral origin confused with verrucous carcinoma. Am J Surg Pathol 6: 357–362

36. Ferlito A 1975 Considerazioni biologiche, morfologiche, immunopatologiche e prognostiche di una variante del carcinoma squamoso della laringe: il carcinoma squamoso verrucoso. Atti XIII Congr Soc Ital Patol, Siena-Chianciano

37. Ferlito A 1976 Histological classification of larynx and hypopharynx cancers and their clinical implications. Pathologic aspects of 2052 malignant neoplasms diagnosed at the ORL Department of Padua University from 1966 to 1976. Acta Otolaryngol 342 (suppl): 1–88

38. Ferlito A 1977 Primary lymphoepithelial carcinoma of the hypopharynx. J Laryngol Otol 91: 361–367

39. Ferlito A 1985 Malignant epithelial tumors of the larynx. In: Ferlito A (ed) Cancer of the larynx, vol I. CRC Press, Boca Raton

40. Ferlito A 1985 Diagnosis and treatment of verrucous squamous cell carcinoma of the larynx: a critical review. Ann Otol Rhinol Laryngol 94: 575–579

41. Ferlito A 1990 Laryngeal fibrosarcoma: an over-diagnosed tumor. ORL J Otorhinolaryngol Relat Spec 52: 194–195

42. Ferlito A 1990 Pathology of malignant tumors of the larynx. In: Inouye T, Fukuda H, Sato T, Hinohara T (eds) Recent advances in bronchoesophagology. Excerpta Medica, Amsterdam

43. Ferlito A, Recher G 1980 Ackerman's tumor (Verrucous carcinoma) of the larynx. A clinicopathologic study of 77 cases. Cancer 46: 1617–1630

44. Ferlito A, Antonutto G, Silvestri F 1976 Histological appearances and nuclear DNA content of verrucous squamous cell carcinoma of the larynx. ORL 38: 65–85

45. Ferlito A, Friedmann I, Recher G 1985 Primary giant cell carcinoma of the larynx. A clinico-pathological study of four cases. ORL J Otorhinolaryngol Relat Spec 47: 105–112

46. Fisher H R 1975 Verrucous carcinoma of the larynx. A study of its pathologic anatomy. Can J Otolaryngol 4: 270–277

47. Fisker A V, Philipsen H P 1984 Verrucous hyperplasia and verrucous carcinoma of the rat oral mucosa. Experimental oral carcinogenesis using 4-nitroquinoline I-oxide. Acta Pathol Microbiol Immunol Scand A 92: 437–445

48. Fliss D M, Hartwick R W J, Noble-Topham S F, Noyek A M, Freeman J L 1992 Laryngeal verrucous carcinoma (LVC) clinico-pathologic review and detection and typing of human papilloma virus by polymerase chain reaction (PCR). Am Laryngol Rhinol Otol Soc, abstract

49. Fonts E A, Greenlaw R H, Rush B F, Rovin S 1969 Verrucous squamous cell carcinoma of the oral cavity. Cancer 23: 152–160

50. Frable W J, Frable M A S 1990 The larynx and trachea. In: Silverberg S G (ed) Principles and practice of surgical pathology, 2nd edn, vol 1. Churchill Livingstone, New York

51. Friedell H L, Rosenthal L M 1941 The etiologic role of chewing tobacco in cancer of the mouth. Report of eight cases treated with radiation. JAMA 116: 2130–2135

52. Friedmann I, Ferlito A 1988 Granulomas and neoplasms of the larynx. Churchill Livingstone, Edinburgh

53. Glanz H, Kleinsasser O 1978 Verrucöse Akanthose (verrucöses Karzinom) des Larynx. Laryngol Rhinol Otol 57: 835–843

54. Glanz H, Kleinsasser O 1987 Verrucous carcinoma of the larynx — a misnomer. Arch Otorhinolaryngol 244: 108–111

55. Goethals P L, Harrison E G, Devine K D 1963 Verrucous squamous carcinoma of the oral cavity. Am J Surg 106: 845–851

56. Hadley G G, Bullock W K 1953 Autopsy reports of pulmonary carcinoma — survey at Los Angeles County Hospital for 1951. Calif Med 79: 431–433

57. Hagen P C, Lyons G D, Haindel C 1992 Verrucous carcinoma of the larynx 1991: role of human papillomavirus, radiation and surgery. Am Laryngol Rhinol Otol Soc, abstract

58. Harada T 1982 Three cases of verrucous carcinoma of the larynx. Otolaryngol (Tokyo) 54: 627–632

59. Harwood A R 1982 Cancer of the larynx — the Toronto experience. J Otolaryngol 11 (suppl): 3–21

60. Heffner D K 1991 Sinonasal and laryngeal salivary gland lesions. In: Ellis G L, Auclair P L, Gnepp D R (eds) Surgical pathology of the salivary glands. Saunders, Philadelphia

61. Hellquist H, Olofsson J 1989 Spindle cell carcinoma of the larynx. APMIS 97: 1103–1113

62. Hertenstein J C, Fechner R E 1986 Acantholytic squamous cell carcinoma. Arch Otolaryngol Head Neck Surg 112: 780–783

63. Hyams V J 1975 Verrucous carcinoma of the larynx. (Discussion). Can J Otolaryngol 4: 280–283

64. Hyams V J, Batsakis J G, Michaels L 1988 Tumors of the upper respiratory tract and ear. In: Atlas of tumor pathology, 2nd series, fasc 25. Armed Forces Institute of Pathology, Washington DC

65. Ibekwe A O, Duvall E 1988 Verrucous carcinoma of the larynx: problems of diagnosis and treatment. J Laryngol Otol 102: 79–82

66. Kashima H K 1990 Human papillomavirus: their etiologic relevance to head and neck cancer. In: Fee W E Jr, Goepfert H, Johns M E, Strong E W, Ward P H (eds). Head and neck cancer, vol 2. Decker, Toronto

67. Klijanienko J, Micheau C, Azli N, Cvitkovic E, Eschwege F, Marandas P, Armand J P, Casiraghi O, Schwaab G, de Vathaire F 1989 Undifferentiated carcinoma of nasopharyngeal type of tonsil. Arch Otolaryngol Head Neck Surg 115: 731–734

68. Kraus F T, Perez-Mesa C 1966 Verrucous carcinoma: clinical and pathologic study of 105 cases involving oral cavity, larynx and genitalia. Cancer 19: 26–38

69. Lawson W, Biller H F, Suen J S 1989 Cancer of the larynx. In: Myers E N, Suen J Y (eds) Cancer of the head and neck, 2nd edn. Churchill Livingstone, New York

70. Lee R J 1988 Verrucous carcinoma of the larynx. Otolaryngol Head Neck Surg 98: 593–509

71. Lekas M D, Kamath C R, Vitavasiri A 1977 Hemoptysis and supraglottic verrucous carcinoma. Ear Nose Throat J 56: 315–319

72. Leuszler R W, Shapshay S M, Strong M S 1984 Conservation

surgery for laryngeal pseudosarcoma. Otolaryngol Head Neck Surg 92: 480–484

73. Leventon G S, Evans H L 1981 Sarcomatoid squamous cell carcinoma of the mucous membranes of the head and neck: a clinico-pathologic study of 20 cases. Cancer 48: 994–1003

74. Lichtiger B, Mackay B, Tessmer C F 1970 Spindle-cell variant of squamous carcinoma. A light and electron microscopic study of 13 cases. Cancer 26: 1311–1320

75. Luna M A, El Naggar A, Parichatikanond P, Weber R S, Batsakis J G 1990 Basaloid squamous carcinoma of the upper aerodigestive tract. Clinicopathologic and DNA flow cytometric analysis. Cancer 66: 537–542

76. Luna M A, Tortoledo M E 1988 Verrucous carcinoma. In: Gnepp D R (ed) Pathology of the head and neck. Churchill Livingstone, New York

77. Lundgren J A V, Van Nostrand A W P, Harwood A R, Cullen R J, Bryce D P 1986 Verrucous carcinoma (Ackerman's tumor) of the larynx: diagnostic and therapeutic considerations. Head Neck Surgery 9: 19–26

78. Mandych A K, Benninger M S, Zarbo R J 1992 Epithelial dedifferentiation in squamous carcinoma of the larynx. Am Laryngol Rhinol Otol Soc, abstract

79. Mark H 1926 Ueber 'lymphoepitheliale' Geschwülste, besonders des Kehlkopfes. Ztschr Hals Nasen Ohrenheil 15: 392–395

80. Mark P A, Lupin A J 1989 Cancer of the larynx: the Northern Alberta experience. J Otolaryngol 18: 344–349

81. Maw A R, Culler R J, Bradfield J W B 1982 Verrucous carcinoma of the larynx. Clin Otolaryngol 7: 305–311

82. McClure D L, Gullane P J, Slinger R P, Wysocki G P 1984 Verrucous carcinoma-changing concepts in management. J Otolaryngol 13: 7–12

83. McCoy J M, Waldron C A 1981 Verrucous carcinoma of the oral cavity. A review of forty-nine cases. Oral Surg 52: 623–629

84. McKay M J, Bilous A M 1989 Basaloid–squamous carcinoma of the hypopharynx. Cancer 63: 2528–2531

85. Medina J E, Dichtel M W, Luna M A 1984 Verrucous-squamous carcinomas of the oral cavity. A clinicopathologic study of 104 cases. Arch Otolaryngol 110: 437–440

86. Meijer J W R, Ramaekers F C S, Manni J J, Sloof J J L, Aldeweireldt J, Vooys G P 1988 Intermediate filament proteins in spindle cell carcinoma of the larynx and tongue. Acta Otolaryngol 106: 306–313

87. Memula N, Ridenhour G, Doss L 1980 Radiotherapeutic management of oral cavity verrucous carcinoma. Am Soc Therap Radiol Texas

88. Meyer-Breiting E, Burkhardt A 1988 Tumours of the larynx. Histopathology and clinical inferences. Springer-Verlag, Berlin

89. Michaels L 1984 Pathology of the larynx. Springer-Verlag, Berlin

90. Michaels L, Cooper J, Brewer C J, Hyams V J 1984 Image analysis in histological diagnosis of verrucous squamous carcinoma of the larynx. J Pathol 143: 329A

91. Micheau C, Luboinski B, Schwaab G, Richard J, Cachin Y 1979 Lymphoepitheliomas of the larynx (undifferentiated carcinomas of the nasopharyngeal type). Clin Otolaryngol 4: 43–48

92. Milford C A, O'Flynn P E 1991 Management of verrucous carcinoma of the larynx. Clin Otolaryngol 16: 160–162

93. Myers E, Sobol S, Ogura J H 1980 Hemilaryngectomy for verrucous carcinoma of the glottis. Laryngoscope 90: 693–698

94. Nash A D, Stout A P 1957 Giant cell carcinoma of the lung. Report of 5 cases. Cancer 11: 369–376

95. Okagaki T, Clark B A, Zachow K R, Twiggs L B, Ostrow R S, Pass F, Faras A J 1984 Presence of human papillomavirus in verrucous carcinoma (Ackerman) of the vagina. Immunocytochemical, ultrastructural, and DNA hybridization studies. Arch Pathol Lab Med 108: 567–570

95a. O'Malley B W Jr 1992 Basaloid–squamous carcinoma of the right pyriform sinus. Arch Otolaryngol Head Neck Surg 118: 212–215

96. Ophir D, Marshak G, Czernobilsky B 1987 Distinctive immunohistochemical labeling of epithelial and mesenchymal elements in laryngeal pseudosarcoma. Laryngoscope 97: 490–494

97. Perez C A, Kraus F T, Evans J C, Powers W E 1966 Anaplastic transformation in verrucous carcinoma of the oral cavity after radiation therapy. Radiology 86: 108–115

98. Pérez-Ayala M, Ruiz-Cabello F, Esteban F, Concha A, Redondo M, Oliva M R, Cabrera T, Garrido F 1990 Presence of HPV 16 sequences in laryngeal carcinomas. Int J Cancer 46: 8–11

99. Prioleau P G, Santa Cruz D J, Meyer J S, Bauer W C 1980 Verrucous carcinoma. A light and electron microscopic, autoradiographic and immunofluorescence study. Cancer 45: 2849–2857

100. Proffitt S D, Spooner T R, Kosek J C 1970 Origin of undifferentiated neoplasm from verrucous epidermal carcinoma of oral cavity following irradiation. Cancer 26: 389–393

101. Recher G 1985 Spindle cell squamous carcinoma of the larynx. Clinico-pathological study of seven cases. J Laryngol Otol 99: 871–879

102. Rider W D 1975 Toronto experience of verrucous carcinoma of the larynx. Can J Otolaryngol 4: 278–279

103. Russo C, Brunelli M, Costantini S 1987 Il carcinoma verrucoso della laringe. Contributo clinico. Otorinolaringologia 37: 39–42

104. Ryan R E, DeSanto L W, Devine K D, Weiland L H 1977 Verrucous carcinoma of the larynx. Laryngoscope 87: 1989–1994

105. Schrader M, Laberke H G 1988 Differential diagnosis of verrucous carcinoma in the oral cavity and larynx. J Laryngol Otol 102: 700–703

106. Schrader M, Laberke H G, Jahnke K 1987 Lymphknotenmetastasen beimverrukösen Karzinom (Ackerman-Tumor). HNO 35: 27–30

107. Schwade J G, Wara M M, Dedo H H, Phillips T L 1976 Radiotherapy for verrucous carcinoma. Radiology 120: 677–679

108. Seidman J D, Berman J J, Yost B A, Iseri O A 1991 Basaloid squamous carcinoma of the hypopharynx and larynx associated with second primary tumors. Cancer 68: 1545–1549

109. Shanmugaratnam K 1991 Histological typing of tumours of the upper respiratory tract and ear. World Health Organization. International Histological Classification of Tumours, 2nd edn. Springer-Verlag, Berlin

110. Sherwin R P, Strong M S, Waughn C W 1963 Polypoid and junctional squamous cell carcinoma of the tongue and larynx with spindle cell carcinoma ('pseudosarcoma'). Cancer 16: 51–60

110a. Shvili Y, Talmi Y T, Gal R, Kessler E, Kolkov Z, Zohar Y 1990 Basaloid–squamous carcinoma of larynx metastatic to the skin of the nasal tip. J Cranio–Max–Fac Surg 18: 322–324

111. Sllamniku B, Bauer W, Painter C, Sessions D 1989 Clinical and histopathological considerations for the diagnosis and treatment of verrucous carcinoma of the larynx. Arch Otorhinolaryngol 246: 126–132

112. Smith R R L, Kuhajda F P, Harris A E 1985 Anaplastic transformation of verrucous carcinoma following radiotherapy. Am J Otolaryngol 6: 448–452

113. Stanley R J, Weiland L H, DeSanto L W, Neel H B III 1985 Lymphoepithelioma (undifferentiated carcinoma) of the laryngohypopharynx. Laryngoscope 95: 1077–1081

114. Stecker R H, Devine K D, Harrison E G 1964 Verrucose 'snuff dipper's' carcinoma of the oral cavity. A case of self-induced carcinogenesis. JAMA 14: 838–840

115. Stinson S F, Reznik-Schüller H M, Reznik G, Donahoe R 1983 Spindle cell carcinoma of the hamster trachea induced by N-methyl-N-nitrosourea. Am J Pathol 111: 21–26

116. Strong M S 1985 Diagnosis and treatment of verrucous squamous cell carcinoma of the larynx: a critical review. (Discussion) Trans Am Laryngol Ass 106: 163–164

117. Thomas J R, Syderman S C, Giffin C S, Goin D W, Wayne F 1973 Verrucous carcinoma of the pyriform sinus. Arch Otolaryngol 97: 488–489

118. Toda S, Yonemitsu N, Miyabara S, Sugihara H, Maehara N 1989 Polypoid squamous cell carcinoma of the larynx. An immuno-histochemical study for ras p21 and cytokeratin. Path Res Pract 185: 860–866

119. Toker C, Peterson D W 1978 Lymphoepithelioma of the vocal cord. Arch Otolaryngol 104: 161–162

119a. Tsang W Y W, Chan J K C, Lee K C, Leung A K F, Fu Y T 1991 Basaloid–squamous carcinoma of the upper aerodigestive tract and so-called adenoid cystic carcinoma of the oesophagus: the same tumour type? Histopathology 19: 35–46

120. Turner J E, Hodge S J, Callen J P 1980 Verrucous carcinoma in a

renal transplant patient after long term immunosuppression. Arch Dermatol 116: 1074–1076

121. Van Nostrand A W P, Olofsson J 1972 Verrucous carcinoma of the larynx. A clinical and pathologic study of 10 cases. Cancer 30: 691–702

122. Vossenberg A 1928 Über lymphoepitheliale Geschwülste, besonders des Kehlkopfes. Z Laryngol Rhinol Otol 17: 153–165

123. Wain S L, Kier R, Vollmer R T, Bossen E H 1986 Basaloid–squamous carcinoma of the tongue, hypopharynx, and larynx: report of 10 cases. Hum Pathol 17: 1158–1166

124. Weidner N 1987 Sarcomatoid carcinoma of the upper aerodigestive tract. Sem Diagn Pathol 4: 157–168

125. Youngberg G A, Thornthwaite J T, Inoshita T 1983 Cytologically malignant squamous cell carcinoma arising in a verrucous carcinoma of the penis. J Dermatol Surg Oncol 9: 474–479

126. Zachow K R, Ostrow R S, Bender M, Watts S, Okagaki T, Pass F, Faras A J 1982 Detection of human papillomavirus DNA in anogenital neoplasias. Nature 300: 771–773

127. Zarbo R J, Crissman J D, Venkat H, Weiss M A 1986 Spindle-cell carcinoma of the upper aerodigestive tract mucosa. An immunohistologic and ultrastructural study of 18 biphasic tumors and comparison with seven monophasic spindle-cell tumors. Am J Surg Pathol 101: 741–753

12. Neuroendocrine neoplasms

A. Ferlito, I. Friedmann

The dispersed or diffuse neuroendocrine cell system comprises a wide variety of cells in the central and peripheral nervous system and in several organs including the larynx. These cells may be identified by silver impregnation, immunohistochemistry, electron microscopy and in situ hybridization histochemistry.[71]

The development of immunohistochemical methods as applied to the study of endocrine cells and tumours of the larynx has greatly enhanced our knowledge of these neoplasms.

Neuroendocrine neoplasms of the larynx constitute a morphologically heterogeneous group recognized only recently. More than 400 cases have been reported,[1–6,8, 9,11–24,26–29,31–43,45,47–50,52–54,57–69,72–75,77–94,96–122,124,126–139, 141–144,146,148–187,189–192,194–198,200–225,227–239,241–255] and the atypical carcinoid tumour represents the most frequent type of neuroendocrine neoplasm of the larynx. The designation 'neuroendocrine' has no relationship to the embryological derivation of the cells and has been used in a morpho-functional sense.[211] Electron microscopy has contributed greatly to the diagnosis of neuroendocrine neoplasms, which often display a complex or mixed morphology under the light microscope, by the demonstration of membrane-bound neurosecretory granules in their cells.

Human neuroendocrine neoplasms arising in various locations can express a great variety of immunoactive peptides which can be identified by the immunoperoxidase technique.

An ever-increasing range of new mono- and poly-clonal antibodies and markers are being developed and made available to the diagnostic histopathologist.[68] This field has been expanding, and the final assessment of the role of the peptide-based neuroendocrine system in health and disease will require further intensive study.

Neuroendocrine neoplastic lesions can be conveniently divided into two main groups: those of epithelial origin (typical carcinoid tumour, atypical carcinoid tumour and small cell neuroendocrine carcinoma) and those of neural type (paraganglioma).

CARCINOID TUMOUR

Introduction

Markel et al[154] take credit for the first description of a typical carcinoid tumour of the larynx in 1980, but the microscopy of this case recently reviewed by Woodruff and Ferlito showed the features of an atypical carcinoid tumour. Gehanno et al[81] reported a case of typical carcinoid of the larynx without histological documentation and the first well-documented case was described by Duvall et al in 1983.[50]

Terminology

Various terms have been applied — such as typical carcinoid, carcinoid tumour, mature carcinoid, well-differentiated neuroendocrine carcinoma, endocrine tumour, and others.

Definition

A carcinoid tumour is an epithelial tumour of low-grade malignancy characterized by histological, histochemical, immunohistochemical and ultrastructural evidence of neuroendocrine differentiation.

Incidence

This represents the rarest neuroendocrine carcinoma of the larynx accounting for 3% of all primary neuroendocrine neoplasms of the larynx and approximately 5% of all carcinoid tumours.[52]

Only 14 cases of typical carcinoid tumour have been reported,[14,23,50,52,72,81,89,133a,149,185,210,217,245].

Clinical features

The tumour affects mainly men of sixty to seventy years of age who have been heavy cigarette smokers. The supraglottic region is the usually affected site, especially the

169

arytenoid and the aryepiglottic fold. The lesion presents as a polypoid or sessile submucosal nodule. The symptoms and signs are similar to those of other laryngeal tumours and depend upon the region involved. Dysphagia, hoarseness, 'lump' and sore throat are the most commonly reported symptoms. Carcinoid tumours of the larynx are typically non-functional. However, one case of carcinoid tumour, identified from the files of the Armed Forces Institute of Pathology in Washington, developed the carcinoid syndrome following liver metastasis. The patient with this neoplasm had increased 5-HIAA levels in the urine and was treated with streptozotocin and 5-FU, producing a subsequent decrease in the 5-HIAA level.[244] The features of the carcinoid syndrome are: episodic flushing of the skin, asthma-like symptoms, diarrhoea, ascites, lacrimation, hypotension, sweating, vomiting. Few patients display all the symptoms, but the most common are flushing, diarrhoea and oedema.

Pathology

Gross pathology

The tumour presents as a submucosal, encapsulated mass.

Histopathology

The neoplastic tissue is composed of nests and sheets of large and uniformly bland cells with abundant granular eosinophilic cytoplasm and centrally-placed, small, round to ovoid nuclei (Fig. 12.1). Ribbon-like and rosette-like formations may be present.[50] Glandular differentiation has been observed.[245]

The stroma is fibrovascular or hyalinized. Occasionally the tumour may produce amyloid.[50] Mitoses are scant and necrosis is lacking (Fig. 12.2). The overlying epithelium is usually intact (Fig. 12.3).

The neoplasm may take on a distinct oncocytic appearance. This variant, called *oncocytic carcinoid tumour*, is composed of large cells with abundant eosinophilic, finely granular cytoplasm with a small, centrally-located hyperchromatic nucleus.[78,219] Ultrastructurally, the cells show marked mitochondrial hyperplasia.[217]

Histochemistry

Argyrophilic stains (Grimelius, Sevier-Munger, Pascual, Chrurukian–Schenk, Bodian, Wilder) are usually positive, while argentaffin stains (Fontana–Masson, Masson–Hamperl, Diazo, Schmorl) are often negative.

Immunocytochemistry

Immunoperoxidase stains for chromogranin, neuron-specific enolase (NSE), serotonin, keratin, somatostatin may reveal cytoplasmic positivity (see Table 12.1).

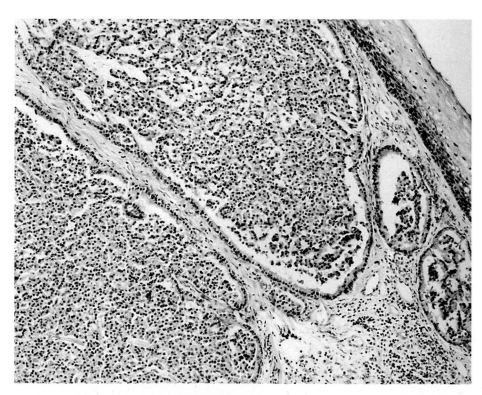

Fig. 12.1 Typical carcinoid tumour of the larynx with a submucosal alignment of organoid groups of uniform gland-like cells. H&E, ×60. (Courtesy of Dr A K El-Naggar, Houston, and the editor of *ORL; Journal for Oto-Rhino-Laryngology and its Related Specialties*.)

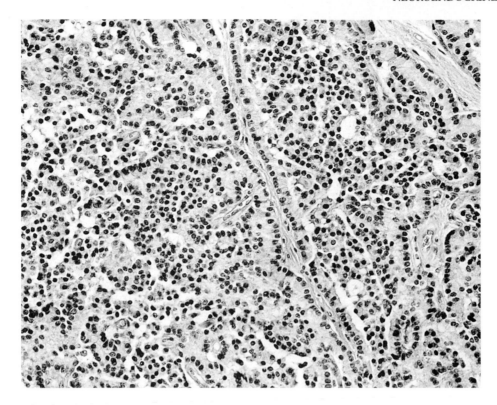

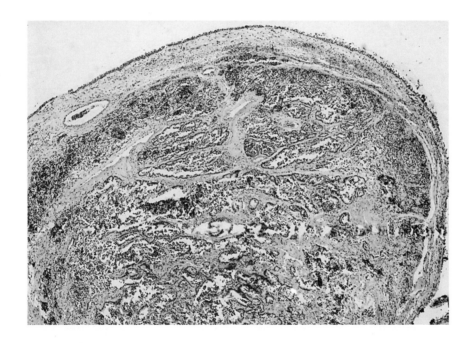

Fig. 12.2 (*top*) Trabecular arrangement of cells of the typical carcinoid shown in Fig. 12.1. Note absence of pleomorphism, mitosis or necrosis. H&E, ×140. (Courtesy of Dr A K El-Naggar, Houston, and the editor of *ORL; Journal for Oto-Rhino-Laryngology and its Related Specialties*.)

Fig. 12.3 (*bottom*) Laryngeal carcinoid tumour infiltrating submucosal tumour with cell nests and glands. H&E, ×40. (Courtesy of Dr B. M. Wenig, Washington, and the editor of *Cancer*.)

Table 12.1 Positive immunohistochemical reactions in typical and atypical carcinoids of the larynx

Antisera	Year	References
Calcitonin, somatostatin, ACTH[1]	1981	91
Calcitonin, somatostatin, ACTH[1]	1982	90
Calcitonin, somatostatin, ACTH[1]	1982	183
CEA, calcitonin[2]	1981	223
Calcitonin, ACTH, α-hCG[3]	1983	34
CEA, calcitonin, VIP[4]	1983	209
Calcitonin[3]	1984	212
ACTH	1983	182
CEA, Leu7, calcitonin, ACTH,	1984	152
NSE, CEA, calcitonin, somatostatin, serotonin, HCG	1985	251
NSE	1986	210
Chromogranin, NSE, serotonin	1987	14
Chromogranin	1987	185
Chromogranin, NSE, cytokeratin, EMA, calcitonin, met-enkephalin, ACTH, serotonin	1987	191
Chromogranin A, NSE, cytokeratin, calcitonin, gastrin, somatostatin, glucagon, GH	1988	72
Chromogranin, NSE, cytokeratin, serotonin	1988	89
Chromogranin	1988	247
Synaptophysin, cytokeratin	1988	243
Chromogranin, NSE, cytokeratin, CEA, S-100 protein, calcitonin, somatostatin, ACTH, HCG, gastrin, glucagon, serotonin, imsulin	1988	245
NSE, EGC	1989	138
Chromogranin, NSE, calcitonin, somatostatin, serotonin[5]	1989	46
Chromogranin A, NSE, neurofilament, S-100 protein, calcitonin, serotonin, ACTH	1989	47
Chromogranin A, calcitonin	1989	150
Chromogranin A, cytokeratin, calcitonin	1989	253
Chromogranin, NSE, PGP 9.5, cytokeratin, calcitonin	1989	164
Chromogranin, NSE, cytokeratin, CEA, neurofilament, calcitonin, somatostatin[5]	1990	207
Chromogranin, NSE	1990	94
NSE, calcitonin, serotonin	1990	118
NSE, cytokeratin, calcitonin	1990	213
NSE[6]	1990	161
Chromogranin, NSE, synaptophysin, PGP 9.5 cytokeratin, calcitonin	1991	165
CGRP, VIP	1991	Milroy (p.c.)
Chromogranin A, synaptophysin, cytokeratin, CEA, S-100 protein, calcitonin	1991	250
Chromogranin A, synaptophysin, cytokeratin, calcitonin	1991	66
Chromogranin, NSE, CEA, calcitonin, serotonin	1991	53
Chromogranin	1991	134
Chromogranin, NSE, cytokeratin, EMA	1991	179
Chromogranin A, cytokeratin, calcitonin, met-enkephalin, serotonin	1991	97
Chromogranin, cytokeratin	1991	150a
Chromogranin A, NSE, cytokeratin, EMA, CEA, calcitonin, somatostatin, glucagon	1992	47a

[1,3,5]Authors refer to the same patient.
[2]Duvall et al[50] and Woodruff et al[251] consider this case as laryngeal atypical carcinoid, while Sweeney et al[223] present it as ectopic thyroid medullary carcinoma of the larynx.
[4]Konowitz et al[128] consider only the second of the two cases of paraganglioma reported by Sneige et al[209] as atypical carcinoid, whereas Wenig and Gnepp[244] consider both as atypical carcinoids.
[6]This case is also enclosed in Milroy's series.[165]
p.c. = personal communication.

Electron microscopy

The neoplasm shows, without exception, the presence of numerous round and oval neurosecretory granules with a mean size of about 110–140 nm, preferentially located in the periphery of the cytoplasm. The membrane-bound granules have an electron-dense core separated from the membrane by a clear space.

Diagnosis and differential diagnosis

The histological diagnosis is not problematic and may be supported by special histochemical reactions and confirmed by immunohistochemical and ultrastructural investigations. The tumour has to be distinguished from the atypical carcinoid tumour and paraganglioma. The lack of pleomorphism, necrosis and mitosis differentiates typical from atypical carcinoid. The distinction between typical carcinoid and paraganglioma may be difficult. The presence of prominent vascularity, the typical 'Zellballen' pattern, negativity on immunostaining for keratin, carcinoembryonic antigen (CEA) and calcitonin indicate a paraganglioma.

Therapy

The treatment of choice for this tumour is surgical excision. However, in spite of attempting conservative treatment in the first instance, laryngectomy may eventually become necessary. Lymph node dissection should not be performed since the likelihood of metastasis occurring is low.[52] Chemotherapy and/or radiotherapy have not been effective in the limited number of patients treated.

Prognosis

The prognosis is favourable and the biological behaviour is less aggressive than that of the more frequent atypical carcinoid tumour; however, late distant metastases, which may involve the liver and cause death, have occurred.[52]

ATYPICAL CARCINOID TUMOUR

Introduction

Although the atypical carcinoid tumour of the larynx is rare, it is the commonest type of non-squamous laryngeal carcinoma.[251]

Terminology

The atypical carcinoid tumour has been reported under various names, e.g., malignant carcinoid, apudoma, neuroendocrine carcinoma, moderately differentiated neuroendocrine carcinoma, large cell neuroendocrine carcinoma, endocrine carcinoma.

Definition

An atypical carcinoid tumour is a malignant epithelial neoplasm characterized by histological, histochemical, immunohistochemical and ultrastructural evidence of neuroendocrine differentiation.

Incidence

Goldman et al[88] presented the first description of an atypical carcinoid tumour of the larynx in 1969. In 1991 Woodruff and Senie, with the assistance of Ferlito,[250] identified approximately 200 reported cases and noted that several of the recorded examples of aggressive and metastasizing laryngeal paraganglioma also proved to be atypical carcinoid tumours.[8,10,244,245,250,251] Other cases have been reported,[5a,47a,133a,150a] or reclassified.[37a]

Clinical features

The sex incidence shows a predilection for men, and there is a peak incidence in the sixth and seventh decades. Most of the patients were heavy smokers.

More than 90% of the tumours occurred in the supraglottic region. The epiglottis is often involved but the hypopharynx is a rare site.[164] Presenting symptoms are hoarseness, dysphagia, sore throat, haemoptysis and ear pain. The tumour may be asymptomatic and seldom causes the carcinoid syndrome.[14]

Pathology

Gross pathology

The tumour appears as a nodular or polypoid submucosal lesion (Figs 12.4–12.8).

Histopathology

This neoplasm displays a variable pattern showing a trabecular or mosaic arrangement of pleomorphic cells of atypical size and shape (Figs 12.9, 12.10). There is enhanced mitotic activity, nuclear irregularity, pleomorphism and focal necrosis. Amyloid may be formed (Fig. 12.11)[10a,31,50,89] and mucin production has been reported.[34,183] Oncocytic and/or oncocytoid changes may occur (Fig. 12.12) and such tumours are called *oncocytic and oncocytoid carcinoid tumours*.[72,217] They are composed of large cells with an abundant eosinophilic, finely granular cytoplasm with small, centrally-located hyperchromatic nuclei (oncocytes). Mucinous changes may sometimes be present (*mucinous carcinoid*). Another variant is formed by spindle cells called *spindle carcinoid tumours*.[242,251] Various patterns may be displayed by the same tumour and perineural, vascular (Fig. 12.13) and lymphatic invasion has been observed.

The atypical carcinoid tumour may be found adjacent to squamous cell carcinoma.[14,164] Dual differentiation (neuroendocrine and epithelial) may occur in laryngeal neoplasms.[245]

Histochemistry

Argyrophil stains are usually positive, while argentaffin stains are often negative. The glandular lumen may contain PAS- and Alcian blue-positive material.

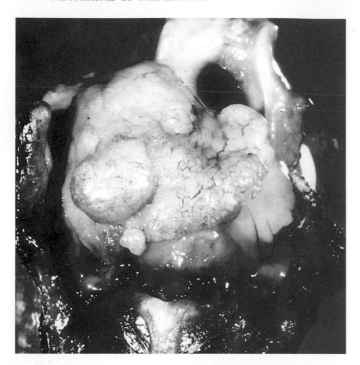

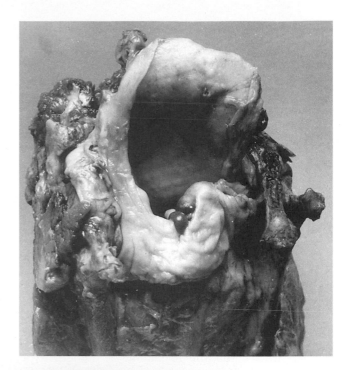

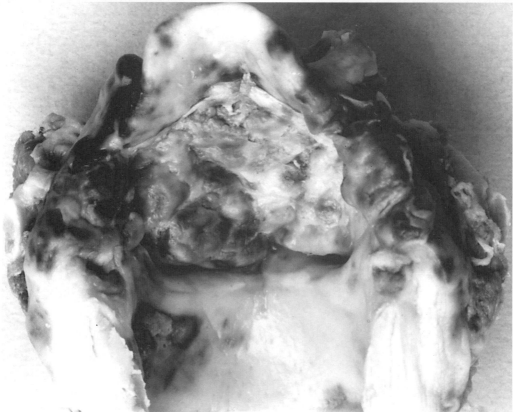

Fig. 12.4 (*top, left*) Laryngectomy specimen showing a large, nodular atypical carcinoid tumour. (Courtesy of Dr B. M. Wenig, Washington, and the editor of *Cancer*.)

Fig. 12.5 (*top, right*) Laryngectomy specimen showing a small, nodular, atypical carcinoid tumour on the aryepiglottic fold. (Courtesy of Dr C. M. Milroy, London, and the editor of *Histopathology*.)

Fig. 12.6 (*bottom*) Laryngectomy specimen showing a large atypical carcinoid tumour involving the supraglottis. (Courtesy of Dr C. M. Milroy, London.)

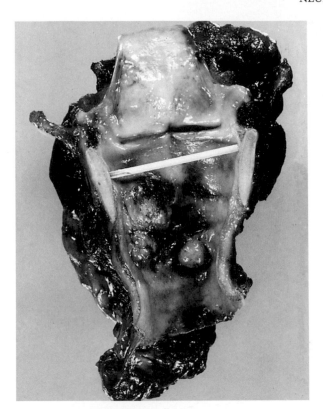

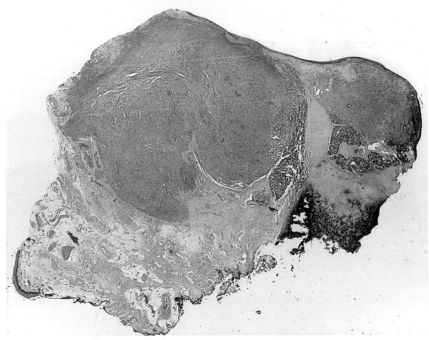

Fig. 12.7 (*top*) Laryngectomy specimen showing a large atypical carcinoid tumour of the subglottis. (Courtesy of Dr J. M. Woodruff, New York, and the editor of *American Journal of Surgical Pathology*.)

Fig. 12.8 (*bottom*) Bulging, 1 cm intramural atypical carcinoid tumour arising in the right aryepiglottic fold. Note clusters of seromucous glands. (Courtesy of Dr J. M. Woodruff, New York, and the editor of *American Journal of Surgical Pathology*.)

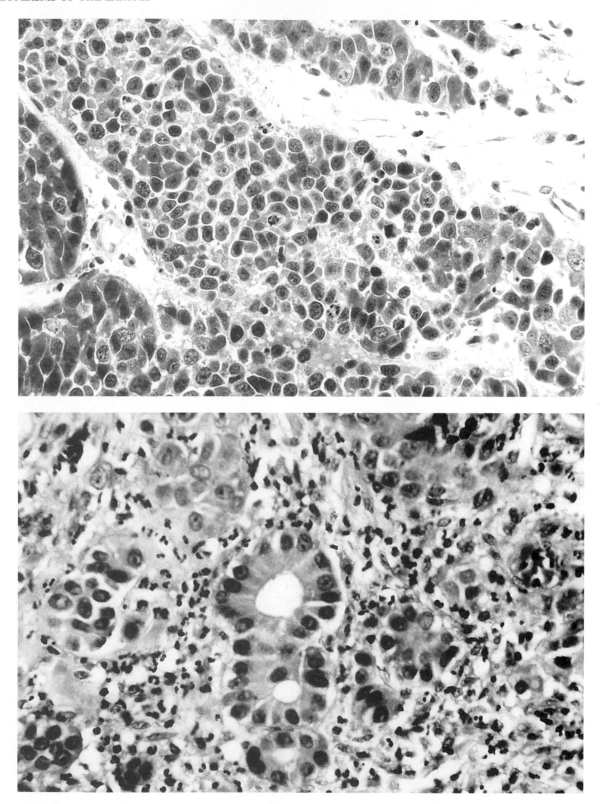

Fig. 12.9 (*top,*) Atypical carcinoid tumour of the larynx. Note the large cells with abundant eosinophilic cytoplasm and centrally-placed, round to ovoid nuclei. H&E, ×100 OM.

Fig. 12.10 (*bottom*) Atypical carcinoid tumour of the larynx displaying a glandular component. This lesion was mistakenly diagnosed as an 'adenocarcinoma'. H&E, ×100 OM.

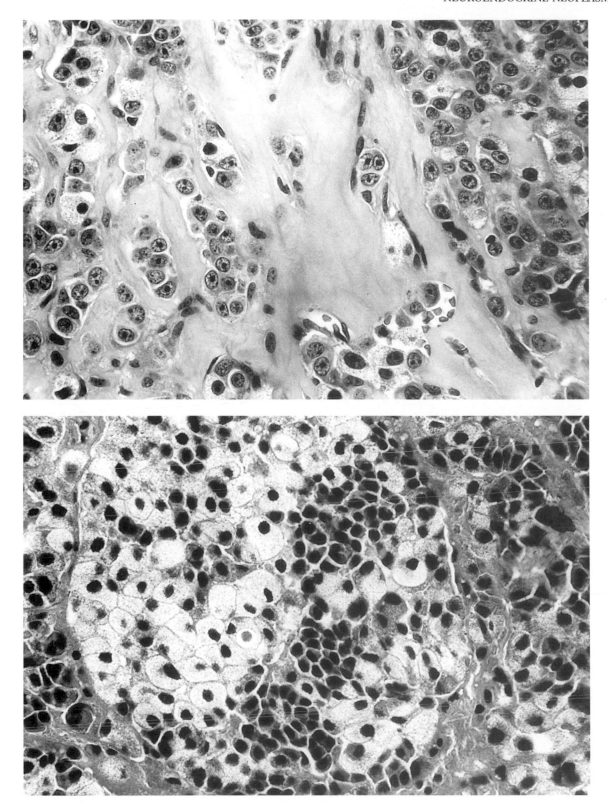

Fig. 12.11 (*top*) Dense, avascular stroma showing the presence of amyloid. H&E, ×100 OM.

Fig. 12.12 (*bottom*) Atypical carcinoid tumour of the larynx showing oncocytoid features. H&E, ×100 OM.

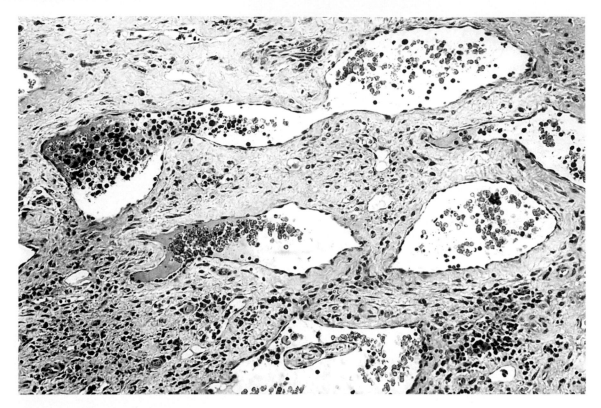

Fig. 12.13 Atypical carcinoid tumour of the larynx showing vascular invasion. H&E, ×40 OM.

Immunocytochemistry

This tumour may show positive staining for chromogranin, NSE, synaptophysin (Fig. 12.14), protein gene product 9.5 (PGP 9.5), Leu 7, endocrine granule constituent (EGC), cytokeratin (Fig. 12.15), neurofilaments (Fig. 12.16), epithelial membrane antigen (EMA), CEA, S-100 protein, calcitonin (Fig. 12.17), serotonin, somatostatin, adrenocorticotropic hormone (ACTH), gastrin, glucagon, growth hormone (GH), α-chain of human chorionic gonadotropin (α-HCG), human chorionic gonadotropin (HCG), and met-enkephalin. These tumours also stain for calcitonin gene-related peptide (CGRP) and vasoactive intestinal peptide (VIP) (Milroy, personal communication).

The positive reaction to different antisera in laryngeal carcinoids is recorded in Table 12.1

DNA image analysis

Aneuploidy is often seen in atypical carcinoid tumours of the larynx, but this has not provided any useful prognostic information.[167]

Electron microscopy

There are many round and oval neurosecretory granules in the cytoplasm but in smaller numbers than in the typical carcinoid tumour. The membrane-bound granules have an electron-dense core separated from the membrane by a clear space (Fig. 12.18).

Diagnosis and differential diagnosis

Morphological diagnosis is based primarily on conventional light microscopy and confirmed by histochemical, immunohistochemical and ultrastructural investigations. The differential diagnosis may be difficult from poorly differentiated squamous cell carcinoma, small cell neuroendocrine carcinoma, acinic cell carcinoma, paraganglioma, medullary carcinoma of the thyroid gland and otherwise unspecified adenocarcinoma. Several of the cases described in the literature had been misdiagnosed as 'undifferentiated' carcinoma and melanoma. Several reported cases diagnosed as laryngeal paragangliomas were, in fact, atypical carcinoids.[8,245,250,251]

The presence of neurosecretory granules assists in distinguishing these neoplasms from a squamous cell carcinoma. The granules in carcinoid tumours are larger and more numerous than those in small cell neuroendocrine carcinomas. A marked elevation of 5-hydroxyindoleacetic acid, caused by impaired tryptophan metabolism, is considered pathognomonic for carcinoid tumour.

Pretreatment evaluation

The propensity of atypical carcinoid tumours of the larynx to metastasize widely makes staging procedures most im-

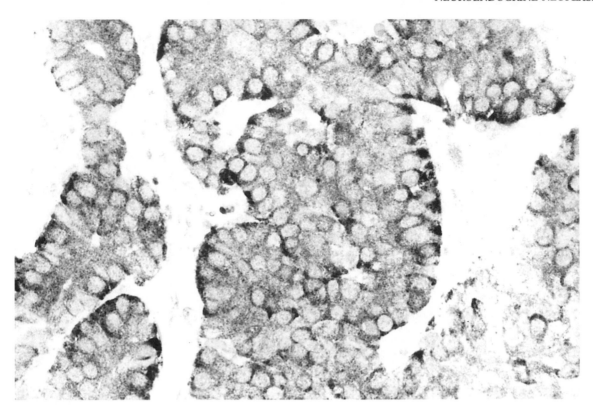

Fig. 12.14   Laryngeal atypical carcinoid tumour showing positive immunostaining for synaptophysin. Immunoperoxidase, ×100 OM.

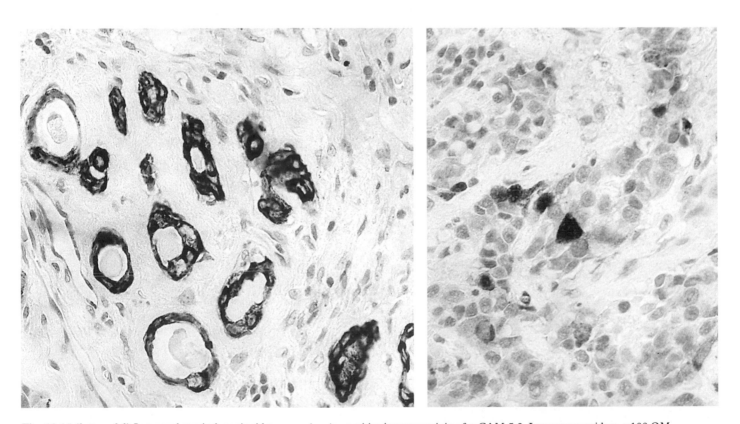

Fig. 12.15 (*bottom, left*) Laryngeal atypical carcinoid tumour showing positive immunostaining for CAM 5.2. Immunoperoxidase, ×100 OM.

Fig. 12.16 (*bottom, right*) Focal positivity for neurofilaments is present. Immunoperoxidase, ×100 OM.

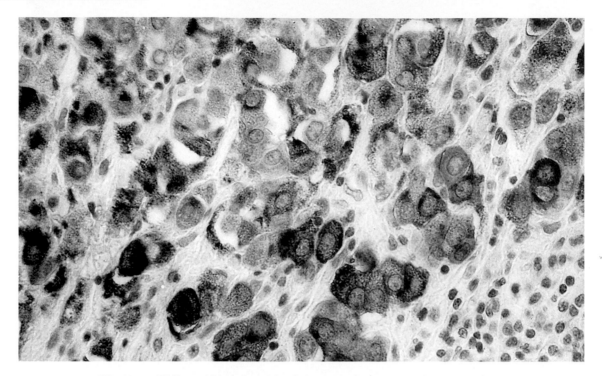

Fig. 12.17   Diffuse positivity for calcitonin is present. Immunoperoxidase, ×100 OM.

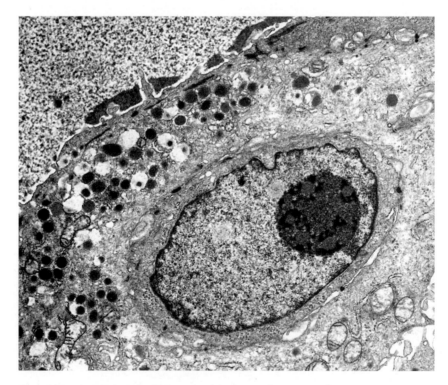

Fig. 12.18   Atypical carcinoid tumour of the larynx displaying neurosecretory granules. ×10 000. (Courtesy of Dr S. Smets, Brussels, and the editor of *Virchows Archiv. A. Pathological Anatomy and Histopathology*.)

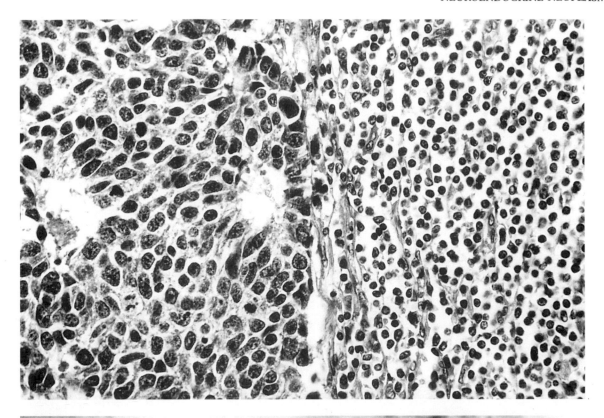

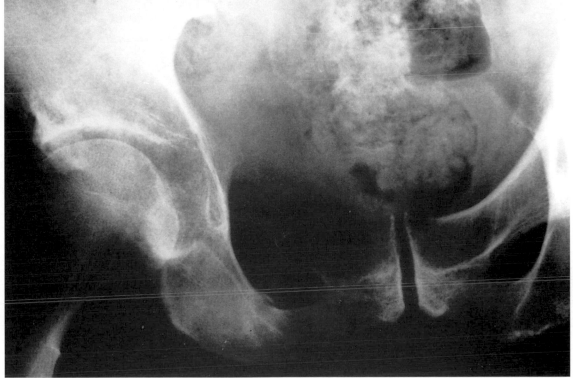

Fig. 12.19 (*top*,) Secondary atypical carcinoid tumour of the larynx in a cervical lymph node. H&E, ×100 OM.

Fig. 12.20 (*bottom*) Classical pattern of pelvic bone metastasis from an atypical carcinoid tumour of the larynx.

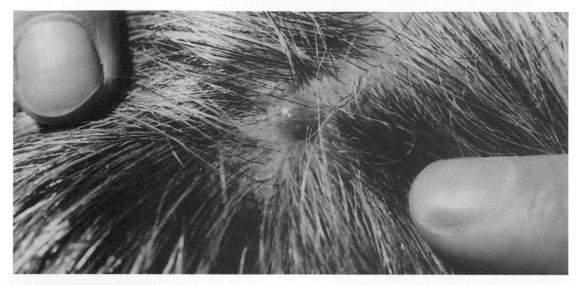

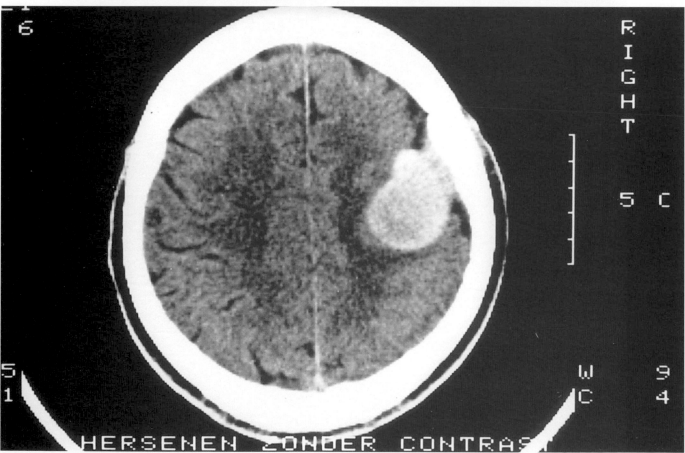

Fig. 12.21 (*top*) Subcutaneous metastasis from atypical carcinoid tumour of the larynx. (Courtesy of Dr G. Zambruno, Modena, and the editor of *Annales de Dermatologie et de Venereologie*.)

Fig. 12.22 (*bottom*) Lateral view of ^{123}I-meta-iodobenzylguanidine planar scintigram showing parietal accumulation of the tracer. (Courtesy of Dr D. Deleu, Brussels, and the editor of *American Journal of Medicine*.)

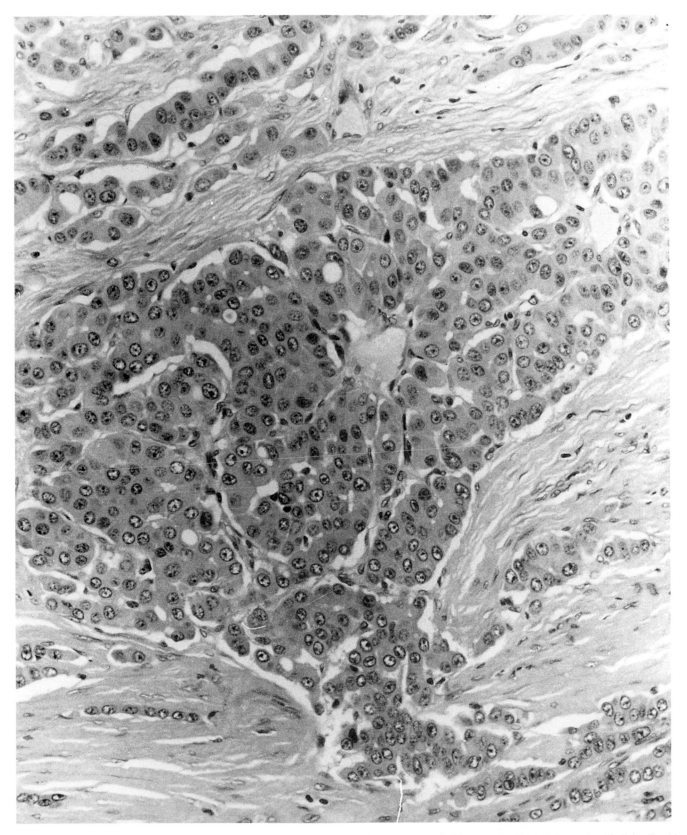

Fig. 12.23 Metastasis from an atypical carcinoid tumour of the larynx in the dura mater. Solid nests of uniform polygonal epithelial cells with round nuclei invade a partly hyalinized fibrous stroma. H&E, ×150 OM. (Courtesy of Dr D. Deleu, Brussels, and the editor of *American Journal of Medicine*.)

portant. Investigation of the patient for distant metastases should be performed, including endoscopic examination of the upper aerodigestive tract, chest radiographs, whole lung tomography, bone scintigraphy, liver echotomography, iliac crest bone marrow aspiration and biopsy, computed tomography of the brain and laboratory investigations.

Hepatic staging is important in the assessment of the prognosis. Hepatic metastases may be diagnosed by computed tomography, isotopic liver scans and ultrasound. Computed tomography-guided fine needle biopsy is useful for ascertaining the nature of the disease. Liver function tests play a limited role in the diagnosis of liver metastases. The skin should be examined carefully and the patient questioned about the presence of subcutaneous nodules,[14] because 22% of reported cases had secondaries to the skin or subcutaneous tissue.[250]

Therapy

Surgical resection is the treatment of choice for laryngeal atypical carcinoid tumours. Conservative laryngeal surgery should be employed if the tumour could be adequately removed.[14,245] Large tumours may require total laryngectomy. Neck dissection should also be performed in atypical carcinoid tumour because of the high likelihood of cervical lymph node metastases; conversely, it is not indicated in typical neoplasms. Local recurrence can be surgically removed by means of a more extensive procedure. The best palliative treatment for distant metastases is surgical excision, whenever possible. It can relieve the pain caused by subcutaneous nodules. Radiotherapy has been used without observable effect in pre-operative, postoperative and primary modalities.[210] Currently available chemotherapeutic options are inadequate. Horikawa and Matsubara[109] have used hyperthermia without success.

Prognosis

The clinical behaviour of an atypical carcinoid tumour is aggressive. Cervical lymph node metastases are often present (Fig. 12.19). Other sites of metastases include bones (Fig. 12.20), the skin, subcutaneous tissues (Fig. 12.21), distant lymph nodes, lung, mediastinum, liver, heart, pancreas, diaphragm, peritoneum, gastrointestinal tract, prostate, breast, brain, dura mater (Figs 12.22, 12.23), pleura, testicle and muscles. Laccourreye et al[134] reported a case of synchronous laryngeal and pancreatic neuroendocrine carcinoma, but Woodruff and we consider this pancreatic lesion as a metastasis from the laryngeal neoplasm.

Death has usually resulted from distant metastases and not from local or regional recurrence.

The survival rate is 48% at 5 years and 30% at 10 years.[250]

SMALL CELL NEUROENDOCRINE CARCINOMA

Introduction

Extrapulmonary primary small cell neuroendocrine carcinoma has been reported with increasing frequency.[58, 90, 91, 112] These neoplasms may arise in the nasal cavity, paranasal sinuses, oral cavity, tongue, larynx, salivary glands, oesophagus, trachea, stomach, pancreas, small and large bowel, uterine cervix, endometrium, breast, prostate, urinary bladder, skin and thymus.

Pulmonary small cell neuroendocrine carcinoma is a highly aggressive neoplasm with a high mortality rate.

Terminology

Various terms have been applied, e.g., small cell carcinoma, oat cell carcinoma, undifferentiated small cell carcinoma, neuroendocrine carcinoma, neuroendocrine neoplasm, endocrine carcinoma, anaplastic small cell carcinoma, small cell endocrine carcinoma, poorly differentiated neuroendocrine carcinoma, neuroendocrine carcinoma with exocrine differentiation, Kultschitzky cell carcinoma, neuroendocrine carcinoma of small cell type, etc.

Definition

Small cell neuroendocrine carcinoma is a highly malignant epithelial neoplasm composed of round, oval or spindle cells with histochemical, immunohistochemical and ultrastructural evidence of neuroendocrine differentiation.

Incidence

The first case in the larynx was reported by Olofsson and van Nostrand in 1972.[180] The total number reported in the world literature may be about 130.[85,150a,251a] The larynx is one of the most common sites of extra pulmonary small cell neuroendocrine carcinoma.

Clinical features

The neoplasm affects mainly men of fifty to seventy years of age who have been heavy cigarette smokers.[63,151] It has not been reported to date in children. The neoplasm may occur in any part of the larynx, although the supraglottic and subglottic regions are the most affected sites.

Symptoms and signs are similar to those of other laryngeal neoplasms and depend upon the region involved. Patients often present with complaints of hoarseness and a neck mass or masses.

Histogenesis

The histogenesis of neuroendocrine carcinomas (carcinoid tumour, atypical carcinoid tumour and small cell neuroendocrine carcinoma) has remained obscure. They are thought to originate from endocrine cells or argyrophilic Kultschitzky cells (K cells) normally found in animal[55, 123,145,226] and human[188] laryngeal mucosa and are therefore included in the group of neoplasms of the diffuse endocrine system.

It is also possible that the neoplasms arise from normally non-argyrophilic but pluripotential indifferent cells situated in the seromucous gland-duct apparatus[251] and in the squamous epithelium. The coexistence of tonofilaments, cilia, desmosomes, neurosecretory granules and mucin granules within single tumour cells supports the hypothesis that the neuroendocrine neoplasms arise from a common primitive and pluripotential stem cell, rather than from a specific neuroendocrine precursor.

Pathology

Gross pathology

The tumour presents as a submucosal lesion (Fig. 12.24).

Histopathology

The tumour is formed by small cells of varied shape with scanty cytoplasm and relatively large, hyperchromatic, oval, round or spindle-shaped nuclei with delicate chromatin and inconspicuous nucleoli (Fig. 12.25). Necrosis is prominent. Typical crush artefact is present. Mitoses are numerous and vascular, perineural (Fig. 12.26) and skeletal muscle invasion is commonly seen. Rosette formation is rare. The stroma is scanty and rarely mucoid. Scattered neoplastic multinucleated giant cells

may be present. Occasionally the cells appear to cluster around alveolar-like spaces containing diastase PAS-positive material. Rarely, glandular structures may be present (Fig. 12.27). Reticulin staining is negative.

Histochemistry

Grimelius and Fontana–Masson stains for argyrophilic and argentaffin cells are frequently negative, probably due to the paucity of neurosecretory granules.

Immunocytochemistry

This tumour may yield positive reactions to chromogranin (Fig. 12.28), NSE, synaptophysin, PGP 9.5, cytokeratin, neurofilaments, CEA, calcitonin, somatostatin, ACTH, C-flanking peptide of human pro-bombesin (CFB), bombesin, serotonin, neurotensin, gastrin-releasing polypeptide (GRP) and β-endorphin (see Table 12.2).

Electron microscopy

There are several dense-core neurosecretory-type granules (Fig. 12.29), preferentially located in the periphery of the cytoplasm.[17,89]

Classification

The small cell neuroendocrine carcinoma may be classified as follows:

Table 12.2 Positive immunohistochemical reactions in laryngeal small cell neuroendocrine carcinomas and carcinoma with neuroendocrine differentiation

Markers	Year	References
Calcitonin[1]	1981	91
Calcitonin, somatostatin[1]	1982	90
NSE, cytokeratin, calcitonin, ACTH, neurotensin, GRP, β-endorphin	1985	19
NSE, calcitonin	1985	241
NSE, CEA, serotonin	1985	251
NSE, PGP 9.5, bombesin, CFB	1986	216
Chromogranin, NSE, cytokeratin, CEA, bombesin, serotonin	1988	89
Chromogranin A, synaptophysin, cytokeratin, neurofilaments	1990	49
Chromogranin, NSE, PGP 9.5, cytokeratin	1991	165
Cytokeratin	1991	150a
NSE, cytokeratin	1991	251a
NSE	1992	127a

[1]Authors refer to the same patient.

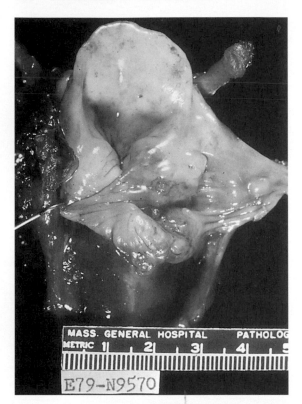

Fig. 12.24 (*top*) Submucosal small cell neuroendocrine carcinoma is present as a mass in the right aryepiglottic fold that insidiously extends into the left arytenoid area and epiglottis (fresh specimen, posterior view). (Courtesy of Dr P. G. Googe, Boston, and the editor of *Archives of Pathology and Laboratory Medicine*.)

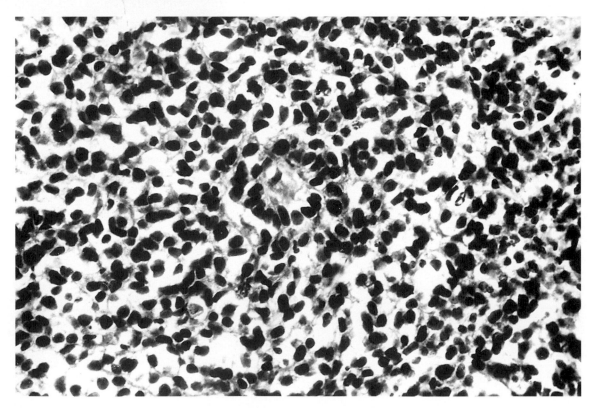

Fig. 12.25   Small cell neuroendocrine carcinoma, oat cell type. Note a typical rosette. H&E, ×100 OM.

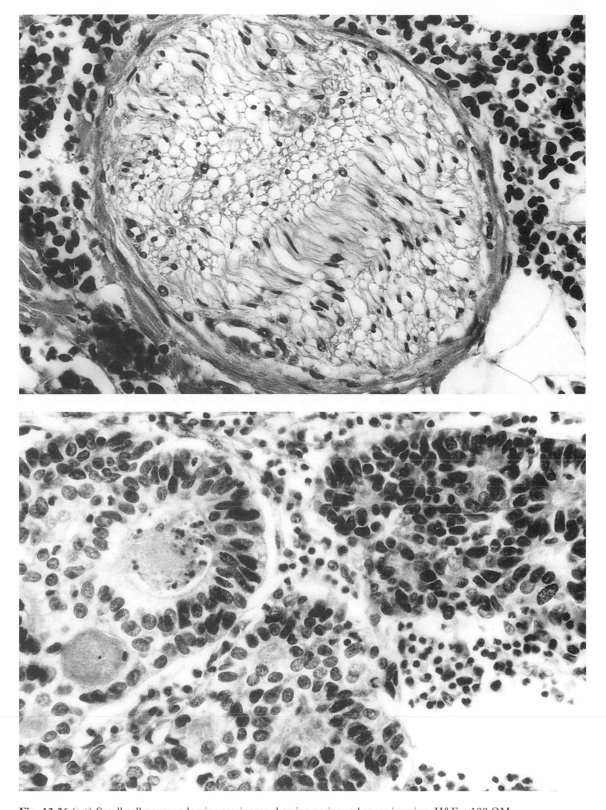

Fig. 12.26 (*top*) Small cell neuroendocrine carcinoma showing perineural space invasion. H&E, ×100 OM.

Fig. 12.27 (*bottom*) Small cell neuroendocrine carcinoma forming glandular structures. H&E, ×100 OM.

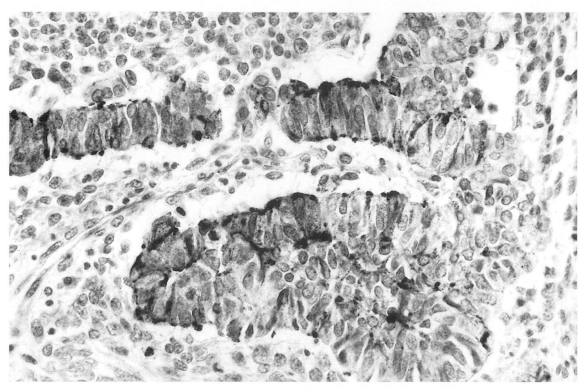

Fig. 12.28   Small cell neuroendocrine carcinoma showing a positive reaction for chromogranin. Immunoperoxidase, ×100 OM.

Oat cell carcinoma. A malignant tumour composed of uniform small cells, generally larger than lymphocytes, having dense round or oval nuclei, diffuse chromatin, inconspicuous nucleoli and very sparse cytoplasm.

Intermediate cell type. A malignant neoplasm composed of small cells, with nuclear characteristics similar to the oat cell type but with more abundant cytoplasm. The cells may be polygonal or fusiform and are less regular in appearance than those of oat cell carcinoma.

Combined cell type. A neoplasm in which there is a definite component of oat cell carcinoma (or intermediate cell type) with squamous cell carcinoma (Fig. 12.30) and/or adenocarcinoma.

Hybrid cell type. A neoplasm rarely shows simultaneous evidence of squamous, glandular and neuroendocrine differentiation. A recently-reported tumour showed squamous, glandular, neuroendocrine and exocrine as well as chondrosarcomatous and rhabdomyosarcomatous differentiation.[49] Another similar tumour has been described.[127a]

Diagnosis and differential diagnosis

The diagnosis presents no major difficulty and is based essentially on the microscopic features of the lesion, confirmed by ultrastructural evidence of neurosecretory granules and assisted by histochemical and immunocytochemical investigations. The differential diagnosis includes the typical carcinoid tumour, atypical carcinoid tumour, small cell squamous carcinoma (or 'pseudo' oat cell carcinoma), lymphoma and mycosis fungoides. It is also important to ascertain whether the small cell neuroendocrine carcinoma is a primary or a secondary from a bronchogenic, tracheal or prostatic neoplasm. This possibility is rare, and only five cases have been reported.[25,76,95,132,193]

There is an overlap in immunoreactivity between carcinoid tumours and small cell neuroendocrine carcinoma. Electron microscopy is useful in distinguishing this tumour from small cell squamous carcinoma. The presence of spindle-shaped cells, rosettes and glandular structures in small cell neuroendocrine carcinoma and the usually high mitotic index may assist in the differential diagnosis with respect to malignant lymphoma. CEA may be expressed by the cells of the small cell neuroendocrine carcinoma but not by the cells of a lymphoma.[192] Leucocyte common antigen is present in lymphomas but is absent in neuroendocrine carcinomas. Besides L-26, a pan B cell marker, or UCHL-1, a pan T cell marker, are negative in small cell neuroendocrine carcinoma.[85] Dense-core granules are not found in lymphomas. Mycosis fungoides involving the larynx[70] may also be difficult to distinguish from this neoplasm. A polymorphic lymphocytic infiltrate, Sézary cells with cerebriform nuclei and Pautrier mucosal microabscesses are distinguishing features of mycosis fungoides.

In classifying laryngeal neuroendocrine carcinomas, the distinction between typical carcinoid tumour, atypical

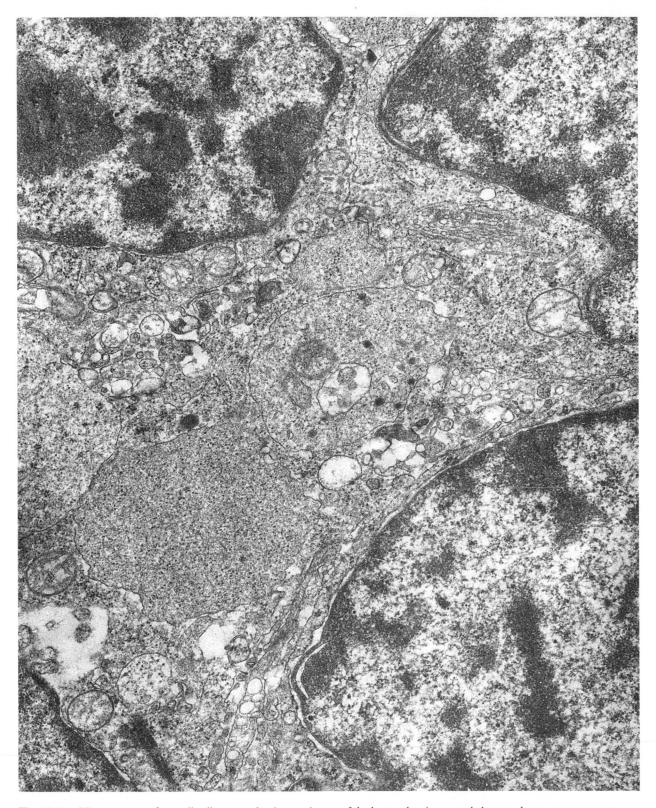

Fig. 12.29 Ultrastructure of a small cell neuroendocrine carcinoma of the larynx showing several electron-dense neurosecretory granules. ×24 000.

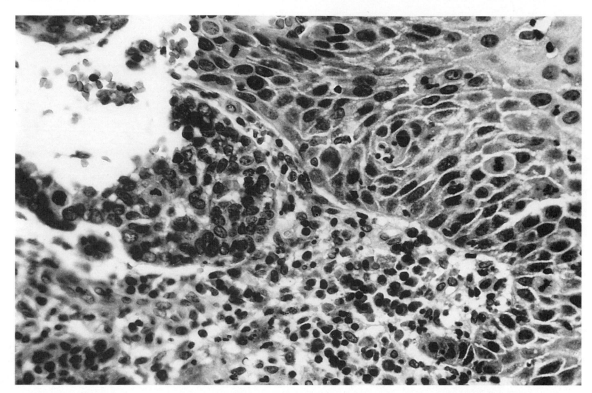

Fig. 12.30   Combined small cell neuroendocrine carcinoma of the larynx. H&E, ×100 OM.

carcinoid tumour, and small cell neuroendocrine carcinoma is of paramount prognostic importance. Typical carcinoid tumours and small cell neuroendocrine carcinomas probably occupy the two ends of a spectrum of neoplasms with differing degrees of neuroendocrine differentiation. Table 12.3 illustrates the comparative differential diagnostic findings of all neuroendocrine neoplasms of the larynx.

Paraneoplastic syndromes

A paraneoplastic syndrome may be the first indication of an underlying laryngeal endocrine carcinoma. These syndromes are not due to direct organ invasion, but they are caused by substances elaborated by the distant neoplasm. Such syndromes may precede the presentation of the cancer by many months, or occasionally by several years. Both the hormones and the antibodies share the property of acting far from their sites of synthesis. Paraneoplastic syndromes associated with small cell neuroendocrine carcinoma have been reported. In 1979, Trotoux et al[233] described the Schwartz–Bartter syndrome (inappropriate secretion of antidiuretic hormone) in a 61-year-old man that led to the detection of a small cell neuroendocrine carcinoma in the subglottic region of the patient. This case confirmed the hormone-secreting property of the neoplastic cells. Diagnostic criteria include hyponatraemia, hypo-osmolar serum, continued urinary sodium excretion with less than maximally diluted urine, normal intravascular volume status,

normal renal and adrenal function, elevated plasma concentrations of vasopressin and hypo-urycaemia because of increased renal clearance. In this syndrome there is a deficiency in re-absorption of sodium in the proximal part of the renal tubules with water retention. The syndrome can be caused by drugs such as vincristine and cyclophosphamide and also by infections like tuberculosis. It has also been described following neck dissection. Fluid restriction can prevent the development of this syndrome and its sequelae. Clinically it is characterized by an altered mental status, confusion, seizures and, occasionally, coma.

In 1989, Takeuchi et al[227] reported a case of small cell neuroendocrine carcinoma of the larynx associated with inappropriate secretion of antidiuretic hormone. In 1984, Medina et al[158] reported a case of primary small cell neuroendocrine carcinoma of the larynx associated with clinical and electromyographic evidence of the myasthenic syndrome, which was first described by Eaton and Lambert in 1957.[51] It is characterized by muscular weakness and easily fatigued proximal muscles, particularly of the lower extremities. The upper extremities may become involved. Ocular and bulbar involvement is rare and, when present, less severe than that of myasthenia gravis. Deep tendon reflexes are hypo-active or absent, but sensory function is preserved. In contrast to myasthenia gravis, muscle strength improves with exercise. Electromyography is essential in the diagnosis of this syndrome and the EMG findings differ from those observed in patients with myasthenia gravis. Electrophysiological diagnosis of the Eaton–Lambert

Table 12.3   Comparison of laryngeal neuroendocrine neoplasms[1]

Features	Carcinoid tumour	Atypical carcinoid tumour	Small cell neuroendocrine carcinoma	Paraganglioma
Clinical features				
Age	6th decade	6th, 7th decades	6th, 7th decades	5th decade
Sex (M:F)	6:1	3:1	3:1	1:3
Location	Supraglottic submucosal	Supraglottic submucosal	Supraglottic submucosal	Supraglottic submucosal
Symptoms	Hoarseness	Hoarseness	Hoarseness	Hoarseness
Behaviour	Usually benign	Malignant	Malignant	Benign
Metastases	Rare	Frequent: neck lymph nodes, lung, bone, liver, skin	Frequent: neck lymph nodes, liver, lung, bone marrow, brain	Extremely rare
Paraneoplastic syndromes	Exceptional	Exceptional	Occasional	Absent
Treatment	Surgery	Surgery	Systemic chemotherapy and irradiation	Surgery
Prognosis	Excellent, with cure following surgery	48% 5-year survival; 30% 10-year survival	16% 2-year survival; 5% 5-year survival	Excellent
Histological features				
Surface involvement	Absent	Generally absent	Absent	Absent
Ulceration	Absent	Commonly absent	Present	Absent
Architecture	Organoid, trabecular	Organoid, trabecular, cribriform, solid	Solid, sheets, ribbons	Organoid
Cellular pattern	Orderly	Disorganized	Disorganized	Orderly
Fibrovascular stroma	Present	Present	Absent	Present
Vascular/lymphatic invasion	Absent	Occasionally present	Commonly present	Exceptional
Perineural infiltration	Absent	May be present	Commonly present	Exceptional
Glands	May be present	Present	Rarely present	Absent
Squamous nests	May be present	May be present	Occasionally present	Absent
Pleomorphism	Absent	Mild to marked	Prominent	Infrequent
Nuclear hyperchromasia	Slight	Marked	Prominent	May be marked
Necrosis	Absent	Uncommon, focal	Prominent	Exceptional
Mitoses	Absent	Scant	Abundant	Rare
Crush phenomenon	Absent	Absent	Prominent	Absent
Oncocytic feature	May be present	May be present	Absent	Absent
Azzopardi's effect	Absent	Absent	Present	Absent
Nuclei	Round to oval; vesicular; central	Round to oval; vesicular to markedly hyperchromatic; central to eccentric	Oval to spindle; intensely hyperchromatic	Round to oval; hyperchromatic
Cytoplasm	Eosinophilic; oncocytic	Eosinophilic to amphophilic; may be oncocytic	Minimal	Eosinophilic to clear
Nucleoli	Absent	Absent to prominent	Absent	Occasionally present
N/C ratio	Low	Variable	High	Variable
Histochemistry				
Epithelial mucin	Commonly present	Commonly present	May be present	Absent
Argyrophilia	Positive	Variable	Sparse	Positive
Argentaffinity	Rarely present	Rarely present	Absent	Absent
Immunocytochemistry				
CK	+	+	+	−
EMA	+	+	+	−
CEA	+	+	+	−
CT	+	+	+	−
CHROM	+	+	+	+
NSE	+	+	+	+
Ultrastructure				
Neurosecretory granules	Abundant; 90–230 nm	Common; 70–420 nm	Rare; 50–200 nm	Abundant; 100–250 nm
Cellular junctional complexes (desmosomes; tonofilaments)	Present	Present	Scant	Infrequent
Sustentacular cells	May be present	May be present	Absent	Present

[1]Modified from Ferlito and Friedmann[67] and Wenig and Gnepp.[244]
Abbreviations: CK, cytokeratin; CT, calcitonin; CHROM, chromogranin.

syndrome rests on the observation of a progressive increase in the amplitude — by 200% or more — of the compound muscle action potential evoked by repetitive supramaximal nerve stimulation. In 1985, Bishop et al[19] reported a case of laryngeal small cell neuroendocrine carcinoma with the ectopic ACTH syndrome. Adrenocorticotropic hormone production may also occur in this tumour. The metastatic syndromes associated with laryngeal neuroendocrine neoplasms are summarized in Table 12.4. Only one patient suffering from a typical carcinoid tumour with liver metastasis has survived (Wenig, personal communication).

Table 12.4 Paraneoplastic syndromes associated with laryngeal neuroendocrine neoplasms

Type of tumour	Syndromes	Year	References
Typical carcinoid	Carcinoid	1989	244
Atypical carcinoid	Carcinoid	1987	14 (case n. 2)
SCNC	SIADH	1979	233
	Eaton–Lambert	1984	158
	ACTH	1985	19
	SIADH	1989	227

SCNC = small cell neuroendocrine carcinoma.
SIADH = syndrome of inappropriate antidiuretic hormone.
ACTH = adrenocorticotropic hormone.

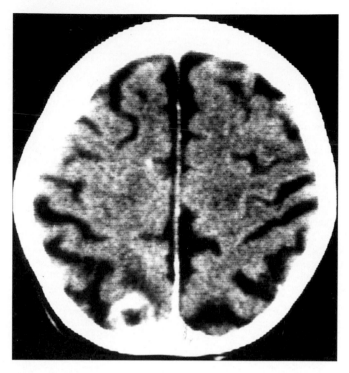

Fig. 12.31 CT scan showing solitary brain metastasis in left occipital lobe.

Pretreatment evaluation

Tumour staging is mandatory for therapeutic and prognostic reasons, and examination should include: pan-endoscopy, chest radiographs, whole lung tomography, bone scintigraphy, liver echotomography, iliac crest bone marrow aspiration and biopsy, computed tomography of the brain and laboratory investigations.

Therapy

The treatment of laryngeal small cell neuroendocrine carcinoma remains a challenge for the surgeon. Radical surgical procedures (total laryngectomy and radical neck dissection) have failed in the majority of cases reported.[83] Total laryngectomy will result in voice loss, and will control only the primary lesion. This is not justifiable if treatment is possible with modalities that preserve the voice and improve the clinical course.

Systemic polychemotherapy with irradiation is the treatment of choice. Commonly-used agents include cyclophosphamide, doxorubicin hydrochloride, vincristine sulphate, methotrexate and lomustine.

Radiotherapy alone has been used successfully to control limited neoplasms. However, in consideration of the early widespread dissemination of the neoplasm, intensive systemic chemotherapy is usually indicated. Some patients may already have a disseminated neoplasm at the time of diagnosis and, in such cases, a course of multi-agent chemotherapy is warranted. Occasionally the disease may appear to be localized, and only rigorous staging procedures can reveal the extent of the tumour. Occult metastases may be present and it is advisable to avoid primary single-modality therapies, such as radiotherapy or surgery alone.

Cerebral metastases (Fig. 12.31) are rare and usually occur as a preterminal event. In small cell lung cancer prophylactic cranial irradiation may reduce the incidence of brain metastases, but does not enhance survival.

Prognosis

The prognosis is poor, and the clinical course is rapidly fatal. The most common sites of metastatic spread of this very aggressive neoplasm are the cervical lymph nodes, liver, lung (Fig. 12.32), bone (Fig. 12.33) and bone marrow. Two- and five-year survivals are 16% and 5%, respectively.[85]

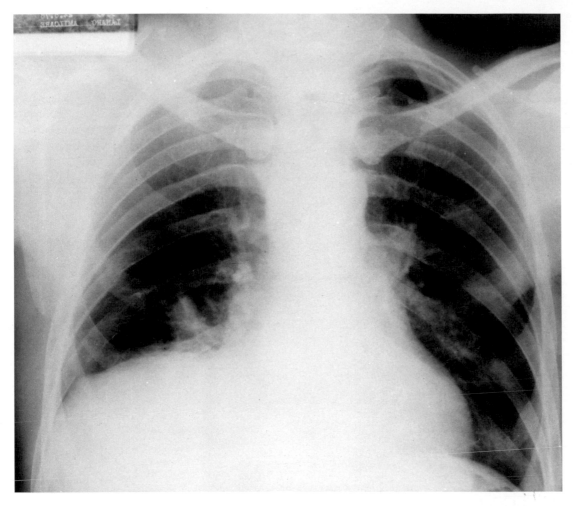

Fig. 12.32   Chest X-ray showing multiple metastases from small cell neuroendocrine carcinoma of the larynx.

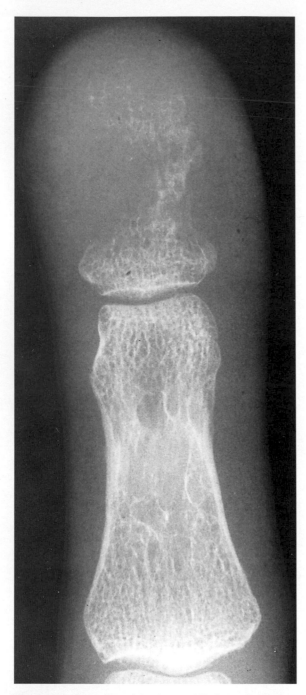

Fig. 12.33 X-ray film of the right middle finger showing metastasis in the distal phalanx.

PARAGANGLIOMA

Anatomy

There are two pairs of paraganglia in the larynx which can give rise to a paraganglioma: one laryngeal glomus in the upper and anterior third of the vestibular fold[240] and another just above the division of the recurrent laryngeal nerve into its anterior and posterior branches, at the level of the inferior border of the thyroid cartilage.[125] The two structures are known as 'glomus laryngicum superior'

(superior laryngeal paraganglia) and 'glomus laryngicum inferior' (inferior laryngeal paraganglia). The superior glomus has a variable and probably multiple distribution in relation to the aryepiglottic fold and the arytenoid region.[140] The superior paraganglia are between 0.1 to 0.3 mm in diameter, while the inferior paraganglia are larger, averaging 0.3 to 0.4 mm in diameter. Minute nests of aberrant paraganglionic tissue may occur anterior and lateral to the cricoid cartilage and posterior in relation to the transverse arytenoid muscle (Fig. 12.34).

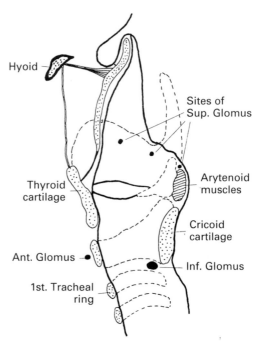

Fig. 12.34 Diagram of sites of glomera of the larynx (Reproduced from Friedmann I, Ferlito A 1988 *Granulomas and Neoplasms of the Larynx* with permission of the publishers, Churchill Livingstone, Edinburgh.)

Terminology

Neoplasms arising from paraganglia have been referred to by a variety of names, including glomus tumour, chromaffin and non-chromaffin paraganglioma, pheochromocytoma, chemodectoma, apudoma. The term glomus tumour is unacceptable since it has been mistaken for — and erroneously assumed as related to — the tumour derived from true glomera, specialized arteriovenous shunts of the skin that regulate temperature.[8] The division of tumours into chromaffin and non-chromaffin types is inadequate. The term paraganglioma, as recommended by the WHO, is preferable.[78]

Definition

Paraganglioma is a tumour derived from paraganglia which tends to reproduce the architecture of a normal paraganglion.

Incidence

The tumour is rare and has been confused with a variety of other primary and secondary laryngeal neoplasms, especially with typical carcinoid and atypical carcinoid tumour. Barnes[8] has critically reviewed the world literature on laryngeal paraganglioma and accepted only 34 cases. Other cases have been reported, one of which occurred in pregnancy.[27a,28a,110,165,234,245a]

Clinical features

This neoplasm is three times more common in women than in men and occurs most often after middle age. The lesion is frequently localized in the supraglottic region, in particular in the right aryepiglottic fold. It may also be present in the subglottic region.[6,27a,28a,89,157,165,181] and may be confused with thyroid neoplasms.[27a]. Some tumours described as 'thyroid paraganglioma' are actually laryngeal paragangliomas derived from inferior laryngeal paraganglia. The major symptom is hoarseness. Other symptoms include dysphagia, dyspnoea, stridor and dysphonia. As a rule these tumours are not functional and they are seldom associated with paragangliomas in other sites. One case report of functional paraganglioma[139] involved a patient with sinus tachycardia and hypertension which disappeared following surgical excision of the tumour. Other reported cases of functional paraganglioma[117,178,238] were probably atypical carcinoids.[9,68,250] Pain has frequently been mentioned as a presenting symptom but the majority of 'pain-inducing' laryngeal paragangliomas were atypical carcinoid tumours.[8] Paraneoplastic or non-metastatic syndromes have not been reported in association with paraganglioma. Biopsy has been associated with brisk, occasionally severe haemorrhage. Milroy et al[165] reported that three out of four biopsies produced catastrophic haemorrhage, which required multiple blood transfusions and ligation of the external carotid artery in one case to arrest the bleeding. Another case of bleeding after biopsy being controlled with difficulty by diathermy was reported by Hussain et al.[110]

Levels of urinary metadrenaline, normetadrenaline and vanillymandelic acid may be raised.[165]

Magnetic resonance imaging is very useful in demonstrating the extent of the lesion (Fig. 12.35).

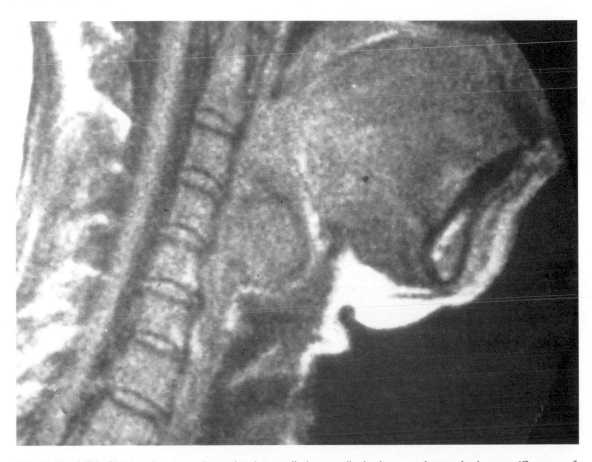

Fig. 12.35   MRI of laryngeal paraganglioma showing a well-circumscribed sub-mucosal supraglottic mass. (Courtesy of Dr C. M. Milroy, London, and the editor of *Histopathology*.)

Aetiology and pathogenesis

The cause of this neoplasm is obscure. Enlarged carotid bodies have been described in relation to chronic hypoxaemia[7] and there are reported increases in the incidence of carotid body tumours at high altitudes.[199]

Histogenesis

The neoplasm arises from paraganglionic tissue normally present in the larynx which has its origin from neural crest cells. This tumour is therefore a neuroendocrine neoplasm of neural type.[71]

Pathology

Gross pathology

The tumours vary in size from a few millimetres to several centimetres (Fig. 12.36) and are almost always encapsulated and of intramucosal location. On cut section (Fig. 12.37), the lesion appears blue or pink, and geographic haemorrhage may be present.

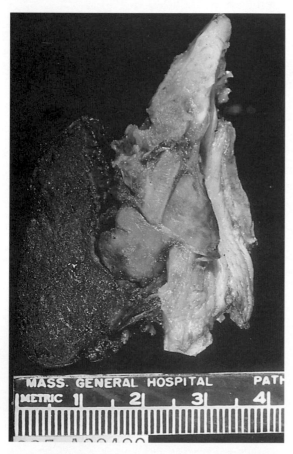

Fig. 12.36 Paraganglioma of the larynx. Submucosal, well-circumscribed, dumbbell-shaped paraganglioma is located between thyroid and cricoid cartilages. It protrudes into and obstructs the subglottic larynx and abuts on the thyroid gland (formalin-fixed specimen, parasagittal section). (Courtesy of Dr P. G. Googe, Boston, and the editor of *Archives of Pathology and Laboratory Medicine*.)

Histopathology

The neoplasm is composed of chief cells arranged in clusters and round cell nests (Zellballen, Fig. 12.38) surrounded by a delicate stroma containing numerous vascular channels. Cell number varies from a few to over 10 cells. The cells have abundant granular eosinophilic cytoplasm and large vesicular nuclei (Figs 12.39, 12.40). Mitoses, necrosis and vascular invasion are infrequent and do not necessarily indicate aggressive or malignant behaviour.[8] Dendritic-like spindle cells or sustentacular cells are found, interspersed among the clusters of polygonal cells. Reticulin stain accentuates the organoid pattern. The tumour contains no mucin. A fibrous capsule might be present.

Histochemistry

Cytoplasmic argyrophilic granules may be demonstrated by the Grimelius stain. The Fontana–Masson stain is negative for argentaffin granules.

Immunocytochemistry

Reactivity has been observed for chromogranin A, synaptophysin, NSE, PGP 9.5, met-enkephalin and serotonin. S-100 protein and glial fibrillary acidic protein (GFAP) are not identified in the tumour cells but may be present in the sustentacular cells[68,165] (see Table 12.5).

Table 12.5 Positive immunohistochemical reactions in paragangliomas of the larynx

Markers	Year	References
NSE	1985	198
Serotonin	1985	251
Chromogranin, NSE, S-100 protein	1988	89
Chromogranin, NSE, S-100 protein, met-enkephalin, GFAP	1989	127
Chromogranin	1989	234
Chromogranin, NSE, S-100 protein	1991	8
Chromogranin, NSE, synaptophysin, PGP 9.5, S-100 protein, met-enkephalin, GFAP	1991	165
NSE, S-100 protein	1992	27a
Chromogranin, NSE, synaptophysin, S-100 protein	1992	245a
Chromogranin, S-100 protein	1992	28a

DNA image analysis

The DNA content has been investigated but nuclear ploidy, whether diploid or aneuploid, cannot be correlated with prognosis.[8,166,167] Aneuploidy per se is not an absolute criterion of malignancy.

Electron microscopy

The neoplastic tissue is formed by large oval or polygonal cells with round to oval nuclei in close apposition to the

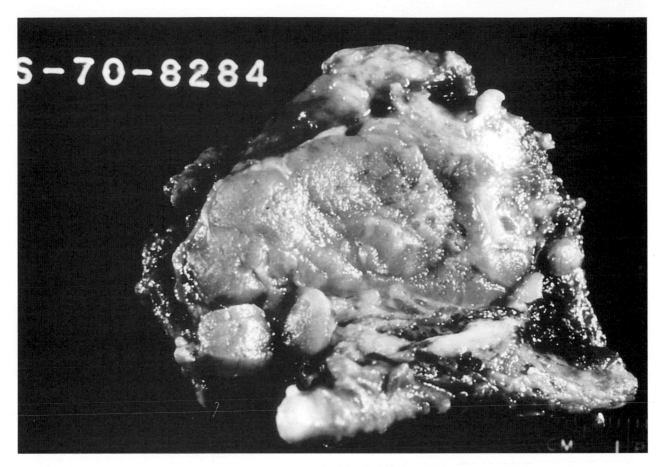

Fig. 12.37   Paraganglioma of the larynx. Cut surface of the lesion. Note the multinodular appearance. (Courtesy of Dr L. Barnes, Pittsburgh and the editor of *ORL; Journal for Oto-Rhino-Laryngology and its Related Specialties*.)

cytoplasmic membranes. These cells contain numerous mitochondria interspersed with strands of rough endoplasmic reticulum. There are large numbers of dense-core neurosecretory granules present in the cytoplasm of neoplastic chief cells (Fig. 12.41). Sustentacular cells have occasionally been described as containing lysosomes but no neurosecretory granules.[89]

Special procedures

Paragangliomas exposed to formalin vapours produce a characteristic green fluorescence due to the reaction of formaldehyde with epinephrine or norepinephrine.[8,44,56]

Diagnosis and differential diagnosis

A survey of the literature indicates that this tumour has often been misdiagnosed — and not only in pre-immunocytochemical times. The diagnostic histological finding is the 'Zellballen' pattern, and the presence of profuse vascular spaces is also characteristic. It is important to make a differential diagnosis from carcinoid tumour (typical or atypical), malignant melanoma (primary or secondary), metastatic renal cell carcinoma and medullary carcinoma of the thyroid.[51a]

The presence of glandular structures, mucus production and positivity for keratin, EMA and CEA are findings incompatible with the diagnosis of paraganglioma. Sustentacular cells may also be present in laryngeal paraganglioma and have been reported in carcinoid tumours of several sites, so this is not a valid element for the differential diagnosis between carcinoids and paraganglioma. The presence of glandular lumina with microvilli argues against a paraganglioma and favours the diagnosis of carcinoid.[30]

As to the differences between paraganglioma and melanoma, paraganglioma is chromogranin-positive but S-100 protein- and HMB-45-negative in the chief cells (only the sustentacular cells are S-100 protein-positive), whereas melanoma is S-100 protein- and HMB-45-positive but chromogranin-negative. Unlike paraganglioma, renal cell carcinoma is negative for chromogranin and NSE.[8] Medullary carcinoma of the thyroid is positive for CEA and calcitonin and generally contains amyloid, while these stains are negative in paraganglioma.[8]

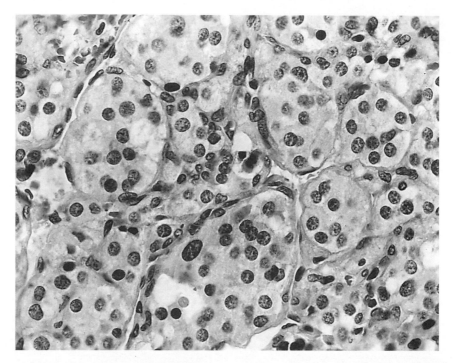

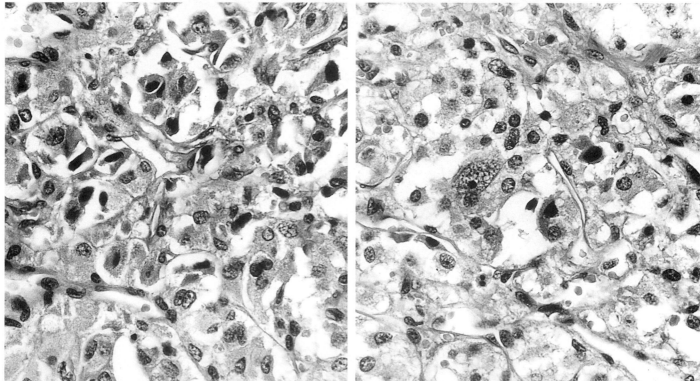

Fig. 12.38 (*top*) Same tumour as in Fig. 12.36. Clusters of chief cells are separated by capillaries producing typical Zellballen of paraganglioma. H&E, ×500. (Courtesy of Dr P. G. Googe, Boston, and the editor of *Archives of Pathology and Laboratory Medicine*.)

Fig. 12.39 (*bottom, left*) Same case as in Fig. 12.37. Typical pattern of paraganglioma. Note the abundant granular cytoplasm of the cells. H&E, ×100 OM. (Slide contributed by Dr L. Barnes, Pittsburgh.)

Fig. 12.40 (*bottom, right*) Same case as in Fig. 12.37. Note in particular the large vesicular nuclei of the lesion. H&E, ×100 OM. (Slide contributed by Dr L. Barnes, Pittsburgh.)

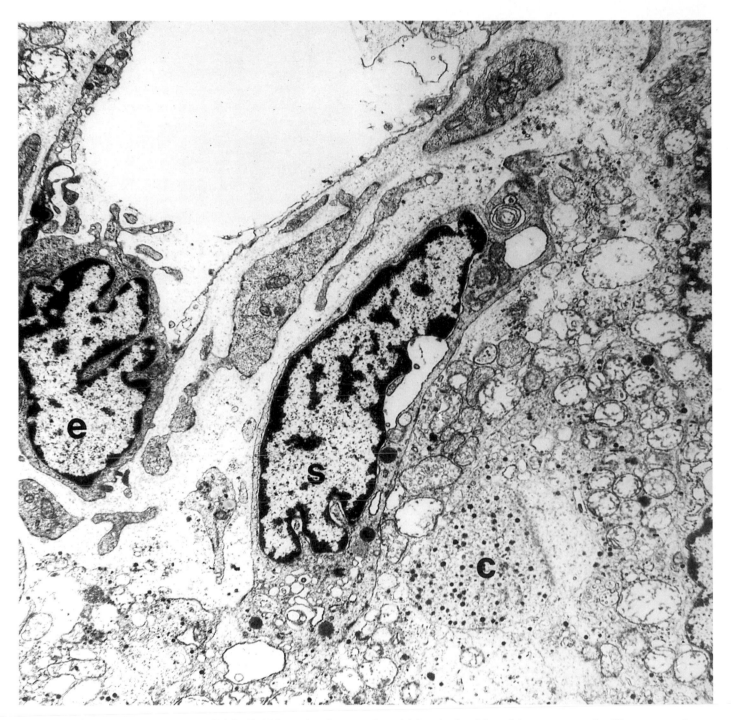

Fig. 12.41   Same case as in Fig. 12.36. Chief cells (c) have abundant cytoplasm rich in mitochondria and dense-core granules. The sustentacular cell (s) is present at the periphery of the nest of chief cells. Delicate capillary network (endothelial cell e) divides tumour cell nests from one another. ×10 260 OM. (Courtesy of Dr P. G. Googe, Boston, and the editor of *Archives of Pathology and Laboratory Medicine.*)

Therapy

Surgery is the treatment of choice for this tumour. Moisa and Silver[171] recommend surgical resection by the lateral pharyngotomy approach, with ligation of the superior thyroid artery as an initial step. Pre-operative angiography and embolization seem unnecessary.[9] Endoscopic excision should be avoided, even for apparently small lesions, since bleeding (which may be profuse even from the biopsy) may be difficult to control.[8,171] Endoscopic excision also makes it difficult to define the margins of excision[9] and local recurrence is common.[128,218] Laser therapy has not been successful[108,128] and there is no proven role for adjuvant radiotherapy in the management of paraganglioma of the larynx.

Prognosis

The biological behaviour of paraganglioma of the larynx is a matter still under discussion, but it seems to be almost exclusively benign. Malignant behaviour has been reported in several cases, but Barnes[8] has accepted only one *possible* case of malignant paraganglioma of the larynx in a 36-year-old woman who developed a metastasis to the lumbar spine 16 years after diagnosis[198] — representing only a 3% incidence of malignancy for laryngeal paraganglioma.

Determination of DNA ploidy fails to provide useful diagnostic or prognostic information.[8,167]

The presence of sustentacular cells indicates benignity and these are usually absent in metastases from paraganglioma of other sites.[127] Histological aspects such as mitoses, nuclear pleomorphism, necrosis and vascular invasion, are of little or no prognostic assistance.[78]

Primary location is often more valuable than histology in assessing prognosis.[127]

REFERENCES

1. Adlington P, Woodhouse M A 1972 The ultrastructure of chemodectoma of the larynx. J Laryngol Otol 86: 1219–1232
2. Aguila Artal A F, Manos Pujol M, Gil Garces E, Soler T, Oncins R, Juan Prada A, Manos Gonzalbo M 1988 Carcinoma neuroendocrino de laringe. A propósito de dos casos. Nota previa. Acta Otorrinolaringol Esp 39: 407–409
3. Aguilar E A III, Robbins K T, Stephens J, Dimery I W, Batsakis J G 1987 Primary oat cell carcinoma of the larynx. Am J Clin Oncol 10: 26–32
4. Ali S, Aird D W, Bihari J 1983 Pain-inducing laryngeal paragangliomas (non-chromaffin). J Laryngol Otol 97: 181–188
5. Andrews A H 1955 Glomus tumors (nonchromaffin paragangliomas) of the larynx. Ann Otol Rhinol Laryngol 97: 181–188
5a. Andrews T M, Myer C M 1992 Malignant (atypical) carcinoid of the larynx occurring in a patient with laryngotracheal papillomatosis. Am J Otolaryngol 13: 238–242
6. Ani A N, Junaid T A, Martinson F D, Adeloye A A 1979 Chemodectoma: a review of 17 cases. Int Surg 64: 43–48
7. Arias-Stella J, Valcarcel J 1976 Chief cell hyperplasia in the human carotid body at high altitude. Physiologic and pathologic significance. Human Pathol 7: 361–373
8. Barnes L 1991 Paraganglioma of the larynx. A critical review of the literature. ORL J Otorhinolaryngol Relat Spec 53: 220–234
9. Basset J M, Paraire F, Francois M, Fleury P 1982 Deux nouvelles tumeurs rares du larynx. Un lipome, un chémodectome. Ann Otolaryngol Chir Cervicofac 99: 151–158
10. Batsakis J G 1979 Tumors of the head and neck. Clinical and pathological considerations, 2nd edn. Williams & Wilkins, Baltimore.
10a. Batsakis J G, El-Naggar A K, Luna M A 1992 Neuroendocrine tumors of larynx. Ann Otol Rhinol Laryngol 101: 710–714
11. Baugh R F, Wolf G T, McClatchey K D 1986 Small cell carcinoma of the head and neck. Head Neck Surg 8: 343–354
12. Baugh R F, McClatchey K D, Sprik S A, Jones H 1987 Laryngeal paraganglioma. J Otolaryngol 16: 167–168
13. Baugh R F, Wolf G T, Beals T, Krause C J, Forastiere A 1986 Small cell carcinoma of the larynx: results of therapy. Laryngoscope 96: 1283–1290
14. Baugh R F, Wolf G T, Lloyd R V, McClatchey K D, Evans D A 1987 Carcinoid (neuroendocrine carcinoma) of the larynx. Ann Otol Rhinol Laryngol 96: 315–321
15. Baxter G D 1965 Glomus tumor (chemodectoma) of the larynx. Ann Otol Rhinol Laryngol 74: 813–820
16. Benevant R G, Bru P, Bompoint J, Boumehdi M 1971 Un nouveau cas de chémodectome laryngé. Cahiers ORL 6: 659–664
17. Benisch B M, Tawfik B, Breitenbach E E 1975 Primary oat cell carcinoma of the larynx: an ultrastructural study. Cancer 36: 145–148
18. Bielawna E, Lubinski J, Sowa J 1982 Przyzojak niechromochlonny krtani. Otolaryngol Pol 36: 261–264
19. Bishop J W, Osamura R Y, Tsutsumi Y 1985 Multiple hormone production in an oat cell carcinoma of the larynx. Acta Pathol Jpn 35: 915–923
20. Bitiutskii P G, Koshanov L G, Baeva A B, Gnucheu E U 1981 Laryngeal carcinoid. Vestn Otorinolaringol 5: 70–71
21. Bitran J D, Toledo-Pereyra L H, Matz G 1978 Oat cell carcinoma of the larynx. Response to combined modality therapy. Cancer 42: 85–87
22. Blanchard Cl, Saunder W H 1955 Chemodectoma of the larynx: case report. Arch Otolaryngol 61: 472–474
23. Blok P H H M, Manni J J, Broek P van den, Haelst U J G M van, Sloof J L 1985 Carcinoid of the larynx: a report of three cases and a review of the literature. Laryngoscope 95: 715–719
24. Boles R 1975 Unusual tumors of the larynx. Canad J Otolaryngol 4: 328–332
25. Bolla A, Cabassa N, Scolari R 1968 Metastasi solitaria al laringe da microcitoma polmonare. Arch Ital Otol 79: 74–82
26. Bone R C, Deer D 1978 Oat cell carcinoma of the larynx. Laryngoscope 88: 1190–1195
27. Bootz F, Helliwell T R, Gärtner H V 1988 Chemodektom des Larynx (Zwei Fallberichte). HNO 36: 166–170
27a. Brandwein M, Levi G, Som P, Urken M L 1992 Paraganglioma of the inferior laryngeal paraganglia. A case report. Arch Otolaryngol Head Neck Surg 118: 994–996
28. Brisigotti M, Fabbretti G, Lanzanova G, Russo Brugneri E, Presutti L, Artoni S 1987 Atypical carcinoid of the larynx: case report. Tumori 73: 427–421
28a. Brownlee R E, Shockley W W 1992 Thyroid paraganglioma. Ann Otol Rhinol Laryngol 101: 293–299
29. Capella G 1989 Paraganglioma laringeo. Acta Otorrinolaringol Esp 40 (suppl 2): 289–294
30. Capella C, Riva C, Cornaggia M, Chiaravalli A M, Frigerio B Solcia E, 1988 Histopathology, cytology and cytochemistry of pheocromocytomas and paragangliomas including chemodectomas. Path Res Pract 183: 176–187
31. Capper J W R, Michaels L, Gregor R T 1981 A malignant

carcinoid tumour of the supraglottic larynx. J Laryngol Otol 95: 963–971

32. Carles D, Devars F, Traissac L, Darasse D, Rinaldo J F, Richir C 1983 Carcinoïde primitif du larynx. Ann Pathol 3: 65–68

33. Casolino D, Caliceti U, Sorrenti G 1990 Carcinoid tumours of the larynx: report of two cases. J Laryngol Otol 104: 264–266

34. Cefis F, Cattaneo M, Carnevale Ricci P M, Frigerio B, Usellini L, Capella C 1983 Primary polypeptide hormones and mucin-producing malignant carcinoid of the larynx. Ultrastruct Pathol 5: 45–53

35. Chen D A, Mandell Brown M, Moore S F, Johnson J T 1986 'Composite' tumour — mixed squamous cell and small-cell anaplastic carcinoma of the larynx. Otolaryngol Head Neck Surg 95: 99–103

36. Coakley J F 1985 Primary oat cell carcinoma of the larynx. J Laryngol Otol 99: 301–303

37. Cosby W N, Babin R W 1988 Simultaneous oat cell and squamous cell carcinoma of the larynx. Milit Med 153: 196–198

37a. Crissman J D, Rosenblatt A 1978 Acinous cell carcinoma of the larynx. Arch Pathol Lab Med 102: 233–236

38. Crowther J A, Colman B H 1987 Chemodectoma of the larynx. J Laryngol Otol 101: 1095–1098

39. D'Agnone N, Ruscito P 1989 Carcinoma a piccole cellule (microcitoma) primitivo della laringe: descrizione di un caso clinico e revisione della letteratura. Otorinolaringologia 39: 561–566

40. Davidge-Pitts K J 1985 Laryngeal paraganglioma. S Afr Med J 68: 971–972

41. De Azevedo-Gamas A, Gloor F 1968 Un cas très rare de tumeur du larynx. Diagnostic anatomo-pathologique inattendu. Ann Otolaryngol Chir Cervicofac 85: 329–335

42. De Barros M C 1962 Neuralgia do laryngeu superior por tumor glomico da arytenoide. Neurobiologica 25: 68–76

43. De la Torre-Rendòn F E, Cisneros-Bernal E, Ochoa-Salas J A, Delfino-Reynoso H A 1979 Carcinoma indiferenciado de celulas pequenas de la laringe. Presentaciòn de un caso con metàstases masivas al hìgado. Patologia 17: 47–57

44. DeLellis R A 1971 Formaldehyde-induced fluorescence technique for the demonstration of biogenic amines in diagnostic histopathology. Cancer 28: 1704–1710

45. Deleu D, De Geeter F 1991 Neurological manifestations of neuroendocrine neoplasms of the larynx. ORL J Otorhinolaryngol Relat Spec 53: 250–258

46. Deleu D, DeGeeter F, Buisseret T, Goossens A,Caemaert J, Ebinger G 1989 Dural metastasis from laryngeal malignant carcinoid. Am J Med 86: 502–505

47. Dellagi K, Jaubert F, Micheau C, Brasnu D, Laccoureye H 1989 Carcinoïdes du larynx. Carcinomes neuroendocrines bien différenciés. A propos de 4 cas. Ann Pathol 9: 284–288

47a. Dictor M, Tennvall J, Akerman M 1992 Moderately differentiated neuroendocrine carcinoma (atypical carcinoid) of the supraglottic larynx. A report of two cases including immunohistochemistry and aspiration cytology. Arch Pathol Lab Med 116: 237–238

48. Dietz R, Wilhelm H J 1978 Therapie des primären 'oat-cell' Karzinoms des Larynx. Laryngol Rhinol Otol 57: 1072–1076

49. Doglioni C, Ferlito A, Chiamenti C, Viale G, Rosai J 1990 Laryngeal carcinoma showing multidirectional epithelial, neuroendocrine and sarcomatous differentiation. ORL J Otorhinolaryngol Relat Spec 52: 316–326

50. Duvall E, Johnston A, McLay K, Piris J 1983 Carcinoid tumour of the larynx. A report of two cases. J Laryngol Otol 97: 1073–1080

51. Eaton L M, Lambert E H 1957 Electromyography and electric stimulation of nerves in diseases of motor unit: observation on the myasthenic syndrome associated with malignant tumors. JAMA 163: 1117–1121

51a. El-Naggar A 1992 Laryngeal neuroendocrine carcinoma. Victims of semantics. Arch Pathol Lab Med 116: 237–238

52. El-Naggar A K, Batsakis J G 1991 Carcinoid tumor of the larynx. A critical review of the literature. ORL J Otorhinolaryngol Relat Spec 53: 188–193

53. El-Naggar A K, Batsakis J G, Vassilopoulou-Sellin R, Ordonez N G, Luna M A 1991 Medullary (thyroid) carcinoma-like carcinoids

of the larynx. J Laryngol Otol 105: 683–686

53a. El-Silimy O, Harvy L 1992 A clinico-pathological classification of laryngeal paraganglioma. J Laryngol Otol 106: 635–639

54. Eusebi V, Betts C M, Giangaspero F 1978 Primary oat-cell carcinoma of the larynx. Virchows Arch 380: 349–354

55. Ewen S W B, Bussolati G, Pearse A G E 1972 Uptake of L-dopa and L-5-hydroxytryptophan by endocrine-like cells in the rat larynx. Histochem J 4: 103–110

56. Falk B, Owman C 1965 A detailed methodological description of the fluorescence method for the cellular demonstration of biogenic monoamines. Acta Univ Lund 7: 5–23

57. Fedorova E N, Böikov V P, Filippova N A 1987 [Carcinoid of the larynx]. Arkh Patol 49: 69–73

58. Fer F M, Levenson R M Jr, Cohen M H, Greco F A 1981 Extrapulmonary small cell carcinoma. In: Greco F A, Oldham R K, Bunn P A Jr (eds) Small cell lung cancer. Grune and Stratton, New York pp 301–325

59. Ferlito A 1974 Oat cell carcinoma of the larynx. Ann Otol Rhinol Laryngol 83: 250–256

60. Ferlito A 1974 Oat cell carcinoma of the larynx (letter to editor). Ann Otol Rhinol Laryngol 83: 834

61. Ferlito A 1976 Histological classification of larynx and hypopharynx cancers and their clinical implications. Pathologic aspects of 2052 malignant neoplasms diagnosed at the ORL Department of Padua University from 1966 to 1976. Acta Otolaryngol 342 (suppl): pp 1–88

62. Ferlito A 1978 Primary oat-cell carcinoma of the larynx following supraglottic laryngectomy for squamous cell carcinoma. J Am Geriatr Soc 26: 278–283

63. Ferlito A 1985 Malignant epithelial tumors of the larynx. In: Ferlito A (ed) Cancer of the larynx, vol I. CRC Press, Boca Raton, pp 91–195

64. Ferlito A 1986 Diagnosis and treatment of small cell carcinoma of the larynx: a critical review. Ann Otol Rhinol Laryngol 95: 590-600

65. Ferlito A 1987 Malignant laryngeal epithelial tumors and lymph node involvement: therapeutic and prognostic considerations. Ann Otol Rhinol Laryngol 96: 542–548

66. Ferlito A cited by Woodruff J M, Senie R T 1991 Atypical carcinoid tumor of the larynx. A critical review of the literature. ORL J Otorhinolaryngol Relat Spec 53: 194–209

67. Ferlito A, Friedmann I 1989 Review of neuroendocrine carcinomas of the larynx. Ann Otol Rhinol Laryngol 98: 780–790

68. Ferlito A, Friedmann I 1991 The contribution of immunohistochemistry in the diagnosis of neuroendocrine neoplasms of the larynx. ORL J Otorhinolaryngol Relat Spec 53: 235–244

69. Ferlito A, Polidoro F 1980 Simultaneous primary oat cell carcinoma (apudoma) and squamous cell carcinoma of the hypopharynx. ORL J Otorhinolaryngol Relat Spec 42: 146–157

70. Ferlito A, Recher G 1986 Laryngeal involvement by mycosis fungoides. Ann Otol Rhinol Laryngol 95: 275–277

71. Ferlito A, Rosai J 1991 Terminology and classification of neuroendocrine neoplasms of the larynx. ORL J Otorhinolaryngol Relat Spec 53: 185–187

72. Ferlito A, Friedmann I, Goldman NC 1988 Primary carcinoid tumour of the larynx. ORL J Otorhinolaryngol Relat Spec 50: 129–149

73. Ferlito A, Recher G, Caruso G 1985 Primary combined small cell carcinoma of the larynx. Am J Otolaryngol 6: 302–308

74. Ferlito A, Caruso G, Nicolai P, Recher G, Silvestri F 1981 Primary small cell ('oat cell') carcinoma of the larynx and hypopharynx. A clinico-pathological study of 8 cases with a review of the literature. ORL J Otorhinolaryngol Relat Spec 43: 204–222

75. Ferlito A, Pesavento G, Recher G, Caruso G, Dal Fior S, Montaguti A, Carraro R, Narne S, Pennelli N 1986 Long-term survival in response to combined chemotherapy and radiotherapy in laryngeal small cell carcinoma. Auris Nasus Larynx 13: 113–123

76. Fiaoni M, Colonna A, Leonardi M Jr, Passamonti G L 1989 Metastasi laringea solitaria di carcinoma a piccole cellule polmonari 'cosiddetto microcitoma': Descrizione di un caso clinico. Valsalva 65: 203–209

77. Fraidooni H 1976 La chimiothèrapie dans un cas de chémodectome du larynx. Ann Otolaryngol Chir Cervicofac 93: 303–305

78. Friedmann I, Ferlito A 1988 Granulomas and neoplasms of the larynx. Churchill Livingstone, Edinburgh, pp 197–222

79. Gallivan M V E, Chun B, Rowden G, Lack E E 1979 Laryngeal paraganglioma: case report with the ultrastructural analysis and literature review. Am J Surg Pathol 3: 85–92

80. Gapany-Gapanavicius V, Kenan S 1981 Carcinoid tumor of the larynx. Ann Otol Rhinol Laryngol 90: 42–47

81. Gehanno P, Lallemant Y, Groussard O, Blanchet F, Veber F, Guedon C, Rame J A 1980 Apudomes en O.R.L. à propos de 6 observations (dont 1 chémodectome et 1 carcinoïde du larynx); critique du concept d'apudome. J Franc Otorhinolaryngol 29: 7–18

82. Gelot R, Rhee T R, Lapidot A 1975 Primary oat-cell carcinoma of head and neck. Ann Otol Rhinol Laryngol 84: 238–244

83. Giddins N A, Kennedy T L, Vrabec D P 1987 Primary small cell carcinoma of the larynx: analysis of treatment. J Otolaryngol 16: 157–65

84. Gignoux M, Martin H, Feroldi J, Lapicorey G 1964 Paragangliome non chromaffine du larynx. Ann Otolaryngol Chir Cervicofac 82: 505–508

85. Gnepp D R 1991 Small cell neuroendocrine carcinoma of the larynx. A critical review of the literature. ORL J Otorhinolaryngol Relat Spec 53: 210–219

86. Gnepp D R, Ferlito A, Hyams V 1983 Primary anaplastic small cell (oat cell) carcinoma of the larynx. Review of the literature and report of 18 cases. Cancer 51: 1731–1745

87. Goldman N C, Hood C I, Singleton G T 1969 Carcinoid of the larynx. Arch Otolaryngol 90: 91–93

88. Goldman N C, Katibah G M, Medina J 1985 Carcinoid tumors of the larynx. Ear Nose Throat J 64: 130–134

89. Googe P B, Ferry J A, Bhan A K, Dickersin G R, Pilch B Z, Goodman M 1988 A comparison of paraganglioma, carcinoid tumor, and small-cell carcinoma of the larynx. Arch Pathol Lab Med 112: 809–815

90. Gould V E 1982 Neuroendocrine tumors in 'miscellaneous' primary sites: clinical, pathologic, and histogenetic implications. In: Fenoglio C M, Wolff M (eds) 1982 Progress in surgical pathology IV, Masson, New York, pp 181–198

91. Gould V E, Banner B F, Baerwaldt M 1981 Neuroendocrine neoplasms in unusual primary sites. Diagn Histopathol 4: 263–277

92. Greenberg E, Uri N, Kelner J 1990 Laryngeal neuroendocrine carcinoma (carcinoid). Harefuah 119: 9–10

93. Greenway R E, Heeneman H 1975 Chemodectoma of the larynx. Can J Otolaryngol 4: 499–504

94. Gregorio A, Sicurella F, Castellano F, Brenna A 1990 Il tumore carcinoide della laringe. A proposito di un caso. Otorinolaringologia 40: 59–62

95. Grignon D J, Ayala A G, Ro J Y, Chong C 1990 Carcinoma of prostate metastasizing to vocal cord. Urology 36: 85–88

96. Guerrier Y, Lallemant J G, Charlin B, Pages A 1985 Carcinoid tumors of the larynx. A case study. ORL J Otorhinolaryngol Relat Spec 47: 113–118

97. Guerzider P, Fiche M, Beauvillain C, Le Bodic M F 1991 Tumeur neuro-endocrine du larynx. A propos d'un cas. Ann Pathol 11: 253–256

98. Hamlyn P J, O' Brien C J, Shaw H J 1986 Uncommon malignant tumours of the larynx. A 35 year review. J Laryngol Otol 100: 1163–1168

99. Hanna G S, Ali M H 1986 Chemodectoma of the larynx. J Laryngol Otol 100: 1081–1087

100. Harrison D F N 1981 Unusual tumors. In: Suen J Y, Myers E N (eds) Cancer of the head and neck. Churchill Livingstone, New York, pp 650–698

101. Hartmann E 1960 Chemodectoma laryngis. Acta Otolaryngol 51: 528–532

102. Hay J H, Busuttil A 1981 Oat-cell carcinoma of the larynx. J Laryngol Otol 95: 1081–1088

103. Helpap B, Koch U 1974 Uber ein Paraganglioma des Kehlkopfes. Laryngol Rhinol Otol 53: 410–415

104. Higazi M T 1979 Primary oat cell carcinoma of the larynx. J Laryngol Otol 93: 835–837

105. Hodge K M, Byers R M, Peters L J 1988 Paragangliomas of the head and neck. Arch Otolaryngol Head Neck Surg 114: 872–877

106. Hohbach C, Mootz W 1978 Chemodectoma of the larynx. Virchows Arch (A) 378: 161–172

107. Hooper R 1972 Chemodectoma of the glomus laryngicum superior. Laryngoscope 82: 686–692

108. Hordijk G J, Ruiter D J, Bosman F T, Mauw B J 1981 Chemodectoma (paraganglioma) of the larynx. Clin Otolaryngol 6: 249–254

109. Horikawa T, Matsubara F 1972 A carcinoid tumor of the epiglottis. Otolaryngology 44: 437–440

110. Hussain S S M, Davis A E, Johnstone C I 1990 Chemodectoma of the larynx. Ear Nose Throat J 69: 627–629

111. Iarlykov S A, Shagova V S, De-Zhorzh I G 1988 Carcinoid tumor of the larynx. Vestn Otorinolaringol 5: 77–78

112. Ibrahim N B N, Briggs J C, Corbishley C M 1984 Extrapulmonary oat cell carcinoma. Cancer 54: 1645–1661

113. Ishida M, Hasegawa S, Sato T, Tateishi R 1971 Glomus tumor (Nonchromaffin-paraganglioma) of the larynx. Laryngoscope 81: 957–961

114. Johnson G D, Abt A B, Mahataphongse V P, Conner G H 1979 Small cell undifferentiated carcinoma of the larynx. Ann Otol Rhinol Laryngol 88: 774–778

115. Jones S R, Myers E N, Barnes L 1984 Benign neoplasms of the larynx. Otolaryngol Clin North Am 17: 151–178

116. José B, Conley J G, Tobin D A, Dorman D W 1981 Primary oat cell carcinoma of the larynx: a case history and literature review. J Surg Oncol 16: 43–47

117. Justrabo E, Michiels R, Calmettes C, Cabanne F, Bastein H, Horiot J C, Guerrin J 1980 An uncommon apudoma: a functional chemodectoma of the larynx. Report of a case and review of the literature. Acta Otolaryngol 89: 135–143

118. Kameya T 1980 Spectrum of neuroendocrine marker substance production in carcinoid tumors revealed by immunohistochemistry. In: Lechago J, Kameya T (eds) Endocrine pathology update, vol I. Field & Wood, New York pp 151–169

119. Kamimura R, Miyata S, Matsui O, Takashima T, Nonomura A 1980 Carcinoid of the larynx: a case report. Gan No Rinsho 26: 1255–1258

120. Khansur T, Subramoni C, Balducci L 1988 Small-cell carcinoma of the larynx (letter to editor). Ear Nose Throat J 7: 126–128

121. Kim K M, Choi E C, Hong W P, Jeong H J 1989 Primary carcinoid tumor of the larynx. Yonsei Med J 30: 193–197

122. Kimmelman C P, Haller D G 1983 Small cell carcinomas of the head and neck. Otolaryngol Head Neck Surg 91: 708–712

123. Kirkeby S, Romert P 1977 Argyrophilic cells in the larynx of the guinea pig demonstrated by the method of Grimelius. J Anat 123: 87–92

124. Klap P, Reizine D, Monteil J P, Despreaux G, Hadjean E, Merland G G, Huy P T B 1984 Tumeurs et malformations vasculaires du larynx: aspects angiographiques et indications therapeutiques. Ann Otolaryngol Chir Cervicofac 101: 579–583

125. Kleinsasser O 1964 Das Glomus laryngicum inferius. Ein bisher unbekanntes, nicht chromaffines Paraganglion vom Bau der sogenannten Carotisdrüse im menschlichen Kehlkopf. Arch Ohrenheilk 184: 214–224

126. Kleinsasser O 1988 Tumors of the larynx and hypopharynx. Thieme, Stuttgart, pp 277–288

127. Kliewer K E, Wen D-R, Cancilla P A, Cochran A J 1989 Paragangliomas: assessment of prognosis by histologic, immunohistochemical, and ultrastructural techniques. Human Pathol 20: 29–39

127a. Klijanienko J, Vielh P, Duvillard P, Luboinski B 1992 True carcinosarcoma of the larynx. J Laryngol Otol 106: 58–60

128. Konowitz P M, Lawson W, Som P M, Urken M L, Breakstone B A, Biller H F 1988 Laryngeal paraganglioma: update on diagnosis and treatment. Laryngoscope 98: 40–49

129. Kos L G, Spiro R H, Hajdu S 1972 Small cell (oat cell) carcinoma of minor salivary gland origin. Cancer 30: 737–741

130. Koshii K, Hirabayashi H, Uno K et al 1987 A case of carcinoid tumor of the larynx. J Jpn Bronchoesophagol Soc 38: 452–456

131. Kozhanov L G, Sergeev S A, Belous T A, Kats V A 1987 Carcinoid of the larynx. Vestn Otorinolaringol 11: 76–78
132. Kyriakos M, Berlin B P, De Schryver-Kecskemeti K 1978 Oat cell carcinoma of the larynx. Arch Otolaryngol 104: 168–176
133. Lablack A, Abdelouahab H 1989 Chemodectomas of the larynx: a case of double localization. XIV World Congr Otorhinolaryngol Head Neck Surg, abstract 862, p 253, Madrid: September 10–15
133a. Laccourreye O, Brasnu D, Carnot F, Fichaux P, Laccourreye H 1991 Carcinoid (neuroendocrine) tumor of the arytenoid. Arch Otolaryngol Head Neck Surg 117: 1395–1399
134. Laccourreye O, Chabardes E, Weinstein G, Carnot F, Brasnu D, Laccourreye H 1991 Synchronous arytenoid and pancreatic neuroendocrine carcinoma. J Laryngol Otol 105: 373–375
135. Lack E E, Cubilla A L, Woodruff J M 1979 Paragangliomas of the head and neck region. Human Pathol 10: 191–218
136. Lack E E, Cubilla A L, Woodruff J M, Farr H W 1977 Paragangliomas of the head and neck region. A clinical study of 69 patients. Cancer 39: 397–409
137. Landry M M, Sarma D P, Haindel C J 1990 Small cell carcinoma of the larynx. J La State Med Soc 142: 24–27
138. Larsen L G, Jacobsen G J 1989 Carcinoid tumor of the larynx. APMIS 97: 748–753
139. Laudadio P 1971 Chemodectoma (paraganglioma non cromaffine) del glomo laringeo superiore. Otorinolaringol Ital 39: 19–31
140. Lawson N, Zak F G 1974 The glomus bodies ('paraganglia') of the human larynx. Laryngoscope 84: 98–111
141. Lechago J, Kameya T (eds) 1990 Endocrine pathology update, vol I. Field & Wood, New York
142. Lehmann W, Widmann J J, Pipard G, Peytremann R, Plattner H, Montandon P 1981 Tumeur carcinoïde du larynx. XIV Congr Soc Franç Carcinol Cervico-fac, Lyon
143. Leonardelli G B, Cova P L, Pignataro O, Sambataro G 1980 Carcinoma anaplastico a piccole cellule (cd. microcitoma) primitivo della laringe (1 caso e revisione della letteratura). Nuovo Arch Ital Otol 8: 175–184
144. Levenson R M, Ihde D C, Matthews M J, Cohen M H, Gazdar A F, Bunn P A, Minna J D 1981 Small cell carcinoma presenting as an extra-pulmonary neoplasm: sites of origin and response to chemotherapy. JNCI 67: 607–612
145. Lewis D J, Prentice D E 1980 The ultrastructure of rat laryngeal epithelia. J Anat 130: 617–632
146. Liang C H 1989 Pathology and biologic behavior of laryngeal carcinoid. Chin J Otorhinolaryngol 24: 98–100
147. Lindell M M Jr, Jing B, Luna M A 1981 Glomus laryngicum superior; a case studied arteriographically. Am J Roentgen 136: 618–619
148. Lindell M M, Jing B, Mackay B 1981 Primary oat cell carcinoma of the larynx. Am J Roentgen 107: 506–509
149. Lippi L, Porzio P 1985 Il carcinoide laringeo: revisione bibliografica e presentazione di un caso. Riv ORL Aud Fon 5: 137–140
150. Lloyd R V 1990 Endocrine pathology. Springer-Verlag, New York
150a. Logue J P, Banerjee S S, Slevin N J, Vasanthan S 1991 Neuroendocrine carcinomas of the larynx. J Laryngol Otol 105: 1031–1035
151. Lorenz S A III, Arena S 1979 Primary oat cell carcinoma of the larynx. Penn Med 82: 41–42
152. Luboinski B, Bosq J M, Marandas P, Domenge C, Hayem M 1984 Tumeurs neuroendocrines du larynx. A propos d'un cas. In: Leroux-Robert J, Pech A (eds) Les chémodectomes (paragangliomes) cervico-céphaliques. Masson, Paris, pp 115–122
153. Mafee M F, Langer B, Valvassori G E, Soboroff B J, Friedman M 1986 Radiologic diagnosis of nonsquamous tumors of the head and neck. Otolaryngol Clin North Am 19: 507–521
154. Markel S F, Magielski J E, Beals T F 1980 Carcinoid tumor of the larynx. Arch Otolaryngol 106: 777–778
155. Markowska A, Wojtala R, Szydlo Z 1976 Chemodectoma laryngis. Patol Polska 27: 75–78
156. Marks PV, Brookes G B 1983 Malignant paraganglioma of the larynx. J Laryngol Otol 97: 1183–1188
157. Martinson F D 1967 Chemodectoma of the 'glomus laryngicum inferior'. Arch Otolaryngol 86: 70–73

158. Medina J E, Moran M, Goepfert H 1984 Oat cell carcinoma of the larynx and Eaton–Lambert syndrome. Arch Otolaryngol 110: 123–126
159. Michaels L 1975 Neurogenic tumors, granular cell tumor, and paraganglioma. Can J Otolaryngol 4: 319–327
160. Michaels L 1984 Pathology of the larynx. Springer-Verlag, Berlin pp 285–300
161. Michaels L 1990 Atlas of ear, nose and throat pathology. In: Gresham G A (ed) 1990 Current histopathology, vol 16. Kluwer Academic Publishers, Dordrecht, pp 108–116
162. Mills S E, Johns M E 1984 Atypical carcinoid tumor of the larynx. A light microscopic and ultrastructural study. Arch Otolaryngol 110: 58–62
163. Mills S E, Cooper P H, Garland T A, Johns M E 1983 Small cell undifferentiated carcinoma of the larynx: report of two patients and review of 13 additional cases. Cancer 51: 116–120
164. Milroy C M, Robinson P J, Grant H R 1989 Primary composite squamous cell carcinoma and large cell neuroendocrine carcinoma of the hypopharynx. J Laryngol Otol 103: 1093–1096
165. Milroy C M, Rode J, Moss E 1991 Laryngeal paragangliomas and neuroendocrine carcinomas. Histopathology 18: 201–209
166. Milroy C M, Williams R A, Charlton I G, Moss E, Rode J 1990 DNA ploidy in laryngeal neuroendocrine carcinomas and paragangliomas. J Pathol 160: 156A
167. Milroy C M, Williams R A, Charlton I G, Moss E, Rode J 1991 Nuclear ploidy in neuroendocrine neoplasms of the larynx. ORL J Otorhinolaryngol Relat Spec 53: 245–249
168. Mirejovsky P, Hrobon M 1975 Small cell carcinoma of the larynx. Cesk Patol 11: 45–49
169. Miyahara H, Sato T, Yoshino K, Umatani K, Tsuruta Y 1988 Carcinoid tumor of the larynx. Pract Otol 81: 1761–1767
170. Moisa II 1991 Neuroendocrine tumors of the larynx. Head Neck 13: 498–508
171. Moisa II, Silver C E 1991 Treatment of neuroendocrine neoplasms of the larynx. ORL J Otorhinolaryngol Relat Spec 53: 259–264
172. Morrison M D, in discussion, Ferlito A 1986 Diagnosis and treatment of small cell carcinoma of the larynx: a critical review. Trans Am Laryngol Ass 107: 159–160
173. Mullins J D, Newman R K, Coltman C A Jr 1979 Primary oat cell carcinoma of the larynx: a case report and review of the literature. Cancer 43: 711–717
174. Myerowitz R L, Barnes E L, Myers E 1978 Small cell anaplastic (oat cell) carcinoma of the larynx: report of a case and review of the literature. Laryngoscope 88: 1697–1702
175. Neto R C 1980 Quimiodectoma da laringe. Rev Ass Med Brasil 26: 61–62
176. Nikolaev M P, Antonova N A 1976 Khemodectoma gortani. Vestn Otorinolaringol 5: 104–105
177. Nonomura A, Shintani T, Kono N, Kamimura R, Ohta G 1983 Primary carcinoid tumor of the larynx and review of the literature. Acta Pathol Jpn 33: 1041–1049
178. Ohsawa M, Kurita Y, Horie A, Kurita K 1983 Malignant chemodectoma (paraganglioma) of the larynx. A case report with electron microscopy and biochemical assay. Acta Pathol Jpn 33: 1279–1288
179. O'Leary T G, Kotecha B, Butterworth D 1991 Carcinoid tumour of the larynx: a case report and clinico-pathological review. Ir J Med Sci 160: 109–111
180. Olofsson J, van Nostrand AWP 1972 Anaplastic small cell carcinoma of larynx. Case report. Ann Otol Rhinol Laryngol 81: 284–287
181. Olofsson J, Gröntoft O, Sökjer H, Risberg B 1984 Paraganglioma involving the larynx. ORL J Otorhinolaryngol Relat Spec 46: 57–65
182. Pages A, Pignodel C, Ramos J 1983 Carcinoïde du larynx. Etude ultra-structurelle et immunofluorescence. Ann Pathol 3: 59–64
183. Paladugu R R, Nathwani B N, Goodstein J, Dardi L E, Memoli V E, Gould V E 1982 Carcinoma of the larynx with mucosubstance production and neuroendocrine differentiation: an ultrastructural and immunohistochemical study. Cancer 49: 343–349
184. Pardo Mindan F J, Algarra S M, Lozano B R, Tapia R G 1989 Oat cell carcinoma of the larynx. A study of six new cases. Histopathology 14: 75–80

185. Patterson S D, Yarington C T Jr 1987 Carcinoid tumor of the larynx: the role of conservative therapy. Ann Otol Rhinol Laryngol 96: 12–14

186. Pedrazzini A, Pedrinis E, Luscieti P, Losa G, Cavalli F 1983 Ein Fall von metastasierendem Paragangliom des Larynx. Schweiz Med Wschr 113: 1363–1366

187. Perrin C, Floquet J, Andre J M, Plenat J F, Petit C 1978 Reflexions à propos d'un chémodectome laryngé. Rev Otoneuroophtalmol 50: 173–179

188. Pesce C, Tobia-Galleli F, Toncini C 1984 APUD cells of the larynx. Acta Otolaryngol 98: 158–162

189. Piquet J J, Dupont A, Houcke M 1976 Les paragangliomes non chromaffines du larynx. Etude clinique et au microscopie electronique. Ann Otolaryngol Chir Cervicofac 93: 255–262

190. Pizzi G B, Sotti G, Zorat P L, Tomio L, Calzavara F, Polidoro F, Ferlito A 1981 Chemo-radiotherapy regimen in the treatment of the oat-cell carcinoma of the larynx. UICC Conference on Clinical Oncology 1981, abstract 02-0104, Lausanne, Switzerland

191. Porto D P, Wick M R, Ewing S L, Adams G L 1987 Neuroendocrine carcinoma of the larynx. Am J Otolaryngol 9: 97–104

192. Posner M R, Weichselbaum R R, Carrol E, Fabian R L, Miller D, Ervin T J 1983 Small cell carcinomas of the larynx: results of combined modality treatments. Laryngoscope 93: 946–948

193. Radici M, Croce A, Leante M, Bicciolo G 1988 Metastasi alla laringe da neoplasie primitive sistemiche. Revisione critica. Valsalva 63: 105–110

194. Reddy G N, Vrabec D P, Bernath A M 1980 Primary oat cell carcinoma of the larynx. Penn Med 83: 22

195. Remick S C, Hafez G R, Carbone P P 1987 Extrapulmonary small-cell carcinoma. A review of the literature with emphasis on therapy and outcome. Medicine 66: 457–471

196. Richardson R L, Weiland L H 1982 Undifferentiated small cell carcinomas in extrapulmonary sites. Semin Oncol 9: 484–496

197. Rubin J S, Silver C E 1988 Surgical approach to vascular tumors of the supraglottis. Proceedings of the Second International Conference on Head and Neck Cancer, Boston, abstract 285

198. Rüfenacht H, Mihatsch M J, Jundt K, Gächter A, Tanner K, Heitz PhU 1985 Gastric epithelioid leiomyomas, pulmonary chondroma, non-functioning metastasizing extra-adrenal paraganglioma and myxoma: a variant of Carney's triad. Report of a patient. Klin Wochenschr 63: 282–284

199. Saldana M J, Salem L E, Travezan R 1973 High altitude hypoxia and chemodectomas. Human Pathol 4: 251–263

200. Sato K, Higaki Y, Sakaguki S, Hirano M, Tanimura A, Sasaguri Y 1991 Carcinoid tumor of the larynx. Auris Nasus Larynx 18: 39–53

201. Schaefer S D, Blend B L, Denton J G 1980 Laryngeal paragangliomas: evaluation and treatment. Am J Otolaryngol 1: 451–455

202. Schall L A 1959 An extralaryngeal approach for certain benign lesions of the larynx. Trans Am Laryngol Assoc 80: 36–47

203. Schild J A, Cohen M H 1985 Laryngeal nonchromaffin paraganglioma. Trans Am Laryngol Assoc 106: 149–152

204. Sesi M, Dierks E, Burns D 1988 Small cell carcinoma of the larynx and hypopharynx. Proceedings of the Second International Conference on Head and Neck Cancer, Boston, abstract 138

205. Shipton E A, van der Linde J C 1984 Paraganglioma of the larynx. S Afr Med J 65: 176–177

206. Sizeland A M, Grey P A, Farrar D T 1989 Laryngeal carcinoid. Otolaryngol Head Neck Surg 101: 480–484

207. Smets G, Warson F, Dehou M F, Storme G, Sacrè R, van Belle S, Somers G, Gepts W, Klöppel G 1990 Metastasizing neuroendocrine carcinoma of the larynx with calcitonin and somatostatin secretion and CEA production, resembling medullary thyroid carcinoma. Virchows Arch (A) 416: 539–543

208. Smith O, Youngs R, Snell D, van Nostrand P 1988 Paraganglioma of the larynx. J Otolaryngol 17: 293–301

209. Sneige N, Mackay B, Ordonez N G, Batsakis J G 1983 Laryngeal paraganglioma. Report of two tumors with immunohistochemical and ultrastructural analysis. Arch Otolaryngol 109: 113–117

210. Snyderman C, Johnson J T, Barnes L 1986 Carcinoid tumor of the larynx: case report and review of the world literature.

Otolaryngol Head Neck Surg 95: 158–164

211. Solcia E, Rindi G, Capella C 1990 Neuroendocrine tumours and hyperplasias. In: Filipe M I, Lake B D (eds) Histochemistry in pathology. Churchill Livingstone, Edinburgh, pp 397–409

212. Solcia E, Capella C, Buffa R, Usellini L, Fiocca R, Sessa F, Tortora O 1984 The contribution of immunohistochemistry to the diagnosis of neuroendocrine tumors. Sem Diagn Pathol 1: 285–296

213. Soussi A C, Benghiat A, Holgate C S, Majumdar B 1990 Neuroendocrine tumours of the head and neck. J Laryngol Otol 104: 504–507

214. Spagnolo D V, Paradinas F J 1985 Laryngeal neuroendocrine tumour with features of a paraganglioma, intracytoplasmic lumina and acinar formation. Histopathology 9: 117–131

215. Spiro R H 1986 Salivary neoplasms: overview of a 35-year experience with 2807 patients. Head Neck Surg 8: 177–184

216. Springall D R, Ibrahim N B N, Rode J, Sharpe M S, Bloom S R, Polak J M 1986 Endocrine differentiation of extrapulmonary small cell carcinoma demonstrated by immunohistochemistry using antibodies to PGP 9.5, neuron-specific enolase and the C-flanking peptide of human pro-bombesin. J Pathol 150: 151–162

217. Stanley R J, DeSanto L W, Weiland L H 1986 Oncocytic and oncocytoid carcinoid tumors (well-differentiated neuroendocrine carcinomas) of the larynx. Arch Otolaryngol Head Neck Surg 112: 529–535

218. Stanley R J, Weiland L H, Neel H B III 1986 Pain-inducing laryngeal paraganglioma: report of the ninth case and review of the literature. Otolaryngol Head Neck Surg 95: 107–112

219. Stanley R J, Scheithauer B W, Weiland L H, Neel H B III 1987 Neural and neuroendocrine tumors of the larynx. Ann Otol Rhinol Laryngol 96: 630–638

220. Stearns M P 1982 Chemodectoma of the larynx. J Laryngol Otol 96: 1181–1185

221. Sterba J 1968 Metastazujici achromafinni paragangliom. Plezn Lek Sborn 30: 81–84

222. Sun C J, Hall-Craggs M, Adler B 1981 Oat cell carcinoma of larynx. Arch Otolaryngol 107: 506–509

223. Sweeney E C, McDonnell L, O'Brien C 1981 Medullary carcinoma of the thyroid presenting as tumours of the pharynx and larynx. Histopathology 5: 263–275

224. Sykes J M, Ossoff R H 1986 Paragangliomas of the head and neck. Otolaryngol Clin North Am 19: 755–767

225. Tachi T, Tamori M, Kamimura R, Shintani T, Fukushiro R 1981 Laryngeal carcinoid tumor with skin metastasis. Jpn J Clin Dermatol 35: 581–586

226. Taira K 1985 Endocrine-like cells in the laryngeal mucosa of adult rabbits demonstrated by electron microscopy and by the Grimelius silver-impregnation method. Biomed Res 6: 377–385

227. Takeuchi K, Nishii S, Jin C S, Ukai K, Sakakura Y 1989 Anaplastic small cell carcinoma of the larynx. Auris Nasus Larynx 16: 127–132

228. Tamai S, Iri H, Maruyama T, Kasahara M, Akatsura S, Sakurai S, Murakami Y 1981 Laryngeal carcinoid tumor: light and electron microscopic studies. Cancer 48: 2256–2259

229. Tanaka M, Hasegawa T, Kin S, Tamaoki H, Kotou K, Yoshida J 1987 A case of atypical carcinoid of the larynx. Otolaryngology 59: 663–669

230. Thompson D H, Kao Y H, Klos J, Fay J, Fetter T W 1982 Primary small cell (oat cell) carcinoma of the larynx associated with IgD multiple myeloma. Laryngoscope 92: 1239–1244

231. Tobin H A, Harris H H 1972 Nonchromaffin paraganglioma of the larynx: case report and review of the literature. Arch Otolaryngol 96: 154–156

232. Triantafilidi J G, Nasyrov V A 1980 Chemodectomas with an outlet into the parapharyngeal space and larynx. Vestn Otorinolaringol 5: 83

233. Trotoux J, Glickmanas M, Sterkers O, Trousset M, Pinel J 1979 Syndrome de Schwartz-Bartter: révélateur d'un cancer laryngé sous-glottique à petites cellules. Ann Otolaryngol Chir Cervicofac 96: 349–358

234. Urso C, Messerini L, de Meester W, Ferri G 1989 Paraganglioma (chemodectoma). Presentazione di 2 casi. Pathologica 81: 611–616

235. Uvarov A A, Ogol'tsova E S 1983 Zlokachestvennaia paraganglioma gortani. Vestn Otorinolaringol 1: 76–77

236. van Vroonhoven T J, Peutz W H, Tjan T G 1982 Presurgical devascularization of a laryngeal paraganglioma. Arch Otolaryngol 108: 600–602

237. Verzhbitskii G V, Darovskii B G 1975 Malignant chemodectoma of the larynx. Zh Ushn Nos Gorl Bolezn 3: 92–93

238. Vetters J M, Toner P G 1970 Chemodectoma of larynx. J Pathol 101: 259–265

239. Vrabec D P, Bartels L J 1980 Small cell anaplastic carcinoma of the larynx: review of the literature and report of a case. Laryngoscope 90: 1720–1726

240. Watzka M 1963 Über Paraganglien in der Plica ventricularis des menschlichen Kehlkopfes. Dtsch Med Forsch 1: 19–20

241. Weidauer H, Blobel G A, Nemetschek-Gansler H , Gould V E, Mall G 1985 Das neuro-endokrine Larynxkarzinom vom kleinzelligen (oat-cell) Typ. Morphologische und immunohistochemische Befunde und ihre Bedeutung fur die Therapie: Laryngol Rhinol Otol 64: 121–127

242. Weighill J S, Tankel J W, Mene A 1986 Carcinoid tumour of the larynx (a case report and review of the literature). J Laryngol Otol 100: 1421–1426

243. Welkoborsky H J, Sorger K, Moll R, Collo D 1988 Primäres Larynxkarzinoid. Fallvorstellung und Literaturübersicht. Laryngol Rhinol Otol 67: 559–563

244. Wenig B M, Gnepp D R 1989 The spectrum of neuroendocrine carcinoma of the larynx. Semin Diagn Pathol 6: 329–350

245. Wenig B M, Hymas V J, Heffner D K 1988 Moderately differentiated neuroendocrine carcinomas of the larynx: a clinicopathologic study of 54 cases. Cancer 62: 2658–2676

245a. Werner J A, Harismann M-L, Lippert B M, Rudert H 1992 Laryngeal paraganglioma and pregnancy. ORL J Otorhinolaryngol Relat Spec 54:163–167

246. Wetmore R F, Tronzo R D, Lane R J, Lowey L D 1981 Nonfunctional paraganglioma of the larynx: clinical and pathological considerations. Cancer 48: 2717–2723

247. Wick M R, Abenoza P, Manivel J C 1988 Diagnostic immunohistopathology. In: Gnepp DR (ed) Pathology of the head. Churchill Livingstone, New York, pp 191–261

248. Wilhelm H J, Dietz R, Schondorf J 1980 Diagnostik und Therapie seltener Tumoren im Larynx-Pharynx-Bereich. Laryngol Rhinol Otol 59: 137–143

249. Woeckel W, Rose K G, Stanulla H 1965 Zur Kenntnis der Chemodektoma des Kehlkopfes (Z Faelle). Acta Otorhinolaryngol Belg 19: 768–775

250. Woodruff J M, Senie R T 1991 Atypical carcinoid tumor of the larynx. A critical review of the literature. J Otorhinolaryngol Relat Spec 53: 194–209

251. Woodruff J M, Huvos A G, Erlandson R A, Shah J P, Gerold F P 1985 Neuroendocrine carcinomas of the larynx. A study of two types, one of which mimics thyroid medullary carcinoma. Am J Surg Pathol 9: 771–790

251a. Yoshihara T, Kubota I, Narita N, Ishii T 1991 Primary small cell carcinoma of the larynx. Larynx Jpn 3: 103–109

252. Zachariah K J, Shah J H 1972 Chemodectoma of larynx. J Laryngol Otol 86: 1213–1218

253. Zambruno G, Bertazzoni M G, Botticelli A, Manca V, Giannetti A 1989 Carcinome neuro-endocrine du larynx avec métastases cutanées. Ann Dermatol Venereol 116: 855–858

254. Zeitlhofer J 1955 Ungewöhnlicher Tumor im Larynx (chromophobes Paragangliom). Mschr Ohrenheilk 89: 133–136

255. Zikk D, Samuel Y, Jossipohov J, Green I, Bloom J 1987 Paraganglioma of the subglottic larynx. ORL J Otorhinolaryngol Relat Spec 49: 270–275

13. Malignant melanoma*

B. M. Wenig

INTRODUCTION

Malignant melanoma is a ubiquitous neoplasm arising primarily in cutaneous sites. There is a tremendous amount of information in the medical literature detailing the clinicopathological features, treatment protocols and prognostic factors in relation to cutaneous malignant melanomas and their precursor lesions. Similarly, medical professionals are well acquainted with this category of neoplasm. However, the same familiarity does not apply to mucosal-derived malignant melanomas. In the head and neck region, mucosal-derived malignant melanomas are encountered throughout the upper respiratory tract and are most frequently seen within the sinonasal tract and oral cavity.[9,23,25,34,72,85] Primary laryngeal malignant melanomas (LMM) are exceedingly rare neoplasms. This chapter will detail the clinicopathological features of laryngeal malignant melanoma and will also discuss its histogenesis, differential diagnosis, biological behaviour and treatment.

TERMINOLOGY

The terminology of cutaneous malignant melanoma and its precursor lesions is well established and widely accepted. The spectrum of cutaneous malignant melanomas includes both in situ and invasive malignant melanomas. The in situ malignant melanoma group by definition is confined to the epidermis, is described as radial or horizontal growth phase, and includes lentigo maligna and the in situ variants of superficial spreading and acral lentiginous.[21,55,62] The invasive types of malignant melanoma by definition invade the dermis, are referred to as the vertical growth phase, and include lentigo malignant melanoma, superficial spreading malignant melanoma, acral lentiginous malignant melanoma and nodular malignant melanoma. The descriptive terminology for each of these subtypes refers to specific clinical and histopathological appearances.[21] Other rarer types of malignant melanoma include melanomas arising within the dermis from congenital melanocytic nevi or from intradermal nevi, and malignant blue nevus.[55]

In contrast to cutaneous malignant melanomas, the upper respiratory tract mucosal-derived malignant melanomas are not subtyped into specific diagnostic categories. Rather, these neoplasms are simply diagnosed as malignant melanoma. As will be discussed below, the cells comprising these neoplasms vary and, while it is acceptable and often justified for differential diagnostic purposes to indicate the predominant cell type (e.g. epithelioid, spindle-shaped or mixed cell pattern), the cell type has no bearing on prognosis or treatment. The overwhelming majority of the upper respiratory tract mucosal-derived malignant melanomas are invasive at the time of diagnosis. These neoplasms may take origin from melanocytes located either in the basal cell layer of the surface epithelium, the subjacent stroma or from the minor salivary glands.[14,44,53,76] While an in situ component and/or continuity with these structures may be seen, often surface ulceration precludes identification of mucosal derivation. Nevertheless, malignant melanomas of the upper respiratory tract, in the absence of provable metastasis from another site, take origin from the mucosae.

DEFINITION

Melanomas are malignant neoplasms arising from melanocytes. Melanocytes originate from the neural crest, a neuroectodermal-derived structure formed in the fourth week of gestation.[64] Other cellular components taking origin from the neural crest include those of the adrenal medulla, carotid body, ultimobranchial apparatus (thyroid C cells), peripheral nerve sheaths (Schwann cells) and

*The opinions or assertions contained herein are the private views of the author and are not to be construed as official or as reflecting the views of the Department of the Navy, Department of the Army, or the Department of Defense.

sympathetic ganglia. Collectively, this group of cells and their corresponding neoplasms have been referred to as the *a*mine *p*recursor *u*ptake and *d*ecarboxylase system (APUD). Pearse described the APUD cell concept and defined the APUD cell characteristics on the basis of shared common cytochemical (amine-handling capacity) and ultrastructural (membrane-bound secretory vesicles) properties.[74] Pearse concluded that the neural crest cell was the embryological forefather of these APUD cells. This conclusion was based on the common property of formaldehyde-induced fluorescence (FIF) and on the common cytochemical and ultrastructural characteristics of APUD cells and definitive neural crest cells (thyroid C cells). Presently, this group of cells and their corresponding neoplasms derived from the neural crest are referred to as belonging to the *d*ispersed *n*euro*e*ndocrine *c*ell *s*ystem (DNES).[56,75] The cellular derivatives of the DNES are scattered throughout the body, accounting for an array of neoplastic proliferations seen in various viscera.[56,75] The migration of these cellular components from the neural crest to the various target organs explains the presence of a given neoplasm in locations not typical for their occurrence. Such is the case of malignant melanomas occurring in the upper respiratory tract.

INCIDENCE

Primary laryngeal malignant melanoma (LMM) are exceedingly rare neoplasms. A total of 44 cases of LMM have been reported in the literature either as single case reports or as part of large series describing mucosal melanomas of the upper aerodigestive tract.[3,6,7,10,13,15,17,22, 23,28–30,32,37,49,51,52,57,63,67,71,72,73,79, 80,85,87,94,95] Review of the Otolaryngic Tumor Registry at the Armed Forces Institute of Pathology (OTR-AFIP) reveals a total of nine cases of *primary* LMM. This represents 0.09% (9 of 10 270 cases) of all primary laryngeal neoplasms seen at the Armed Forces Institute of Pathology over a 75-year period (1917–1991). In relation to malignant melanomas occurring throughout mucosal sites of the head and neck, which represent from 0.5 to 3% of malignant melanomas of all sites,[10,48,72,85] laryngeal melanomas have been reported to represent from 3.6%[43] to 3.8%[23] to 7.4%[63] of these neoplasms.

While the presence of melanocytes in the larynx has been well established, albeit not in overwhelming numbers, an argument could be put forth as to why laryngeal malignant melanomas are not identified more often. Busuttil, stimulated by identification of melanocytes within the squamous epithelium of a laryngeal biopsy specimen, attempted to identify melanocytes in larynges from fifteen autopsy specimens.[14] While unable to identify melanocytes, he found clear cells in the basal layer of the squamous epithelium. He felt that these cells may represent Langerhan's cells akin to those seen in the epidermis. Although under dispute and presently considered to be in the macrophage/histiocyte family,[41] Masson considered the Langerhan's cells to represent shed or degenerate melanocytes.[60] Busuttil[14] then suggested that the clear cells he identified in the laryngeal specimens represented effete melanocytes, and he further suggested that laryngeal malignant melanomas are not seen more commonly due to degeneration of melanocytes and replacement by the clear (Langerhan's) cells.

When considering a diagnosis of LMM, one should bear in mind the rarity of this neoplasm and its greater frequency in relation to cutaneous sites. Therefore, a metastasis to the larynx should be ruled out. Metastatic neoplasms to the larynx are uncommon. The neoplasms which are most frequently implicated in metastasizing to the larynx are malignant melanoma and renal cell carcinoma.[1,8,38,98] Therefore, as will be discussed later in the chapter, prior to diagnosing a primary LMM, evaluation for and exclusion of a metastasis to the larynx from a separate/distant malignant melanoma must be accomplished.

CLINICAL FEATURES

Primary LMM is a disease of older men. From the reported cases of LMM in the literature documenting the age of the patient and those cases identified from the OTR-AFIP, >80% were identified in men. The age range of all patients was from 35 to 86 years of age, with >62% presenting in the sixth to seventh decades of life. This contrasts with cutaneous melanomas which affect women more frequently and are seen in an age group approximately a decade younger than is the case for malignant melanomas of the larynx.[2,21,43,61] When recorded, LMM occurs almost exclusively in Caucasians with no reported occurrences in Blacks and a single occurrence in an Asian man.[52] However, the case of the lentigo in the larynx coexisting with an oral cavity malignant melanoma, and the case of the intralaryngeal nevus, did occur in Black patients.[84,92] Nevertheless, the predilection for laryngeal malignant melanomas to be more common in Caucasians than in Blacks and possibly in other races, is consistent with the documentation in the literature which indicates that mucosal malignant melanomas of the upper aerodigestive tract occur more commonly in Caucasians than in other races.[10,17,19,63,85] The exception to this statement may be the apparent higher incidence of oral cavity malignant melanoma in Japanese people.[90]

The anatomical confines of the larynx are divided into three compartments: supraglottis, glottis and subglottis. The majority of LMM occur in supraglottic locations and include the following sites: epiglottis, arytenoids, aryepiglottic folds, ventricle, false vocal cord and pyriform fossa. When recorded, laryngeal malignant melanomas were identified in supraglottic locations in >60%

of cases. The other site specific LMM involved the glottic region and were identified along the true vocal cord and posterior commissure. A few of the reported cases did not have a specific site of occurrence and no subglottic malignant melanomas were identified.

The symptoms associated with LMM vary; they include hoarseness, dysphagia, sore throat, sensation of a 'lump' in the throat, neck or jaw pain and a neck mass. Symptoms generally occurred over a short period of time within the range 3 to 6 months. Occasionally, the patients claimed that their symptoms had been present for up to 2 years. There are no known definitive aetiological factors correlated with the development of laryngeal malignant melanoma. Perhaps, as with other head and neck primary mucosal malignant neoplasms, in particular squamous-cell malignancies, direct insult to the mucosa by oncogenic stimuli associated with these neoplasms (excess tobacco and/or alcohol) may also contribute to the development of LMM.[44] To this end, Reuter and Woodruff[79] speculate that tobacco smoking plays an important factor in the development of LMM. They support this contention on the basis of identifying a smoking history in a limited number of patients reported with LMM as well as stating that, when recorded, a smoking history was identified in 70% of patients with mucosal melanoma of the head and neck identified at Memorial Hospital.[79]

HISTOGENESIS

Melanoblasts, the precursor cells to melanocytes, form in the early part of fetal life and following migration to peripheral sites differentiate into melanocytes.[65] Melanocytes are primarily identified in the basal portions of the epidermis at the dermo-epidermal junction.[65] However, primary malignant melanomas have been described in virtually every organ system, and they take origin from the neural crest-derived melanocytes which have migrated to those specific body sites.[27,84] Among the target organs included in this peripheral migration of melanocytes are the mucosae of the upper respiratory tract. Laryngeal melanomas arise from melanocytes which have migrated from the neural crest during embryogenesis to the laryngeal mucosae. Evidence for the presence of melanocytes, as well as argyrophilic and/or APUD cells in the larynx has been documented in animal and human models.[14,36,44,53,76,91] Additional manifestations of melanocytic migration to the larynx include melanin pigmentation or melanosis of the larynx,[44,77] intralaryngeal naevi (Fig. 13.1)[83,84] and lentigo of the larynx.[92] The latter case coexisted with an oral cavity malignant melanoma. Given the development of malignant melanoma from melanocytes as well as the fact, previously mentioned, that malignant melanomas may arise from congenital melanocytic naevi or from intradermal naevi, there is overwhelming evidence for the development of LMM from neural crest-derived melanocytes which have migrated to this region. For completion, it should be mentioned that some authors have attempted to explain the existence of respiratory tract malignant melanomas as representing metastasis from occult malignant melanomas arising from separate sites which have undergone spontaneous regression.[16] While certainly plausible, especially in the light of the well-known capability of cutaneous malignant melanomas to regress spontaneously,[21,61] given the previous evidence it is justified to state that laryngeal malignant melanoma arises in the larynx from malignant degeneration of melanocytes or melanocytic lesions.

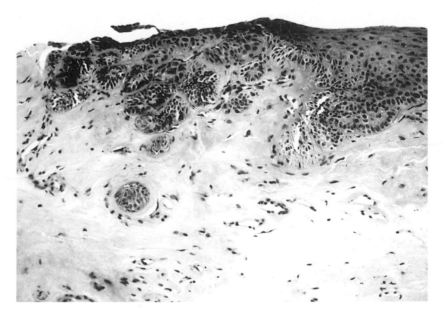

Fig. 13.1   Intralaryngeal benign naevus arising from the squamous epithelium. ×150.

As detailed previously, the majority of laryngeal melanomas arise in the supraglottic compartment. A similar localization to the supraglottis is seen with laryngeal neuroendocrine carcinomas.[96,97] Explanations for the supraglottic preference for laryngeal neuroendocrine carcinomas were based on (i) the different embryogenesis of the supraglottic versus glottic and subglottic regions, with the supraglottis arising from the third and fourth branchial arches (buccopharyngeal anlage), and the glottis and subglottis arising from the sixth branchial arch (pulmonary anlage),[66] and (ii) the number and distribution of mucous glands in the adult human laryngeal mucosa with the greatest number of mucous glands found in the supraglottic region.[70] These findings, coupled with evidence of argyrophilic-positive cells within the laryngeal mucoserous glands, could explain the predominant supraglottic location of laryngeal neuroendocrine carcinomas. Similar speculations could be applied to LMM. However, they are not as plausible in explaining the supraglottic preference of LMM when compared to similar localization of laryngeal neuroendocrine carcinomas. In contrast to neuroendocrine neoplasms, the majority of LMM are not confined to the submucosal compartment. Therefore, the association of argyrophilic-positive cells in the laryngeal mucoserous glands and the prevalence of mucoserous glands in the supraglottis and submucosal growth—all strongly supporting the supraglottic localization of laryngeal neuroendocrine carcinomas does not readily apply to LMM. Nevertheless, the majority of LMM occur in the supraglottic area. The literature detailing the presence of melanocytes in animal or human larynges describes their occurrence in the squamous epithelium, ciliated respiratory epithelium and/or mucoserous glands.[14,36,44,53,76,91] These studies specifically document sampling from the supraglottic region, thus suggesting that there is a greater percentage of these cells normally residing in the supraglottic compartment. This would then lend support for the predominance of LMM occurring in the supraglottic larynx. However, other studies clearly identify pigmented cells within the glottic area (true vocal cord).[14,77] While there is circumstantial evidence to explain the supraglottic preference of LMM there is no clear reason as to why this occurs. Additional studies, specifically detailing the localization of melanocytes within the larynx, are needed to allow for a more definitive explanation to account for this phenomenon.

Reuter and Woodruff specifically comment on the absence of documentation in many of the reported cases of LMM of an in situ component.[79] Their feeling was that, without documentation of an in situ component, primary origin from the laryngeal epithelium could not be validated. To justify this contention, they and other authors[23,29] use the criterion of junctional change as the sine qua non for assuring primary derivation in the larynx. Allen and Spitz defined the criteria for diagnosing a primary lesion for cutaneous as well as mucosal malignant melanomas.[2] However, given the identification of melanocytes in both the mucoserous glands and the submucosal compartment of the larynx,[44,53,91] it is entirely possible that a malignant melanoma arising in the larynx may take origin from melanocytes in one or both of these areas and *not* arise from the surface epithelium. Therefore, the presence of an in situ or junctional component, seen in all the cases from the AFIP with an intact epithelium and representing positive proof of primary laryngeal origin, is not necessarily required in order to postulate origin or lack thereof from the larynx. Certainly in cases where an intact epithelium is seen, and there is no junctional activity, a metastasis must be ruled out.

PATHOLOGY

Gross pathology

The macroscopic descriptions of LMM are varied, and they include nodular, mulberry-like, sessile, pedunculated, polypoid and exophytic growth patterns (Fig. 13.2). The neoplasms may or may not have associated

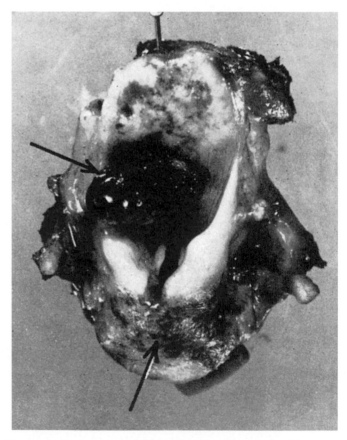

Fig. 13.2 Laryngectomy specimen showing a black, polypoid supraglottic (epiglottic) malignant melanoma (upper arrow). Melanosis is seen in the superior portion of the epiglottis as well as in the posterior cricoid area (lower arrow). (Reproduced with permission from D. Catlin 1967 Mucosal melanomas of the head and neck. *American Journal of Roentgenology* 99: 809–816.)

ulceration. Equally varied are the range of colours associated with the masses described as black, brown, red-pink, tan-grey and white. The size of the neoplasms ranges from as small as 3–4 mm to growths measuring up to 8 cm in greatest dimension.

Histopathology

The histological appearance of LMM is that of a cellular, infiltrating neoplasm (Fig. 13.3). Often, surface ulceration supervenes, obliterating identification of derivation from the laryngeal epithelium. However, when not ulcerated, the surface epithelium may be unremarkable, hyperplastic or atrophic with identification of in situ or junctional changes (continuity with the mucosal epithelium) (Fig. 13.4). In addition, upward extension of the tumour cells into the epithelium may be seen. The neoplastic growth pattern is usually solid, with an absence of cellular cohesiveness; however, pseudoglandular, alveolar, and nested foci may be seen. The majority of LMM are categorized as epithelioid, being composed of large round cells with large, round to oval, hyperchromatic to vesicular nuclei, prominent eosinophilic nucleoli, and a variable amount of eosinophilic cytoplasm. Marked cellular pleomorphism, increased mitotic activity and necrosis are commonly seen (Fig. 13.5).

Occasionally, the neoplastic cells have a plasmacytoid appearance composed of cells with round, eccentrically located, vesicular to basophilic appearing nuclei and an eosinophilic cytoplasm (Fig. 13.5). These cells lack a paranuclear clear zone (hof) seen in plasma cell proliferations. As previously mentioned, foci of apparent glandular (pseudoglands) differentiation may be seen but are usually limited in extent (Fig. 13.6). Similarly, on occasion, squamous cell differentiation may be an integral part of the neoplasm but, like the glandular differentiation, represents only a minimal portion of a neoplasm otherwise predominantly composed of cells indicative of malignant melanoma. The other major type of cytomorphology identified is a spindle-shaped cell proliferation (spindle cell malignant melanoma) with a fascicular to storiform growth (Fig. 13.7). The spindle cells are elongated to oval and are marked by cellular pleomorphism, multinucleation and increased mitotic activity. Nuclei are large, vesicular to hyperchromatic, with prominent nucleoli and a variable amount of eosinophilic cytoplasm (Fig. 13.7). This cytological appearance may represent the only cell type seen or, more commonly, is admixed in a neoplasm with both spindle and epithelioid cells (Fig. 13.8). A lymphocytic cell infiltrate may be identified varying in intensity from mild to marked.

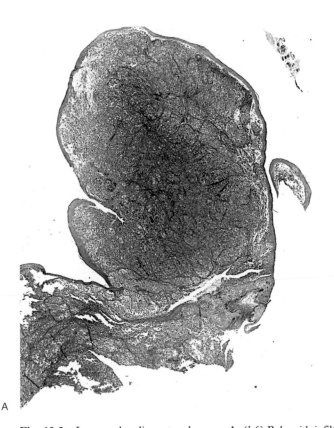

A

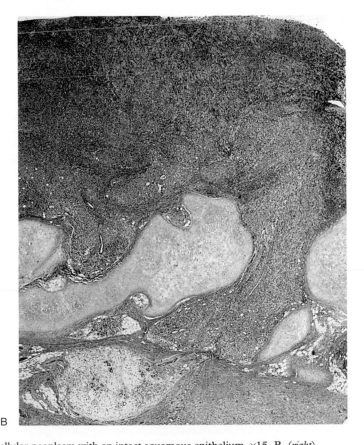

B

Fig. 13.3 Laryngeal malignant melanoma. A. (*left*) Polypoid, infiltrating cellular neoplasm with an intact squamous epithelium. ×15. B. (*right*) cellular neoplasm associated with epithelial ulceration and extensive infiltration. ×30.

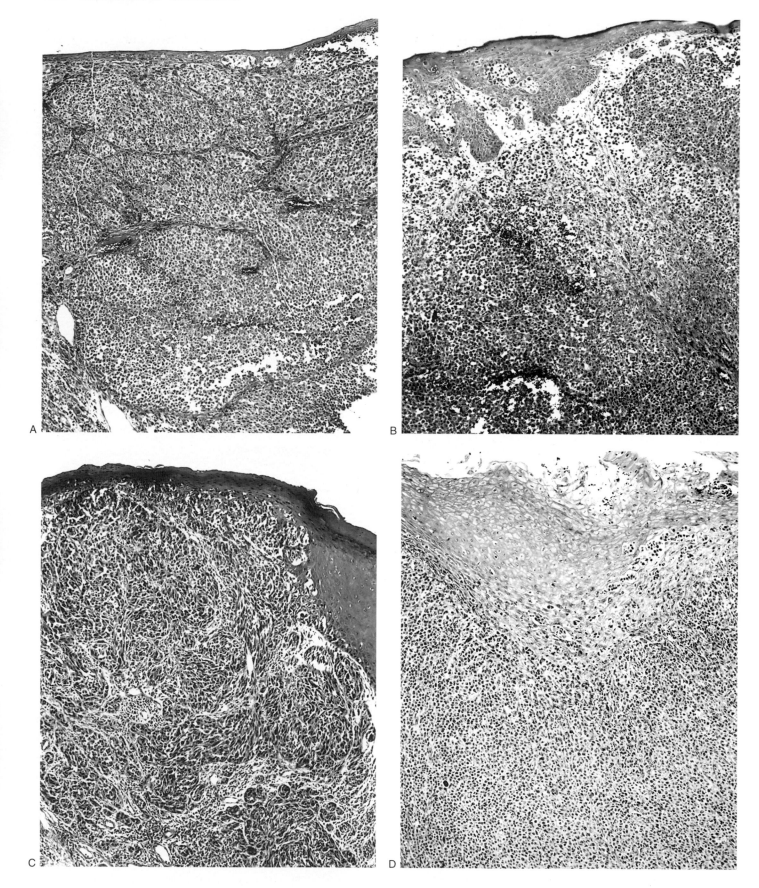

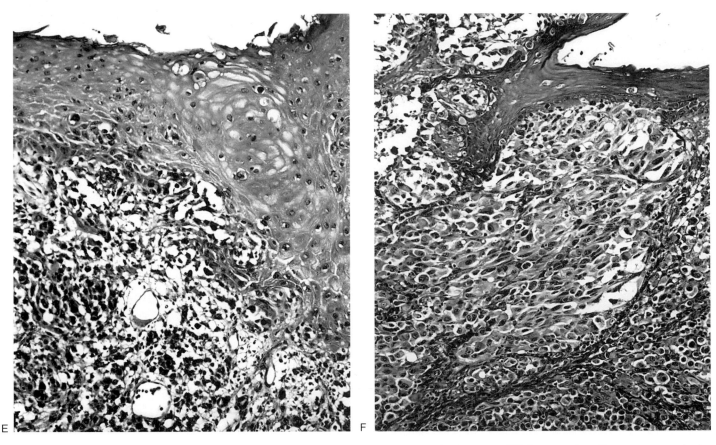

E   F

Fig. 13.4 A–D (*opposite page*) and E, F (*above*). Junctional changes as demonstrated by nests and/or individual neoplastic cell continuity with the mucosal epithelium seen arising from the basal epithelial layer in association with atrophic, normal or hyperplastic squamous epithelia. Solid, alveolar and pseudoglandular growth patterns can be seen as well as upward extension into the superficial layers of the epithelium by the neoplastic cells. A–D ×75; E, F ×150.

LMM are invasive neoplasms which may demonstrate invasion and obliteration of mucoserous glands as well as invasion of laryngeal mesenchymal structures such as nerves, cartilage, muscle and adipose tissue (Fig. 13.9). Vascular and/or lymphatic invasion may occur. Given the propensity for invasion, metastases are often seen, and among the organs targeted for metastatic foci are regional lymph nodes, lung and liver (Fig. 13.10).

Histochemistry

The identification of melanin may be seen by light microscopy in any given neoplasm, and it is an invaluable aid in diagnosis. This pigment appears as intracytoplasmic brown to black granularity (Fig. 13.11). While melanin deposition may be obvious and readily apparent, this varies from case to case, and identification of melanin may be difficult—requiring an extensive search of many sections; melanin may, in fact, be absent. In such instances the term amelanotic melanoma may be used. Caution should be exercised in interpreting all apparent pigmentation as melanin. Other endogenous or exogenous intracytoplasmic substances which may be confused with melanin deposition include iron as well as formalin

pigment—an artifactual deposition resulting from the normal processing of tissue. The presence of melanin in a malignant melanoma can be documented by argentaffin and/or argyrophil stains. The argentaffin stain used is the Fontana–Masson, and the argyrophil stain is either the Grimelius or its modification the Churukian–Schenk stain.[20] These staining qualities are based on the ability of a cell to reduce ammoniacal silver to its metallic state either endogenously (argentaffinity) or through the addition of an exogenous reducing agent (argyrophilia).[88] Melanin is identified by the presence of fine, black intracytoplasmic granules by the Fontana–Masson stain, and as black or brown intracytoplasmic granules by the Churukian–Schenk stain (Fig. 13.11). Mucin, as demonstrated by mucicarmine and/or periodic acid–Schiff (PAS) stains, occasionally may be seen as intracytoplasmic material which appears red to pink. The presence of intracytoplasmic (red) granules identified in plasma cells by the methyl green pyronine (MGP) stain, are not seen in melanomas. In differentiating iron from melanin, an iron stain (Prussian blue) may be used. Iron deposition, resulting from haemorrhage, will be seen by the presence of blue cytoplasmic granularity; melanin will not be stained by iron stains.

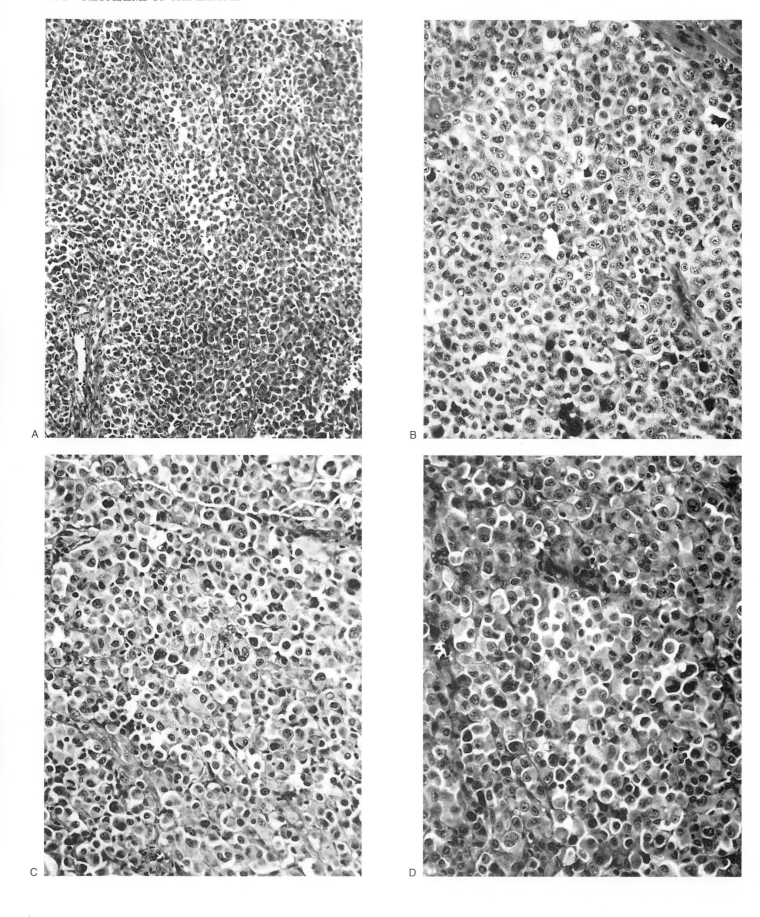

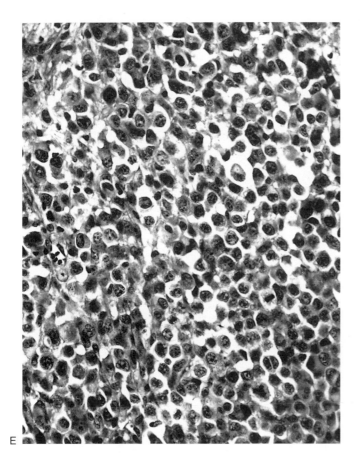

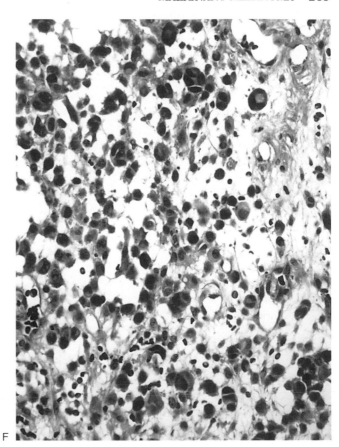

E

F

Fig. 13.5 A–D (*opposite page*) and E, F (*above*). Laryngeal malignant melanoma composed of a solid but dyscohesive epithelioid cell population with large, round to oval cells, hyperchromatic to vesicular nuclei, prominent eosinophilic nucleoli and a variable amount of eosinophilic cytoplasm. Marked cellular pleomorphism and increased mitotic activity are evident; neoplastic cells may have a plasmacytoid appearance composed of cells with round, eccentrically located, vesicular to basophilic appearing nuclei. A ×75; B, C ×150; D–F ×300.

Immunocytochemistry

The immunocytochemical profile of malignant melanomas include positive reactivity with both S-100 protein[68] and HMB-45. Both positive reactions are seen as intra-cytoplasmic brown granularity, and the S-100 protein will also demonstrate nuclear staining (Fig. 13.12). The marked intensity and diffuse staining pattern with *both* of these antibodies is diagnostic for malignant melanomas. While S-100 protein positive immunoreactivity is not specific for malignant melanomas, and can be seen in a wide variety of neoplasms,[31,93,99] HMB-45 is a melanocytic specific tumour marker assuring a diagnosis of malignant melanoma.[46,99] While considered virtually specific for melanocytic tumours, recent evidence has shown HMB-45 reactivity in other neoplasms.[54] Further, HMB-45 is not positive in all cases of malignant melanoma. This is especially true for the spindle cell malignant melanoma.[99] In addition, neuron specific enolase (NSE) is positive, but this antibody is neither specific for not diagnostic of malignant melanoma. Additional antibodies which should be included in the immunocytochemical evaluation of LMM are those formed against cytokeratin, chromogranin, synaptophysin, calcitonin, leukocyte common antigen (LCA), B- and T-cell markers (L-26, UCHL), kappa and lambda light-chain immunoglobulins, vimentin, actin and desmin. All of these antibodies are generally non-reactive with melanocytic cells, although melanocytic cells may demonstrate immunoreactivity with vimentin,[99] and should be used in differentiating malignant melanoma from other histologically similar appearing neoplasms (Table 13.1). Chromogranin, a sensitive and specific marker of neuroendocrine differentiation[100] has not been reported in melanocytic lesions; one of the AFIP cases of LMM showed positive, albeit focal, chromogranin immunoreactivity (Fig. 13.13). This latter finding may be explained by the synchronous production of immuno-reactive peptides and melanin, a hypothesis previously proposed by Gould et al.[45]

Electron microscopy

The diagnosis of malignant melanoma is generally made by light microscopic and immunocytochemical evalu-

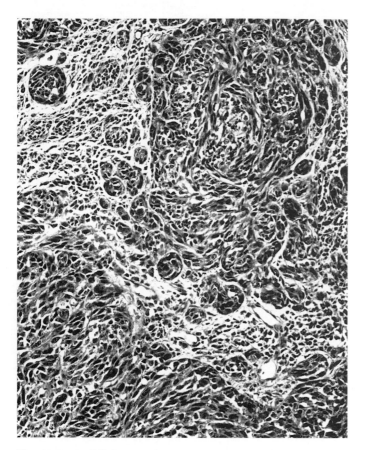 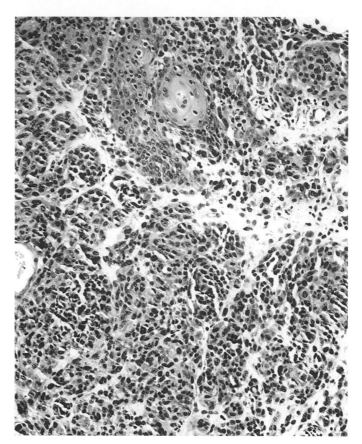

Fig. 13.6 A. (*left*) Laryngeal malignant melanoma with pseudoglandular formation. B. (*right*) Laryngeal malignant melanoma with squamous cell differentiation. ×150.

ation. With the advent and extensive use of immuno-cytochemistry in the realm of tumour diagnosis, the role of electron microscopy has ebbed almost to the point of non-utilization. However, ultrastructural analysis may yield diagnostic information otherwise not seen either by light microscopy or immunocytochemistry.

The ultrastructural findings in malignant melanomas include the presence of melanosomes and/or premela-nosomes, organelles characteristic of melanocytic differ-entiation.[35,50] Melanosomes and premelanosomes are membrane-limited vesicles with a distinctive internal structure varying from parallel lamellae to helical to zig-zag structures with a periodicity of 8–10 nm (Fig. 13.14). Cytoplasmic organelles identified (other than melanosomes and premelanosomes) include Golgi apparatus and polyribosomes. Thin intracytoplasmic intermediate fila-ments may occasionally be seen; however, tonofilaments are not seen. Intermediate cell junctions and desmosome-like formations are infrequently identified; true desmo-somes are not present. Basal laminae may be seen but are either poorly developed or absent. When seen, it is usually at the periphery of neoplastic cell nests but not surrounding individual cells.

DIAGNOSIS AND DIFFERENTIAL DIAGNOSIS

The diagnosis of LMM is generally not clinically deter-mined but is dependent on histopathological evaluation. From a clinical standpoint, by laryngoscopy and radiographic studies (CT, MRI), the presence, local-ization and extent of a mass will be determined. However, unless deeply pigmented, there are no specific macroscopic features which will indicate the presence of a laryngeal malignant melanoma. The pathological diag-nostic criteria for LMM are detailed above, and, given these findings, a diagnosis can be determined. Never-theless, because there are pathological features of laryngeal malignant melanoma which overlap with other primary laryngeal malignant neoplasms, detailed patho-logical evaluation of a laryngeal pleomorphic/anaplastic and/or spindle cell neoplasm is necessary prior to rendering a diagnosis of LMM. In this way, LMM could be considered a diagnosis of exclusion.

Among the laryngeal neoplasms included in the differ-ential diagnosis of LMM are squamous cell carcinoma (conventional and spindle cell squamous carcinoma), neuroendocrine carcinoma, extramedullary plasma-cytoma, paraganglioma, non-Hodgkin's malignant lym-phomas and sarcomas (malignant fibrous histiocytoma,

Table 13.1 Immunocytochemical differential diagnostic profile for laryngeal malignant melanoma

	S-100	HMB-45	CK	CG	SYN	LCA	Lymphocyte cell markers (B- or T-cell)	Light chain Ig	ACT	DES
LMM	+	+	–	–	–	–	–	–	–	–
SCC	–	–	+	–	–	–	–	–	–	–
SCSC	–	–	+	–	–	–	–	–	–	–
NEC	+	–	+	+	+	–	–	–	–	–
LP	+	–	–	+	+	–	–	–	–	–
LEP	–	–	–	–	–	+	+ for B-cell markers	+ (monotypic)	–	–
ML	–	–	–	–	–	+	+ (monoclonal)	–	–	–
MFH	–	–	–	–	–	–	–	–	–	–
FS	–	–	–	–	–	–	–	–	–	–
MS	+	–	–	–	–	–	–	–	–	–
LMS	–	–	–	–	–	–	–	–	+	+

LMM = laryngeal malignant melanoma; SCC = squamous cell carcinoma; SCSC = spindle cell squamous carcinoma; NEC = neuroendocrine carcinoma; LP = laryngeal paraganglioma; LEP = laryngeal extramedullary plasmacytoma; ML = non-Hodgkin's malignant lymphoma; MFH/FS = malignant fibrous histiocytoma and fibrosarcoma; MS = malignant Schwannoma; LMS = leiomyosarcoma.
S-100 = S-100 protein; CK = cytokeratin; CG = chromogranin; SYN = synaptophysin; LCA = leukocyte common antigen; Light chain Ig = kappa and lambda light chain immunoglobulins; ACT = actin; DES = desmin.

fibrosarcoma and malignant Schwannoma). Certainly, when considering a diagnosis of LMM, metastasis from a separate/distant primary source to the larynx must be ruled out. The following discussion details the essential pathological features which help in differentiating LMM from neoplasms with similar histological features. The definitive method of differentiation may depend on the immunocytochemical findings detailed in the text and highlighted in Table 13.1.

In general, when considering the differential diagnosis of laryngeal squamous cell carcinoma, malignant melanoma is seldom considered. However, in poorly-differentiated squamous cell carcinomas predominantly or exclusively composed by a non-keratinizing anaplastic cell population, or those squamous cell carcinomas composed of a spindle cell population, differentiation from a malignant melanoma may be considered. Poorly differentiated squamous cell carcinomas are non-keratinizing neoplasms composed of cohesive cells marked by pleomorphism, mitoses and necrosis. An in situ carcinomatous component is common, and this may be extensive and may be seen adjacent to the invasive carcinoma. Keratinization may be present but is usually focal. Histochemical evaluation is non-contributory. Despite its poor differentiation, immunocytochemical evaluation for cytokeratin is at least focally positive. In contrast to LMM, no immunoreactivity will be seen with S-100 protein or HMB-45.

Spindle cell squamous carcinoma (SCSC) or 'sarcomatoid' carcinoma consists of foci of conventional squamous cell carcinoma (in situ or invasive carcinoma) associated with a spindle cell stromal component. Histologically, these neoplasms are predominantly or exclusively characterized by a spindle cell proliferation. The spindle cell component is extensively infiltrative and varies from a bland to an overtly pleomorphic-appearing infiltrate. The growth patterns include fascicular, storiform or palisading, and may be associated with a myxomatous stroma. These are generally hypercellular and pleomorphic neoplasms with large, hyperchromatic nuclei, prominent nucleoli, many mitoses (typical and atypical) and multinucleated giant cells. Unequivocal diagnosis of a spindle cell carcinoma can be made in the presence of an in situ and/or frankly invasive squamous cell carcinoma. Typically, the squamous carcinoma is keratinizing and of varying differentiation (well to poorly differentiated). It should be noted that this component may be limited and may require multiple sectioning for identification. In addition to the malignant spindle and squamous cell components, heterologous elements can be seen — including bone and cartilage. The latter may be benign or may be malignant (osteosarcomatous and chondrosarcomatous foci). Necrosis is not uncommon. The differentiation from LMM is entertained in those cases composed entirely of a malignant pleomorphic spindle cell infiltrate. Immunocytochemistry is an invaluable aid in the differential diagnosis in that the spindle cells are at least focally cytokeratin positive in the majority of cases. However, the spindle cells may be keratin-negative in as many as 40% of the cases.[33] Despite the absence of cytokeratin immunoreactivity, a diagnosis of spindle cell carcinoma is not excluded. In general, a polypoid, superficially-located laryngeal malignant spindle cell neoplasm is a spindle cell carcinoma until proven otherwise. Therefore, a full immunocytochemical antigenic profile must be performed, including S-100 protein and HMB-45. The presence or absence of these antibodies will assist in differentiating these neoplasms.

Laryngeal neuroendocrine carcinomas are composed of three distinct lesions, including carcinoid tumours, atypical carcinoid tumours and small cell neuroendocrine carcinomas.[39,86,96,97] A more standardized classification scheme has been proposed.[96,97] The laryngeal classification includes well-differentiated neuroendocrine carcinoma synonymous with carcinoid tumour; moderately differentiated neuroendocrine carcinoma (MDNEC)

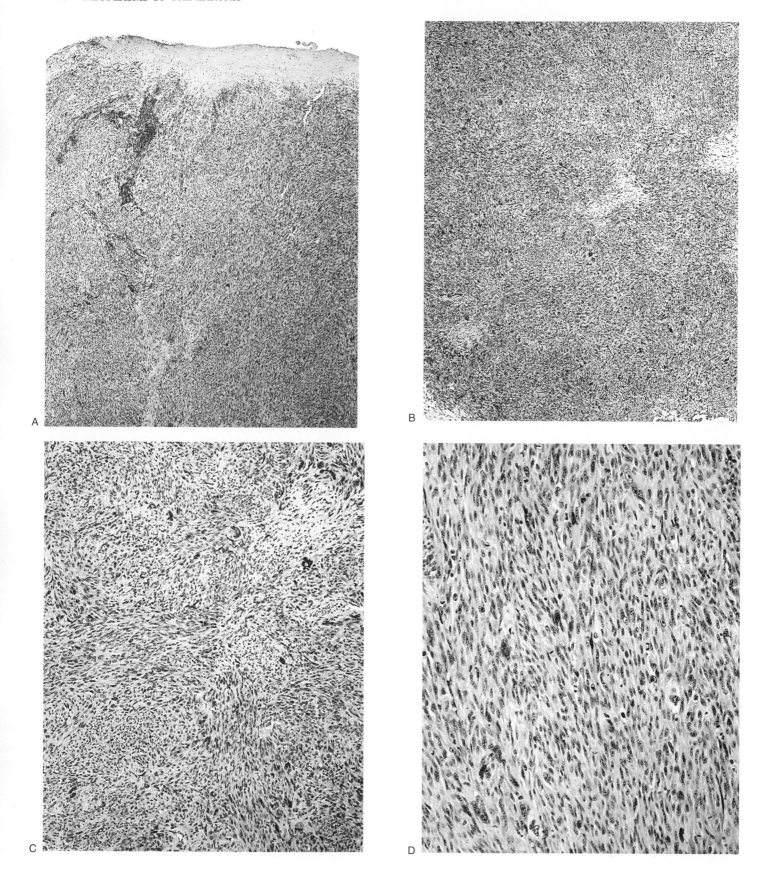

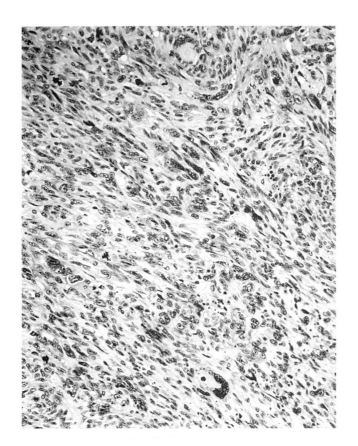 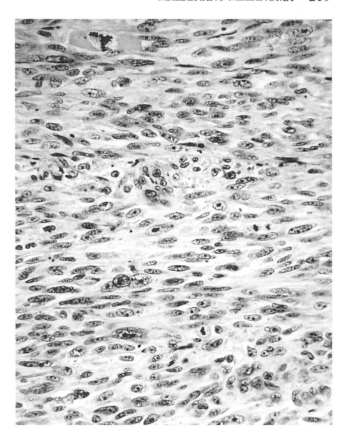

Fig. 13.7 Spindle cell malignant melanoma. A, B. (*opposite page: top left, right*) Infiltrating spindle cell neoplasm associated with surface ulceration, numerous multinucleated cells and a storiform growth pattern ×30. C–F. (*opposite page: bottom left, right; above: left, right*) Spindle cells are elongated, marked by cellular pleomorphism, vesicular to hyperchromatic nuclei, prominent nucleoli, variable amount of eosinophilic cytoplasm, the presence of multinucleated cells and increased mitotic activity including many bizarre forms. C ×75; D, E ×150; F ×300.

includes those entities previously designated as atypical, pleomorphic, malignant, or anaplastic carcinoid tumours. Poorly differentiated neuroendocrine carcinoma (PDNEC) includes small cell carcinoma, both the 'oat' cell and intermediate cell variants.

The differential diagnosis of LMM is generally readily accomplished with both the well-differentiated (carcinoid) and poorly differentiated (small cell) types of NEC. Therefore, this discussion will be limited to the moderately differentiated NEC. MDNEC are malignant neoplasms demonstrating differentiation along both epithelial and neuroendocrine cell lines. Like LMM, MDNEC are most frequently identified in the supra-glottic region with the arytenoids and epiglottis being the most frequent locations.[96,97] Grossly, the masses are predominantly polypoid or nodular varying in size from 0.2 to 4.0 cm in greatest dimension. Microscopically, the tumours are submucosal in origin, infiltrative, with a varied growth pattern including glandular, organoid, acinar, trabecular, solid and nesting architectures. Glands or partial glands are seen in a majority of the cases. Both the absence of epithelial junctional change and the presence of glands are valuable diagnostic findings in differentiating MDNEC from LMM. However, these features are not always found and, therefore, cannot be

relied upon. Cytologically, MDNEC are characterized by large polyhedral to round cells in which non-cohesive cells are occasionally prominent. A varying amount of cytoplasm can be seen in all cases; the cytoplasm stains lightly to deeply eosinophilic. Nuclei are round to oval, often eccentrically located, and in all cases display pleomorphism ranging from mild to severe. The chromatin pattern is generally stippled. Nucleoli, when present, are eosinophilic and multiple. All tumours display a fibrovascular and/or hyaline stroma separating tumour nests. Necrosis and mitoses are generally not prominent features.

The differentiation of MDNEC from LMM can usually be made by light microscopy. However, histo-chemical and immunocytochemical analysis may be required, and these procedures assist in differentiating these neoplasms. MDNEC demonstrate both epithelial (adenocarcinoma) and neuroendocrine differentiation by histochemical, immunocytochemical and ultrastructural analyses. Epithelial mucin (PAS with and without enzyme digestion) shows both intracytoplasmic and luminal positivity. Argyrophilic staining (Churukian–Schenk) is positive, but while Fontana–Masson positivity may be seen in rare examples of MDNEC it is usually absent. The immunocytochemical profile for MDNEC includes

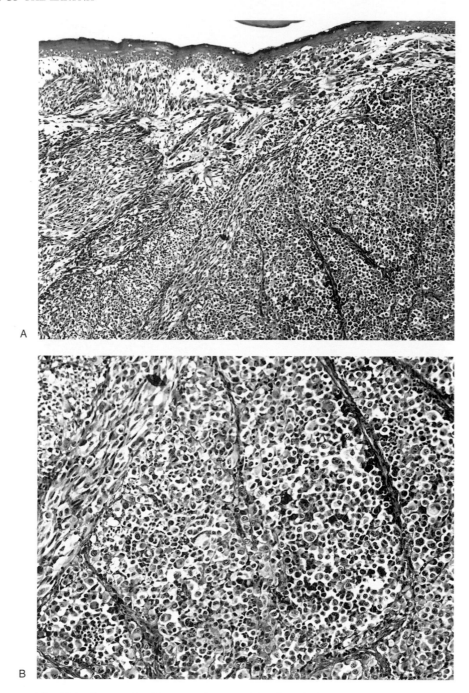

Fig. 13.8   Laryngeal malignant melanoma arising from the basal layer of the squamous epithelium composed of an admixture of epithelioid and spindle cells. A. (*top*) ×75; B (*bottom*) ×150.

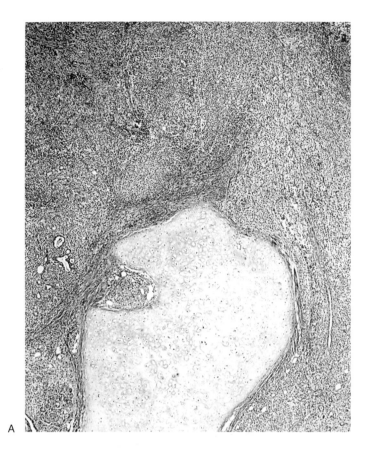 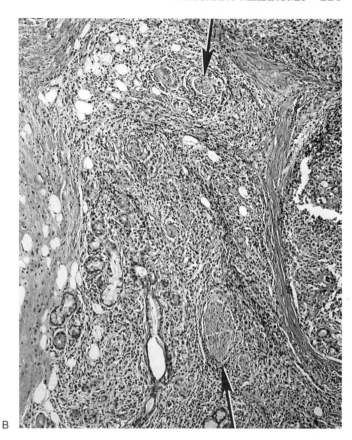

Fig. 13.9   Invasive laryngeal malignant melanoma with (A, *left*) obliteration of mucoserous glands and extension to the perichondrium (×30), and (B, *right*) perineural invasion (arrows) (×75). Residual minor salivary glands can be seen.

cytokeratin, chromogranin and calcitonin reactivity in the majority of cases.[96,97] While S-100 protein immunoreactivity may be seen, it is, in contrast to LMM, usually focal and not as intensely positive. Further, HMB-45 is negative in MDNEC.

Laryngeal (non-chromaffin) paragangliomas (LP) are histologically characterized by cell nests (Zellballen) with a highly vascular stroma. Cellular pleomorphism, mitoses or necrosis are not prominent features. LP do not form glands nor contain PAS-positive material. LP are argyrophilic but do not stain with argentaffin stains. Definitive differentiation from LMM can be accomplished by immunocytochemistry which, for LP, will demonstrate intense and diffuse chromogranin immunoreactivity in the chief cells and characteristic S-100 protein staining identified *only* in the sustentacular cell population. HMB-45 is negative.

Similarities between LMM and laryngeal extramedullary plasmacytomas (LEP) include round cells with abundant eosinophilic cytoplasm and eccentrically located nuclei with a stippled chromatin pattern and occasional presence of a prominent eosinophilic nucleolus. However, in contrast to LMM, LEP typically have a clear zone around the nuclei—referred to as a paranuclear halo—which corresponds to the Golgi

apparatus. Further, LEP demonstrate intracytoplasmic methyl green pyroninophilia. These latter two features are not seen in LMM. In addition, LEP do not display the cellular pleomorphism, mitotic activity, argyrophilia, argentaffinity or the immunoreactivity (S-100 protein and HMB-45) staining seen with LMM.

Primary laryngeal sarcomas are rare, and by far the most common laryngeal sarcoma is the chondrosarcoma.[69] Malignant fibrous histiocytoma (MFH), fibrosarcoma, malignant Schwannoma and leiomyosarcoma arising in the larynx are decidedly uncommon neoplasms. Nevertheless, because of their cellular appearance—consisting of spindle-shaped cells and/or an epithelioid cell population often associated with marked cellular pleomorphism and increased mitotic activity—differentiation from LMM may be necessary. While cytomorphological features may be similar, immunocytochemical evaluation will differentiate these sarcomas from LMM. In contrast to LMM, MFH and fibrosarcoma do not demonstrate S-100 protein and HMB-45 reactivity but will show reactivity with non-specific markers such as vimentin. KP1, a histiocytic cell marker, can be seen in MFH. Malignant Schwannomas do react with S-100 protein but typically are less intensely and not as diffusely positive as compared to LMM; malignant Schwannomas

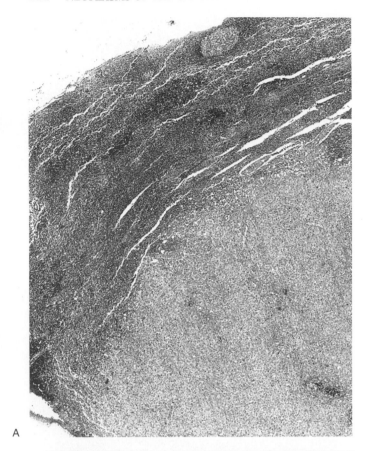

A

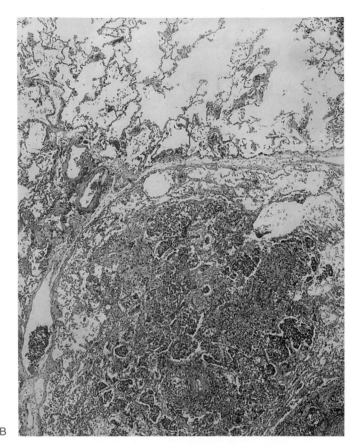

B

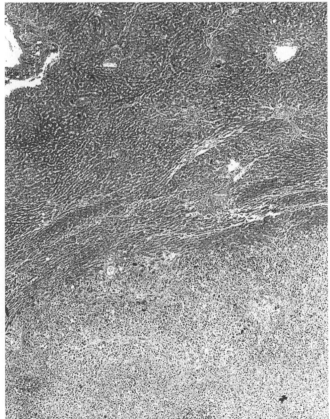

C

Fig. 13.10 Metastatic laryngeal malignant melanoma to the regional cervical lymph nodes (A, *top left*), lung (B, *top right*) and liver (C, *bottom*). ×30.

will not react with HMB-45. Leiomyosarcomas are positive with vimentin, desmin and actin but do not demonstrate S-100 protein and HMB-45 reactivity. However, Wick et al reported four of five cutaneous leiomyosarcomas to demonstrate S-100 protein reactivity.[99]

While, in the broad sense, non-Hodgkin's malignant lymphoma is considered in the differential diagnosis of LMM, the light-microscopic appearance usually allows for the differentiation of these neoplasms. Malignant lymphoma of the larynx (MLL) is rare and may be seen as an isolated process or as part of systemic disease. In differentiating (MLL) from LMM, lymphoma cells will be leukocyte common antigen (LCA)-positive and, depending on their cell lineage, will demonstrate immunoreactivity with either B-cell (L-26) or T-cell (UCHL) markers. MLL are neither S-100 protein nor HMB-45 positive.

Prior to establishing a diagnosis of LMM, it is essential to rule out a metastasis to the larynx from a separate cutaneous or mucosal-based malignant melanoma.[1,8,18,36,38,40,42,58,59,98] Along with renal cell carcinoma, metastatic malignant melanoma represents the most common malignant neoplasm to metastasize to the larynx.[1,8,26,38] This fact, coupled with the rarity of primary laryngeal malignant melanoma, behooves the physicians involved to consider, evaluate for, and rule out the presence of a primary malignant melanoma arising in a separate site. Once this has been adequately accomplished, a diagnosis of primary laryngeal malignant melanoma can be confidently rendered.

THERAPY

The treatment of choice for laryngeal malignant melanoma is complete surgical excision.[9,15,25,26,72,89] The surgical treatment of LMM depends on the stage of the disease. In the absence of regional or distant metastases, surgical eradication of the disease may be accomplished by local resection (partial[87] or total laryngectomy). Any treatment modality short of complete surgical excision will result in local recurrence of the neoplasm. This was borne out by several cases cited in the literature in which the patients had incomplete surgical excision or were treated by non-surgical therapy resulting in recurrent tumour.[7,32,52,71,85,94] Reuter and Woodruff comment on the relatively low incidence of local recurrence of LMM as compared to mucosal melanomas of other head and neck sites.[79] They suggested that the laryngeal tumours are more likely to be delimited and, therefore, more amenable to surgical excision. Given the fact that LMM are amenable to surgical resection, thus limiting the potential of the neoplasms to recur, the incidence of regional lymph node metastasis is considered low.[89] Therefore, elective neck dissection is not recommended.[10,72] However, as will be detailed later, mucosal melanomas of the head and neck tend to present with more advanced (invasive) disease as compared to their cutaneous counterparts, thereby, allowing for greater accessibility of the neoplasm to vascular channels and increasing the likelihood of metastatic disease. This is illustrated by documentation of a large percentage of LMM demonstrating regional and distant metastases.[79] As such, detailed clinical evaluation of the neck is indicated and, if clinically warranted, neck dissection should be performed.

The utility of radiotherapy and/or chemotherapy in the treatment of mucosal malignant melanomas is by and large felt to have no effect on local or distant disease[9,17,24,71,85] and is presently used as adjuvant therapy.[9,10] Malignant melanomas are felt to be radioresistant tumours.[9,10,24,51,72,85] However, studies on cutaneous melanomas suggest that melanoma cell lines may not be intrinsically radioresistant, and to overcome their capacity to resist sublethal radiation doses, high-dose per-fraction therapy (minimal dose per fraction of 400 cGy) should be administered.[47,48] In this way, radiotherapy may offer a greater chance of local control of the primary neoplasm resulting in longer remission periods. At this time, surgery remains the treatment of choice; however, additional testing is needed to validate the utility of radiotherapy in the treatment of malignant melanoma. Certainly, the previous held dogma that malignant melanomas are radioresistant tumours has been challenged by the recent studies.[47,48] An argument can be made for using radiotherapy as the initial mode of treatment in mucosal melanomas. Typically, the clinical presentation of mucosal melanoma is with advanced disease which would require surgery resulting in unacceptable mutilations.[25] Surgical intervention could be reserved for those patients who fail radiation therapy and still have localized disease. The use of postoperative radiotherapy may be warranted in either localized or systemic disease based on evidence that some melanomas respond temporarily to irradiation.[25] Alternative therapeutic modalities used in the treatment of malignant melanoma include cryosurgery,[7] immunotherapy,[78] and the administration of vitamins.[11] The philosophy behind these therapeutic modalities is to function as immunopotentiators boosting the immunological status of the patient by provoking a lymphocytic response to the neoplasm. Despite this 'shot in the arm' to the patient's immune status, it does not appear that there is a decided benefit to these modes of treatment.

PROGNOSIS

The prognosis of mucosal malignant melanomas in general, and laryngeal malignant melanomas in particular, is not good. The average survival rates are usually less than 3.5 years,[19,43,79,94] with 5-year survival rates of less than 20%.[24,43,63,72,79] Cure rates are equally

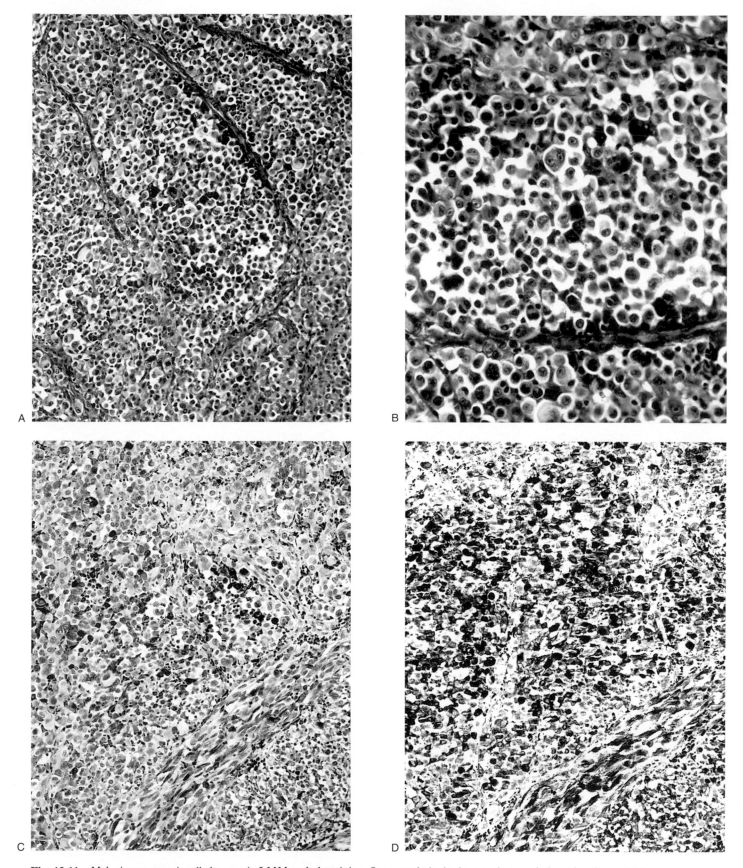

Fig. 13.11   Melanin can occasionally be seen in LMM as dark staining, fine granularity in the cytoplasm and obscuring the nuclei in scattered neoplastic cells. A (*top left*) ×150; B (*top right*) ×300. Histochemistry and laryngeal malignant melanoma as demonstrated by argentaffin-positive staining (C, *bottom, left*) and argyrophilic-positive staining (D, *bottom, right*) in both the epithelioid and spindle cells. ×150.

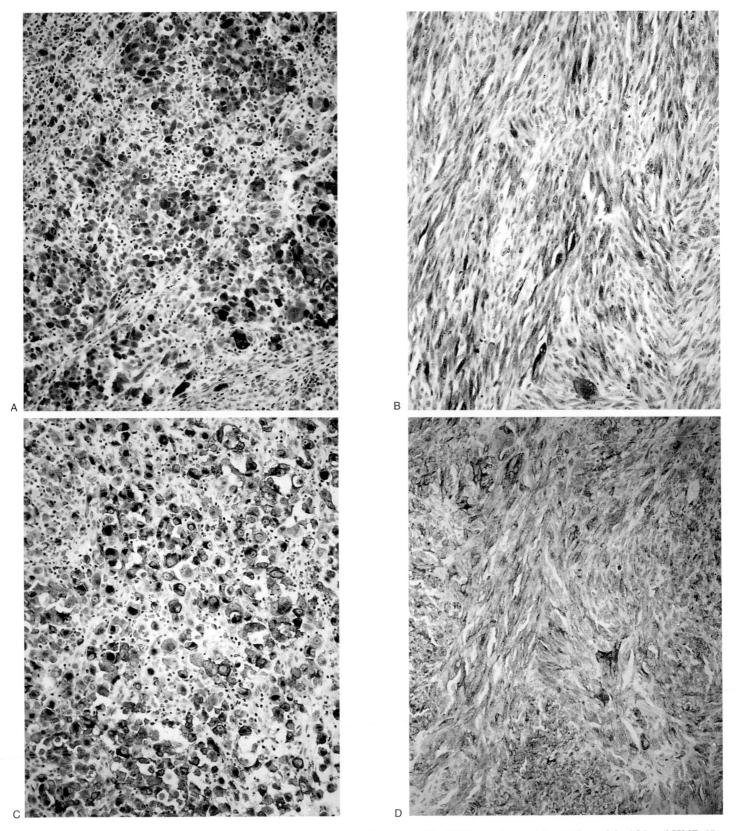

Fig. 13.12 Immunocytochemistry of laryngeal malignant melanoma as demonstrated by S-100 protein reactivity (A, B: *top left, right*) and HMB-45 reactivity (C, D: *bottom left, right*) in both the epithelioid and spindle cells. ×150.

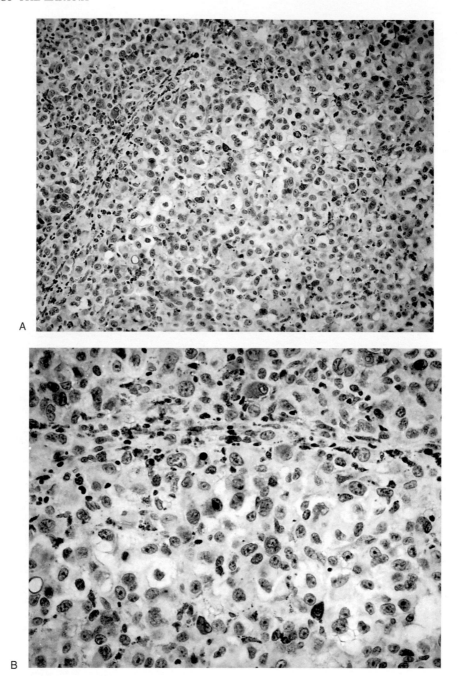

Fig. 13.13 Although malignant melanomas are not associated with chromogranin immunoreactivity, this case of laryngeal malignant melanoma demonstrated scattered cells with positive chromogranin staining. A (*top*) ×150; B (*bottom*) ×300.

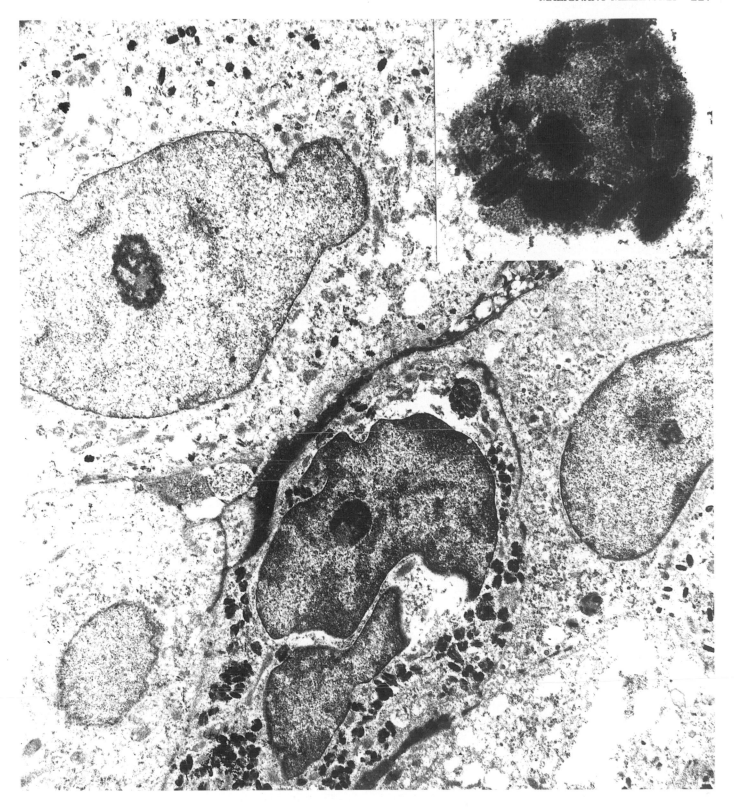

Fig. 13.14 Ultrastructural appearance of laryngeal malignant melanoma. Epithelioid cells with irregularly shaped nuclei, prominent nucleoli, incomplete basal laminae and intracytoplasmic bundles of melanosomes seen in three separate cells. ×3000. *Inset.* Melanosomes are oblong, dark-staining, with some fibrillary arrangements ×20 000.

low, and include 8%[24] and 15%.[23] Overall, recurrence rates for mucosal melanomas vary, and include 40%,[23] 42%[89], 64%[85] and 69%.[72] In contrast, LMM have a lower incidence of recurrence—reported by Conley and Pack in their series to be 32%.[23] The poor behaviour of LMM is seen despite the lower incidence of local recurrence and, like mucosal malignant melanomas of other sites, can be attributed to a tendency of these neoplasms to remain occult until the appearance of symptoms—which usually indicates an advanced stage of disease. This is particularly true of LMM, the majority of which are identified in supraglottic locations away from the glottic region. The importance of this phenomenon is that if these neoplasms had a predilection for occurring in the glottic region, symptoms such as hoarseness or change in voice would occur earlier in the disease (smaller neoplasm, lower clinical stage). This might then prompt the patient to seek medical attention, lead to earlier detection, and make the neoplasm more amenable to surgical treatment with less likelihood for local recurrence or distant metastasis. These findings contrast with those of cutaneous malignant melanomas which occur in exposed areas of the body, making them readily visible and detectable earlier—resulting in a better prognosis as compared with mucosal melanomas.[10,34] Other features seen in mucosal malignant melanomas which differ from cutaneous malignant melanomas, and which may influence prognosis, include: (i) occurrence in an older age group,[34,43] (ii) histologically higher grade with greater anaplasia, pleomorphism and mitotic activity,[2,34] and (iii) less accessibility and greater anatomic hindrances, precluding the ability to completely resect the neoplasm.[10,63,72]

Contributing to the poor prognosis in patients with LMM is a tendency of these neoplasms to metastasize. Reuter and Woodruff in their review of the literature identified metastatic disease to regional lymph nodes or to distant sites in 80% of the patients.[79] Most of the metastatic deposits were seen at periods following the initial diagnosis; however, in 27% of the patients metastatic tumour was identified at the time of diagnosis. Metastases occur to virtually every organ system, and their identification generally portends the imminent demise of the patient. However, with continued advances in the field of immunotherapy and molecular biology, therapeutic modalities are being implemented which may alter the dire consequences normally associated with advanced disease. Rosenberg et al[81] have demonstrated regression of metastatic malignant melanoma in humans using immunotherapy with infusion into the patients of tumour-infiltrating lymphocytes (TIL) plus interleukin-2. Recently, Rosenberg et al[82] have incorporated gene transfer experiments in humans using tumour-infiltrating lymphocytes modified by retroviral-mediated gene trans-

duction to optimize the immunotherapy treatments allowing for in vivo gene markers to define the distribution and survival of TIL. Although these studies included only a limited number of patients followed for short periods of time, they potentially offer hope to individuals who have previously been viewed as having 'one foot in the grave'.

A tremendous contribution to understanding the biology of cutaneous malignant melanoma is the measurement of tumour thickness which represents the single most important factor in predicting survival.[61] Two schemas have been developed for cutaneous malignant melanomas which measure tumour depth based on: (i) the level (extent through the skin) of invasion (Clark levels I –V),[21] and (ii) measurement of tumour thickness with a micrometer (Breslow classification).[12] Five-year mortality figures and the likelihood of regional lymph node metastasis correlate with the depth of invasion, as defined by both Clark and Breslow. Other histological parameters implicated in adverse prognosis include ulceration, absence of a lymphocytic infiltrate, cellular anaplasia, increased mitotic activity, presence of vascular or lymphatic invasion and absence of melanin.[5,55,61] However, these histological findings adversely affect prognosis largely because thay correlate with tumour thickness.[4] Application of the above detailed prognostic parameters, developed for cutaneous malignant melanomas, cannot be applied to mucosal melanomas of the head and neck and, in fact, some authors state that there is a lack of correlation between the depth of invasion and prognosis.[51,72] In contrast to the neat compartmentalization of the skin, similar histological landmarks —such as the papillary and reticular dermis—do not exist in the mucosae of the upper aerodigestive tract. Therefore, it would seem that prognosis of LMM is based on the clinical stage of the tumour and, following biopsy diagnosis, appropriate work-up should be instituted to establish the clinical stage of the neoplasm. To this end, a staging system to define the extent of disease has been proposed; this includes stage I: disease confined to the primary site; stage II: presence of regional metastasis; stage III: presence of distant metastasis.[48] Finally, clinical parameters have been identified for cutaneous melanomas which relate to favourable prognosis; these include occurrence in women, younger age, and location on hair-bearing portions of the extremities.[55,61] However, although LMM tend to occur in men more frequently than in women, there appear to be no clinical parameters which will have a bearing on prognosis.[85] Rather, prognosis for mucosal melanomas of the head and neck will be the same for equally matched clinical stages irrespective of age, sex or location of the malignant melanoma.[25]

REFERENCES

1. Abemayor E, Cochran A J, Calcaterra T C 1983 Metastatic cancer to the larynx: diagnosis and management. Cancer 52: 1944–1948
2. Allen A C, Spitz S 1953 Malignant melanoma: a clinicopathological analysis of the criteria for diagnosis and prognosis. Cancer 6: 1–45
3. Ash J E, Raum M 1949 An atlas of otolaryngic pathology. Armed Forces Institute of Pathology, Washington DC, p 340
4. Balch C M, Murad T M, Soong S J, Ingalls A L, Richards P C, Maddox W A 1979 Tumor thickness as a guide to surgical management of clinical stage I melanoma patients. Cancer 43: 883–888
5. Balch C M, Wilkerson J A, Murad T M, Soong S J, Ingalls A L, Maddox W A 1980 The prognostic significance of ulceration of cutaneous melanoma. Cancer 45: 3012–3017
6. Baron F, Legent F, Mussini M, Le Neel M, Bruneau Y, Seite P 1971 Un noveau cas de mélanome malin du larynx. Rev Laryngol Otol Rhinol 92: 331–337
7. Barton R T 1975 Mucosal melanomas of the head and neck. Laryngoscope 85: 93–99
8. Batsakis J G, Luna M A, Byers R M 1985 Metastases to the larynx. Head Neck Surg 7: 458–460
9. Berthelsen A, Andersen A P, Jensen T S, Hansen H S 1984 Melanomas of the mucosa in the oral cavity and upper respiratory passages. Cancer 54: 907–912
10. Blatchford S J, Koopmann C F, Coulthard S W 1986 Mucosal melanoma of the head and neck. Laryngoscope 96: 929–934
11. Bregman M D, Myskens F L 1984 Modulation of malignant melanoma growth with vitamins and other chemically refined biologic modifiers. In: Costanzi J J (ed) Clinical management of malignant melanoma. Martinus Niihoff, Boston, pp 179–182
12. Breslow A 1970 Thickness, cross-sectional area and depth of invasion in the prognosis of cutaneous melanoma. Ann Surg 172: 902–908
13. Buchholz W 1958 Über Melanoblastome im bereich der oberen luft- und soeisewege. Z Laryng Rhinol 37: 549–554
14. Busuttil A 1976 Dendritic pigmented cells within the human laryngeal mucosa. Arch Otolaryngol 102: 43–44
15. Cady B, Rippey J H, Frazell E L 1968 Non-epidermoid cancer of the larynx. Ann Surg 167: 116–120
16. Campbell C F 1968 Surgical management of melanoma of lung, trachea, and bronchi. Tex Med 64: 62–66
17. Catlin D 1967 Mucosal melanoma of the head and neck. Am J Roentgenol 99: 809–816
18. Chamberlain D 1966 Malignant melanoma, metastatic to the larynx. Arch Otolaryngol 83: 63–64
19. Chaudhry A P, Hampel A, Gorlin R J 1958 Primary malignant melanoma of the oral cavity. Cancer 11: 923–928
20. Churukian C J, Schenk E A 1979 A modification of Pascual's argyrophil method. J Histotechnol 2: 102–103
21. Clarke W H, From L, Bernardino E A, Mihm M C 1969 The histogenesis and biologic behavior of primary human malignant melanoma of the skin. Cancer Res 29: 705–726
22. Claux J, Ané P, Durroux R, Chamayou P 1977 Le naevocarcinome endolaryngé. J Fr Otorhinolaryngol 26: 381–385
23. Conley J, Pack G T 1974 Melanoma of the mucous membranes of the head and neck. Arch Otolaryngol 99: 315–319
24. Conley J, Hamaker R C 1977 Melanoma of the head and neck. Laryngoscope 87: 760–764
25. Conley J J 1989 Melanomas of the mucous membranes of the head and neck. Laryngoscope 99: 1248–1254
26. Conley J 1990 The melanocyte and melanoma. Laryngoscope 100: 1310–1312
27. Cove H 1979 Melanosis, melanocytic hyperplasia, and primary malignant melanoma of the nasal cavity. Cancer 44: 1424–1433
28. Cremonesi G 1956 Su un eccezionale reperto di sarcoma melanotico primitivo della laringe. Minerva Otorinolaringol 6: 333–340
29. Curtiss C, Kosinski A A 1955 Primary malignant melanoma of the larynx: report of a case and review of the literature. Cancer 8: 961–963
30. De Juan P 1955 Melanosarcoma laringeo y otras consideraciones. Acta Otorrinolaringol Ibero Am 7: 296–308
31. Drier J K, Swanson P E, Cherwitz D L, Wick M R 1987 S100 protein immunoreactivity in poorly differentiated carcinomas: immunohistochemical comparison with malignant melanoma. Arch Pathol Lab Med 111: 447–452
32. El-Barbary A E, Fouad H A, El-Sayed A F 1968 Malignant melanoma involving the larynx: report of two cases. Ann Otol Rhinol Laryngol 77: 338–343
33. Ellis G L, Langloss J M, Heffner D K, Hyams V J 1987 Spindle-cell carcinoma of the aerodigestive tract: an immunohistochemical analysis of 21 cases. Am J Surg Pathol 11: 335–342
34. Eneroth C M, Lundberg C 1975 Mucosal malignant melanoma of the head and neck: with special reference to cases having a prolonged clinical course. Acta Otolaryngol 80: 452–458
35. Espinoza C G, Lavallee-Grey M C 1988 Malignant melanoma. In: Azar H A (ed) Pathology of human neoplasms. Raven Press, New York, pp 405–427
36. Ewen S W B, Bussolati G, Pearse A G E 1972 Uptake of 1-dopa and 1–5–hydroxytryptophan by endocrine-like cells in the rat larynx. Histochem J 4: 103–110
37. Fenning F R 1955 Malignant melanoma of the larynx. Ann Otol Rhinol Laryngol 64: 1281–1283
38. Ferlito A, Caruso G, Recher G 1988 Secondary laryngeal tumors: report of seven cases with review of the literature. Arch Otolaryngol Head Neck Surg 114: 635–639
39. Ferlito A, Rosai J 1991 Terminology and classification of neuroendocrine neoplasms of the larynx. ORL J Otorhinolaryngol Relat Spec 53: 185–187
40. Fisher G E, Odess J S 1951 Metastatic malignant melanoma of the larynx. Arch Otolaryngol 54: 639–642
41. Foucar K, Foucar E 1990 The mononuclear phagocytic and immunoregulatory effector (m-pire) system: evolving concepts. Semin Diagn Pathol 7: 4–18
42. Freeland A P, van Nostrand A W P, Jahn A F 1979 Metastases to the larynx. J Otolaryngol 8: 448–456
43. Gallagher J C 1970 Upper respiratory melanoma pathology and growth rate. Ann Otol Rhinol Laryngol 79: 551–556
44. Goldman J L, Lawson W, Zak F G, Roffman J D 1972 The presence of melanocytes in the human larynx. Laryngoscope 82: 824–835
45. Gould V E, Memoli V A, Dardi L E, Sobel J H, Somers S C, Johannessen J V 1981 Neuroendocrine carcinomas with multiple immunoreactive peptides and melanin production. Ultrastruct Pathol 2: 199–217
46. Gown A M, Vogel A M, Hoak D, Gough F, McNutt M A 1986 Monoclonal antibodies specific for melanocytic tumors distinguish subpopulations of melanocytes. Am J Pathol 123: 195–203
47. Harwood A R, Dancuart F, Fitzpatrick P J, Brown T 1981 Radiotherapy in nonlentiginous melanoma of the head and neck. Cancer 47: 2599–2605
48. Harwood A R 1984 Melanoma of the head and neck. In: Million R R, Cassisi N J (eds) Management of head and neck cancer. Lippincott, Philadelphia, pp 513–528
49. Havens F Z, Parkhill E M 1941 Tumors of the larynx other than squamous cell epithelioma. Arch Otolaryngol 34: 1113–1122
50. Henderson D W, Papadimitrou J M 1982 Melanocytic tumors. In: Henderson D W, Papadimitrou J M (eds) Ultrastructural appearances of tumours: a diagnostic atlas. Churchill Livingstone, Edinburgh, pp 100–107
51. Hussain S S M, Whitehead E 1989 Malignant melanoma of the larynx. J Laryngol Otol 103: 533–536
52. Kim H, Park C I 1982 Primary malignant laryngeal melanoma: report of a case with review of literature. Ynsei Med J 23: 118–122

53. Kirkeby S, Romert P 1977 Argyrophilic cells in the larynx of the guinea-pig demonstrated by the method of grimelius. J Anat 123: 87–92
54. Kornstein M J, Franco A P 1990 Specificity to HM B-45. Arch Pathol Lab Med 114: 450
55. Lever W F, Schaumberg-Lever G 1990 Benign melanocytic tumors and malignant melanoma. In: Lever W F, Schaumberg-Lever G (eds) Histopathology of the skin. Lippincott, Philadelphia, pp 756–804
56. Lloyd R V 1989 The neuroendocrine and paracrine systems. In: Sternberg S S (ed) Diagnostic surgical pathology. Raven Press, New York, pp 435–443
57. Lorentz E 1979 Das maligne Melanom des Kehlkopfes. HNO 27: 275–277
58. Loughhead J R 1952 Malignant melanoma of larynx. Ann Otol Rhinol Laryngol 61: 154–158
59. Loughhead J R, Bushnell J 1954 Metastasis of malignant melanoma to the larynx. Laryngoscope 60: 50–52
60. Masson P 1948 Pigmented cells in man. In: Biology of melanomas, vol 4, New York Academy of Sciences, New York, pp 15–81
61. McGovern V J 1982 The nature of melanoma: a critical review. J Cutan Pathol 9: 61–81
62. Mihm M C, Imber M J 1989 Melanocytic lesions. In: Sternberg S S (ed) Diagnostic surgical pathology. Raven Press, New York pp 103–118
63. Moore E S, Martin H 1955 Melanoma of the upper respiratory tract and oral cavity. Cancer 8: 1167–1176
64. Moore K L 1988 The nervous system. In: Moore K L (ed) The developing human: clinically oriented embryology. Saunders, Philadelphia, pp 364–401
65. Moore K L 1988 The integumentry system: the skin and related structures. In: Moore K L (ed) The developing human: clinically oriented embryology. Saunders, Philadelphia, pp 421–436
66. Moore K L 1988 The respiratory system: In: Moore K L (ed) The developing human: clinically oriented embryology. Saunders, Philadelphia, pp 207–216
67. Müller E 1968 Melanoblastome in Kehlkopf und Mittelohr. HNO 16: 133–136
68. Nakajima T, Watanabe S, Sato Y, Kameya T, Shimosato Y, Ishihara K 1982 Immunohistochemical demonstration of S100 protein in malignant melanoma and pigmented nevus, and its diagnostic application. Cancer 50: 912–918
69. Nicolai P, Ferlito A, Sasaki C T, Kirchner J A 1990 Laryngeal chondrosarcoma: incidence, pathology, biological behavior, and treatment. Ann Otol Rhinol Laryngol 99: 515–523
70. Nielsen K O, Bak-Petersen K 1985 Intra-epithelial mucous glands in the adult human laryngeal mucosa. Acta Otolaryngol 100: 470–476
71. Nsamba C 1966 A case of malignant melanoma of the larynx. J Laryngol Otol 80: 1178–1181
72. Panje W R, Moran W J 1986 Melanoma of the upper aerodigestive tract: a review of 21 cases. Head Neck Surg 8: 309–312
73. Pantazopoulos P E 1964 Primary malignant melanoma of the larynx. Laryngoscope 74: 95–102
74. Pearse A G E 1969 The cytochemistry and ultrastructure of polypeptide hormone-producing cells of the APUD series and the embryologic and pathologic implications of the concept. J Histochem Cytochem 17: 303–313
75. Pearse A G E, Takor-Takor T 1979 Embryology of the diffuse neuroendocrine system and its relationship to the common peptides. Fed Proc 38: 2288–2294
76. Pesce C, Toncini C 1983 Melanin pigmentation of the larynx. Acta Otolaryngol 96: 189–192
77. Pesce C, Tobia-Gallelli F, Toncini C 1984 APUD cells of the larynx. Acta Otolaryngol 98: 158–162
78. Pinsky C M 1984 The immunology and immunotherapy of malignant melanoma. In: Costanzi J J (ed) Clinical management of malignant melanoma. Martinus Niihoff, Boston pp 101–118
79. Reuter V E, Woodruff J M 1986 Melanoma of the larynx. Laryngoscope 96: 389–393
80. Romero L, Scola B, Arangüez G, Garro J, Sacristán T 1982 Melanoma maligno laringeo. Acta Otorrinolaringol Esp 33: 168–172
81. Rosenberg S A, Packard B S, Aebersold P et al 1988 Use of tumor-infiltrating lymphocytes and interleukin-2 in the immunotherapy of patients with metastatic melanoma: a preliminary report. N Engl J Med 319: 1676–1680
82. Rosenberg S A, Aebersold P, Cornetta K et al 1990 Gene transfer into humans — immunotherapy of patients with advanced melanoma, using tumor-infiltrating lymphocytes modified by retroviral gene transduction. N Engl J Med 323: 570–578
83. Schimpf A, Musebeck K, Mootz W 1969 Naevuszellnaevus (compoundnaevus) im Larynxbereich (plica ventricularis). Z Haut Geschlechtskr 44: 137–144
84. Seals J L, Shenefelt R E, Babin R W 1986 Intralaryngeal nevus in a child: a case report. Int J Ped Otorhinolaryngol 12: 55–58
85. Shah J P, Huvos A G, Strong E W 1977 Mucosal melanomas of the head and neck. Am J Surg 134: 531–535
86. Shanmugaratnam K 1991 Histological typing of tumours of the upper aerodigestive tract and ear. World Health Organization. International histological classification of tumours, 2nd edn. Springer-Verlag, Berlin
87. Shanon E, Covo J, Loeventhal M 1970 Melanoma of the epiglottis: a case treated by supraglottic laryngectomy. Arch Otolaryngol 91: 304–305
88. Smith D M, Haggitt R C 1983 A comparative study of generic stains for carcinoid secretory granules. Am J Surg Pathol 7: 61–68
89. Snow G B, VanDer Esch E P, van Sloaten E A 1978 Mucosal melanoma of the head and neck. Head Neck Surg 1: 24–30
90. Tagaki M, Ishikawa G, Movi W 1974 Primary malignant melanoma of the oral cavity in Japan: with special reference to mucosal melanoma. Cancer 34: 358–370
91. Taira K 1985 Endocrine-like cells in the laryngeal mucosa of adult rabbits demonstrated by electron microscopy and by the Grimelius silver-impregnation method. Biomedical Res 6: 377–385
92. Travis L W, Sutherland C 1980 Coexisting lentigo of the larynx and melanoma of the oral cavity: report of a case. Otolaryngol Head Neck Surg 88: 218–220
93. Vanstapel M J, Gatter K C, de Wolf-Peeters C, Mason D Y, Desmet V D 1986 New sites of human S-100 immunoreactivity detected with monoclonal antibodies. Am J Clin Pathol 85: 160–168
94. Vouri E E J, Hormia M 1969 Primary malignant melanoma of the larynx and pharynx. J Laryngol Otol 83: 281–287
95. Welsh L W, Welsh J J 1961 Malignant melanoma of the larynx. Laryngoscope 71: 185–191
96. Wenig B M, Hyams V J, Heffner D K 1988 Moderately differentiated neuroendocrine carcinoma of the larynx: a clinicopathologic study of 54 cases. Cancer 62: 2658–2676
97. Wenig B M, Gnepp D R 1989 The spectrum of neuroendocrine tumors of the larynx. Semin Diagn Pathol 6: 329–350
98. Whicker J H, Carder G A, Devine K D 1972 Metastasis to the larynx: report of a case and review of the literature. Arch Otolaryngol 96: 182–184
99. Wick M R, Swanson P E, Rocamora A 1988 Recognition of malignant melanoma by monoclonal antibody HMB-45: an immunohistochemical study of 200 paraffin-embedded cutaneous tumors. J Cutan Pathol 15: 201–207
100. Wilson B S, Lloyd R V 1984 Detection of chromogranin in neuroendocrine cells with a monoclonal antibody. Am J Pathol 115: 458–468

14. Salivary gland neoplasms

J. N. El-Jabbour, A. Ferlito, I. Friedmann

INCIDENCE

The incidence of salivary gland neoplasms of the larynx cannot be assessed accurately because of the confusion with other neoplasms. Their frequency has been estimated at less than 1% of all laryngeal tumours.[13,28,57,130,134,151,180] A survey of 2569 salivary gland tumours studied by the British Salivary Gland Tumour Panel recorded no salivary neoplasms of the larynx;[56] Heffner[89] mentioned 46 cases of laryngeal salivary gland tumours collected at the Armed Forces Institute of Pathology between 1976 and 1985 (excluding oncocytic lesions).

It is also difficult to estimate the incidence of the different types of laryngeal salivary neoplasms. The lack of a uniform terminology and definition of some of these tumours contributes to the difficulty. Furthermore, changes in diagnostic criteria and the recognition of recently described entities, such as salivary duct carcinoma[69] and epithelial–myoepithelial carcinoma[120] in the larynx, have added to the difficulty and have made it almost impossible to assess independently the accuracy of reported cases.

The difference in the relative incidence of various types of salivary gland neoplasms among the major series may not be due to some diagnostic 'bias' in favour of certain entities, but rather to prevailing geographical or racial factors. For example, it is interesting to note the high incidence of laryngeal malignant tumours in Italy.

CLINICAL FEATURES

The clinical presentation of these tumours does not differ substantially from that of squamous cell carcinomas, which may present as ulcerated or non-ulcerated swellings, and unless relevant we will not elaborate on it in the description of each neoplasm. The laryngeal seromucinous minor salivary glands are concentrated in decreasing frequency in the vestibular folds and in the aryepiglottic folds. The symptoms depend on tumour location in the larynx in relation to the glottis (i.e., supraglottic tumours most commonly present with dysphagia and hoarseness, whereas subglottic tumours tend to produce shortness of breath, exertional dyspnoea and cough) and are due mainly to narrowing and/or obstruction of the larynx, involvement of the vestibular folds and vocal cords and compression of adjacent structures, e.g., the oesophagus. The presenting symptoms are of a progressive nature and, in addition to those mentioned, may include dysphonia, haemoptysis, stridor, sore throat or 'lumpy sensation'. Pain caused by the infiltration of nerves may be present as in adenoid cystic carcinoma.

DIAGNOSTIC METHODS

The diagnosis is based on endoscopic biopsies. Frequently these are too small and fragmented for a definite diagnosis to be made, and the final histological diagnosis may have to await the detailed examination of the resection specimen. Descriptive light microscopy remains the basic tool, the mainstay of the pathologist's diagnostic nomenclature. New techniques such as immunocytochemistry and electron microscopy have contributed considerably to the diagnosis and more precise classification of various tumours reported as 'undifferentiated' by light microscopy. Immunocytochemistry has assisted in the detection of structural differentiation of the cytoskeleton (intermediate filaments) and in demonstrating multidirectional differentiation in pleomorphic adenoma, adenoid cystic carcinoma and epithelial–myoepithelial carcinoma. Electron microscopy has been useful in the differential diagnosis of squamous cell carcinoma and adenocarcinoma: tonofilaments are distinctive of squamous cell carcinoma while microvilli, intercellular lumina and secretory granules are characteristic of adenocarcinoma. Other new techniques such as in situ hybridization may have a role in clarifying the aetiology of some tumours; studies of cell kinetics using flow cytometry, proliferation markers and bromodeoxyuridine incorporation may provide information about the proliferative activity of tumours. This information may help to tailor the therapeutical protocols to the needs of individual tumours. Flow cytometry detects abnormal nuclear DNA content (i.e., aneuploidy) and measures the various phases of the cell cycle, providing additional information about some tumours with a borderline or equivocal histological appearance (see myoepithelioma).

CLASSIFICATION

The classification of salivary gland tumours, based primarily on their histogenesis, has not been successful. Electron microscopy and immunocytochemistry have revealed a similar histogenetic basis for several of the apparently distinct types and have highlighted the role of the myoepithelial cell in their origin; however, neither has replaced light microscopy in the classification of tumours. Sobin discussed how new techniques influence tumour nomenclature,[157] recognizing that pathologists are obliged to provide consistent data for those who depend on standardized terms, e.g., clinical trials, tumour registries and practising physicians and surgeons. There is the dilemma of when to replace a standard term with a recent term. The recognition that conceptual terms and descriptive terms have separate functions may help pathologists in dealing with terminological changes. In this chapter, we have followed the updated WHO terminology and classifications given in *Histological Typing of Tumours of the Upper Respiratory Tract and Ear*[152] and *Histological Typing of Salivary Gland Tumours*,[148] both published in 1991, which offer a more reliable basis and uniformity of diagnostic terminology to be applied to similar studies in the future. We have discussed some tumour-like lesions because they might be misinterpreted as malignant neoplasms.

NEOPLASMS

Pleomorphic adenoma

Introduction and incidence

Pleomorphic adenoma of the larynx is rare, in complete contrast to its major salivary gland counterpart, where it is the most frequently encountered tumour.

The true incidence of pleomorphic adenoma cannot be accurately assessed. There are several reported cases in the earlier literature;[124,145,164] however, some of these reports are poorly illustrated and do not allow an independent judgement to be made. Furthermore, the distinction between benign and malignant mixed tumours was not sufficiently clear in past reports.

Pleomorphic adenoma of the larynx was first mentioned by Cunning,[34] but it seems that the first well-documented account was published in 1955 by Abercromby and Rewell.[2] Since then, a number of cases have been reported.[3,8a,14,16,] 31,71,78,82,98,107,112,139,158,167a,170,174,178,182,183 The case described by Pinel et al, however, has been reported twice.[139,178]

Heffner[89] has seen only three cases of laryngeal salivary mixed tumour at the Armed Forces Intitute of Pathology, Washington DC, in the period between 1976 and 1985.

Definition and terminology

According to the WHO classification, pleomorphic adenoma is a tumour of pleomorphic structure containing luminal type ductal epithelial cells, myoepithelial cells and tissues of mucomyxoid or chondroid appearance.[152] Due to its diverse histological elements and patterns, this neoplasm has also been called benign mixed tumour. Both terms are currently widely accepted.

Histogenesis

It is postulated that the tumour arises from the neoplastic proliferation of the complete ductal-acinar unit.[39]

Clinical features

There is no sex predilection, and equally there is no age preponderance. The majority of cases occur in the epiglottis, aryepiglottic fold and vestibular fold.[31]

Pathology

Grossly, the tumour forms a firm, well-defined, sessile, slightly lobulated mass. Its size ranges from 1 to 5 cm.[31] On sectioning, the tumour displays various patterns: solid, myxoid or chondroid. Ossification is uncommon.

Microscopically, it resembles pleomorphic adenoma of the major salivary glands. The tumour may be sharply demarcated, and has a fibrous pseudocapsule with several satellite nodules. It consists of varying proportions of epithelial and myoepithelial cells lying in a mixed stroma. The proportion of epithelial and mesenchymal components bears no relationship to behaviour. The epithelial and myoepithelial cells may be arranged in adenomatous, ductal or cribriform structures. Squamous metaplasia and oncocytic changes may occur in the epithelial component. The stroma may consist predominantly of fibrous, myxomatous, myxochondroid, chondroid—or even osseous—tissues, or of a mixture of these tissues.

Two types of crystalline inclusion have been described in pleomorphic adenoma: tyrosine-rich crystalloids and radially arranged collagen fibre crystalloids.[24]

Immunocytochemistry. Studies performed on pleomorphic adenomas of the major salivary glands[91,125,129] have confirmed the bipolar differentiation in this neoplasm and revealed great variations in the immunoreactivity of the tumour cells for various antibodies, as well as multiple and co-expressions of these antibodies.

The ductal luminal tumour cells are immunoreactive for carcinoembryonic antigen (CEA), various types of cytokeratin and epithelial membrane antigen (EMA), suggesting an origin from the intercalated duct cells; the outer tumour cells of the tubulo-ductal structures and neoplastic myoepithelial cells are positive with vimentin, S-100 protein, actin, myosin and, to a lesser extent, some types of cytokeratin, suggesting that the outer cells are derived from the ductal basal cells. Perhaps the most remarkable finding is the consistent demonstration of focal immunoreactivity for glial fibrillary acidic protein (GFAP) in the periductal and stromal cells, specifically those in which ultrastructural features indicative of myoepithelial origin are either scant or absent.[6,129]

Electron microscopy. Various studies[39,40,135] have shown that both epithelial and myoepithelial cells play a part in the neoplastic proliferation of pleomorphic adenoma. The principal proliferating tumour cell is a structurally modified myoepithelial cell that frequently shows squamous differentiation.

Diagnosis and differential diagnosis

The histological features of pleomorphic adenoma are characteristic. Nevertheless, due to the diverse patterns and their patchy distribution, confusion with other tumours may occur. Squamous metaplasia in pleomorphic adenoma has been misdiagnosed as squamous cell carcinoma;[112] the cribriform pattern may be confused with adenoid cystic carcinoma. If the biopsy consisted entirely of cartilaginous tissue, an incorrect diagnosis of chondroma may be made. The tumour has been misdiagnosed as mucoepidermoid carcinoma.[183]

Therapy and prognosis

The treatment of choice is complete surgical excision. These tumours are benign, but malignant transformation in the form of carcinoma in pleomorphic adenoma[121] or malignant myoepithelioma[43,155] is well documented. Occasionally, malignant transformation occurred more than twenty years after the first excision.

Myoepithelioma

Myoepitheliomas are composed in their entirety of myoepithelial cells with no ductal epithelial component.[152] Usually of benign nature, they may be locally aggressive.[12] However, malignant myoepitheliomas (myoepithelial carcinomas) have been described.[95]

Myoepitheliomas, though rare, occur more frequently in the major rather than in the minor salivary glands. Only two cases have been reported in the larynx, one of myoepithelioma[12] and one of malignant myoepithelioma.[95] This limits our ability to draw meaningful conclusions regarding behaviour and appropriate treatment.

The case reported by Batsakis (as myoepithelioma) was of a 52-year-old male who presented with acute respiratory obstruction; laryngoscopy showed an ovoid mass almost completely filling the supraglottis and occupying the laryngeal surface of the epiglottis; no nodal metastases were found.[12] The case reported by Ibrahim et al (as malignant myoepithelioma) was that of a 71-year-old male who presented with a neck mass and massive metastatic involvement of the liver.[95]

Grossly, there are no distinctive features.

Microscopically, myoepitheliomas display various growth patterns: solid (non-myxoid), myxoid (pleomorphic adenoma-like), reticular (canalicular-like) and mixed. The cell types encountered are plasmacytoid (hyaline), spindle, epithelial and clear cells.[38] The different cellular compositions do not reflect differences in behaviour, recurrence rate, frequency, patient's age or site. Solid tumours may be arranged in discrete nests separated by fibrous or hyalinized stroma or in featureless sheets. The myxoid tumours mimic pleomorphic adenoma. The growth pattern in reticular myoepitheliomas resembles that of canalicular adenoma. Other patterns, such as pseudomicrocystic and neuroendocrine patterns, may also be encountered. Cellular and nuclear pleomorphism is not prominent except in the occasional examples of plasmacytoid (hyaline) myoepitheliomas, and perhaps in spindle cell myoepitheliomas. The case of malignant myoepithelioma referred to by Ibrahim et al[95] consisted of solid sheets lacking any particular pattern immersed in a myxoid stroma; the tumour cells were of round, oval, or spindle shape with hyperchromatic nuclei, inconspicuous nucleoli and scant eosinophilic cytoplasm.[95] Malignant myoepithelioma may also arise in a pleomorphic adenoma.[43, 155]

Immunocytochemistry. The tumour cells display varying degrees of immunoreactivity for S-100 protein, cytokeratin, GFAP, myosin, actin (including smooth muscle actin), vimentin and CEA.

Electron microscopy. The tumour cells exhibit epithelial features: tonofilaments, desmosomes and hemidesmosomes, and myofilaments of smooth muscle type, including focal densities and a well-formed basal lamina.[12,38,95]

Differential diagnosis. This includes neuroendocrine carcinoma, plasma cell lesions, clear cell carcinoma, pleomorphic adenoma, mucoepidermoid carcinoma and malignant mixed tumour. Histological diagnosis is hindered by the many patterns which this tumour may display. Immunocytochemistry and electron microscopy may be useful in the differential diagnosis, especially in metastatic deposits.[95]

Therapy. This should be designed as for a benign salivary gland tumour: surgical excision with an appropriate margin of uninvolved tissue. Batsakis' patient was treated by total laryngectomy and unilateral neck dissection because of an initial diagnosis of clear cell carcinoma.

Except for local recurrence, the *prognosis* is good, provided that the tumour had been completely excised and there were no nodal metastases at presentation. Batsakis' patient was alive and well with no evidence of disease two years after the diagnosis.[12] The patient with a malignant myoepithelioma of the larynx, reported by Ibrahim et al, had liver metastases at presentation and died three months later. Post mortem examination revealed disseminated malignancy in the lymph nodes, pleura, vertebral bone, and peritoneum.[95]

Histological indicators of malignancy have not been consistent and reliable, and the search for predictors of aggressive behaviour has continued. In a study of the DNA content and proliferative capacity (S-phase fraction) of 16 myoepitheliomas of salivary glands using flow cytometry, El-Naggar et al[52] found that 13 tumours were diploid and three were aneuploid, and that high proliferative capacity was associated with an abnormal DNA content. They also concluded that the S-phase fraction appears to be a better indicator of aggressiveness.

Mucoepidermoid carcinoma

Introduction

This tumour was first described in a major salivary gland by Masson and Berger,[117] but it is Arcidiacono and Lomeo[7] who are credited with reporting the first laryngeal occurrence.

Terminology

Synonyms include double-metaplasia epithelioma,[117] mixed epidermoid and mucus-secreting carcinoma[42] and Schleimbildendes epithelioma.[156] The term mucoepidermoid tumour has been used by some authors to encompass all benign and malignant types of this neoplasm.[149,165,172] Since we consider all mucoepidermoid tumours as malignant, we have been using the term mucoepidermoid carcinoma, as preferred by the WHO Classification,[152] Foote and Frazell,[72] Eneroth,[53] Spiro[161] and Batsakis.[10]

Definition

Mucoepidermoid carcinoma is a malignant epithelial tumour composed of a mixture of squamous cells, mucin-secreting cells and cells of intermediate type, present in varying proportions. Both squamous cells and mucin-secreting cells should be demonstrable in any neoplasm placed in this category.

Incidence

Approximately 100 cases have been reported in the literature to date.[7,8,18–20,23,33,37,41,44,59,70,75,77,80,84,85,89,92,100,103,106,108,109,114,122,127,132,143,150,151,153,159,161,167,169,173,175,176,180,185] However, the true incidence of this carcinoma may be higher, or even lower, than is believed since confusion with squamous cell carcinoma or adenosquamous carcinoma may contribute to under- or over-diagnosis.[37,70,183]

Histogenesis

It is believed that mucoepidermoid carcinomas arise from the intercalated ducts of the seromucinous glands.[92] The evidence as listed by Ho et al[92] includes multidirectional differentiation of tumour cells, formation of cystic spaces and ductular structures, intermingling of neoplastic cells with submucosal seromucinous glands, dilatation of non-neoplastic ductules and atrophy of acini proximal to the tumour, in the presence of the benign intact surface mucosa.

Clinical features

Males are affected six times more than females. The mean age at presentation was the seventh decade for males and the sixth decade for females[33] but, as in extra-laryngeal sites,[51] it has also been reported in children.[122] The epiglottis, which is rich in glandular structures, is the most commonly affected site, though involvement of other laryngeal regions has been reported.[70,80,173] Hoarseness and dysphagia are the most common symptoms.

Pathology

Grossly, the neoplasm is indistinguishable from the more common squamous cell carcinoma or any other type of laryngeal carcinoma. However, the tumour may be partially cystic.

Microscopically, the tumour exhibits features similar to those encountered in the major salivary glands. It is characterized by both solid and glandular components (Fig. 14.1) with micro- and macro-cystic spaces filled with mucin staining positively with mucicarmine, Alcian blue, PAS and PAS/D; myxoid or chondroid stroma is notably lacking.

Three cell types can be identified in the tumour: epidermoid cells, mucous cells and intermediate cells. Most of the glandular and cystic areas consist of tall columnar cells and mucous cells; the cells lining the cystic spaces are usually flattened. These spaces and the glands are surrounded by sheets of squamous and intermediate cells. The squamous cells may have intercellular bridges and show occasional keratinization; epithelial pearls are

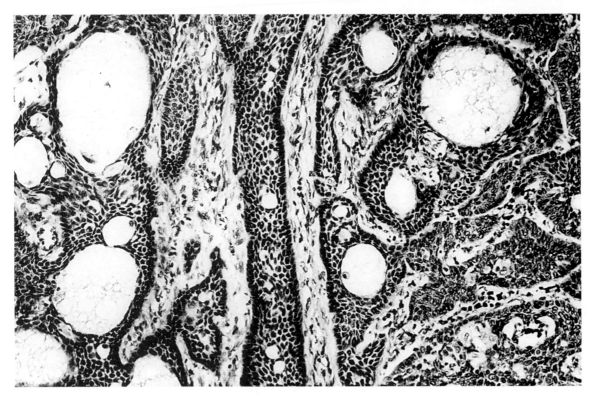

Fig. 14.1   Mucoepidermoid carcinoma showing solid areas composed of squamous cells and some cysts containing mucous secretion. H&E, ×40 OM.

uncommon. Oncocytes, sebaceous or spindle cells may also be present, and clear cells may be abundant.[84,150] The change in clear cells is caused by hydropic degeneration in the squamous cells. There is only moderate nuclear anaplasia, cellular pleomorphism and mitotic activity in a mucoepidermoid carcinoma, mainly in high-grade types; these features may vary from region to region in any single tumour, and from tumour to tumour.[54]

Mucoepidermoid carcinomas are divided into two categories: low- and high-grade carcinomas. In a study of 69 cases of mucoepidermoid carcinomas of major and minor salivary glands, Evans[54] considered a tumour to be histologically high-grade when 90% or more of its area was made up of tumour cells and 10% or less of intracystic spaces, and low-grade when the ratio was lower. The proportion of cell types was not considered in the grading system although intermediate, epidermoid and clear cells (Fig. 14.2) usually predominated in high-grade tumours. Evans' histological grading system correlated significantly with survival.

Immunocytochemistry. The tumour cells show co- and triple expression of cytokeratin, vimentin and GFAP, as well as positive staining with antibodies to EMA, non-specific CEA, and Leu-M1.[86] Regezi et al[141] demonstrated that myoepithelial differentiation appears to be minimal (as evidenced by the limited expression of S-100 protein, GFAP, smooth muscle actin and myosin) and that immunocytochemistry is not useful in the sub-classification of mucoepidermoid carcinomas.

Electron microscopy. Six types of tumour cells with special ultrastructural features have been identified,[92] although not all of them can be recognized by light microscopy; they include: undifferentiated intermediate cells, intermediate cells with glandular differentiation (Fig. 14.3), mature mucus-secreting cells (Fig. 14.4), intermediate cells with squamous differentiation (Fig. 14.5), squamous cells (Fig. 14.6) and non-secreting lumen-lining cells (Fig. 14.5). Some of the cells forming glands may be rich in either mitochondria, glycogen or both. Tonofilaments are abundant. Membrane-bound electron-dense granules of varying sizes have also been reported.[126,176] In contrast to adenoid cystic carcinoma, myoepithelial cells are seldom seen.[92,102,126]

Diagnosis and differential diagnosis

Mucoepidermoid carcinoma is a distinct entity with a characteristic clinical behaviour; it is therefore important to establish the diagnosis before any treatment is undertaken. If the initial biopsy lacks glandular elements, or the larger resection specimen contains large squamous areas, the tumour may be misdiagnosed as squamous cell carcinoma. Histochemical stains for mucin can be useful.

As regards distinguishing it from adenoid cystic carcinoma, the cribriform pattern with basement membrane-like hyaline material surrounding the cribriform sheets of

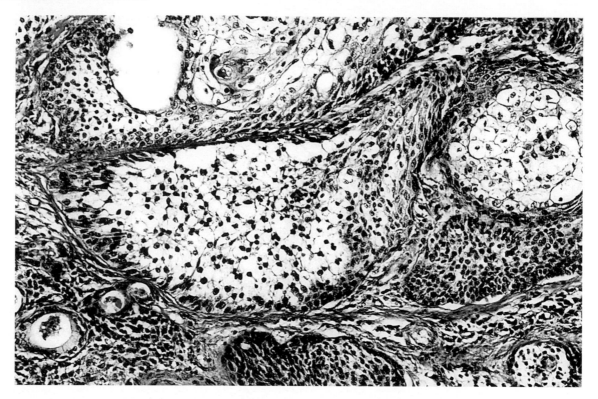

Fig. 14.2 Mucoepidermoid carcinoma, clear cell variant. H&E, ×40 OM.

tumour cells is usually diagnostic of adenoid cystic carcinoma; these features are lacking in mucoepidermoid carcinoma.

Adenosquamous carcinoma contains areas that are unequivocally adenocarcinoma and distinct areas of squamous carcinoma. The distinction is worthwhile since adenosquamous carcinoma is clinically more aggressive than mucoepidermoid carcinoma.

The presence of both more- or less-differentiated epidermoid elements and mucin-secreting cells in muco-epidermoid carcinoma facilitates its distinction from acinic cell carcinoma. Occasionally, mucoepidermoid carcinoma has to be distinguished from pleomophic adenoma[183] and necrotizing sialometaplasia which may occur, though rarely, in the larynx.[179]

Therapy

This tumour is moderately responsive to radiotherapy; partial regression is the most that could be expected. Therefore, the treatment of choice is complete surgical removal. Radical neck dissection would only be justified for cases in which the clinical picture[63] or imaging techniques suggested lymph node involvement.

Prognosis

The biological behaviour of mucoepidermoid carcinoma is less aggressive than that of squamous cell carcinoma. It may, however, recur and/or metastasize to the cervical lymph nodes and lungs. Incomplete initial resection enhances the chances of local recurrence. The prognosis depends on both the histological grading and stage. Evans' histological grading[54] correlated significantly with survival, local recurrence and cervical nodal metastases. Patients with high-grade mucoepidermoid carcinomas had a poorer survival rate, with a higher risk of local recurrence and cervical node metastases.

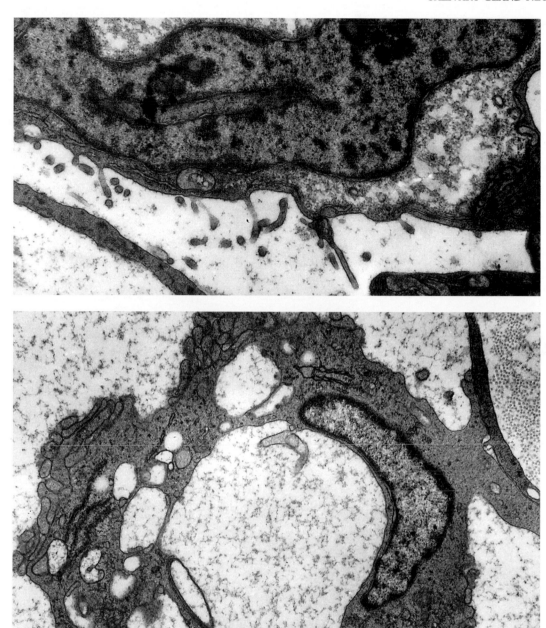

Fig. 14.3 (*top*) Mucoepidermoid carcinoma. Ultrastructure of tumour cells. Intermediate cells with glandular differentiation. Notice formation of lumen, microvilli and scanty intracytoplasmic mucus. ×15 350 OM. (Courtesy of Dr K.-J. Ho, Birmingham, Alabama, and the editor of *Southern Medical Journal*.)

Fig. 14.4 (*bottom*) Mucoepidermoid carcinoma. Mature mucus-secreting cell with membrane-bound intracytoplasmic mucus and abundant dilated rough endoplasmic reticulum. ×7500 OM. (Courtesy of Dr K.-J. Ho, Birmingham, Alabama, and the editor of *Southern Medical Journal*.)

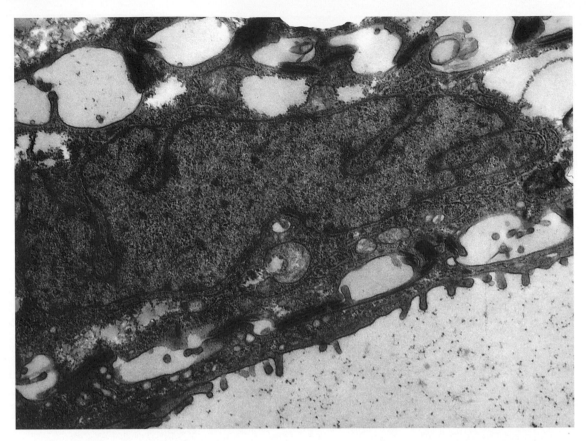

Fig. 14.5   Mucoepidermoid carcinoma. Ultrastructure of intermediate cells with squamous differentiation and non-secretory lining cell with microvilli. ×16 610 OM. (Courtesy of Dr K.-J. Ho, Birmingham, Alabama, and the editor of *Southern Medical Journal.*)

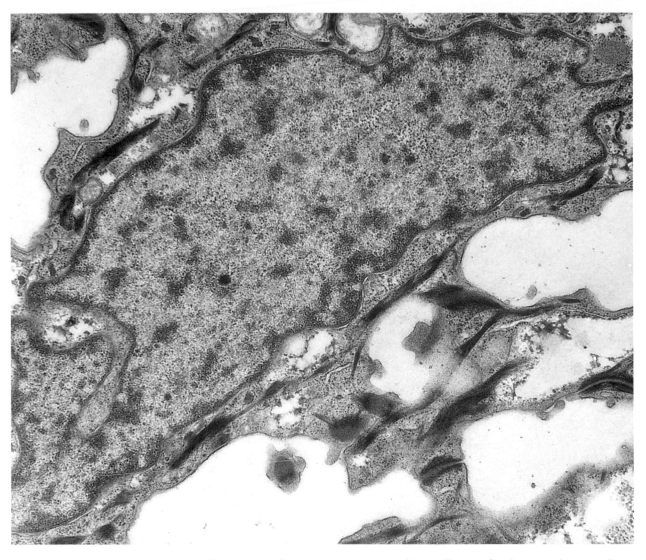

Fig. 14.6   Mucoepidermoid carcinoma. Ultrastructure of maturing squamous cell with tonofilaments forming network surrounding nucleus. ×12 950 OM. (Courtesy of Dr. K. J. Ho, Birmingham, Alabama, and the editor of *Southern Medical Journal*.)

Adenoid cystic carcinoma

Introduction

Robin and Laboulbene[144] were the first to describe this tumour, but the term 'Zylindrome' (cylindroma) was first proposed by Billroth in 1856.[17] The term 'adenoid cystic carcinoma' was first used by Spies in 1930.[160]

Terminology

Synonyms include cylindroma, adenocarcinoma of cylindroma type, cylindromatous carcinoma, and cribriform adenocarcinoma. The term adenoid cystic carcinoma is now widely accepted and recommended by the WHO.[152]

Definition

Adenoid cystic carcinoma is a distinctive form of adenocarcinoma composed mainly of small uniform basaloid cells forming tubules, cords and/or compact masses surrounded and intersected by cylinders of hyaline or mucoid material typically giving a cribriform or lace-like pattern.[152]

Incidence

Adenoid cystic carcinoma is one of the most common salivary gland neoplasms of the larynx. Although its true incidence has not been accurately documented, it is believed to be less than 0.25% of all laryngeal carcinomas.[47] Since the literature review of 76 cases of adenoid cystic carcinoma of the larynx by Ferlito and Caruso,[64] several more cases have been published, and there is now a total of about 120 cases.[28,36,47,49,67,85,94,96,104,109,110,113,118,119,136,138,140,160,163,166,171,184]

Aetiology and histogenesis

The aetiology is unknown, but the tumour is not related to smoking. Hormonal factors may be important in the genesis of this neoplasm.[15]

Histogenetically, the tumour appears to originate from the intercalated duct reserve cells or the terminal tubule complex.

Clinical features

There is no significant sex difference, which is unusual in laryngeal neoplasms. The tumour occurs more frequently between the ages of 50 and 70 years. Approximately, two-thirds of the neoplasms arise in the subglottic region, with the remainder occurring mainly in the supraglottic area and a few involving the glottis.

The history is usually longer than in squamous cell carcinoma, but the symptoms are similar. Patients with subglottic tumours may complain of shortness of breath, exertional dyspnoea and cough, occasionally accompanied by haemoptysis. Supraglottic tumours produce dysphagia,

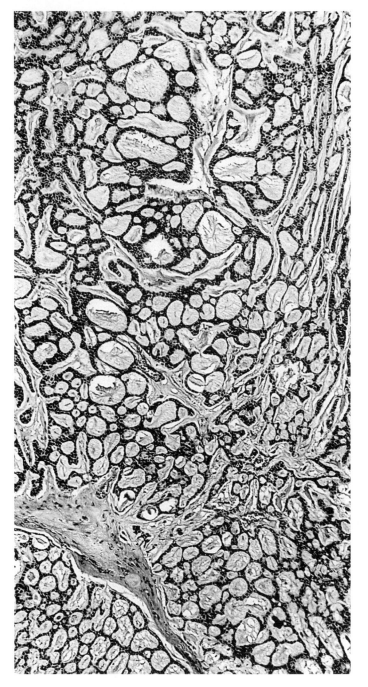

Fig. 14.7 Adenoid cystic carcinoma of the epiglottis showing the classical cribriform pattern. H&E, ×40 OM.

sore throat and hoarseness. Pain may be a prominent symptom in some adenoid cystic carcinomas of the larynx, regardless of their site, due to the propensity of the tumour to invade nerves. Paralysis of the recurrent laryngeal nerve is frequently present.

Pathology

Grossly, the tumour is well defined and sharply circumscribed, but not encapsulated. The overlying mucosa may

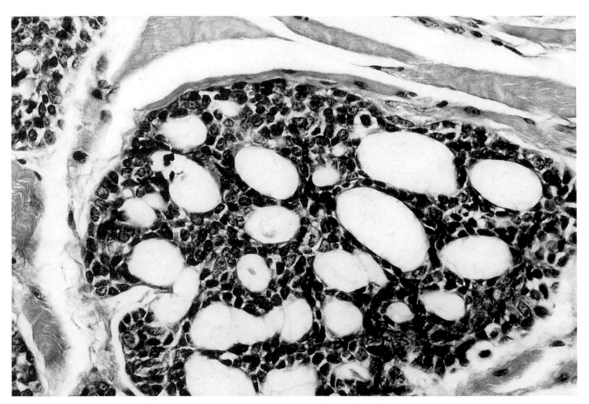

Fig. 14.8   Another case of adenoid cystic carcinoma showing variable-sized cribriform spaces formed by small, basophilic cells. H&E, ×100 OM.

be intact, but is usually ulcerated. The cut surface is homogeneous and pale grey to pink in colour. Cyst formation and haemorrhage are unusual.

Microscopically, the tumour is predominantly composed of uniform, small, basaloid cells with large, deeply-staining ovoid nuclei and scanty, indistinct cytoplasm arranged in anastomosing cords or islands in which there are sharply-defined cylindrical cores of mucoid and/or hyaline material giving a characteristic cribriform (Figs 14.7, 14.8), pseudocystic appearance (cribriform or cylindromatous type—grade I). Small ductal-type epithelial cells with vesicular nuclei and eosinophilic cytoplasm with well-defined cell margins may also be present. Occasionally, the tumour consists of tubules or trabeculae (tubular or trabecular type—grade II) or solid nests (solid or basaloid type—grade III; Figs 14.9, 14.10) that are typically ensheathed by pale hyaline material. The hyaline material around and within the pseudocystic spaces consists mainly of proteoglycans and basement membrane-like material. The tubular spaces may contain diastase-resistant PAS-positive and mucicarmine-positive mucin. The solid variant often shows areas of necrosis. Sometimes the tumour shows a lattice appearance (Fig. 14.11). Mitoses are generally scanty. A typical histological finding is the tendency for perineural infiltration (Fig. 14.12), haematogeneous

spread, and submucosal invasion. Muscle and thyroid invasion is common (Figs 14.13, 14.14).

Immunocytochemistry. Investigations have confirmed the dual (epithelial and myoepithelial) differentiation in adenoid cystic carcinoma and have demonstrated the heterogeneity of its immunophenotype.[25,27,168] The duct luminal cells may be immunoreactive for cytokeratin, CEA, EMA, alpha-1-antichymotrypsin and S-100 protein, but negative for alpha-1-antitrypsin. The non-luminal cells may express muscle-specific actin, vimentin and neuron-specific enolase (NSE) typical of myoepithelial cells. Muscle-specific actin has also been demonstrated in the lining cells of pseudocysts. The basal lamina stains positively with laminin and type IV collagen. Hashimura et al[87] have shown that the myoepithelial tumour cells are positive for proteoglycans, whereas the luminal cells are negative.

Electron microscopy. There are both myoepithelial and intercalated duct cells present. Furthermore, fine myofilaments of smooth-muscle type and dense bodies have been demonstrated in the cells lining the small true glandular lumina and pseudolumina, while many cells exhibit desmosomal attachments. The lumina of the cystic spaces are filled with amorphous, occasionally fibrillary material.[135]

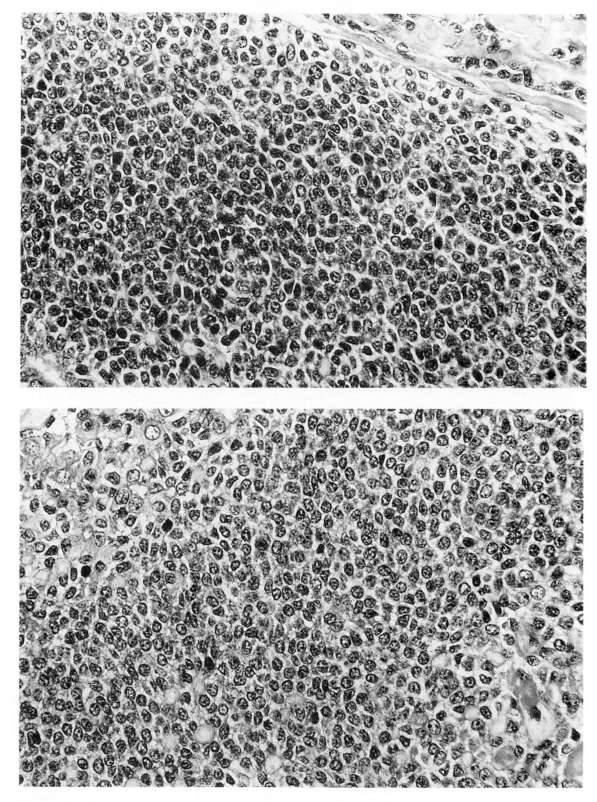

Fig. 14.9 (*top*) Another area of the tumour in Fig. 14.7, showing solid nests. H&E, ×100 OM.

Fig. 14.10 (*bottom*) Another area of the tumour in Fig. 14.7. Note the absence of microcystic spaces and tubules, though mucoid material is present. H&E, ×100 OM.

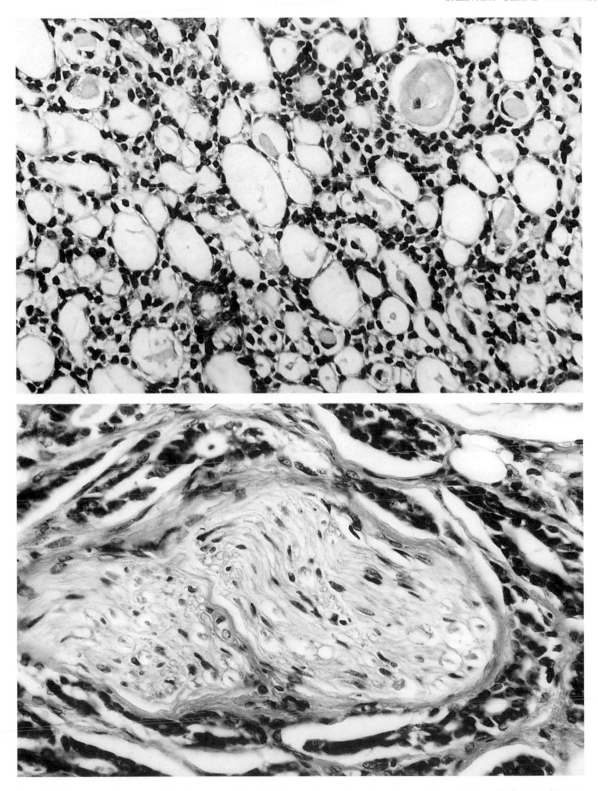

Fig. 14.11 (*top*) Another area of the tumour in Fig. 14.7. Sometimes adenoid cystic carcinoma shows a lattice appearance. H&E, ×100 OM.

Fig. 14.12 (*bottom*) Adenoid cystic carcinoma of the subglottic region showing perineural space invasion. H&E, ×100 OM.

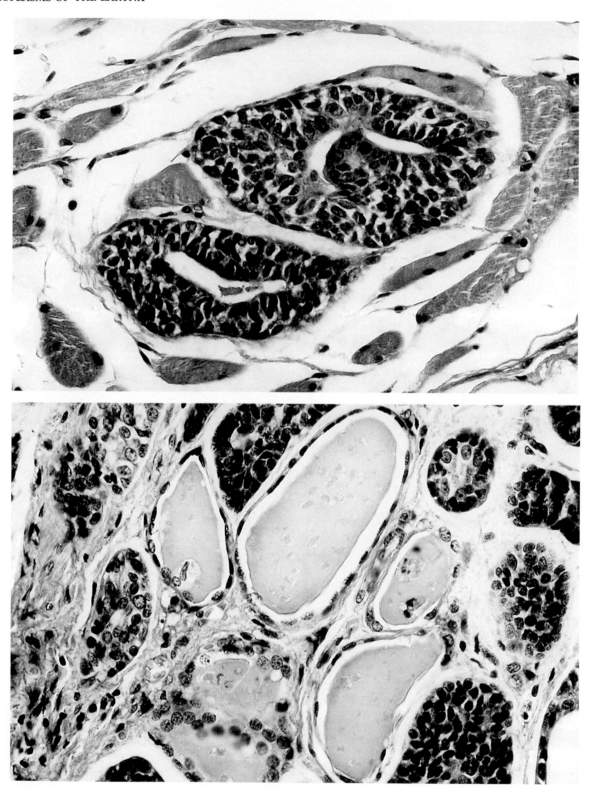

Fig. 14.13 (*top*) Same case as in Fig. 14.12, showing muscle invasion. H&E, ×100 OM.

Fig. 14.14 (*bottom*) Same case as in Fig. 14.12. Note the invasion of the thyroid gland. H&E, ×100 OM.

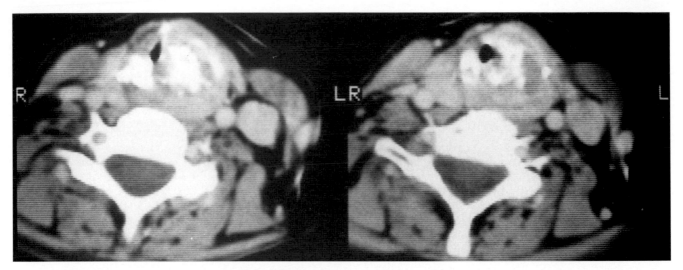

Fig. 14.15 (*top*) Same patient as in Fig. 14.12. CT scan reveals an obstructing subglottic lesion.

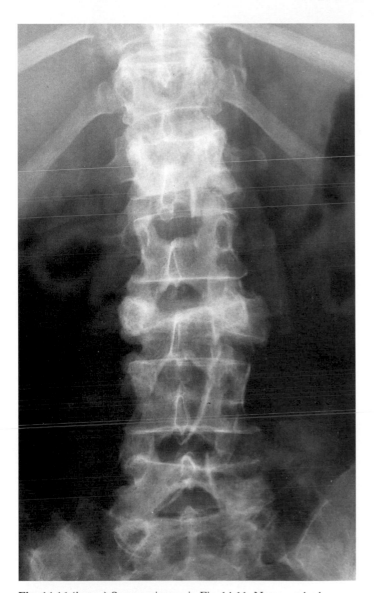

Fig. 14.16 (*bottom*) Same patient as in Fig. 14.11. Note vertebral metastases. No lymph node metastases were present.

Diagnostic imaging

Computed tomography (Fig. 14.15) and magnetic resonance imaging allow localization and quantification of this tumour. Radiological imaging is important in the pretreatment assessment and follow-up of patients with adenoid cystic carcinoma.[131]

Diagnosis and differential diagnosis

The differential diagnosis includes pleomorphic adenoma, mucoepidermoid carcinoma, adenoid and basaloid types of squamous cell carcinoma, small cell neuroendocrine carcinoma, malignant myoepithelioma and salivary duct carcinoma which may produce a pseudocribriform pattern. The distinction may be difficult in a biopsy specimen lacking the characteristic cribriform pattern, but immunohistochemical studies are very useful in making a correct diagnosis when the differential diagnosis is with small cell neuroendocrine carcinoma.

Pretreatment evaluation

The propensity of this tumour to metastasize widely without lymph node involvement makes staging procedures important. Evaluation for distant metastases should be carried out in all cases. Pretreatment evaluation for metastatic disease should include panendoscopy, chest X-ray, whole lung tomography, liver echotomography, computed tomography of the brain, bone scintigraphy and laboratory tests.

Therapy

There seems to be no consensus regarding the best treatment for adenoid cystic carcinoma. It has been treated by local excision, by radical excision and by radiotherapy,

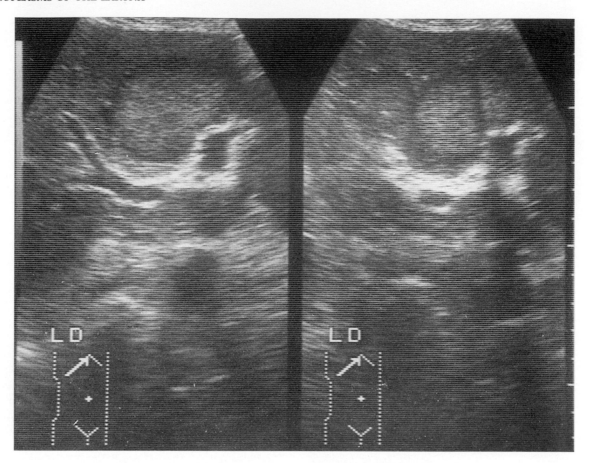

Fig. 14.17   Same case as in Fig. 14.12. Ultrasound pictures of metastases to the liver.

alone or in combination with a local or radical excision. The role of chemotherapy in the management of this neoplasm is still undefined. At present, the treatment of choice remains surgical removal—partial or total laryngectomy according to the size and location of the neoplasm.[67] Total laryngectomy should always be combined with subtotal thyroidectomy. Large subglottic tumours may necessitate resection of the pharynx and of the cervical oesophagus. Pulmonary metastases, often symptomless, should not discourage surgical eradication of the primary tumour, since single or multiple metastases may remain dormant for a decade or more. Neck dissection, however, is indicated only if the patient has clinically enlarged and/or histologically confirmed nodal metastases. A cervical mass is not always a lymph node secondary, it may be a recurrence or persistence of the primary tumour,[64,67] or a metastasis from a basaloid squamous cell carcinoma that is sometimes misdiagnosed as adenoid cystic carcinoma.[89] We agree with Conley and Dingman[29] that radical neck dissection needs only to be included in the primary operation when there are gross metastases or when there is need for a large cuff of soft tissue. No lymph node metastases were found in the series reported by Ferlito et al.[67] This tumour does not usually metastasize to the cervical lymph nodes.[76]

Prognosis

The tumour is slow-growing but is markedly infiltrative and has a special tendency to grow along nerves. The success of treatment and ultimate prognosis is best assessed in terms of a 15–20-year survival rate. Histological subtypes may have important prognostic significance, as the solid type behaves more aggressively.[67] Haematogeneous spread is much more common than lymphatic spread— the lung, bone (Fig. 14.16) and liver (Fig. 14.17) being the most common sites of metastases. In fact, this neoplasm metastasizes more like a sarcoma than a carcinoma.[62] The absence of cervical lymph node metastases cannot be considered a favourable prognostic sign (as in squamous cell carcinoma) because multiple visceral metastases may be present.

Carcinoma in pleomorphic adenoma

Carcinoma in pleomorphic adenoma is a carcinoma arising in a pre-existing pleomorphic adenoma. It repre-

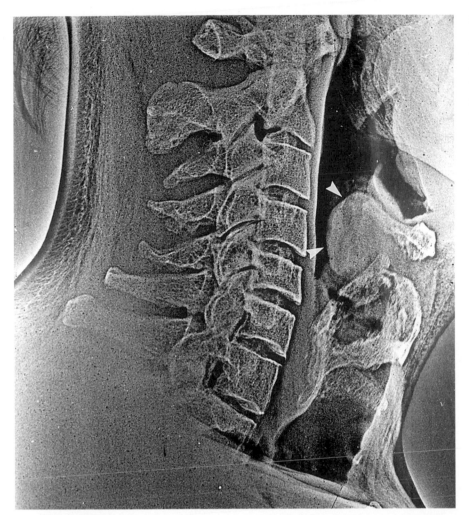

Fig. 14.18 (*top*) Carcinoma in pleomorphic adenoma. Lateral xerogram of the neck showing the neoplasm arising from the laryngeal surface of the epiglottis (arrow heads). (Courtesy of Dr C. A. Milford, London, and the editor of *Journal of Laryngology and Otology*.)

Fig. 14.19 (*bottom*) Carcinoma in pleomorphic adenoma. Area of the tumour showing characteristic appearance of a pleomorphic adenoma adjacent to intact squamous epithelium of the epiglottis. H&E, ×50 OM. (Courtesy of Dr C. A. Milford, London, and the editor of *Journal of Laryngology and Otology*.)

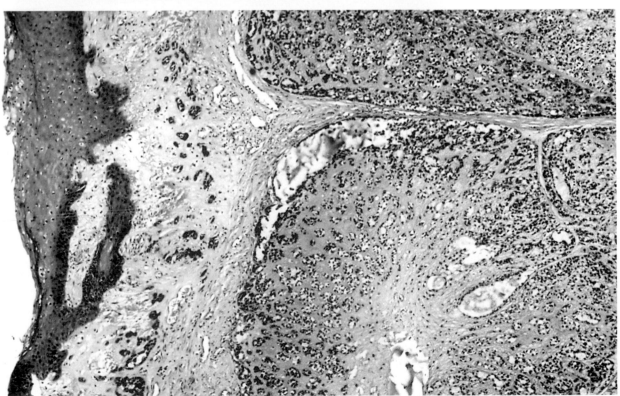

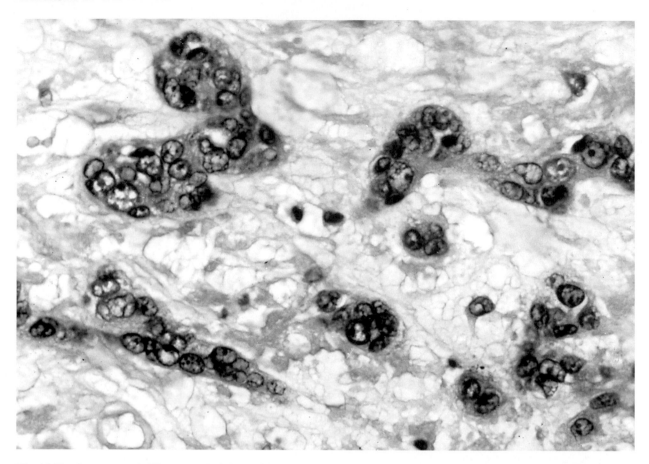

Fig. 14.20   Same case as in Fig. 14.19. Periphery of the tumour showing marked cytological atypia characteristic of malignant change. H&E, ×500 OM. (Courtesy of Dr C. A. Milford, London, and the editor of *Journal of Laryngology and Otology*.)

sents a single variant of malignant mixed tumour, the other being the true malignant mixed tumour (which is divided into two subtypes: metastasizing pleomorphic adenoma and carcinosarcoma). These terms have been used synonymously but ought to be applied more rigidly and only when the diagnostic criteria have been fulfilled. All of these types are extremely rare,[21,62,89,101,121,145] and meaningful conclusions regarding any differences in clinical behaviour cannot be drawn. Only one case of true malignant mixed tumour of the carcinosarcoma type was found in the AFIP series.[89] Carcinoma in pleomorphic adenoma is common in the submandibular and sublingual glands.[56]

Microscopically, carcinoma in pleomorphic adenoma (Figs 14.18–14.22) displays the typical features of pleomorphic adenoma, which may predominate or may be limited to a small focus; there is also a malignant component present, with features of adenocarcinoma or of a specific type of salivary gland carcinoma. Solid cords of atypical squamous cells, tubular structures and small cysts may be present. Mitoses are numerous. The metastatic deposits contain only the carcinomatous component.

True malignant mixed tumours show either benign-looking epithelial and stromal components, with a well-documented metastatic capability (i.e., metastasizing pleomorphic adenoma), or malignant epithelial and stromal components (i.e., carcinosarcoma). Metastatic deposits contain both epithelial and stromal components.

Carcinoma in pleomorphic adenoma must be distinguished from pleomorphic adenoma, malignant myoepithelioma arising in pleomorphic adenoma and mucoepidermoid carcinoma.

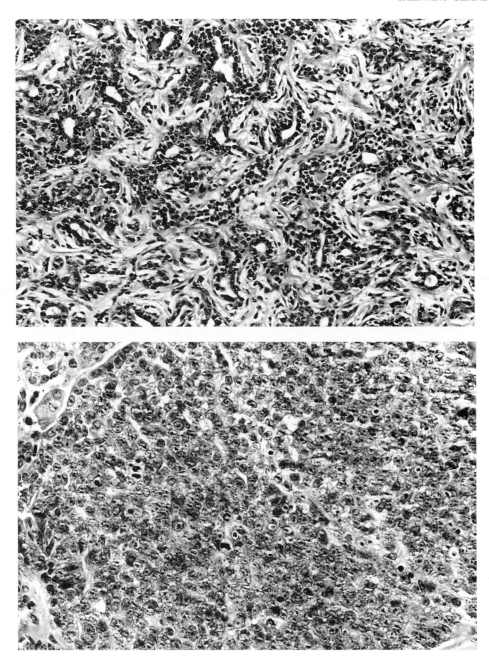

Fig. 14.21 (*top*) Carcinoma in pleomorphic adenoma. This area shows the epithelial–myoepithelial differentiation of a benign mixed tumour. (Courtesy of Dr D. Carter, New Haven.)

Fig. 14.22 (*bottom*) Same case as Fig. 14.21. Anaplastic carcinoma is associated with the benign mixed tumour shown in Fig. 14.21. (Courtesy of Dr D. Carter, New Haven.)

Adenosquamous carcinoma

Introduction

Adenosquamous carcinoma has been recognized as a separate and distinct clinicopathological entity by the WHO Histological Typing of Tumours of the Upper Respiratory Tract and Ear.[152] Although adenosquamous carcinoma has been mentioned by New and Erich[130] and by Havens and Parkhill,[88] the first detailed account of this neoplasm was published by Gerughty et al.[81]

Terminology

Several synonyms have been used. These include adenosquamous (mixed) carcinoma, glassy cell carcinoma, mixed adenosquamous carcinoma, combined adenosquamous carcinoma and adenoepidermoid carcinoma.

Definition

Adenosquamous carcinoma is a malignant epithelial tumour composed of malignant squamous and glandular elements occurring in varying proportions.[152]

Incidence

The reported incidence may be significantly lower than its actual occurrence. The diagnostic criteria are not uniformly applied, and some authors do not distinguish between adenosquamous carcinoma and poorly differentiated (high-grade) mucoepidermoid carcinoma.[37] To date, about 40 cases have been described.[5,37,60,81,83, 89,115,147,186]

Histogenesis

There is a suggestion that adenosquamous carcinomas arise from a multipotential stem cell within the intercalated ducts.

Clinical features

The clinical presentation is not different from that of the squamous cell carcinoma.

Pathology

Grossly, there are no features which distinguish this carcinoma from squamous cell carcinoma.

Microscopically, the tumour consists of a mixture of squamous carcinoma and adenocarcinoma which are more separate and distinct than in a mucoepidermoid carcinoma, where they are closely intermingled (Fig. 14.23). Three basic types of tumour cells are identified: squamous, basal and undifferentiated cells (Fig. 14.24) which form tubular, alveolar or ductal structures lying in a fibrous or myxoid stroma. Areas of in situ ductal carcinoma may also be noted. Sheets of glassy cells lying in a fibrous stroma may be present. These cells have an abundant, clear, PAS-negative cytoplasm with a prominent hyperchromatic nucleus. Numerous scattered giant cells may be found, and some tumours contain masses of keratin. Mucin-secreting cells staining positive with PAS/D and mucicarmine may occur in the lumen of several glandular structures. The surface epithelium may be normal or frankly malignant. Malignancy and stromal invasion, however, are more likely to originate from the submucosal glandular epithelium and to extend to the surface epithelium. Perineural infiltration is frequent.

Immunocytochemistry. Immunostaining for high-molecular-weight cytokeratins (KL1) has been found positive in both squamous and glandular tumour cells, whereas antibodies against low-molecular-weight cytokeratins (K19) and carcino-embryonic antigen have proved positive only in the glandular component.[115]

Diagnosis and differential diagnosis

The diagnosis may not become apparent until a detailed examination of the resection specimen is performed, the biopsy specimen being too small for an adequate assessment. The distinction between adenosquamous carcinoma and poorly differentiated mucoepidermoid carcinoma may be difficult: the areas of adeno- and squamous carcinomas are more separate and distinct in adenosquamous carcinoma. The tumour should also be distinguished from adenoid squamous cell carcinoma, in which the gland-like pattern results from acantholysis and disassociation of the central regions of the tumour cell clusters and groups. True gland formation is not found, and no mucin is detected in adenoid squamous cell carcinoma.

Therapy and prognosis

Complete surgical excision is the treatment of choice.[60,147] Radiotherapy is not advised.

This tumour possesses an aggressive behaviour with a propensity to local recurrence and metastasis. Wide metastatic dissemination to the lungs, liver, bone, brain, kidneys, colon, adrenals, subcutaneous tissue and other organs has been reported.[37,60,81,147] The prognosis is poor.

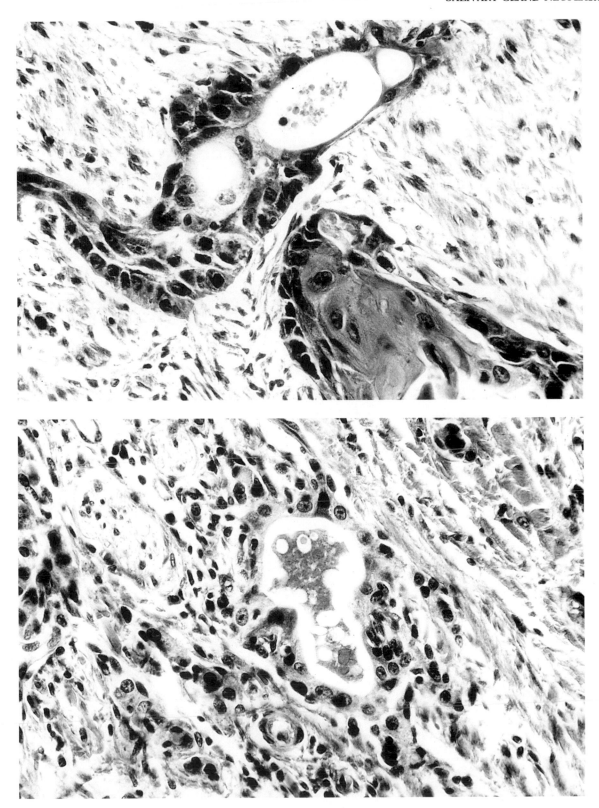

Fig. 14.23 (*top*) Typical adenosquamous carcinoma. Mixed squamous and glandular proliferation are present in the same tumour. H&E, ×100 OM.

Fig. 14.24 (*bottom*) Same case as in Fig. 14.23, showing undifferentiated cells and a glandular structure containing PAS/D and mucicarmine-positive material in the lumen. H&E, ×100 OM.

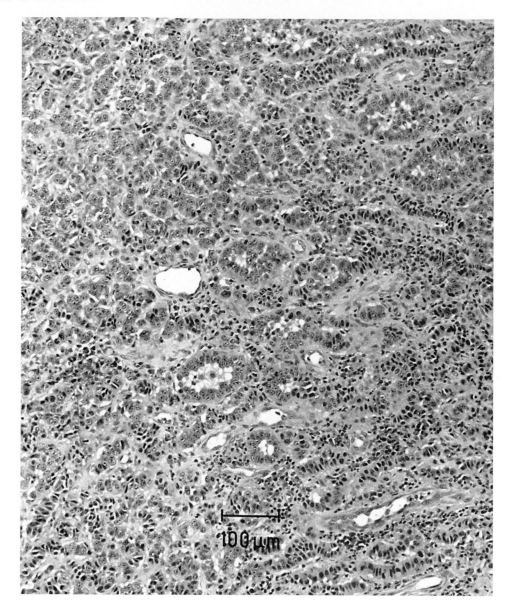

Fig. 14.25   Acinic cell carcinoma. Lower-power view shows diffuse infiltration by tumour cells as well as acinar differentiation. H&E, × Low. (Courtesy of Dr D. J. Stevens, Saskatoon, and the editor of *Journal of Laryngology and Otology*.)

Acinic cell carcinoma

This is an extremely rare tumour which, according to the British Salivary Gland Tumour Panel Review,[56] accounts for 2.5% of all parotid neoplasms. Five cases of acinic cell carcinoma of the larynx have so far been reported[32,61,99, 123,162] but the case reported by Crissman and Rosenblatt[32] was probably a neuroendocrine carcinoma.[42a] The association between this tumour and irradiation has been suggested in a 54-year-old female patient whose neck was irradiated for hyperthyroidism 46 years prior to the development of an acinic-cell carcinoma in the neck (this case has been reported twice).[142,162] The

association is not well substantiated and needs to be further investigated, since a coincidental relationship between this tumour and irradiation cannot be ruled out.

Synonyms include acinic cell adenocarcinoma, acinous cell adenocarcinoma, acinar cell adenocarcinoma, acinic cell tumour and acinous cell carcinoma.

The tumour is composed mainly of cells resembling the serous cells of salivary glands.[152] It is believed to arise from a stem cell of the salivary gland duct system, which is normally engaged in tissue renewal.[9,26,99]

The clinical presentation and the gross appearance of the tumour are not unlike those of squamous cell carcinoma.

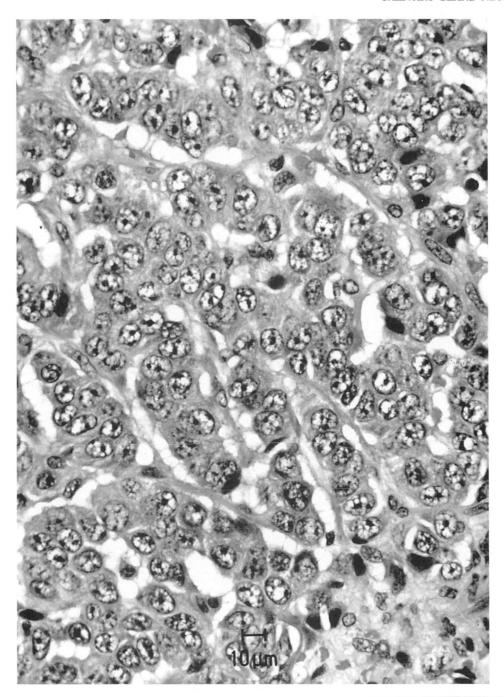

Fig. 14.26 Recurrent acinic cell carcinoma. Cords of tumour cells with oval nuclei, one or two distinct nucleoli and eosinophilic cytoplasm. H&E, × High. (Courtesy of Dr D. J. Stevens, Saskatoon, and the editor of *Journal of Laryngology and Otology.*)

Microscopically, the tumour occurs in the submucosa and displays various histological patterns (solid, microcystic, papillary cystic or acinar). Most tumours consist of groups of tumour cells with an abundant granular basophilic cytoplasm and peripheral nuclei (Figs 14.25, 14.26), resembling normal serous acini. Calcified laminated psammomatous spherules may be seen among the tumour cells and within the scanty fibrovascular stroma. Some groups show central necrosis. Cysts result from the dilatation of the ducts by accumulated secretion. Mitoses are scanty, and nuclear anaplasia is not a feature. In some cases, the tumour cells possess a clear cytoplasm mimicking a clear cell carcinoma of the kidney. Histochemically, the tumour cells stain positively with PAS/D but not with Alcian blue or mucicarmine.

Immunocytochemistry. The tumour cells are positive with cytokeratin and EMA; some cases show either double expression for cytokeratin and vimentin or triple expression for cytokeratin, vimentin and GFAP. Immunoreactivity has also been demonstrated for (monospecific) CEA, S-100 protein, actin, alpha-1-antichymotrypsin, and Leu-M1. Focal dendritic stromal cells staining positive with S-100 protein may be found.[86] Abenoza and Wick[1] demonstrated that the immunophenotype of acinic cell carcinomas closely mirrors that of intercalated ductal elements in the normal salivary gland tissue, concluding that there is differentiation towards an intercalated duct cell pathway in these carcinomas, including a potential for myoepithelial differentiation.

Electron microscopy. This shows groups of tumour cells surrounded by fibrovascular stroma with prominent basal laminae. The tumour cells have microvilli protruding into the lumina.[26] The numerous intracytoplasmic secretory granules resemble those of normal salivary serous cells. The granules are surrounded by a single membrane and contain variable amounts of finely fibrillogranular material. There is a prominent rough endoplasmic reticulum and mitochondria are numerous. Cells with mucous globules have been identified.[26]

Diagnosis and differential diagnosis. The histological appearances are characteristic, and confusion with other salivary gland tumours is unlikely. However, confusion with metastatic clear cell carcinoma of the kidney is more likely when the laryngeal tumour is wholly or predominantly of the clear cell variant. A laryngeal salivary origin is suggested by the demonstration of serous secretory granules in the tumour cells (and clinical exclusion of a renal carcinoma).

Therapy and prognosis. Acinic cell carcinomas of the major and other minor salivary glands are treated by complete excision;[26] they are not radiosensitive. The number of cases reported in the literature is too small to draw meaningful conclusions, so it is mandatory to follow up patients with acinic cell carcinoma for an extended period in order to assess adequately its behaviour.

Salivary duct carcinoma

Kleinsasser et al[105] are credited with describing the first group of cases of this distinct carcinoma of the major salivary glands, but it was only in 1981 that the only case of laryngeal salivary duct carcinoma was described by Ferlito et al.[69]

Kleinsasser et al[105] called this tumour 'Speichelgangcarcinome' — which corresponds, in the English-language literature, to salivary duct carcinoma. Other terms in general use include duct(al) carcinoma and cribriform carcinoma of the excretory ducts.

This is an unusual group of salivary gland tumours with a characteristic histological appearance strikingly similar to invasive ductal carcinomas of the breast. It is believed to arise from the ductal epithelium.

Neither the clinical presentation nor the findings at examination are distinguishable from the conventional squamous cell carcinoma. The prognosis is poor.

Grossly, the tumour exhibits no specific features, although cysts and necrosis may be noted.

Microscopically, three distinct intraductal histological patterns have been described, and several patterns may be recognized in varying proportions, i.e., cribriform, papillary and comedo (Figs 14.27, 14.28), all of which resemble their respective counterparts in an invasive ductal carcinoma of the breast. The ducts are usually extremely dilated and are surrounded by desmoplastic fibrous stroma containing lymphocytes, histiocytes and plasma cells. Foam cells and PAS/D-positive mucous material may be present in the lumen of some ducts. The tumour cells are moderately enlarged and show nuclear pleomorphism and hyperchromasia and an increased nuclear/cytoplasmic ratio.

Immunocytochemistry. In a study of salivary duct carcinoma of the parotid and normal salivary tissue, Brandwein et al[22] demonstrated immunoreactivity for B72.3 and Lewis Y (antibodies known to mark adenocarcinoma) and for low- and high-molecular-weight cytokeratins. These authors noted immunoreactivity for B72.3 in the parotid ductal system adjacent to the salivary duct carcinoma, but not in normal ducts adjacent to pleomorphic adenomas; the presence of B72.3 in the parotid ducts may imply the presence of a malignant tumour nearby. Other studies showed positivity for cytokeratin and CEA and were negative for S-100 protein.[154]

Electron microscopy. The tumour cells may have an increased endoplasmic reticulum with dilated cisternae, showing a concentric arrangement. Tonofilaments may be numerous. Myofibroblasts may be present surrounding the duct formations with their nuclei running parallel to the ductal basal lamina. These cells must be distinguished from myoepithelial cells. The basal lamina of the ducts is of variable thickness and may be multilayered.

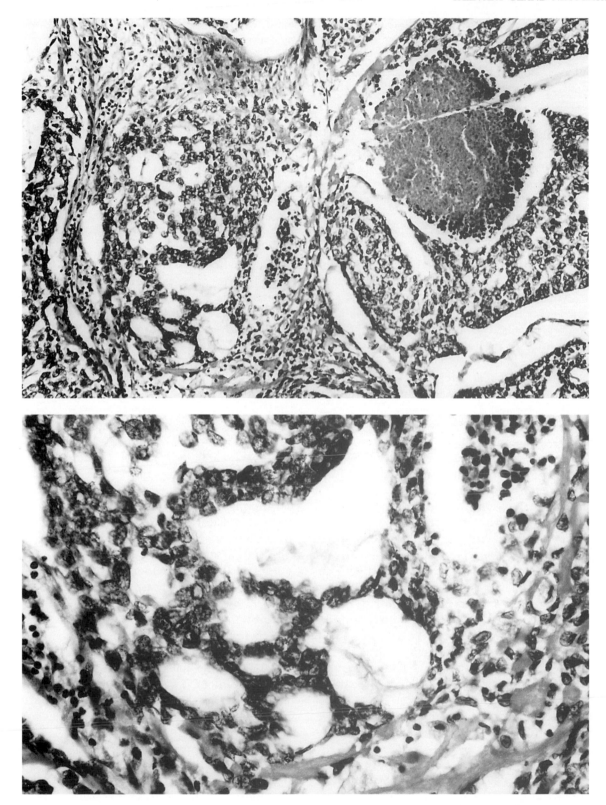

Fig. 14.27 (*top*) Salivary duct carcinoma. Note papillary, cribriform and comedo patterns. H&E, ×40 OM.

Fig. 14.28 (*bottom*) Same case as in Fig. 14.27, showing details of the neoplastic cells. H&E, ×100 OM.

Differential diagnosis. This must be made from adenoid cystic carcinoma, mucoepidermoid carcinoma, acinic cell carcinoma and metastatic carcinoma from a breast or prostate primary.[68] Special histochemical stains (PAS and PAS/D) and electron microscopy may help in establishing a correct diagnosis.

Extended follow-up is warranted to establish the behaviour of this neoplasm. Salivary duct carcinoma of the major salivary glands metastasizes via lymphatic and haematogeneous channels. The most common sites of metastases are the lung, bone and brain.

Epithelial–myoepithelial carcinoma

Epithelial–myoepithelial carcinoma was first described by Donath et al[46] in the parotid gland, where it predominantly occurs.[30] Only one case has been reported in the larynx, by Mikaelian et al.[120]

The tumour is composed of ducts lined by cuboidal or columnar epithelial cells surrounded by myoepithelial cells which are frequently multilayered.[152]

Synonyms include epithelial–myoepithelial duct carcinoma, epithelial–myoepithelial carcinoma of intercalated ducts, and intercalated duct carcinoma. It is believed to arise from the salivary gland duct epithelium.

The clinical presentation appears to be similar to that of a conventional squamous cell carcinoma.

Grossly, the tumour is lobulated, usually of a firm consistency. It has a greyish-pink colour and is covered by a smooth mucous membrane.

Microscopically, the tumour demonstrates a multinodular growth pattern with the formation of satellite nodules, typically displaying tubular structures composed of cystic spaces lined by two types of cells: an inner row of dark cuboidal to low columnar duct-like cells with an eosinophilic cytoplasm, and an outer row composed of ovoid myoepithelial-type cells containing round nuclei and abundant clear cytoplasm overlying some hyalinized basement membrane material. The clear cells are PAS-positive and PAS/D sensitive due to the presence of large amounts of glycogen in their cytoplasm. The proportion of the two cell types varies, with the clear cell element frequently constituting the predominant cell type. There may be necrosis or papillary proliferations in the lumen of the duct-like structures. Cellular anaplasia is moderate, and mitoses are scanty.

In some cases, the biphasic tubular nature of the tumour is less evident, so that the appearance is dominated by solid groups of clear cells separated by fibrous septa, or cords and trabeculae of clear cells separated by thick hyaline basement membrane material. A fibrous connective tissue capsule may be present, often compromised by tumour satellite nodules.

Immunocytochemistry. The clear cells are immunoreactive for S-100 protein and smooth muscle specific actin; the ductal cells are immunoreactive for EMA and cytokeratin, and occasionally for S-100 protein. This confirms the biphasic nature of the tumour.

Electron microscopy. This usually confirms the presence of two cellular components (ductal cells and myoepithelial cells) with their corresponding characteristic features.

Differential diagnosis. This includes pleomorphic adenoma, clear cell carcinoma, the clear cell variant of mucoepidermoid carcinoma, acinic cell carcinoma, salivary duct carcinoma, acinic cell carcinoma, adenoid cystic carcinoma and metastatic clear cell carcinomas from the kidney or thyroid. Hui et al[93] demonstrated ultrastructurally that myoepithelial cells are present in epithelial–myoepithelial carcinoma, but not in salivary duct carcinoma.

The treatment of choice is surgery, with neck dissection restricted to patients with nodal metastases. Radiation therapy may be helpful.

The tumour is regarded as being of low-grade malignancy. Local recurrence is much more common than distant metastasis.

Clear cell carcinoma

Clear cells occur in a variety of primary laryngeal tumours such as squamous cell carcinoma, the clear cell variant of mucoepidermoid carcinoma, epithelial–myoepithelial carcinoma, carcinoid tumours, squamous cell carcinoma with sebaceous differentiation, basaloid squamous cell carcinoma, adenosquamous carcinoma, clear cell variant of pleomorphic adenoma and secondary renal cell carcinoma. Clear cell carcinoma is a descriptive term, and great care must be taken before diagnosing a true primary clear cell carcinoma of the larynx.

Pure clear cell carcinoma is extremely rare in the larynx, and the first case was described by Ferlito,[59] followed by a detailed account of three clear cell carcinomas by Ferlito's team.[137] A fourth case was treated at the ENT Department of Padua University.[35] The WHO Classification of Tumours of the Upper Respiratory Tract and Ear defines clear cell carcinoma as a malignant epithelial tumour composed of cells with clear cytoplasm that stain negatively for mucin and lipid.[152] Most probably this tumour is a poorly differentiated adenocarcinoma of ductal origin.

The clinical presentation resembles that of a conventional squamous cell carcinoma. All reported cases had nodal metastases at presentation.[35,137]

Grossly, there are no particular features distinguishing it from other laryngeal neoplasms.

Microscopically, the neoplasm is composed of nests or clusters of clear cells intersected by fibrous stroma. The clear cells are large and round, with a pale cytoplasm, small vesicular nuclei and prominent nucleoli. The abundant cytoplasm is clear, vacuolated, amphophilic

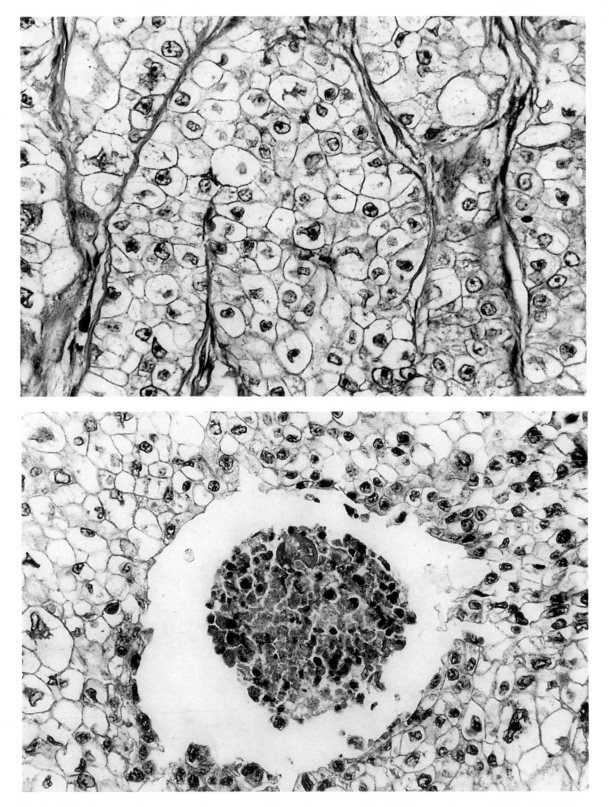

Fig. 14.29 (*top*) Clear cell carcinoma. Note groups of clear cells separated by thin fibrovascular septa. H&E, ×100 OM.

Fig. 14.30 (*bottom*) Same case as in Fig. 14.29. A large area of necrosis is present. H&E, ×100 OM.

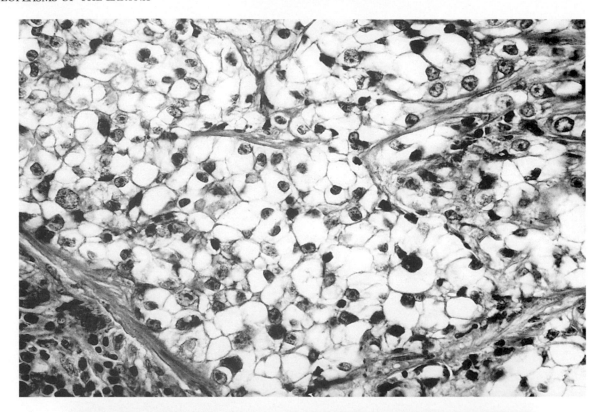

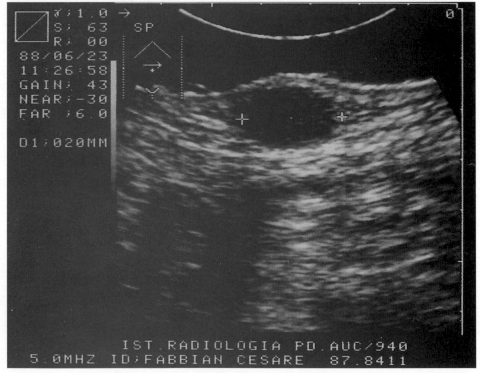

Fig. 14.31 (*top*) Same case as in Fig. 14.29. Lymph node metastasis from clear cell carcinoma of the larynx. The histological pattern is the same as for the primary neoplasm. H&E, ×100 OM.

Fig. 14.32 (*bottom*) Same case as in Fig. 14.29. Ultrasound picture of metastasis to the skin.

and appears to be empty (Fig. 14.29). There may be multinucleated cells with markedly atypical bizarre nuclei and also areas of necrosis (Fig. 14.30). There is no evidence of squamous differentiation, but some abortive glandular differentiation may be encountered. No glycogen, mucin or lipid is usually identified in the cytoplasm of the clear cells.

Immunocytochemistry. The tumour cells are immuno-reactive for cytokeratin, EMA and CEA.

Clear cell carcinoma must be distinguished from tumours with areas of clear cell morphology, such as those mentioned above.

The behaviour of this neoplasm cannot be evaluated accurately (because of its rarity). The cases reported by Ferlito's team[137] had an aggressive course, all presenting with nodal metastases (Fig. 14.31) and one with disseminated disease in the liver, bones and skin (Fig. 14.32); they died within a comparatively short period of the initial diagnosis. Ferlito's cases were treated by total laryngectomy and neck dissection.

Sebaceous carcinoma

Martinez-Madrigal et al[116] have recently described a single case of sebaceous carcinoma of the hypopharynx. This tumour consisted of a mixture of sebaceous, squamous and basaloid cells. The sebaceous cells contained fat in their cytoplasm, as demonstrated by the positive reaction with Oil red O on frozen sections. The squamous cells displayed varying degrees of immunoreactivity for cytokeratin. There was patchy immunostaining for S-100 protein and vimentin in scattered cells showing cytoplasmic processes indicative of myoepithelial cells. The metastatic carcinoma in the lymph nodes exhibited similar features.

Mucoid adenocarcinoma

A recent report by Tsang et al[177] described a single case of mucoid adenocarcinoma in the larynx. The patient was a 46-year-old female presenting with a two-year history of progressive hoarseness. A sessile nodular transglottic mass was found on direct laryngoscopy, and a total laryngectomy was performed without radical neck dissection. Four years after surgery, the patient was alive and well, with no evidence of disease. Histologically, the tumour resembled mucoid adenocarcinomas described in other organs, such as the breast, stomach and rectum; the possibility of a metastatic origin must be excluded before this diagnosis is made.

Adenocarcinoma

'Adenocarcinoma' is used as a generic term for those malignant gland- or duct-forming tumours that do not display characteristic features of the specific types. This category should be distinguished from metastatic adenocarcinomas which may present in the larynx.[68]

Neuroendocrine carcinomas of intermediate differentiation (atypical carcinoids) may be confused as so-called adenocarcinomas,[89] but immunocytochemistry[65] and electron microscopy are useful in making a correct diagnosis.

TUMOUR-LIKE LESIONS

Necrotizing sialometaplasia (salivary gland infarction)

This is a benign, self-healing inflammatory condition which most commonly affects the minor salivary glands of the palate,[4] the importance of which lies in its possible histological confusion with malignancy, particularly with mucoepidermoid and squamous cell carcinoma.[50,58,128] The lesion may occur in almost all minor and major salivary gland tissues,[11,45,73,97] including those in the larynx.[179] Histologically, it is characterized by lobular necrosis of salivary glands, mixed acute and chronic inflammation and regenerative squamous metaplasia of acini and/or ducts. Fibrosis, as the end-product of the hyaline process, may be present. The cause of this lesion remains obscure, although an ischaemic process is blamed.[179] The laryngeal case reported by Walker et al[179] occurred after surgical manipulation of an atherosclerotic aneurysm of the right common carotid artery. The patient was a 69-year-old male who developed malaise, dysphagia and a low-grade fever ten days after operation. Indirect laryngoscopy revealed laryngeal oedema and an exudate over the supraglottic larynx, which later developed into necrotic membrane covering the aryepiglottic folds, vestibular folds and epiglottis with no destruction of cartilage. *Serratia marcescens* were grown in sputum cultures but not in blood cultures. The patient was maintained on supportive treatment. By the end of three months the symptoms had disappeared completely.

Histological confusion with malignancy is a real possibility and may result in unnecessary radical surgery. The preservation of the overall lobular architecture is a feature of benignity and aids in distinguishing necrotizing sialometaplasia from mucoepidermoid and squamous cell carcinomas.

Oncocytic lesions

Oncocytic lesions of the larynx have been described by various authors,[48,55,66,74,79,90,111,133,146,181] but their biological nature has remained controversial. Since they are considered as neoplastic, hyperplastic, metaplastic or degenerative in nature, such lesions have been reported under a variety of names, e.g., oncocytic papillary

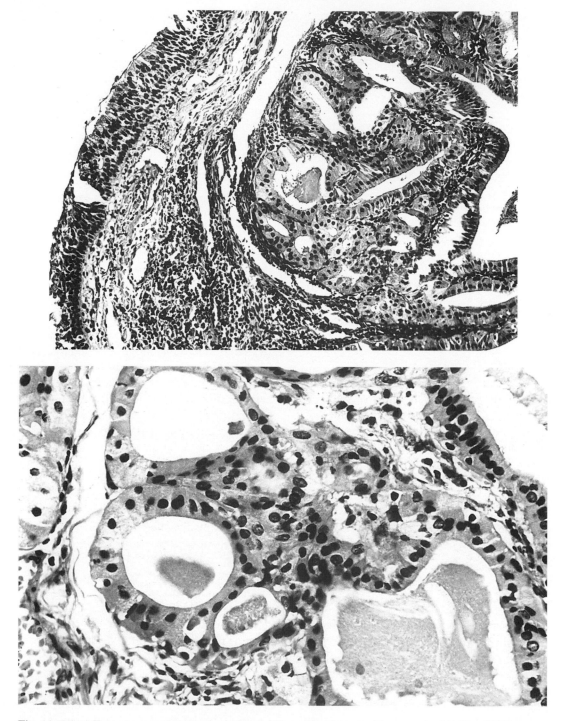

Fig. 14.33 (*top*) Typical oncocytic lesion in the larynx. The surface is covered by normal epithelium. H&E, ×40 OM.

Fig. 14.34 (*bottom*) Same case as in Fig. 14.33. Higher magnification shows more clearly the cytological features of the oncocytes. H&E, ×100 OM.

cystadenoma, oxyphilic granular cell adenoma, oncocytoma, oncocytic cyst, eosinophilic granular cyst, etc.

Oncocytic lesions are probably more common than has been proposed. Estimating their true incidence is difficult because of the confusing terminology used by different authors, although a figure of 0.5–1% of all laryngeal specimens received in histopathology laboratories was suggested by Lundgren et al.[111] Heffner mentions that 12 cases were collected between 1976 and 1985 at the AFIP.[89] Patients aged 50 years and above are commonly affected, suggesting that development of the lesion may be attributed to a long-standing irritation of the larynx. There is a slight predominance of male patients. The presenting symptoms are related to narrowing and/or obstruction of the laryngeal lumen. The most common site is the vestibular fold and the wall of the laryngeal ventricle; the vocal cord is rarely involved.

Grossly, the lesion may be polypoid or cystic, or both, and is often multifocal. On section, it may be wholly cystic, partially cystic or solid; the solid form is much rarer than the other two. The cysts may contain some proteinaceous material.

Microscopically, the cystic areas are lined by oncocytes with abundant eosinophilic granular cytoplasm and a small, dark-staining nucleus near the luminal border of the cells (Figs 14.33, 14.34). There may be adjacent groups of seromucinous glands also showing some oncocytic change. The cystic areas may occasionally form complex papillary processes, filling the cavity.

The solid lesions consist of small acini and ducts lined by up to two layers of oncocytes, with a surrounding layer of myoepithelial cells. Occasionally, the lesion consists of large, solid sheets of small polygonal cells with relatively large nuclei, prominent nucleoli and finely granular eosinophilic cytoplasm. Variable amounts of fibrous stroma may be identified. Dense lymphocytic infiltration may occur in these lesions; a potential source of misdiagnosis is adenolymphoma.[48,55,74,90] Judging by the illustrations, none of the reported cases deserve the diagnosis of adenolymphoma. These lesions may be associated with squamous cell carcinoma of the larynx.[66,79,111,133] They must be distinguished from granular cell tumours, metastatic carcinomas from the thyroid or kidney (which show a well-differentiated oncocytic morphology).

Surgery is the treatment of choice. In most cases, eradication may be obtained by direct laryngoscopy, whereas laryngofissure is sometimes necessary for adequate excision. Recurrence is due mainly to incomplete excision, but may also be caused by the development of a new lesion from a previously clinically undetectable focus of oncocytic change.

REFERENCES

1. Abenoza P, Wick M R 1985 Acinic cell carcinoma of salivary glands: an immunohistochemical study (abstract). Lab Invest 52: 1A
2. Abercromby B M L, Rewell R E 1955 Pleomorphic salivary adenoma ('mixed parotid tumour') of the larynx. J Laryngol Otol 69: 424–429
3. Aboulker P, Demaldent J-E 1966 Tumeur mixte du larynx. Ann Otolaryngol 83: 89–90
4. Abrams A M, Melrose R J, Howell F V 1973 Necrotizing sialometaplasia. A disease simulating malignancy. Cancer 32: 130–135
5. Aden K K, Adams G L, Niehans G, Abdel-Fattah H M M 1988 Adenosquamous carcinoma of the larynx and hypopharynx with five new case presentations. Trans Am Laryngol Ass 109: 216–221
6. Anderson C, Knibbs D R, Abbott S J, Pedersen C, Krutchkoff D 1990 Glial fibrillary acidic protein expression in pleomorphic adenoma of salivary gland: an immunoelectron microscopic study. Ultrastruct Pathol 14: 263–271
7. Arcidiacono G, Lomeo G 1963 I tumori muco-epidermoidali salivari. A proposito di un caso a localizzazione laringea. Clin ORL 15: 95–108
8. Bahadur S, Amatya R C, Kacker S K 1983/84 Muco-epidermoid carcinoma of the larynx. J Otolaryngol Soc Austral 5: 236–238
8a. Baptista P M, Garcia-Tapia R, Vazquez J J 1992 Pleomorphic adenoma of the epiglottis. J Otolaryngol 21: 355–357
9. Batsakis J G 1979 Tumors of the head and neck. Clinical and pathological considerations, 2nd edn. Williams & Wilkins, Baltimore
10. Batsakis J G 1980 Mucoepidermoid and acinous cell carcinoma of salivary tissues. Ann Otol Rhinol Laryngol 89: 91–92
11. Batsakis J G, Manning J T 1987 Necrotizing sialometaplasia of major salivary glands. J Laryngol Otol 101: 962–966
12. Batsakis J G, Hyams V J, Morales A R 1983 Special tumors of the head and neck. Proc Forty-eighth Ann Sem ASCP. ASCP Press, Chicago
13. Batsakis J G, Rice D H, Solomon A R 1980 The pathology of head and neck tumours: squamous and mucous-gland carcinomas of the nasal cavity, paranasal sinuses, and larynx, part 6. Head Neck Surg 2: 497–508
14. Behrendt W 1965 Pleomorphe Adenome (sog. Mischtumoren) ausserhalb der grossen Kopfspeicheldüsen. Arch Ohrenheilk 184: 358–366
15. Belson T P, Toohill R J, Lehman R H, Chobanian S L, Grossman T W, Malin T C 1982 Adenoid cystic carcinoma of the submaxillary gland. Laryngoscope 92: 497–501
16. Berger Z, Luszynska L, Chetnik K C H 1972 Case of mixed laryngeal tumor. Otolaryngol Pol 26: 349–351
17. Billroth T 1856 Die Cylindergeschwulst (Cylindroma) in Untersuchungen uber die Entwicklung der Blutgefasse: nebst Beobachtungen aus der Koniglichen Chirurgischen Universitats-Klinik zu Berlin. Reimer, Berlin
18. Binder W J, Som P, Kaneko M, Biller H F 1980 Mucoepidermoid carcinoma of the larynx. A case report and review of the literature. Ann Otol Rhinol Laryngol 89: 103–107
19. Bitiutskii P G, Finkel'shtern M R 1979 Mucoepidermoid tumours of the larynx. Vestn Otorinolaringol 2: 82–83
20. Boikov V P, Olisaev A D, Abdullin N A 1985 Mucoepidermoid tumor of the larynx. Vestn Otorinolaringol 2: 63–64
21. Bomer D L, Arnold G E 1971 Malignant tumors of the minor salivary glands. Acta Otolaryngol 289 (suppl): 16–17
22. Brandwein M S, Jagirdar J, Patil J, Biller H, Kaneko M 1990 Salivary duct carcinoma (cribriform salivary carcinoma of excretory ducts). A clininicopathologic and immunohistochemical study of 12 cases. Cancer 65: 2307–2314
23. Cady B, Rippey J H, Frazell E L 1968 Non-epidermoid cancer of the larynx. Ann Surg 167: 116–120
24. Campbell W G, Priest R E, Weathers D R 1985 Characterization

of two types of crystalloids in pleomorphic adenomas of minor salivary glands. A light-microscopic, electron-microscopic, and histochemical study. Am J Pathol 118: 194–202

25. Chen J C, Gnepp D R, Bedrossian C W 1988 Adenoid cystic carcinoma of the salivary glands: an immunohistochemical analysis. Oral Surg Oral Med Oral Pathol 65: 316–326

26. Chen S-Y, Brannon R B, Miller A S, White D K, Hooker S P 1978 Acinic cell adenocarcinoma of minor salivary glands. Cancer 42: 678–685

27. Chomette G, Auriol M, Vaillant J M, Kasai T, Okada Y, Mori M 1991 Heterogeneity and co-expression of intermediate filament proteins in adenoid cystic carcinoma of salivary glands. Pathol Biol (Paris) 39: 110–116

28. Cohen J, Guillamondegui O M, Batsakis J G, Medina J E 1985 Cancer of the minor salivary glands of the larynx. Am J Surg 150: 513–518

29. Conley J, Dingman D L 1974 Adenoid cystic carcinoma in the head and neck (cylindroma). Arch Otolaryngol 100: 81–90

30. Corio R L, Sciubba J J, Brannon R B, Batsakis J G 1982 Epithelial–myoepithelial carcinoma of intercalated duct origin. A clinicopathological and ultrastructural assessment of sixteen cases. Oral Surg Oral Med Oral Pathol 53: 280–287

31. Cotelingam J D, Barnes L, Nixon V B 1977 Pleomorphic adenoma of the epiglottis: report of a case. Arch Otolaryngol 103: 245–247

32. Crissman J D, Rosenblatt A 1978 Acinous cell carcinoma of the larynx. Arch Pathol Lab Med 102: 233–236

33. Cumberworth V L, Narula A, MacLennan K A, Bradley P J 1989 Mucoepidermoid carcinoma of the larynx. J Laryngol Otol 103: 420–423

34. Cunning D S 1950 Diagnosis and treatment of laryngeal tumors. JAMA 142: 73–77

35. Dalla Palma P, Blandamura S 1989 Clear cell carcinoma of the larynx: immunocytochemical study. Tumori 75: 594–596

36. Dal Maso M, Lippi L 1985 Adenoid cystic carcinoma of the head and neck: a clinical study of 37 cases. Laryngoscope 95: 177–181

37. Damiani J M, Damiani K K, Hauck K, Hyams V J 1981 Mucoepidermoid–adenosquamous carcinoma of the larynx and hypopharynx: a report of 21 cases and a review of the literature. Otolaryngol Head Neck Surg 89: 235–243

38. Dardick I, Thomas M J, van Nostrand A W P 1989 Myoepithelioma — new concepts of histology and classification: a light and electron microscopic study. Ultrastruct Pathol 13: 187–224

39. Dardick I, van Nostrand A W P, Jeans M T D, Rippstein P, Edwards V 1983 Pleomorphic adenoma, I: ultrastructural organization of 'epithelial' regions. Hum Pathol 14: 780–797

40. Dardick I, van Nostrand A W P, Jeans M T D, Rippstein P, Edwards V 1983 Pleomorphic adenoma, II: ultrastructural organization of 'stromal' regions. Hum Pathol 14: 798–809

41. Davis W E, Beck M R 1975 Mucoepidermoid carcinoma of the larynx — a case report. Eye Ear Nose Throat Month 54: 394–396

42. De M N, Tribedi B P 1939 A mixed epidermoid and mucus-secreting carcinoma of the parotid gland. J Pathol Bacteriol 49: 432–433

42a. Dictor M, Tennvall J, Akerman M 1992 Moderately differentiated neuroendocrine carcinoma (atypical carcinoid) of the supraglottic larynx. A report of two cases including immunohistochemistry and aspiration cytology. Arch Pathol Lab Med 116: 253–257

43. Di Palma S, Pilotti S, Rilke F 1991 Malignant myo-epithelioma of the parotid gland arising in a pleomorphic adenoma. Histopathology 19: 273–275

44. Dogra T S 1973 Adenocarcinoma of the larynx. J Laryngol Otol 87: 685–689

45. Donath K 1979 Pathohistologie des Parotisinfarktes (necrotizing sialometaplasia). Laryngol Rhinol Otol 58: 70–76

46. Donath K, Seifert G, Schmitz R 1972 Zur Diagnose and Ultrastruktur des Tubularen Speichelgangcarcinoms: epithelial–myoepitheliales Schaltstuckcarcinom. Virchows Arch [A] 356: 16–31

47. Donovan D T, Conley J 1983 Adenoid cystic carcinoma of the subglottic region. Ann Otol Rhinol Laryngol 92: 491–495

48. Drut R, Di Rago C A 1975 Cistoadenoma papilar linfomatosa (tumour de Wartin) de laringe. An Otorrinolaringol Ibero Am 3: 207–211

49. Duenas Parrilla J M, Alvarez Bautista A, Sanchez Gomes S, Tirado Zamora I 1991 Cystic adenoid carcinoma of the larynx. Presentation of a case and review of the literature. Acta Otorrinolaringol Esp 42: 67–70

50. Dunlap C L, Barker B F 1974 Necrotizing sialometaplasia. Oral Surg Oral Med Oral Pathol 37: 722–727

51. El-Jabbour J N, Slim M S, Bekdash B, Allam C K, Mansour A, Fahl M H, Issa P 1986 Bronchial mucoepidermoid tumor in childhood. A report of two cases and review of the English literature. Pediatr Surg Int 1: 63–67

52. El-Naggar A, Batsakis J G, Luna M A, Goepfert H, Tortoledo ME 1989 DNA content and proliferative activity of myoepitheliomas. J Laryngol Otol 103: 1192–1197

53. Eneroth C-M 1976 Die Klinik der Kopfspeicheldrusentumoren. Arch Otorhinolaryngol 213: 61–110

54. Evans H L 1984 Mucoepidermoid carcinoma of salivary glands: a study of 69 cases with special attention to histologic grading. Am J Clin Pathol 81: 696–701

55. Evans R A, Cassidy M T, Russell T S 1989 Adenolymphoma of the larynx. J R Coll Surg Edinb 34: 47

56. Eveson J W, Cawson R A 1985 Salivary gland tumours. A review of 2410 cases with particular reference to histological types, site, age and sex distribution. J Pathol 146: 51–58

57. Fechner R E 1975 Adenocarcinoma of the larynx. Can J Otolaryngol 4: 284–289

58. Fechner R E 1977 Necrotizing sialometaplasia. A source of confusion with carcinoma of the palate. Am J Clin Pathol 67: 315–317

59. Ferlito A 1976 Histological classification of larynx and hypopharynx cancers and their clinical implications. Pathologic aspects of 2052 malignant neoplasms diagnosed at the ORL Department of Padua University from 1966 to 1976. Acta Otolaryngol 342 (suppl): 1–88

60. Ferlito A 1976 A pathologic and clinical study of adenosquamous carcinoma of the larynx. Report of four cases and review of the literature. Acta Otorhinolaryngol Belg 30: 379–389

61. Ferlito A 1980 Acinic cell carcinoma of minor salivary glands. Histopathology 4: 331–343

62. Ferlito A 1985 Malignant epithelial tumors of the larynx. In: Ferlito A (ed) Cancer of the larynx, vol I. CRC Press, Boca Raton

63. Ferlito A 1987 Malignant laryngeal epithelial tumors and lymph node involvement: therapeutic and prognostic considerations. Ann Otol Rhinol Laryngol 96: 542–548

64. Ferlito A, Caruso G 1983 Biological behaviour of laryngeal adenoid cystic carcinoma. Therapeutic considerations. ORL J Otorhinolaryngol Relat Spec 45: 245–256

65. Ferlito A, Friedmann I 1991 Contribution of immunohistochemistry in the diagnosis of neuroendocrine neoplasms of the larynx. ORL J Otorhinolaryngol Relat Spec 53: 235–244

66. Ferlito A, Recher G 1981 Oncocytic lesions of the larynx. Arch Otorhinolaryngol 232: 107–115

67. Ferlito A, Barnes L, Myers E N 1990 Neck dissection for laryngeal adenoid cystic carcinoma: is it indicated? Ann Otol Rhinol Laryngol 99: 277–280

68. Ferlito A, Caruso G, Recher G 1988 Secondary laryngeal tumours. Report of seven cases with review of the literature. Arch Otolaryngol Head Neck Surg 114: 635–639

69. Ferlito A, Gale N, Hvala A 1981 Laryngeal salivary duct carcinoma. A light and electron microscopic study. J Laryngol Otol 95: 731–738

70. Ferlito A, Recher G, Bottin R 1981 Mucoepidermoid carcinoma of the larynx. A clinicopathological study of 11 cases with review of the literature. ORL J Otorhinolaryngol Relat Spec 43: 280–299

71. Fleischer K 1956 Drei Seltene Kehlkopftumoren: Speicheldrüsenmischtumor, Teratom, Granuloblastom. Z Laryngol Rhinol Otol 35: 346–356

72. Foote F W Jr, Frazell F W 1953 Tumors of the major salivary glands. Cancer 6: 1065–1131

73. Forney SK, Foley JM, Sugg W E Jr, Oatis G W Jr 1977 Necrotizing sialometaplasia of the mandible. Oral Surg Oral Med Oral Pathol 43: 720–726

74. Foulsham C K, Snyder G G, Carpenter R J 1981 Papillary cystadenoma lymphomatosum of the larynx. Otolaryngol Head Neck Surg 89: 960–964

75. Frable W J, Elzay R P 1970 Tumors of minor salivary glands. A

report of 73 cases. Cancer 25: 932–941

76. Friedmann I, Ferlito A 1988 Granulomas and neoplasms of the larynx. Churchill Livingstone, Edinburgh

77. Gadomski S P, Zwillenberg D A, Choi H Y 1986 Non-epidermoid carcinoma of the larynx: the Thomas Jefferson University experience. Otolaryngol Head Neck Surg 95: 558–565

78. Gaillard J, Haguenauer J P, Dubreuil C, Romanet P 1978 Les tumeurs rares de la cord vocale. A propos de 2 cas: un adénome pléomorphe et un neurinome. J Fr Otorhinolaryngol 27: 714, 716–718

79. Gallagher J C, Puzon B Q 1969 Oncocytic lesions of the larynx. Ann Otol Rhinol Laryngol 78: 307–318

80. Gatti W M, Erkman-Balis B 1980 Mucoepidermoid carcinoma of the larynx. Arch Otolaryngol 106: 52–53

81. Gerughty R M, Hennigar G R, Brown F M 1968 Adenosquamouscarcinoma of the nasal, oral, and laryngeal cavities: a clinico-pathologic survey of ten cases. Cancer 22: 1140–1155

82. Gierek T, Namysowski G, Kamienski J 1990 Pleomorphic adenoma of atypical localisation. Otolaryngol Pol 44: 249–251

83. Glossop L P, Griffiths M, Grant H R 1984 Combined adenocarcinoma and squamous carcinoma of the hypopharynx. A case report. J Laryngol Otol 98: 1161–1166

84. Gomes V, Costarelli L, Cimino G, Magaldi L, Bisceglia M 1990 Mucoepidermoid carcinoma of the larynx. Eur Arch Otolaryngol 248: 31–34

85. Hamlyn P J, O'Brien C J, Shaw H J 1986 Uncommon malignant tumours of the larynx. A 35 year review. J Laryngol Otol 100: 1163–1168

86. Hamper K, Schmitz-Watjen W, Mausch H-E, Caselitz J, Seifert G 1989 Multiple expression of tissue markers in mucoepidermoid carcinomas and acinic cell carcinomas of the salivary glands. Virchows Arch (A) 414: 407–413

87. Hashimura K, Kasai T, Yamada K, Mori M, Chomette G, Auriol M, Vaillant JM 1990 Proteoglycans detected by monoclonal antibodies in adenoid cystic carcinoma of salivary glands. Anticancer Res 10: 1083–1089

88. Havens F Z, Parkhill E M 1941 Tumors of the larynx other than squamous cell epithelioma. Arch Otolaryngol 34: 1113–1122

89. Heffner D K 1991 Sinonasal and laryngeal salivary gland lesions. In: Ellis G L, Auclair P L, Gnepp D R (eds) Surgical pathology of the salivary glands. Saunders, Philadelphia

90. Heinz J 1951 The adenolymphomata. Aust NZ Surg 21: 47–51

91. Hirano T, Kashiwado I, Suzuki I, Yoshihiro T, Yuge K, Asano G 1990 Immunohistopathological properties of pleomorphic adenoma in salivary gland. J Nippon Med Sch 57: 172–179

92. Ho K-J, Jones J M, Herrera G A 1984 Mucoepidermoid carcinoma of the larynx: a light and electron microscopic study with emphasis on histogenesis. South Med J 77: 190–195

93. Hui K K, Batsakis J G, Luna M A, Mackay B, Byers R M 1986 Salivary duct adenocarcinoma: a high grade malignancy. J Laryngol Otol 100: 105–114

94. Hyams V J, Batsakis J G, Michaels L 1988 Tumors of the upper respiratory tract and ear. In: Atlas of tumor pathology, 2nd series, fasc 25. Armed Forces Institute of Pathology, Washington DC, 90–95

95. Ibrahim R, Bird D J, Sieler M W 1991 Malignant myoepithelioma of the larynx with massive metastatic spread to the liver: an ultrastructural and immunocytochemical study. Ultrastruct Pathol 15: 69–76

96. Ishizu Y, Yokoyama M, Takaoka M 1985 A case of adenoid cystic carcinoma occurring in the larynx. Pract Otol (Kyoto) 78 (suppl): 1852–1855

97. Johnston W H 1977 Necrotizing sialometaplasia involving the mucous glands of the nasal cavity. Hum Pathol 8: 589–592

98. Jokinen K, Seppala A, Palva A 1974 Laryngeal pleomorphic adenoma. J Laryngol Otol 88: 1131–1134

99. Kallis S, Stevens D J 1989 Acinous cell carcinoma of the larynx. J Laryngol Otol 103: 638–641

100. Kaznelson D J, Schindel J 1979 Mucoepidermoid carcinoma of the air passages: Report of three cases. Laryngoscope 89: 115–121

101. Kirchner J A, Carter D 1989 The larynx. In: Sternberg S S (ed) Diagnostic surgical pathology, vol 1. Raven Press, New York

102. Klacsmann P G, Olson J L, Eggleston J C 1979 Mucoepidermoid carcinoma of the bronchus. An electron microscopic study of the

low grade and the high grade variants. Cancer 43: 1720–1733

103. Kleinsasser O 1969 Mucoepidermoidtumoren der Speicheldrüsen. Arch Klin Exp Ohrenheilk 193: 171–189

104. Kleinsasser O 1988 Tumors of the larynx and hypopharynx. Thieme, Stuttgart

105. Kleinsasser O, Klein H J, Hübner G 1968 Speichelgangcarcinome. Arch Klin Exp Ohrenheilk 192: 100–115

106. Koike S, Ogawara I, Moriwaki S, Aoki T, Watanabe S 1978 Three cases of adenocarcinoma of the larynx. Pract Otol (Kyoto) 71: 1101–1107

107. Kurandv N I, Mikaelian B A, Ershow U N 1974 Case of mixed tumor of the larynx. Vestn Otorinolaringol 5: 95–96

108. Lebedeva Z P 1979 Adenoma-type of mucoepidermoid tumor of the larynx. Vestn Otorinolaringol 2: 84–85

109. Levine H L, Tubbs R 1986 Nonsquamous neoplasms of the larynx. Otolaryngol Clin North Am 19: 475–488

110. Li T S 1988 Adenoid cystic carcinoma of the larynx. Chung Hua Chung Liu Tsa Chih 10: 465–466

111. Lundgren J, Olofsson J, Hellquist H 1982 Oncocytic lesions of the larynx. Acta Otolaryngol 94: 335–344

112. MacMillan R H III, Fechner R E 1986 Pleomorphic adenoma of the larynx. Arch Pathol Lab Med 110: 245–247

113. Marin I, Tudose N, Cotulbea S, Sarau M, Lupescu A, Anghel I 1986 Adenoid cystic carcinoma: 3 clinical cases with different localizations in the ENT area. Rev Chir (Otorinolaringol) 31: 131–136

114. Martinez-Barona T, Regadera J, Gavilan J, Vicandi B, Patron M 1986 Mucoepidermoid carcinoma of the larynx of a high grade malignancy. Clinico-pathologic study of a case and a review of the literature. An Otorrinolaringol Ibero Am 13: 455–470

115. Martinez-Madrigal F, Baden E, Casiraghi O, Micheau C 1991 Oral and pharyngeal adenosquamous carcinoma. Report of four cases with immunohistochemical studies. Eur Arch Otorhinolaryngol 248: 255–258.

116. Martinez-Madrigal F, Casiraghi O, Khattech A, Ben Nasr-Khattech R, Richard J-M, Micheau C 1991 Hypopharyngeal sebaceous carcinoma: a case report. Hum Pathol 22: 929–931

117. Masson P, Berger L 1924 Epitheliomas a double metaplasie de la parotide. Bull Ass Fr Cancer 13: 366–373

118. Michaels L 1984 Pathology of the larynx. Springer-Verlag, Berlin

119. Miglianico L, Eschwege F, Marandas P, Wibault P 1987 Cervico-facial adenoid cystic carcinoma: study of 102 cases. Influence of radiation therapy. Int J Radiat Oncol Biol Phys 13: 673–678

120. Mikaelian D O, Contrucci R B, Batsakis J G 1986 Epithelial-myoepithelial carcinoma of the subglottic region: a case presentation and review of the literature. Otolaryngol Head Neck Surg 95: 104–106

121. Milford C A, Mugliston T A, O'Flynn P, McCarthy K 1989 Carcinoma arising in pleomorphic adenoma of the epiglottis. J Laryngol Otol 103: 324–327

122. Mitchell D B, Humphreys S, Kearns D B 1988 Mucoepidermoid carcinoma of the larynx in a child. Int J Pediatr Otorhinolaryngol 15: 211–215

123. Montes Noriega B 1974 Adenomas de laringe. An Otorrinolaringol Ibero Am 1: 98–105

124. Moore I 1920 Adenomata (glandular tumours) of the larynx. J Laryngol Otol 35: 65–75

125. Mori M, Yamada K, Tanaka T, Okada Y 1990 Multiple expression of keratins, vimentin, and S-100 protein in pleomorphic salivary adenomas. Virchows Arch (Cell Pathol) 58: 435–444

126. Mullins J D, Barnes R P 1979 Childhood bronchial mucoepidermoid tumors. A case report and review of the literature. Cancer 44: 315–322

127. Muratti G 1969 Epitelioma muco-epidermoide della laringe. Arch Ital Otol Rinol Laringol 80: 131–153

128. Myers E N, Bankaci M, Barnes E L 1975 Necrotizing sialometaplasia. Report of a case: Arch Otolaryngol 101: 628–629

129. Nakazato Y, Ishida Y, Takahashi K, Suzuki K 1985 Immunohistochemical distribution of S-100 protein and glial fibrillary acidic protein in normal and neoplastic salivary glands. Virchows Arch (A) 405: 299–310

130. New G B, Erich J B 1941 Adenocarcinoma of the larynx. Ann Otol Rhinol Laryngol 50: 706–714

131. Noyek A M, Shulman H S 1987 Diagnostic imaging of the larynx. In: Tucker H M (ed) The larynx. Thieme, New York

132. Okinaka Y, Sekitani T 1984 Mucoepidermoid carcinoma of the vocal cord. Report of a case. ORL J Otorhinolaryngol Relat Spec 46: 139–146

133. Oliveira C A, Roth J A, Adams G L 1977 Oncocytic lesions of the larynx. Laryngoscope 87: 1718–1725

134. Olofsson J, van Nostrand A W P 1977 Adenoid cystic carcinoma of the larynx. A report of four cases and a review of the literature. Cancer 40: 1307–1313

135. Orenstein J M, Dardick I, von Nostrand A W P 1985 Ultrastructural similarities of adenoid cystic carcinoma and pleomorphic adenoma. Histopathology 9: 623–638

136. Paredes Osado J R, Cerdan Baeza F J, Talavera Sanchez J 1990 Adenoid cystic subglottic carcinoma. A case report. Acta Otorrinolaringol Esp 41: 245–248

137. Pesavento G, Ferlito A, Recher G 1980 Primary clear cell carcinoma of the larynx. J Clin Pathol 33: 1160–1164.

138. Pignataro L, Brambilla D, Scotti A 1991 Carcinoma adenoideo cistico della laringe e dell'ipofaringe. Relazione su di un caso clinico e revisione della letteratura. Otorinolaringologia 41: 141–144

139. Pinel J, Trotoux J, Vilde F, Werner A 1975 Tumeur mixte de l'epiglotte. Ann Otolaryngol Chir Cervicofac 92: 692–695

140. Piquet J J, Onimus G, Chevalier D, Malard T, Piedor P, Vaneecloo F M 1988 Les cylindromes de l'extrémité céphalique. Rev Laryngol Otol Rhinol 109: 25–27

141. Regezi J A, Zabro R J, Batsakis J G 1991 Immunoprofile of mucoepidermoid carcinomas of minor salivary glands. Oral Surg Oral Med Oral Pathol 71: 189–192

142. Reibel J F, McLean W C, Cantrell R W 1981 Laryngeal acinic cell carcinoma following thyroid irradiation. Otolaryngol Head Neck Surg 89: 398–401

143. Reynolds C T, McAuley R L, Rogers W P 1966 Experience with tumors of minor salivary glands. Am J Surg 111: 168–174

144. Robin C, Laboulbene R C 1853 Comptes rendus de seances. Memoire sur trois productions morbides non decrites. C R Soc Biol 5: 185–196

145. Sabri J A, Hajjar M A 1967 Malignant mixed tumor of the vocal cord. Report of a case. Arch Otolaryngol 85: 118–120

146. Samuel J, Chrystal V, Akerman B S 1986 Oncocytic cyst of the larynx. S Afr Med J 70: 695–696

147. Sanderson R J, Rivron R P, Wallace W A 1991 Adenosquamous carcinoma of the hypopharynx. J Laryngol Otol 105: 678–680

148. Seifert G 1991 Histological typing of salivary gland tumours. World Health Organization. International histological classification of tumours, 2nd edn. Springer-Verlag, Berlin

149. Seifert G, Okabe H, Caselitz J 1986 Epithelial salivary gland tumours in children and adolescents. Analysis of 80 cases (Salivary Gland Register 1965–1984). ORL J Otorhinolaryngol Relat Spec 48: 137–149

150. Seo I S, Tomich C E, Warfel K A, Hull M T 1980 Clear cell carcinoma of the larynx. A variant of mucoepidermoid carcinoma. Ann Otol Rhinol Laryngol 89: 168–172

151. Session D G, Murray J P, Bauer W C, Ogura J H 1975 Adenocarcinoma of the larynx. Can J Otolaryngol 4: 293–296

152. Shanmugaratnam K 1991 Histological typing of tumours of the upper respiratory tract and ear. World Health Organization. International histological classification of tumours, 2nd edn. Springer-Verlag, Berlin

153. Shaw H 1979 Tumours of the larynx. In: Ballantyne J, Groves J (eds) Scott-Brown's diseases of the ear, nose & throat, 4th edn. Butterworth, London

154. Simpson R H, Clarke T J, Sarsfield P T L, Babajews A V 1991 Salivary duct adenocarcinoma. Histopathology 18: 229–235

155. Singh R, Cawson R A 1988 Malignant myoepithelial carcinoma (myoepithelioma) arising in a pleomorphic adenoma of the parotid. Oral Surg Oral Med Oral Pathol 66: 65–70

156. Skorpil F 1940 Uber das schleimbildende Epitheliom der Speicheldrusen. Virchows Arch (A) 305: 661–684

157. Sobin L H 1991 New techniques and tumor nomenclature. APMIS 23 (suppl): 9–12

158. Som P M, Nagel B D, Feuerstein S S, Strauss L 1979 Benign pleomorphic adenoma of the larynx. A case report. Ann Otol Rhinol Laryngol 88: 112–114

159. Snow R T, Fox A R 1991 Mucoepidermoid carcinoma of the larynx. J Am Osteopath Assoc 91: 182–184, 187–189

160. Spies J W 1930 Adenoid cystic carcinoma. Generalised metastases in three cases of basal cell type. Arch Surg 21: 365–404

161. Spiro R H, Lewis J S, Hajdu S I, Strong E W 1976 Mucus gland tumors of the larynx and laryngopharynx. Ann Otol Rhinol Laryngol 85: 498–503

162. Squires J E, Mills S E, Cooper P H, Innes D J Jr, McLean W C 1981 Acinic cell carcinoma: its occurrence in the laryngotracheal junction after thyroid radiation. Arch Pathol Lab Med 105: 266–268

163. Stell P M, Cruickshank A H, Stoney P J, McCormick M S 1985 Lymph node metastases in adenoid cystic carcinoma. Am J Otolaryngol 6: 433–436

164. Stewart E F 1960 Cystadenoma of the larynx. J Laryngol Otol 74: 325–330

165. Stewart F W, Foote F W, Becker W F 1945 Mucoepidermoid tumors of salivary glands. Ann Surg 122: 820–844

166. Stillwagon G B, Smith R R L, Highstein C, Lee D-J 1985 Adenoid cystic carcinoma of the supraglottic larynx: report of a case and review of the literature. Am J Otolaryngol 6: 309–314

167. Supiyaphun P, Vaewvichit K, Pongsupat T, Yenrudi S, Boonyapipat P 1986 Mucoepidermoid carcinoma of the larynx: report of two cases. J Med Assoc Thai 69: 500–504

167a. Suttner H-J, Stöss H, Iro H 1992 Pleomorphes Adenom der Epiglottis. Kasuistik und Literaturbersicht. HNO 40: 453–455

168. Takahashi H, Tsuda N, Fujita S, Tezuka F, Okabe H 1990 Immunohistochemical investigation of vimentin, neuro-specific enolase, alpha 1-antichymotrypsin and alpha 1-antitrypsin in adenoid cystic carcinoma of the salivary gland. Acta Pathol Jpn 40: 655–664

169. Tandon D A, Deka R C, Chowdhury C 1985 Mucoepidermoid carcinoma of the larynx. Ear Nose Throat J 64: 555–557

170. Terracol J 1965 So-called mixed salivary tumors of the larynx. Ann Otolaryngol Chir Cervicofac 82: 959–960

171. Tewfik T L, Novick W H, Schipper H M 1983 Adenoid cystic carcinoma of the larynx. J Otolaryngol 12: 151–154

172. Thackray A C, Sobin L H 1972 Histological typing of salivary gland tumours. International histological classification of tumours, no 7. World Health Organization, Geneva

173. Thomas K 1971 Mucoepidermoid carcinoma of the larynx. J Laryngol Otol 85: 261–267

174. Tobin H A 1981 Mixed tumor of the epiglottis: case report. Otolaryngol Head Neck Surg 89: 953–955

175. Tom L W C, Wurzel J M, Wetmore R F, Lowry L D 1981 Mucoepidermoid carcinoma of the hypopharynx. Otolaryngol Head Neck Surg 89: 753–757

176. Tomita T, Lotuaco L, Talbott L, Watanabe I 1977 Mucoepidermoid carcinoma of the subglottis. An ultrastructural study. Arch Pathol Lab Med 101: 145–148

177. Tsang Y W, Ngan K C 1991 Primary mucoid adenocarcinoma of the larynx. J Laryngol Otol 105: 315–317

178. Vilde F, Werner A, Trotoux J, Pinel J 1976 Mixed tumors of the epiglottis. Arch Anat Cytol Pathol 24: 57–62

179. Walker G K, Fechner R E, Johns M E, Teja K 1982 Necrotizing sialometaplasia of the larynx secondary to atheromatous embolization. Am J Clin Pathol 77: 221–223

180. Whicker J H, Neel H B III, Weiland L H, Devine K D 1974 Adenocarcinoma of the larynx. Ann Otol Rhinol Laryngol 83: 487–490

181. Yamase H T, Putman H C 1979 Oncocytic papillary cystadenomatosis of the larynx. A clinicopathologic entity. Cancer 44: 2306–2311

182. Yoshida T, Kuratomi K, Mitsumasu T 1983 Benign neoplasms of the larynx. A 10-year review of 38 patients. Auris, Nasus, Larynx 10 (suppl): S61–71

183. Zakzouk M S 1985 Pleomorphic adenoma of the larynx. J Laryngol Otol 99: 611–616

184. Zalewski P, Zielinski K W, Baj R 1986 A rare case of adenoid cystic carcinoma of the larynx and trachea. Otolaryngol Pol 40: 462–467

185. Zhumabaev A R, Boikov V P 1990 Mucoepidermoid cancer of the larynx. Vestn Otorinolaringol 3: 66–67

186. Zieske L A, Myers E N, Brown B M 1988 Pulmonary lymphangitic carcinomatosis from hypopharyngeal adenosquamous carcinoma. Head Neck Surg 10: 195–198

15. Soft tissue neoplasms

L. Barnes, A. Ferlito

The new version of the World Health Organization's blue book, *Histological Typing of Tumours of the Upper Respiratory Tract and Ear*,[180] which naturally includes the larynx, proposes the following oncotypes:

Benign tumours

Aggressive fibromatosis
Myxoma
Fibrous histiocytoma
Lipoma
Leiomyoma
Rhabdomyoma
Haemangioma
Haemangiopericytoma
Lymphangioma
Neurilemmoma
Neurofibroma
Granular cell tumour
Paraganglioma

Malignant tumours

Fibrosarcoma
Malignant fibrous histiocytoma
Liposarcoma
Leiomyosarcoma
Rhabdomyosarcoma
Angiosarcoma
Kaposi sarcoma
Malignant haemangiopericytoma
Malignant nerve sheath tumour
Alveolar soft part sarcoma
Synovial sarcoma
Ewing sarcoma

Soft tissue tumours of the larynx are rare.[60] As a whole, they comprise no more than 2% of all benign and malignant neoplasms and less than 1% of malignant laryngeal neoplasms.[84, 199]

This chapter discusses benign and malignant soft tissue neoplasms of the larynx, relying on the terminology of the above-mentioned WHO classification. Nodular fasciitis is also discussed as it is a tumour-like lesion which might be misinterpreted as a malignant soft tissue neoplasm.

BENIGN SOFT TISSUE NEOPLASMS

Aggressive fibromatosis

Fibromatosis of the larynx is distinctly uncommon and may be primary (intrinsic) or secondary (extrinsic), the latter occurring when cervical fibromatosis surrounds or extends into the larynx. Although it has been described in adults up to 67 years of age, primary fibromatosis of the larynx is basically a disease of the newborn and children.[41,103,131,169] It may involve any area of the larynx and presents as a nodular 'cobblestone' mucosal abnormality or as a pedunculated localized growth. A case of congenital solitary fibromatosis of the larynx with areas of fibrosarcomatous change that was treated by total laryngopharyngectomy has been reported (Figs 15.1–15.4).[131]

Hoarseness and breathing difficulties are the most common symptoms. In some instances, there may even be a palpable neck mass.

In a collective review of 14 patients with laryngeal fibromatosis, 11 had disease confined to the larynx and three had laryngeal involvement associated with generalized fibromatosis.[41,103,131,169] The three patients with generalized disease died of disease at 1.5, 3 and 22 days of age.[169] Of the 11 individuals with localized disease, at least five experienced either persistent or recurrent disease following treatment and one died of disease (respiratory failure) 17 weeks later.

Microscopically, fibromatosis is composed of elongated fibroblasts and/or myofibroblasts separated by ample amounts of collagen. The fibroblast nuclei are characteristically vesicular, long and slender; they contain one or

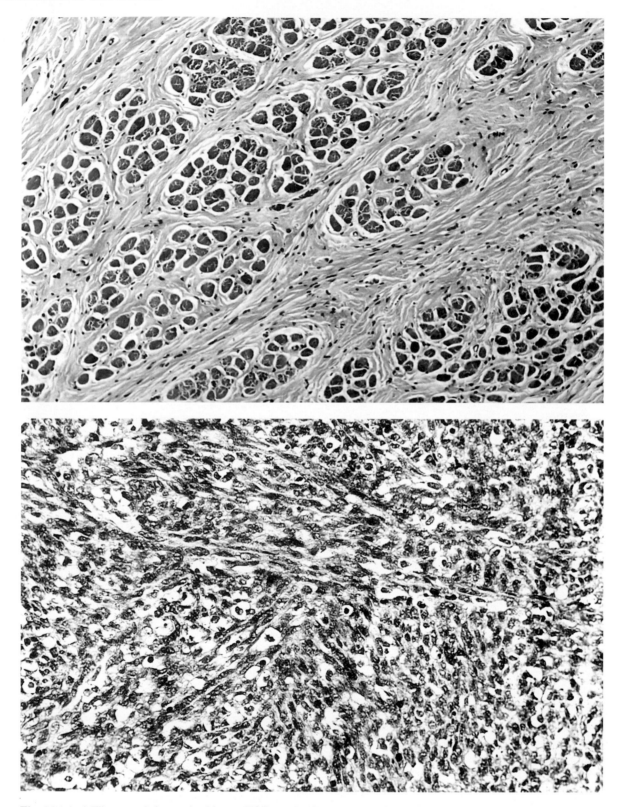

Fig. 15.1 (*top*) Fibromatosis in retrohyoid area. H&E, ×180. (Courtesy of Professor W. A. McIntosh, Johannesburg, and the editor of *Archives of Otolaryngology Head and Neck Surgery*.)

Fig. 15.2 (*bottom*) Same case as in Fig. 15.1. Fibrosarcomatous area. H&E, ×288. (Courtesy of Professor W. A. McIntosh, Johannesburg, and the editor of *Archives of Otolaryngology Head and Neck Surgery*.)

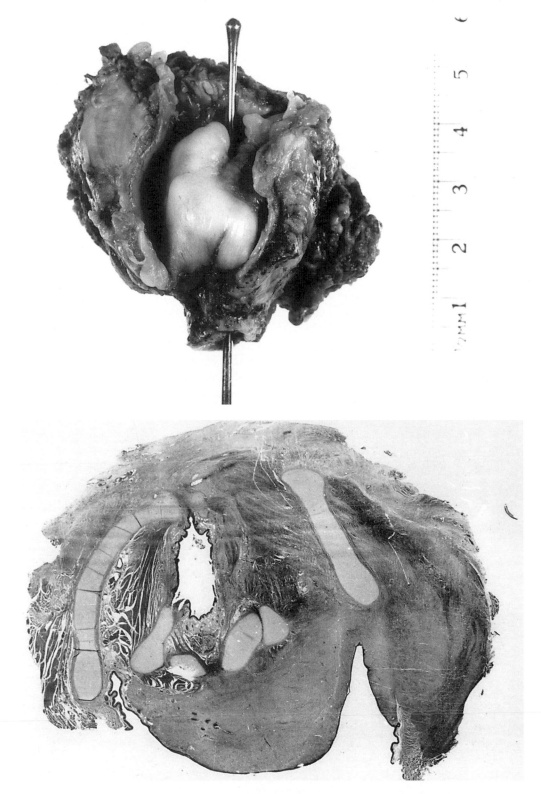

Fig. 15.3 (*top*) Same case as in Fig 15.1. Laryngopharyngectomy specimen of a 14-month-old infant. (Courtesy of Professor W. A. McIntosh, Johannesburg, and the editor of *Archives of Otolaryngology Head and Neck Surgery*.)

Fig. 15.4 (*bottom*) Same case as in Fig. 15.1. Transverse section of larynx showing extensive fibromatosis. H&E, ×4. Level 640 of 1268 transverse serial sections of larynx. (Courtesy of Professor W. A. McIntosh, Johannesburg and the editor of *Archives of Otolaryngology Head and Neck Surgery*.)

more barely discernible nucleoli. The nuclei may occasionally be plump, ovoid or stellate. Mitoses are rare and never atypical. Tumour margins are usually poorly defined and infiltrative (Fig. 15.5). Collagen typing has proved of no diagnostic value.[51]

Fibromatosis must be distinguished from fibrosarcoma because of the latter's tendency to metastasize.[65] The presence of increased cellularity, one or more mitoses per high-power field, atypical mitoses, and a 'herringbone' arrangement of fibroblasts should arouse suspicion of fibrosarcoma.

The clinical course is highly variable. Some patients are cured by initial treatment while others experience numerous recurrences over the course of many years. Although Enzinger and Weiss[51] state that prognosis cannot be correlated with histological appearance, Yokoyama et al[222] indicate that lesions containing an increased number of small vessels in the central portion of the tumour and composed of plump, stellate cells and/or myxomatous foci are more likely to recur.

Surgery continues to be the preferred treatment for fibromatosis. In the case of the larynx, Rosenberg et al recommend that initial clinical management be restricted to local excision.[169] Radiation and chemotherapy may also be useful in selected patients.[11,111,212] However, if radiation is used, periods of more than two years may be required for complete regression.[111]

Nodular fasciitis

Nodular fasciitis, albeit rare, is the most common pseudosarcoma of the soft tissues.[43] It is a benign, self-limited fibroblastic growth that is often mistaken histologically for a malignant mesenchymal tumour. It occurs primarily in individuals between 20 and 40 years of age and affects both sexes equally,[14] but it has also been observed in the paediatric ENT population.[43] The forearm is the site of predilection, but it may occur in any site, including the mucous membranes.[14,214] Approximately 10–20% of cases occur in the head and neck, where the most frequent sites are the neck and face.

The lesion grows rapidly, reaching its maximum size of 1 to 3 cm within a few weeks. Lesions larger than 5 cm are distinctly unusual. Because of its alarming growth, most patients seek medical attention within three months of the onset of the lesion. Although trauma has been implicated as an aetiological factor, only 5–15% of patients actually indicate a history of trauma.

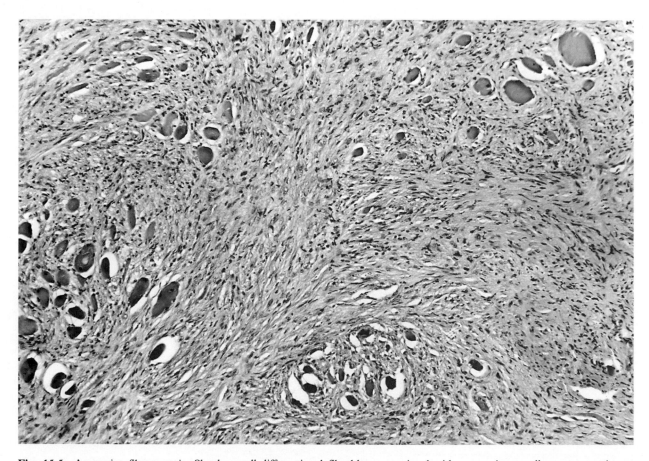

Fig. 15.5 Aggressive fibromatosis. Slender, well-differentiated fibroblasts associated with a prominent collagenous matrix are invading the vocalis muscle. Mitoses are absent. H&E, ×100.

Nodular fasciitis arises typically from the superficial fascia (86% of cases) and occasionally intramuscularly or from the periosteum.[5] It is usually grey-white and focally myxoid and may be either circumscribed or poorly defined. Although numerous histological variants of nodular fasciitis have been described, none have prognostic significance.[5] The following features are common to most cases: (i) proliferation of elongated fibroblasts or myofibroblasts that often have an S-shaped configuration; (ii) small clefts between fibroblasts; (iii) extravasated erythrocytes; (iv) myxoid ground substance; (v) prominent blood vessels that are occasionally radially arranged at the periphery; (vi) mononuclear inflammatory cells; and (vii) mitoses (which average one or more per high-power field and are almost invariably normal).

Simple local excision is usually curative. Recurrences are distinctly unusual, even when the lesion has been incompletely excised. According to Bernstein and Lattes,[14] histological reappraisal has shown that most cases of alleged recurrent nodular fasciitis are examples of other pathological entities.

Stout[189] described two cases of nodular fasciitis involving the trachea. Jones et al[103] reported the first instance of laryngeal nodular fasciitis. The patient, a 61-year-old man, presented with hoarseness of one year's duration. Examination revealed a 1.5 cm submucosal mass of the true vocal cord which was excised via laryngofissure. The patient was followed-up for seven years after surgery and no recurrences were found, despite positive margins.

Another case of what appeared to be a fasciitis-like pseudotumour of the larynx reported in a 65-year-old man[17] subsequently proved to be a malignancy, and the patient died of extensive recurrence (Dr G. Pretto, personal communication, 1992).

Differential diagnosis includes neurofibroma, neurilemmoma, fibrous histiocytoma, aggressive fibromatosis, fibrosarcoma, leiomyosarcoma and liposarcoma.

Myxoma

Myxoma is a relatively rare type of soft tissue tumour. It is not common in the head and neck and has an equal incidence in men and women, in the third and fourth decades of life. It is extremely rare in the larynx and only a handful of cases have been reported.[27,127,177,204]

Grossly, myxoma is grey-white and appears encapsulated. Microscopically it is composed of spindle or stellate cells with small irregular nuclei embedded in an inflammation-free myxoid stroma (Fig. 15.6). Mitotic figures are usually absent.

Differential diagnosis includes laryngeal polyps and several malignant mesenchymal neoplasms showing myxoid features.

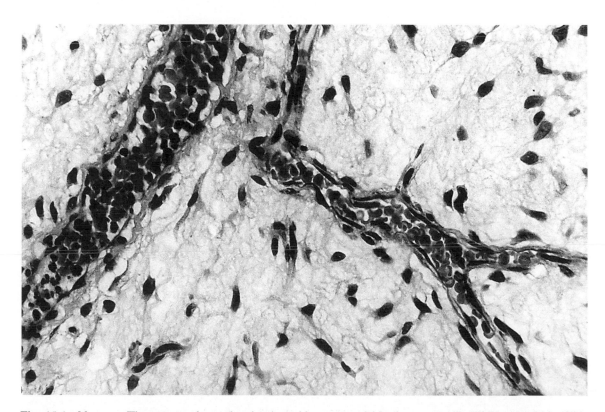

Fig. 15.6 Myxoma. The tumour shows abundant myxoid stroma and bland tumour cells. H&E, ×100 OM. (Slide contributed by Dr K. T. K. Chen, Fresno.)

Simple excision is not an adequate treatment; excision should include a margin of normal tissue around the tumour.[177]

Fibrous histiocytoma

Benign fibrous histiocytoma of the larynx is so rare that such a diagnosis should be made only after the tumour has been totally excised and thoroughly sampled microscopically. This is because malignant fibrous histiocytoma occasionally exhibits a marked regional variation in histological composition and can mimic a benign lesion. Even then, the distinction between benign and malignant fibrous histiocytoma cannot always be made with absolute confidence.

Benign fibrous histiocytoma of the larynx occurs primarily in children. Jones et al[103] described a case involving the true vocal cord in a 13-year-old girl who complained of progressive hoarseness of 6 months' duration (Fig. 15.7). The tumour was removed endoscopically, and nine years of follow-up revealed no recurrence. Heffner[95] mentioned another case occurring in the subglottis of a child of unknown age and sex; no follow-up was provided. Wetmore[215] described another

possible case in the subglottis of a six-year-old girl. The tumour was removed endoscopically with a laser. Unfortunately, she failed to return for follow-up evaluation.

Benign fibrous histiocytoma is distinguishable from malignant variants by the absence of significant stromal atypia. Although local recurrences may develop, metastases, by definition, are not expected.

Lipoma

Lipoma of the larynx is uncommon, and about 80 cases have been reported.[28,44,45,49,152,164,174,224] In a review of 270 benign tumours of the larynx at the University of Pittsburgh, Jones et al identified only one case (Fig. 15.8).[103]

Although the tumour has been described in an eight-year-old child, the majority of patients are over the age of 50 at the time of diagnosis, and almost 70% are males.[224] Lipoma is usually solitary but may sometimes coexist with lipomas in other areas of the body. At least one case has been associated with benign symmetric lipomatosis (Madelung's disease).[140]

Lipoma typically arises in the supraglottic larynx, in the vicinity of the aryepiglottic fold, false vocal cord or ven-

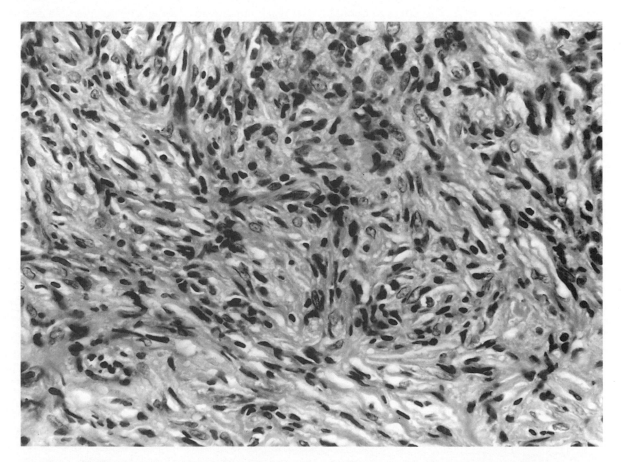

Fig. 15.7   Fibrous histiocytoma. Notice the storiform pattern. Spindle-shaped fibroblasts, histiocytes with round to oval vesicular nuclei, collagenous stroma and a sprinkling of mononuclear inflammatory cells are present. H&E, ×400.

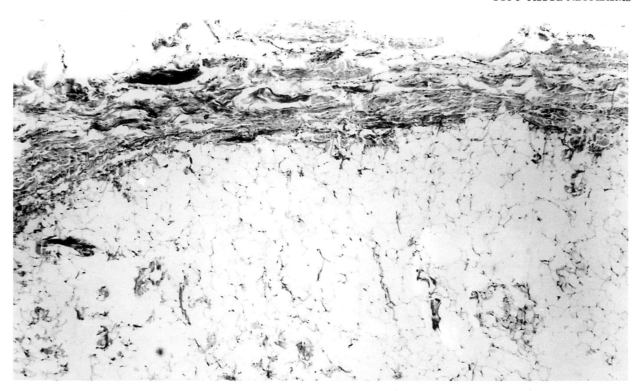

Fig. 15.8   Encapsulated laryngeal lipoma composed of mature adipose tissue. H&E, ×50.

tricle, i.e. areas that normally contain fat. In some in-stances it may occur in the hypopharynx or oropharynx and project into the larynx. The tumour presents as a submucosal mass and varies from sessile to polypoid. Voice changes and dyspnoea are the usual symptoms. Polypoid tumours may even cause acute airway ob-struction through a 'ball-valve' effect, and the patient may be suffocated. Since lipoma is rather deep-seated, biopsies must also be deep or the lesion will be overlooked.

CT scan may be useful in pre-operative diagnosis;[152,174] it not only reveals the extent of the neoplasm but also establishes its lipomatous nature with a high degree of probability. This is because fat is the only soft tissue with a lower density than water (zero Hounsfield units) that can be imaged.[152,174]

As in other areas of the body, lipoma of the larynx is most often circumscribed and encapsulated. Intramuscular and infiltrating lipomas are unusual.[28] When small, the tumour can be effectively removed endoscopically; larger ones may require an external approach (lateral pharyn-gotomy, laryngofissure, subhyoid pharyngotomy).

Leiomyoma

Leiomyomas can be divided into four histological types: conventional, vascular (angiomyoma), epithelioid (leiomyo-blastoma) and mesectodermal. The mesectodermal leiomyoma occurs primarily, not to say exclusively, in the eye.[9,101] Epithelioid leiomyoma (leiomyoblastoma) has only recently been described in the larynx.[140a]

Conventional leiomyoma of the larynx is rare, and approximately 20 cases have been reported in the literature.[100,106,109,115] Not a single case was identified in a review of 270 benign laryngeal tumours by Jones et al.[103] Tumours thus described have occurred in all age groups (range 10–85 years) and have been fairly evenly distributed between the two sexes.[93,100,106,109,115,219] Most have arisen in the supraglottic larynx, particularly from the aryepiglottic fold and ventricle. Subglottic leiomyoma is uncommon. Although Harris et al[93] have described a 5 cm leiomyoma of the larynx, most are 3 cm or less, and they are often attached by a broad-based pedicle. Ob-structive airway symptoms and hoarseness are the usual presenting symptoms.

Microscopically, leiomyoma is composed of interlacing bundles of spindle cells with pink cytoplasm and elongated vesicular nuclei with blunt ends. On small biopsies, it may be difficult to distinguish a leiomyoma from a neurofibroma or neurilemmoma. With the aid of immunoperoxidase stains, however, this is relatively easy. Leiomyoma is both desmin and muscle-specific actin positive and S-100 protein negative, whereas neurofibroma and neurilemmoma are S-100 protein positive and desmin- and muscle-specific actin negative. Leiomyoma is dis-tinguished from leiomyosarcoma by the absence of promi-nent mitotic activity, necrosis and cellular pleomorphism.

Treatment has ranged from simple endoscopic removal for small tumours to local excision via an external approach for larger ones. Kaya et al[109] described an 11-year-old girl who had a 1 cm subglottic tumour that was removed endoscopically and recurred (? persisted) 7 months later. The tumour was described initially as having 'numerous mitoses in each field'. Whether this is actually a bona fide leiomyoma is uncertain.

Vascular leiomyoma (angiomyoma) of the larynx is more rare than the conventional type, and only seven cases have been reported.[115,145,147,160,181,194] It occurs primarily in males, usually over 50 years of age. About half the reported cases have occurred in the supraglottic larynx[145,160,181,194] and the other half in the subglottis.[115,147,181]

Histologically, vascular leiomyoma is encapsulated and composed of blood vessels with thick muscular walls of various sizes and shapes. The vascular component ordinarily comprises from a third to a half of the bulk of the tumour. The intervascular stroma is similar to conventional leiomyoma.

Hoarseness and dyspnoea are the most common symptoms. A few patients have even presented with acute airway obstruction. Although vascular leiomyoma is known to be a painful tumour, none of those described in the larynx to date have been associated with this feature.

The tumour rarely exceeds a maximum dimension of 2 cm and is therefore usually removed endoscopically. Bleeding may be brisk, however, so some advocate that excision via an external approach is always preferable to ensure a better control of haemostasis.[181]

Rhabdomyoma

Rhabdomyoma is an uncommon, benign tumour of either cardiac or skeletal muscle origin; it can be divided into two clinical groups: cardiac and extracardiac. Cardiac rhabdomyoma, as the name implies, occurs in the heart. It is probably a hamartomatous growth, generally multiple, and often associated with tuberous sclerosis.[21,56] Extracardiac rhabdomyoma, in contrast, is usually (but not invariably) a solitary lesion, virtually never associated with a phacomatosis; it occurs primarily in the head and neck.[52]

Rhabdomyoma can also be divided pathologically into two histological types: *adult*[16,19,96,206] and *fetal*.[36,63,85,170] The more common adult type is circumscribed, coarsely nodular and pale to deep brown. It is composed of large rounded or polygonal cells with abundant acidophilic and granular cytoplasm (Fig. 15.9). Sometimes, large strap cells may also be seen. The nuclei are round and vesicular, centrally to eccentrically located, containing prominent nucleoli. The cytoplasm is often vacuolated due to glycogen deposition. In some instances, the glycogen vacuoles may be so extensive that only thin wisps of cytoplasm are seen between vacuoles (spider cells). Cross striations are usually detectable (Fig. 15.10), but often require close scrutiny or special stains for their identification. Some tumours also contain intracytoplasmic crystals (jackstraw crystals) which probably represent Z-band material (Fig. 15.11).

Fetal rhabdomyoma is also circumscribed, but brownish pink to grey-white. It presents as either a non-specific mass or a polyp; on cross-sectioning, it often has a myxoid appearance. Microscopically, fetal rhabdomyoma recapitulates the early stages of muscle development and, as such, is composed of primitive spindle cells. Fetal rhabdomyoma can be further divided into *myxoid* (Figs 15.12, 15.13) and *cellular* variants, based upon the degree of cellularity. The myxoid type has no capsule and is composed of a loose oedematous and myxoid stroma which contains scattered, small spindle cells with scanty cytoplasm and occasionally larger 'strap' and 'ribbon' cells with abundant acidophilic cytoplasm. Many of the strap cells display distinct cross-striations, best shown in sections stained with PTAH or under the electron microscope.[46,63,170]

The cellular type consists of immature elongated spindle cells with a paucity of stroma forming interlacing bundles arranged haphazardly. A 'herringbone' pattern may be seen in some areas. Occasional large, round, mature cells are found, admixed with the spindle cells. Cross striations are scanty. A moderate nuclear hyperchromasia and a variety of cellular shapes and sizes may be present.[46,138]

Striations can be demonstrated with Mallory's phosphotungstic acid haematoxylin or under the electron microscope.[12,85,118]

Although adult rhabdomyoma has been described in infants,[158] it occurs mainly in patients over 40 years of age. It is also more common in males by a 5:1 ratio and over 90% of cases occur in the head and neck.[46] It is multifocal in 5–15% of cases and may recur if it is not totally excised.[18,176]

Fetal rhabdomyoma was initially described as occurring in children, usually under 3 years of age, with a predilection for the post-auricular tissue.[37] It has since been described in patients aged 50 to 60 or more and in head and neck sites other than the post-auricular subcutaneous tissue.[46,85] It is rarely multifocal and seldom recurs following local excision.

In a review of 17 cases in the larynx, Granich et al noted that the tumour typically presented as a 1–2 cm submucosal, polypoid or cyst-like lesion and most often involved the true vocal cords.[85] The average age of diagnosis was 49 years (range 16–82 years), and 11 cases were males. The majority were treated by endoscopic excision. At least three of the patients developed local recurrences,[63,91,138,218] even after a lengthy period of time (15 years), and two were known to have an additional

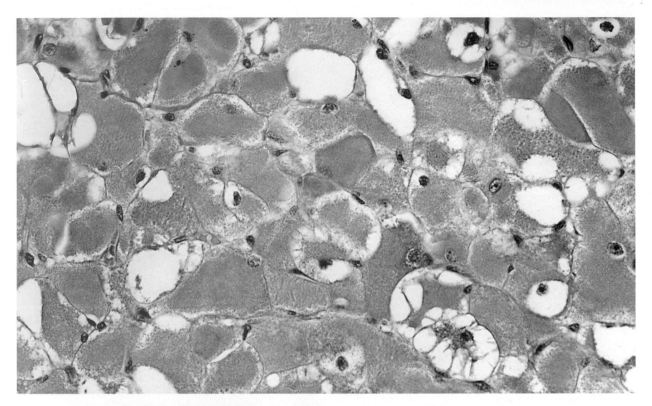

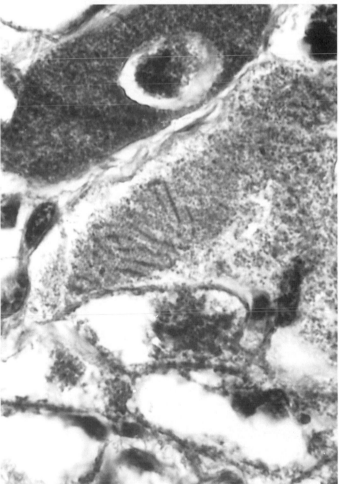

Fig. 15.9 (*above*) Rhabdomyoma, adult type, composed of large polygonal cells with a deeply eosinophilic, occasionally vacuolated cytoplasm. H&E, ×315.

Fig. 15.10 (*left*) Cross-striation in single tumour cells demonstrated by the Masson–Goldner stain. Oil immersion, ×900. (Courtesy of Dr K. Hamper, Hamburg, and the editor of *Archives of Otorhinolaryngology*.)

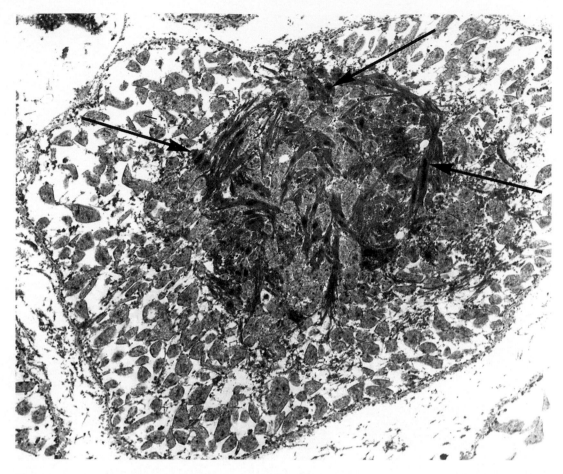

Fig. 15.11 Electron micrograph of another case of adult rhabdomyoma. Cytoplasmic fibrils arranged haphazardly are present, some containing electron-dense areas resembling Z line material (arrows). (Courtesy of Dr T. R. Helliwell, Liverpool, and the editor of *Journal of Clinical Pathology*.)

rhabdomyoma in other sites (floor of mouth and sternocleidomastoid muscle). Eleven out of 17 tumours were of the adult type and six were fetal (3 cellular, 2 myxoid and 1 unspecified).

Although rhabdomyoma has no malignant potential, it may be very difficult to distinguish the fetal cellular type from an embryonal rhabdomyosarcoma.[116] Fetal rhabdomyoma is a circumscribed, non-infiltrating lesion that shows sparse to absent mitoses and no necrosis. Rhabdomyosarcoma is mitotically active, infiltrative, and can often show areas of necrosis.

Adult rhabdomyoma is commonly mistaken for a granular cell tumour.[63] In contrast with granular cell tumour, adult rhabdomyoma never induces pseudo-epitheliomatous hyperplasia of the overlying mucosa. Rhabdomyoma vacuoles are PAS-positive and diastase-sensitive, whereas the granules of a granular cell tumour are PAS-positive but diastase-resistant. Rhabdomyoma is also positive for actin (Fig. 15.14), desmin (Fig. 15.15) and myoglobin, and is generally negative for S-100 protein. Granular cell tumour is S-100 protein-positive and negative for muscle markers.

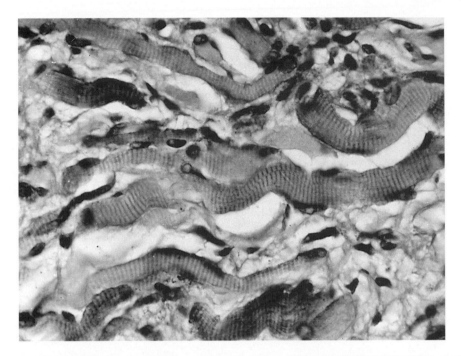

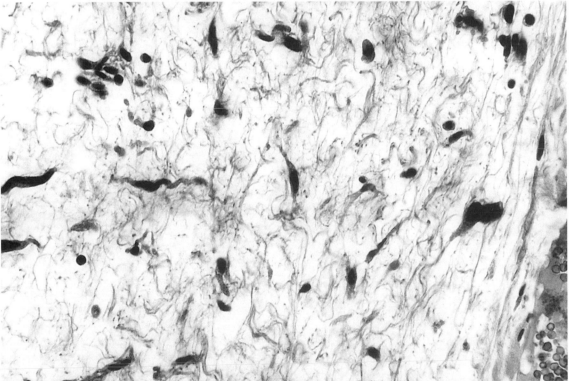

Fig. 15.12 (*top*) Fetal rhabdomyoma, myxoid variant. Notice numerous well-outlined muscle fibres. PAS, ×160 OM.

Fig. 15.13 (*bottom*) Same patient as in Fig. 15.12. Fetal rhabdomyoma, myxoid variant, recurring after 15 years. H&E, ×100 OM.

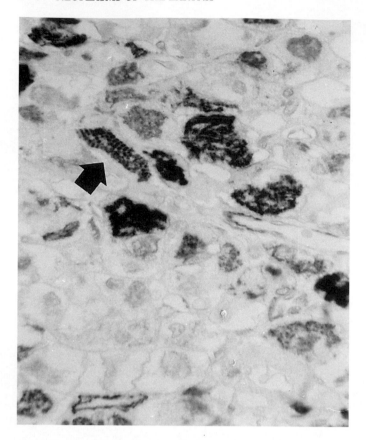

Fig. 15.14 Same case as in Fig. 15.10. Immunocytochemistry of rhabdomyoma positive for actin and showing cross-striation (arrow). ABC method, ×480. (Courtesy of Dr K. Hamper, Hamburg, and the editor of *Archives of Otorhinolaryngology*.)

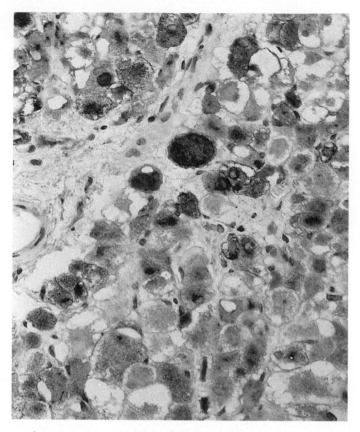

Fig. 15.15 Same case as in Fig. 15.10 Immunocytochemistry of rhabdomyoma positive for desmin. ABC method, ×480. (Courtesy of Dr K. Hamper, Hamburg, and the editor of *Archives of Otorhinolaryngology*.)

Haemangioma

Laryngeal haemangiomas have been divided into two groups: the infantile type and the adult type. The former comprises only 10% of all laryngeal haemangiomas[199] and usually occurs in the newborn and in children under the age of six months; it is twice as common in females. Shikhani et al recently reviewed 333 cases of infantile subglottic haemangioma reported in the English literature.[182]

It is not clear whether this lesion is a hamartoma or a neoplasm, but probably congenital haemangioma is a malformation.

It is usually located in the subglottic region. Dyspnoea and stridor are the most common presenting symptoms of congenital subglottic haemangioma, but it may be asymptomatic at birth and overlooked at tracheostomy, resulting in fatal haemorrhage and suffocation. Some haemangiomas disappear spontaneously or following steroid treatment.[113]

Multicentric lesions and diffuse haemangioma of the upper respiratory tract are extremely rare variants, but are well documented.[117]

Haemangioma in adults may present as an isolated, localized lesion in the supraglottic area, or it may be associated with an extensive cervico-facial angiodysplasia.[113,141] It is more frequent in males and usually manifests as dysphagia or odynophagia.

Histologically, haemangiomas of the larynx can be divided into capillary and cavernous types (Fig. 15.16). The lesion should be distinguished from vascular vocal cord polyp.

Various treatment modalities have been used in the past (such as corticosteroids, radiation therapy, tracheotomy, radioactive implant therapy, surgical excision, cryotherapy) with inadequate results. Laser excision has provided good results in infantile haemangioma. Selective embolization of diffuse laryngeal haemangioma appears to provide another valid therapeutic option in the management of this lesion.[117] The CO_2 laser is not usually advised for adult cavernous haemangioma in view of the greater diameter of the vascular spaces. Surgery is the best treatment and is particularly indicated when the lesion progressively involves additional parts of the larynx. Cryotherapy has also produced excellent results in the treatment of extensive submucosal neoplasms.

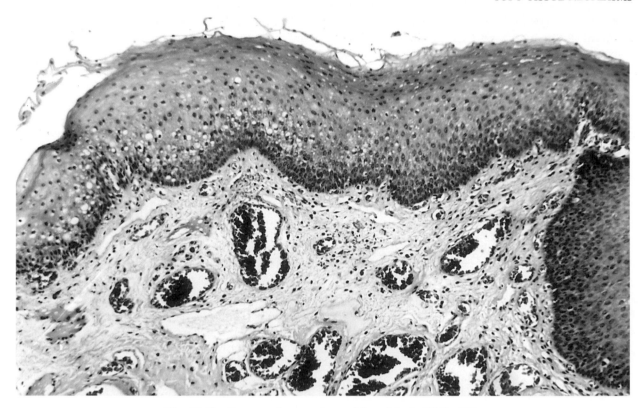

Fig. 15.16 Cavernous haemangioma of the epiglottis. H&E, ×315.

Haemangiopericytoma

The WHO placed this tumour in both the benign and the malignant groups.[180] It is discussed as part of the malignant group because all haemangiopericytomas should be considered as potentially malignant.

Lymphangioma

This lesion most often forms part of a larger cystic hygroma involving the larynx (secondary extrinsic lymphangioma) as well as the neck.[205] It is present at birth and often reaches a considerable size in the first years of life. It is considered as a congenital benign malformation of the lymphatic system rather than as a true neoplasm.[31,180] Lymphangioma is rare in the larynx, particularly isolated laryngeal lymphangioma (primary intrinsic lymphangioma).[50,142] There is a report of lymphangioma of the larynx as a cause of progressive dyspnoea in a 16-year-old girl with Down's syndrome.[30] The combination of a cystic hygroma of the neck with a haemangioma of the larynx has also been described,[53] indicating the close relationship between the two different congenital anomalies.[114] Cohen and Thompson recently reviewed 160 patients with cystic hygroma, 10 of whom had extensive laryngeal involvement.[31]

Lymphangioma is usually localized in the supraglottis, but it also occurs in the glottis, subglottis and postcricoid area.[185] It is histologically divided into capillary, cavernous and cystic types.

Surgery is the best treatment, and tracheostomy is usually necessary.

Neurilemmoma and neurofibroma

Neurilemmoma, or Schwannoma, is 'a benign tumour of Schwann cells', and neurofibroma is 'a benign tumour consisting of a mixture of neurites, Schwann cells and fibroblasts in a collagenous or mucoid matrix'. These are the definitions recently accepted by the WHO experts;[180] however, in small biopsy specimens it may be difficult to establish whether a particular tumour belongs histologically to one or the other of these categories, because intermediate and mixed forms have been found.[135] They are therefore often referred to simply as 'neurogenic tumours' or 'nerve sheath tumours'. Peripheral nerve sheath tumours of the larynx are not very common, and are often of the neurofibroma type, but neurilemmomas have been reported. Laryngeal neurofibromas may occur as an isolated lesion (the majority of cases) or as part of multiple neurofibromatosis (von Recklinghausen's disease).[25,35] A review of the neurogenic tumours of the larynx observed over a 30-year period at the Massachusetts General Hospital noted only nine cases.[35] Approximately 130 cases of laryngeal tumours of neural origin have been reported to date,[114,134,192,207] but it is difficult to distinguish the exact number of neurilemmomas and neurofibromas.

Neurilemmomas are usually seen in females. Neurofibromas involve both sexes in equal proportions, but these patients are generally younger than those with neurilemmoma and they may also include children.[187]

The symptoms are those associated with any slow-growing tumour of the larynx, i.e., gradual changes in voice, the development of inspiratory dyspnoea and foreign body sensation during swallowing. There are some fast-growing cases, however, in which the onset of symptoms can be acute and require prompt treatment. Others are symptom-free and may be discovered only incidentally.[71]

The lesion is often situated in the aryepiglottic fold, probably because the branch of the superior laryngeal nerve is involved. Rarely, the vocal cord is also concerned.[134,211b]

CT scanning can confirm the extent of the lesion. Neurilemmoma (originally called neurinoma) is usually a firm swelling and truly encapsulated (Fig. 15.17). The tumour is composed of spindle cells, often arranged in compact bundles. The nuclei are usually tapered and may be arranged in palisades with a distinct space between rows, forming characteristic Verocay bodies. This solid pattern, which may be interspersed with round or oval foam cells, is designated as type A (Antoni A); a looser arrangement with more cellular pleomorphism is indicated as type B (Antoni B). Nerve fibres may be present in the capsule, but axons are usually not detected within the lesion. Cellular, cystic, ancient (hyalinized) and pleomorphic neurilemmomas have been described, but the distinction has no clinical relevance.[103]

Melanin pigment may be found in neurilemmoma. It shows immunoreactivity to S-100 protein, Leu 7, calcineurin, basal lamina components, nerve growth factor receptors and vimentin.

Electron microscopy has shown that this neoplasm is composed almost entirely of Schwann cells possessing elongated cytoplasmic processes lined with a continuous basal lamina. Long-spaced collagen fibres (Luse bodies) may be present. Neurofibroma is poorly demarcated, uncapsulated and composed of a combined proliferation of axons, fibroblasts and Schwann cells (Fig. 15.18). Unlike neurilemmoma, it sometimes produces an interstitial mucopolysaccharide. It is reactive for S-100 protein. Electron microscopic studies on neurofibromas demonstrate a variety of cell types (fibroblasts, Schwann cells, perineural cells).

Plexiform neurofibroma differs from the non-plexiform lesion in that it is diffuse, poorly localized and highly infiltrating. Several cases of plexiform neurofibroma of the larynx have been reported.[184,187] A plexiform neurofibroma may be mistaken for a plexiform neurilemmoma, as both are S-100 protein positive, but electron microscopy can overcome any doubts. Another variant of

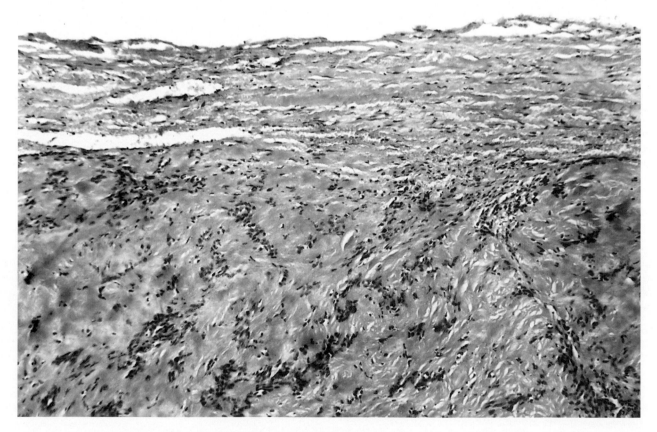

Fig. 15.17 Neurilemmoma. Observe the surrounding fibrous capsule. H&E, ×315.

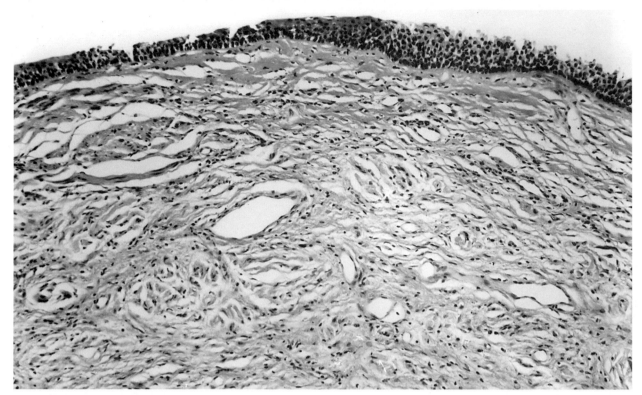

Fig. 15.18 Neurofibroma composed of collagen fibres and Schwann cells. Notice the overlying mucosa and absence of a fibrous capsule. H&E, ×100.

neurofibroma is called 'cellular neurofibroma' and has also been reported in the larynx.[187]

Neonatal laryngeal plexiform neurofibromatosis is very rare, but is well documented in the literature.[148] Surgical excision is an adequate treatment; in particular cases, a lateral pharyngotomy may be indicated.

Neurilemmoma almost never becomes malignant, whereas there is a risk of malignant transformation of neurofibroma. Endoscopic removal can be performed for selective small tumours, while lateral pharyngotomy is indicated for large supraglottic lesions. Thyrotomy offers the best exposure when the tumour occurs at glottic level.[173] The outcome of surgery is generally excellent.

Granular cell tumour

This is the most common benign, non-epithelial neoplasm listed in the AFIP Otolaryngic Tumour Registry.[98] Approximately 200 cases have been reported in the larynx.[4,76,83,92,98,114,167,187,202] The sex incidence shows a moderate male preponderance (2:1). It most commonly occurs in the third to sixth decades of life, but has also been reported in children.[76,83,92]

The majority of granular cell tumours have been located in the posterior third of the vocal cords, many occurring in the posterior larynx;[187] it is occasionally found in the subglottic and supraglottic areas.[71,167] Synchronous multiple granular cell tumours of the laryngotracheo-bronchial tree have been reported.[125]

Macroscopically, the tumour has a nodular or polypoid appearance and is covered by normal mucosa. It measures about 0.5 to 2.5 cm in diameter.

Microscopically, the lesion consists of tightly-packed masses of large, moderately eosinophilic cells with abundant granular cytoplasm (Figs 15.19, 15.20) containing diastase-resistant, PAS-positive granules which also stain red with Masson trichrome. The nuclei are small, hyperchromatic, usually centrally placed, and may contain nucleoli. Large strap-like cells may be seen. Pseudoepitheliomatous hyperplasia of the surface epithelium is often present. The tumour is not encapsulated. It is reactive for S-100 protein, neuron-specific enolase and nerve growth factor receptor.

Electron microscopy reveals numerous lysosomes with 'angulate bodies' and complex granular phagosomes.

The histogenesis of granular cell tumour is still a matter for debate, but there are data to support the hypothesis that granular cell tumour derives from Schwann cells. Ultrastructural and immunohistochemical studies may prove helpful in making the diagnosis in cases where routine histology is inconclusive.[4]

Differential diagnosis includes squamous cell carcinoma, paraganglioma and rhabdomyoma, but some patients also have a concomitant squamous cell carcinoma.[187]

Treatment by endoscopic removal is usually adequate. The lesion rarely recurs.

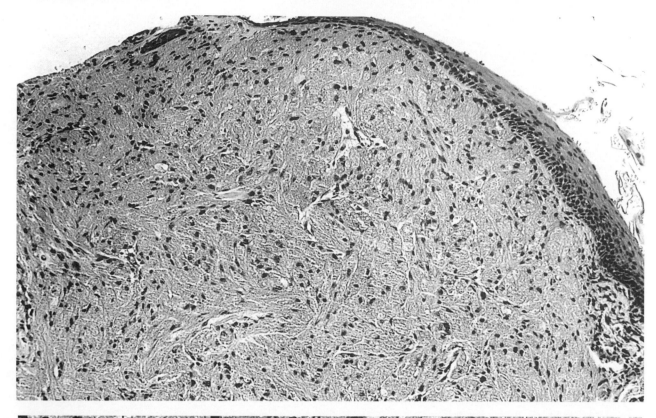

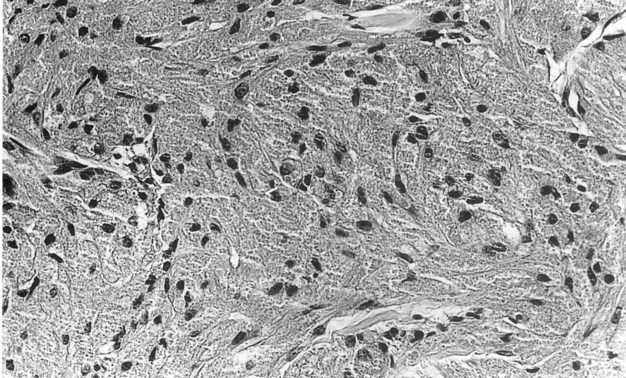

Fig. 15.19 (*top*) Granular cell tumour. The overlying squamous epithelium is ulcerated. There is no evidence of pseudo-epitheliomatous hyperplasia. H&E, ×125. (Courtesy of Dr P. J. Robb, London, and the editor of *Journal of Laryngology and Otology*.)

Fig. 15.20 (*bottom*) Same case as in Fig. 15.19. The tumour cells are large, with indistinct margins, abundant granular eosinophilic cytoplasm and small nuclei. H&E, ×312. (Courtesy of Dr P. J. Robb, London, and the editor of *Journal of Laryngology and Otology*.)

Paraganglioma

Paraganglioma is considered in Chapter 12 because it is basically a neuroendocrine neoplasm.

MALIGNANT SOFT TISSUE NEOPLASMS

Fibrosarcoma

Fibrosarcoma was once regarded as the most common malignant mesenchymal neoplasm of the larynx and it was generally held that at least one-half of laryngeal sarcomas were fibrosarcomas. With the advent of immunoperoxidase stains, it is now apparent that most cases of alleged fibrosarcoma of the larynx are in fact spindle cell squamous carcinomas[61,65,84,225] or other malignant mesenchymal neoplasms[69] such as malignant fibrous histiocytoma and monophasic synovial sarcoma. Any reports dated before 1980 on series of laryngeal fibrosarcomas are therefore unreliable; moreover, it is difficult in more recent literature to find a case of laryngeal fibrosarcoma supported by immunocytochemical and/or ultrastructural investigations. Many of the approximately 35 cases of laryngeal fibrosarcoma collected by Gorenstein et al[84] are more likely to be examples of spindle cell squamous carcinoma. On the other hand, some cases of congenital or infantile fibrosarcoma previously reported ought to be reclassified as fibromatosis.[169] Ferlito[61] found no example of this tumour in a series of about 4000 malignant tumours of the larynx observed at the ENT Department of Padua University, neither did he encounter any cases of pure fibroma of the larynx. Fibromas of the larynx are extremely rare, if indeed they exist at all. In fact, the revised edition of the WHO *Histological Typing of Tumours of the Upper Respiratory Tract and Ear*[180] which naturally includes the larynx, has not included this category.

In our experience, all alleged fibromas of the larynx have been unrecognized cases of the fibrous stage of vocal cord polyps, neurofibromas, fibromatosis, reparative changes (secondary to previous inflammation, surgical biopsies, or radiotherapy) or non-representative biopsies of spindle cell squamous carcinoma or fibrous histiocytoma. Examples of pure fibrosarcoma of the larynx do exist, but they are so rare and (in most reports) so poorly documented histologically that it is impossible to assess the natural history of this oncotype.

Fibrosarcoma has the following histological features: it has an overall, highly cellular, spindle cell pattern in a 'herringbone' arrangement; it stains positive for collagen and negative for muscle markers; it is intracytoplasmically PAS-negative; reticulin preparation usually reveals a dense mesh of fibres between individual cells. Immunocytochemically, a true fibrosarcoma is a marker-negative tumour (apart from vimentin) and the ultrastructural cell composition is fibroblastic.[183,200]

A diagnosis of fibrosarcoma of the larynx should never be made without first thoroughly sectioning the tumour for microscopic evaluation in order to avoid missing small foci of squamous carcinoma. Second, several sections should be immunostained for keratin and/or other epithelial markers. Third, electron microscopy should be performed for ultrastructural evidence of epithelial differentiation; and fourth, there should be no significant dysplasia or merging of the tumour with the overlying mucosa.

Malignant fibrous histiocytoma

According to Barnes and Kanbour,[10] 3–10% of all malignant fibrous histiocytomas (MFH) occur in the head and neck, and of all MFHs of the head and neck, 10–15% arise in the larynx.

More than 35 cases of MFH of the larynx and hypopharynx have been reported in the literature.[10,13,24,32,40, 57,66,67,82,102,104,110,112,114,121,124,126,130,144,149,161,166,168,172,178, 209,211a,221] It is not clear whether the so-called giant cell tumour of the larynx described by Hall-Jones,[90] Coyas et al[33] and Ribari et al[165] is actually MFH, an unusual variant of a carcinoma, or a tumour similar to giant cell tumour of the bone, but they probably represent a distinct subtype of MFH.[66]

All ages may be affected, but the tumour is most prevalent in the sixth and seventh decades.

It is interesting (as pointed out by Godoy et al[82]) that four of the six patients with subglottic tumours were under 30 years of age, whereas patients with glottic or supraglottic tumours tended to be over 50 years old. The significance of this finding, however, remains uncertain in such a small series.

Most patients with MFH of the larynx present with hoarseness or airway obstruction and only infrequently with haemoptysis. The tumours are typically polypoid or sessile with foci of surface ulceration (Figs 15.21–15.23). They average 2.9 cm in greatest dimension (range 0.8 to 5 cm).

Microscopically, MFH shows a spectrum of histological changes that usually include several of the following features: histiocyte-like cells, fibroblasts, collagen production, a storiform pattern that may be focal or diffuse, multinucleated giant cells, tumour giant cells, foam cells, plasma cells, lymphocytes, neutrophils, myxoid areas, normal and/or abnormal mitoses and vascular spaces that vary from curvilinear to cystic.

On the basis of histological composition, MFH can be divided into five types: *storiform-pleomorphic* (Figs 15.24, 15.25), *myxoid* (Fig. 15.26), *inflammatory*, *giant cell* and *angiomatoid*. In general, the best prognosis is associated with the myxoid and angiomatoid variants. The storiform-pleomorphic type is not only the most common form as a whole, but also the most common variant seen

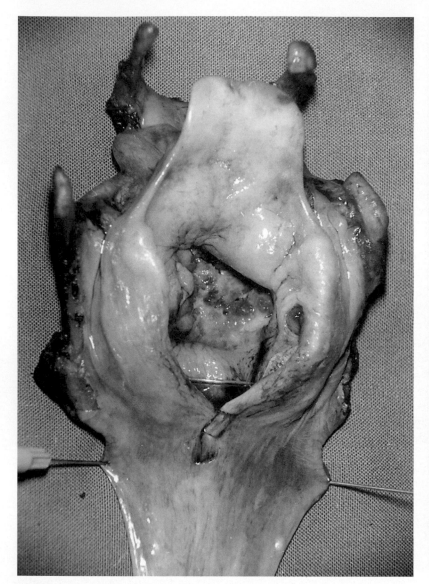 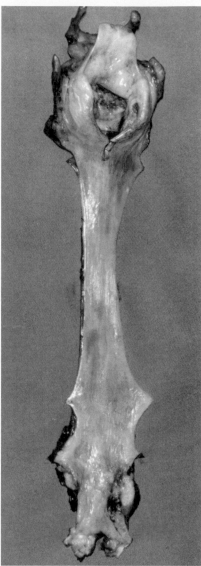

Fig. 15.21 (*left*) Malignant fibrous histiocytoma. Surgical specimen from a 63-year-old-man with malignant fibrous histiocytoma of the larynx and a squamous cell carcinoma of the oesophagus.

Fig. 15.22 (*right*) Detail of Fig. 15.21 in which the extensive laryngeal neoplasm can be seen.

in the larynx.[66] Metastases to the lungs are not unusual (Fig. 15.27). Since MFH is relatively resistant to radiation and chemotherapy, surgery continues to be the most effective treatment modality. The extent of surgical procedures, however, depends on the location and stage of the tumour. Neck dissection does not appear to be indicated unless clinical examination suggests metastatic lymph node involvement.[66]

It is worth bearing in mind that some spindle cell squamous carcinomas of the larynx may appear mono-phasic in biopsies and bear a remarkable resemblance to MFH, even to the extent of exhibiting a storiform pattern and containing multinucleated tumour cells and foam cells. So a diagnosis of laryngeal MFH should never be made without first obtaining an immunoperoxidase stain for cytokeratin and/or employing electron microscopy in order to rule out a spindle cell squamous carcinoma. MFH is also positive on immunostaining for alpha-1-antichymotrypsin.

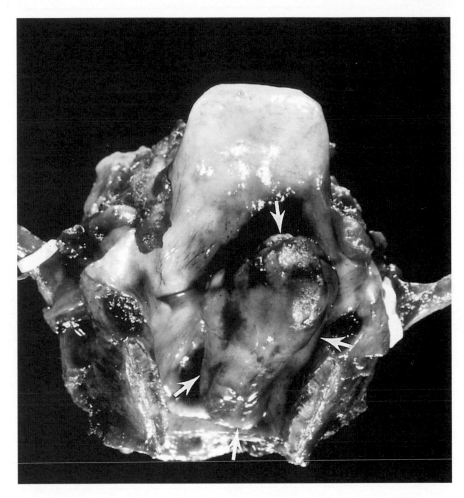

Fig. 15.23   Polypoid malignant fibrous histiocytoma attached primarily to the right true vocal cord (arrows).

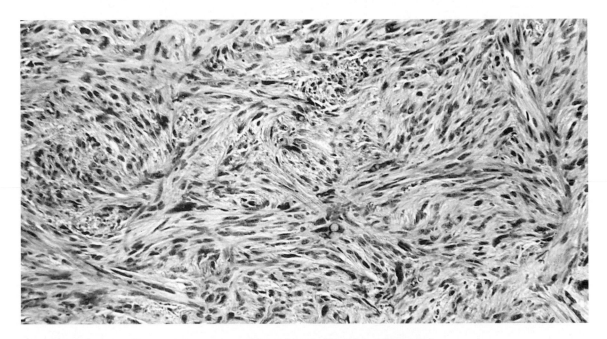

Fig. 15.24   Malignant fibrous histiocytoma, storiform-pleomorphic variant. H&E, ×315.

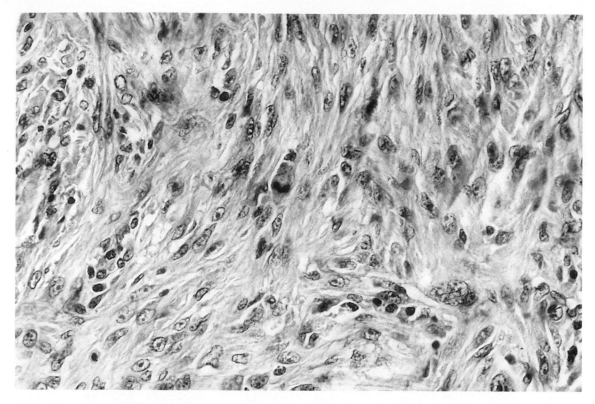

Fig. 15.25 Malignant fibrous histiocytoma containing bizarre cells. H&E, ×100 OM.

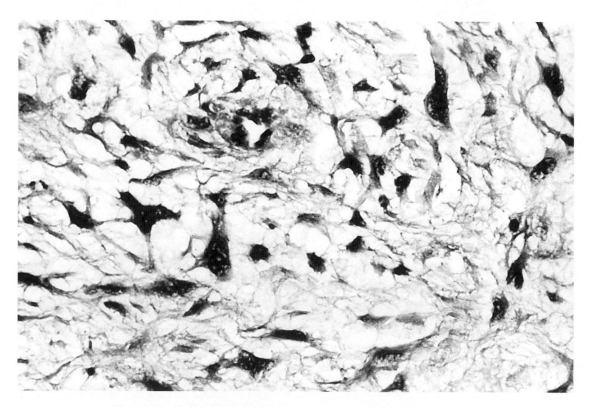

Fig. 15.26 Malignant fibrous histiocytoma, myxoid variant. H&E, ×100 OM.

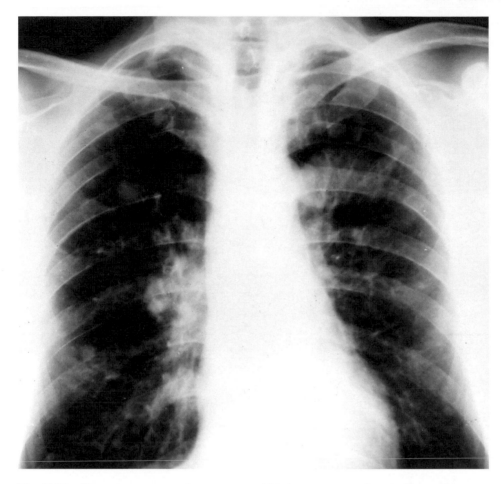

Fig. 15.27   Chest roentgenogram demonstrates multiple lung metastases from malignant fibrous histiocytoma. This pulmonary pattern was present in the terminal stage of the disease.

Liposarcoma

Only about 3% of all liposarcomas occur in the head and neck, most of which are found in the neck.

Liposarcomas of the larynx and pyriform sinus are distinctly unusual. The first case was observed by von Urfer,[210] who described a 'myxolipoma' of the aryepiglottic fold with focal sarcomatous changes. This must be considered a true liposarcoma, not unlike the one described later by Kapur[105] as recurrent lipomata of the larynx and pharynx with late malignant changes. To date, about 30 cases of laryngeal and hypopharyngeal liposarcoma have been reported.[6,47,58,70,75,78,79,105,119,133, 136,143,167a,178,179,200,208,210,213]

The case reported by Tobey et al[200] as 'malignant mesenchymoma with a lipomatous component' has also been included because that tumour might be better classified as a de-differentiated liposarcoma.[213] Narula and Jefferis[143] described a case of liposarcoma occurring metachronously with a squamous cell carcinoma of the larynx. In the larynx, liposarcoma occurs primarily in adult males over 40 years of age and usually arises in the supraglottic larynx or pyriform sinus. It may be exophytic or may infiltrate deeply. The tumour presents as a submucosal or polypoid mass and has ranged in size up to 9 cm in greatest dimension. Airway obstruction, dysphagia and occasional hoarseness are the usual presenting symptoms.

The patients reported in the literature underwent different treatments: simple excision, transoral epiglottectomy, hemilaryngectomy, supraglottic laryngectomy and total laryngectomy. Some patients received postoperative irradiation. Several developed one or more local recurrences, with the interval from initial diagnosis and treatment to first recurrence ranging from 3 months to 30 years. All recurrences were managed by either simple re-excision or total laryngectomy. A few patients are known to have developed distant metastases. One revealed cutaneous and spinal metastasis 2 years after therapy,[119] and another developed paraspinal metastasis after 1 year.[143] Another patient died with pulmonary metastases.[47]

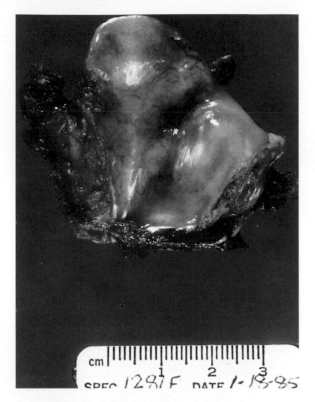

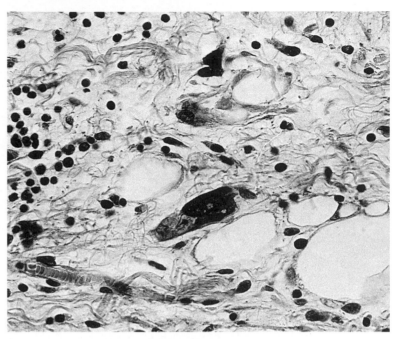

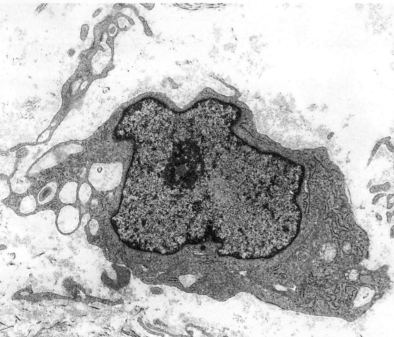

Fig. 15.28 (*top, left*) Liposarcoma. Supraglottic laryngectomy specimen with 2-cm nodule in the right aryepiglottic fold. (Courtesy of Dr B. Mackay, Houston, and the editor of *Archives of Otolaryngology Head and Neck Surgery*.)

Fig. 15.29 (*top, right*) Same case as in Fig. 15.28. Well-differentiated liposarcoma with pleomorphic lipoblasts adjacent to mature adipocytes (left) and lymphoid aggregate (right). H&E, ×400. (Courtesy of Dr B. Mackay, Houston, and the editor of *Archives of Otolaryngology Head and Neck Surgery*.)

Fig. 15.30 (*bottom*) Same case as in Fig. 15.28. Electron micrograph showing spindle-shaped cell resembling a fibroblast with rough endoplasmic reticulum in the cytoplasm. (Courtesy of Dr B. Mackay, Houston, and the editor of *Archives of Otolaryngology Head and Neck Surgery*.)

Pathologically, liposarcomas are divided into four types: well-differentiated (Figs 15.28–15.30), myxoid, round cell and pleomorphic. The well-differentiated type can be further divided into lipoma-like and sclerosing variants. The lipoma-like liposarcoma is usually mistaken initially for an ordinary lipoma, but close scrutiny reveals scattered lipoblasts. The sclerosing variant contains areas of normal adipose tissue alternating with dense fibrous tissue that contains lipoblasts. Myxoid liposarcomas are composed of lipoblasts in various stages of development (particularly signet-ring lipoblasts) and numerous delicate, branching capillaries that lie in a myxoid stroma. Round-cell liposarcoma, as the name implies, contains small round lipoblasts and is often associated with foci of necrosis, haemorrhage and frequent mitoses. In pleomorphic liposarcoma, the lipoblasts are large and multi-nucleated. The most frequent type of liposarcoma of the larynx is the well-differentiated type, followed by the myxoid type. Prognosis is somewhat better for the round-cell variant than for the pleomorphic type.

Differential diagnosis between lipoma and well-differentiated liposarcoma may be difficult. The absence of the characteristic storiform pattern in liposarcoma and the content of neutral fat in the cells distinguish it from malignant fibrous histiocytoma, the cells of which contain mucopolysaccharides.[71]

Surgical therapy with ample excision is the treatment of choice. Elective neck dissection is not indicated, given the absence of cervical metastases in the laryngeal liposarcomas observed in the literature to date.

Leiomyosarcoma

Leiomyosarcomas comprise 5–6% of all soft tissue sarcomas and occur primarily in the uterus, gastro-intestinal tract and retroperitoneum; only 3–10% of cases occur in the head and neck[9] and it is rare in the trachea[198] and larynx. The first leiomyosarcoma of the larynx was reported by Frank[68] in 1941. About 20 cases of leiomyosarcoma of the larynx and hypopharynx have been reported in the literature.[7,15,24a,26,29,39,68,73,74,80,88,107,115,123,128,129,156,186,196,197,201,219,223] The tumour occurs mainly in middle-aged males, but any age may be affected. Chizh[29] described a case in an 8-year-old girl. The most affected areas are the supraglottic and glottic regions. Symptoms vary according to location but usually include hoarseness, dysphagia and progressive airway obstruction and sometimes haemoptysis.

Pathologically, leiomyosarcomas are composed of fascicles of spindle-shaped cells having pink cytoplasm and elongated nuclei with blunt ends (Fig. 15.31). They are distinguished from leiomyomas by a greater mitotic activity, necrosis, cellular pleomorphism and sometimes larger size. The use of immunostains for muscle-specific actin and desmin is often helpful in distinguishing these tumours from other spindle cell malignancies.[8,26,163] Ultra-structurally the neoplastic cells present some features of smooth muscle cells.[15]

Of the patients reported thus far with some degree of follow-up, about 70% have remained free of disease following therapy over an interval of 2 months to 10 years. Local recurrences were experienced by 30%. Two patients are known to have died of their disease, either of massive local recurrence and/or distant metastases.

Treatment has varied from endoscopic excision to laryngofissure, hemilaryngectomy and total laryngectomy. The majority of patients who experienced local recurrences had been treated initially by local excision.

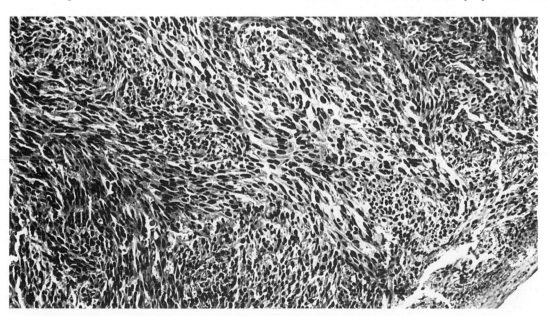

Fig. 15.31 Leiomyosarcoma. The neoplasm shows interlacing bundles of spindle-shaped cells with blunt-ended nuclei. H&E, ×40 OM.

Rhabdomyosarcoma

When rhabdomyosarcoma occurs in the head and neck, the most common site of origin is the orbit (36% of cases), followed by the nasopharynx (15% of cases), middle-ear/mastoid (14% of cases) and sinonasal tract (8% of cases).[9] Only about 3–4% of cases occur in the larynx.[9,55]

In 1987 Dodd-O et al[48] reviewed the literature on laryngeal rhabdomyosarcomas and identified only 48 cases. Of these, 33 occurred in males and 13 in females; the gender was not specified in two cases. The age range at diagnosis was from 1 to 76 years. Half of the patients were over 30 years of age.

The tumour may be bulky, polypoid or sessile, and can arise in any area of the larynx, but with a preference for the glottic region.[23]

Pathologically, it is divided into four types: embryonal, botryoid, alveolar and pleomorphic. The embryonal variant is composed of round, short spindle cells with amphophilic to pink cytoplasm and hyperchromatic nuclei; it is often associated with a myxoid stroma. The botryoid type is generally regarded by most authorities as a variant of embryonal rhabdomyosarcoma, differing from the latter only in its polypoid appearance. The alveolar variant is characterized by small, non-cohesive rhabdomyoblasts arranged in a generally alveolar (but sometimes solid) pattern. Pleomorphic rhabdomyosarcomas are composed of large, often deeply eosinophilic rhabdomyoblasts that vary from round, to spindly, to racquet-shaped (Figs 15.32, 15.33). In general, embryonal, botryoid and alveolar types occur in children or young adults while the pleomorphic variant is found in older adults, usually over 40 years of age, though exceptions do occur. All histological variants of laryngeal rhabdomyosarcoma have been described in the larynx, but about 65–75% are of embryonal and/or botryoid type as opposed to 5–10% of the alveolar and 15–30% of the pleomorphic variants.[48,72,89]

The distinction of rhabdomyosarcoma from other small, round cell neoplasms may be difficult on haematoxylin and eosin sections, but this has become easier with the use of immunoperoxidase stains. Of the various muscle markers, desmin and muscle-specific actin are more sensitive than either myoglobin or creatine kinase M subunit.[153]

Treatment of rhabdomyosarcoma of the larynx has ranged over the years from surgery (often total laryngectomy) to radiation therapy, to combined therapy utilizing surgery, radiation and chemotherapy. According to Dodd-O et al[48], the 5-year survival of 38 of the 48 patients mentioned above (disregarding histological type or method of treatment) was 42%. Recent reports employing triple therapy (i.e. surgery, radiation and chemotherapy), as advocated by the Intergroup Rhabdomyosarcoma Study (IRS), have been most encouraging.[193,216,217] In fact, surgery (once radical) is now often relegated to the role of obtaining a biopsy or debulking the tumour. With this approach, patients with rhabdomyosarcoma of the larynx are often able to retain their larynx and still achieve cure.[42, 87]

The IRS now reports a 3-year actuarial survival rate of 83% for non-orbital, non-parameningeal rhabdomyosarcomas of the head and neck treated according to protocol.[217] Embryonal and botryoid types are more sensitive to this therapy, whereas alveolar and pleomorphic variants are unfavourable histological types.

The incidence of cervical lymph node metastases is about 5–20%[23,216,217] and is an ominous sign. According to Lawrence et al,[122] patients with positive lymph nodes have a 90% higher risk of dying of disease than do those who have negative lymph nodes. Relapse after complete remission is also a poor sign.[162]

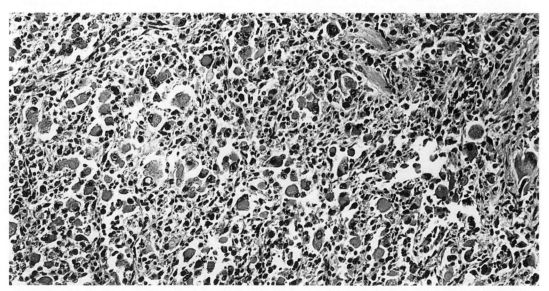

Fig. 15.32 Pleomorphic rhabdomyosarcoma. The neoplasm shows a great variety of cells. H&E, ×40 OM.

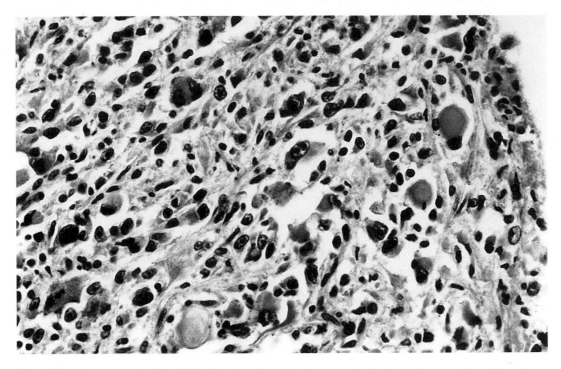

Fig. 15.33 Same case as in Fig. 15.32. Note the giant cells with eccentrically located large nuclei and abundant acidophilic granular cytoplasm. H&E, ×100 OM.

Angiosarcoma

The terms malignant haemangioendothelioma and angiosarcoma are synonymous and describe a malignant vascular neoplasm characterized by the formation of vessels and capillary-like structures of an anastomosing nature, lined with atypical endothelial cells.

Angiosarcomas in the head and neck region tend to involve the scalp and facial soft tissues. The larynx may also occasionally be involved,[60] but the true incidence of angiosarcoma is difficult to ascertain because it has been confused with other vascular neoplasms (e.g. haemangiopericytoma, Kaposi sarcoma and haemangioma) and with non-neoplastic diseases (e.g. intubation granuloma). The

first case of laryngeal angiosarcoma reported in the literature dates back to Yankauer in 1924.[220] The neoplasm was removed by indirect laryngoscopy and presented as a pedunculated growth implanted on a vocal cord. Other cases have since been reported. While reviewing the English medical literature over a period of 30 years, Havens and Parkhill[94] found three cases of laryngeal haemangioendothelioma. They also reported 26 cases of malignant tumour other than squamous cell carcinoma observed during the same period in the Mayo Clinic, eight of which were haemangioendothelioma: seven were adults and one was an infant of 2 months in whom autopsy revealed a vascular tumour involving the under-surfaces of both vocal cords. Pratt and Goodof[159] reported a well-documented case occurring in a 66-year-old man. The neoplasm had metastasized to the lung and spread to the neck and the skin of the cheek. These authors reviewed the literature and collected only 15 previously reported cases.

Only sporadic cases of laryngeal angiosarcoma have been reported in the recent literature.[64,199,203] McRae et al reported the first documented case of laryngeal angiosarcoma arising in a pre-existing benign haemangioma.[132]

Macroscopically, the tumour appears as a white or pink pedunculated mass of friable consistency, often with areas of haemorrhage.

It is composed of non-cohesive cells forming vascular channels (Figs 15.34, 15.35). The latter are lined by large pleomorphic, often multinucleated endothelial cells. Numerous mitotic figures are seen, and necrosis may be present. Reticulin impregnation shows well-defined sheaths containing atypical neoplastic cells.

The immunoperoxidase technique usually reveals factor VIII related antigen and *Ulex europaeus* lectin.[132]

Electron microscopy may reveal Weibel–Palade bodies and intracellular lumina.

The histological diagnosis may be difficult, particularly in poorly differentiated neoplasms. Differential diagnosis must be made particularly from haemangiopericytoma and Kaposi sarcoma. The cellular elements of angiosarcoma grow within the lumen of vessels, whereas haemangiopericytoma displays a perivascular proliferation of tumour cells. Kaposi sarcoma is characterized by a proliferation of spindle-shaped cells, often separated by erythrocytes and foci of haemosiderin pigment.

Surgery is the preferred treatment, with radiation as an adjuvant.

The limited number of reports (which are not always reliable) does not allow conclusions to be drawn about prognosis. In general, the clinical course is very aggressive. The tumour metastasizes preferably via the bloodstream to the lung.[159] One patient was free from recurrence or metastases about 6 years after diagnosis.[64]

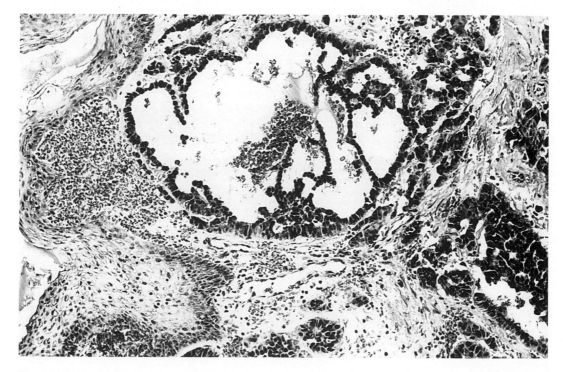

Fig. 15.34 Angiosarcoma. The neoplasm is composed of tortuous and anastomosing vascular channels filled with red blood cells and lined by endothelial cells. H&E, ×16 OM.

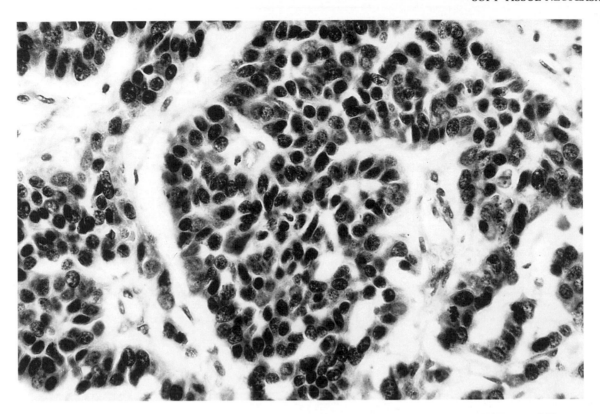

Fig. 15.35   Same case as in Fig. 15.34. Notice atypical and hyperchromatic endothelial cells. H&E, ×100 OM.

Kaposi sarcoma

Kaposi sarcoma occasionally involves the larynx and surrounding tissues.[1,20] The epiglottis is the commonest location of this tumour, which is nearly always associated with classical skin lesions. Only one patient presented with a laryngeal lesion without generalized manifestations.[34] The disease is now seen in a much younger population than previously reported.[81]

Macroscopically, the neoplasm forms a nodular or pedunculated mass and is covered by intact or ulcerated mucosa.

Microscopically, the tumour is composed of a simultaneous proliferation of spindle cells and vascular channels and spaces, frequently lined with abnormal endothelial cells (Figs 15.36, 15.37). The stroma is infiltrated by chronic inflammatory cells and large deposits of haemosiderin pigment are present.

The tumour is often associated with acquired immune deficiency syndrome (AIDS). A virus (HTLV III (HIV)—human T-cell lymphotropic virus) has been identified as the causative agent, and the full clinical picture of AIDS is characterized by opportunistic infections, Kaposi sarcoma occurring as the end stage of an infection with this virus.[3] The histogenesis of this lesion is still controversial.

Correct diagnosis is guided by the presence of multiple lesions occurring in the skin (particularly of the lower extremities) as well as in lymph nodes and the viscera, together with the histological aspect of the tumour. Differential diagnosis must be made from angiosarcoma, fibrosarcoma, vascular leiomyosarcoma, fibrous histiocytoma containing haemosiderin deposits and pyogenic granuloma.

The clinical course of Kaposi sarcoma is variable, but very often patients may live for many years. The prognosis depends upon the clinical patterns of the disease (involvement of the lymph nodes and bones is a poor prognostic sign). In elderly males, Kaposi sarcoma is prolonged, and death occurs only infrequently as a direct result of the tumour.

Kaposi sarcoma has been found in association with lymphomas. There has been an increased incidence of Kaposi sarcoma in homosexual men.[99] Complete regression of laryngeal involvement by classic Kaposi sarcoma with low doses of alpha 2-b interferon has recently been reported.[86]

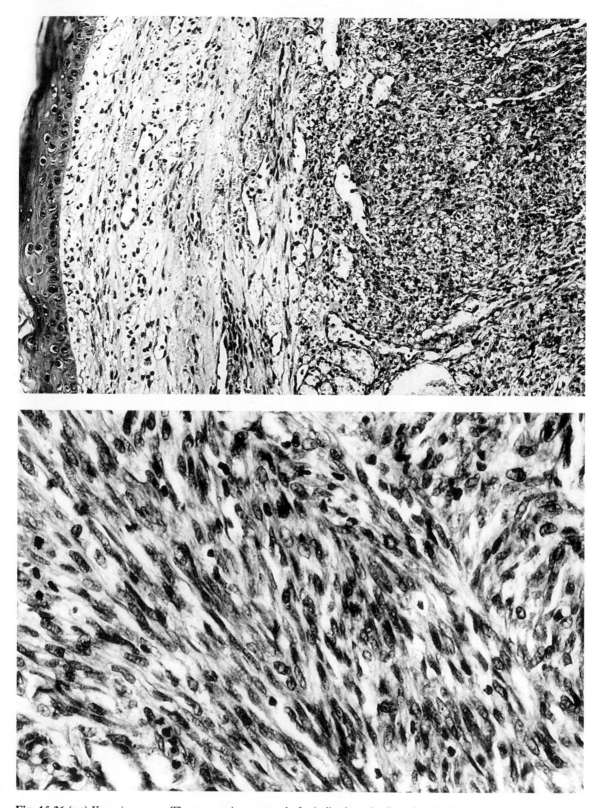

Fig. 15.36 (*top*) Kaposi sarcoma. The tumour is composed of spindle-shaped cells and multiple vascular channels. H&E, ×16 OM.

Fig. 15.37 (*bottom*) Same case as in Fig. 15.36. Notice the spindle cellular part of the tumour. H&E, ×100 OM.

Haemangiopericytoma

Haemangiopericytoma is an uncommon soft tissue neoplasm first described by Stout and Murray in 1942.[190] It usually occurs in the extremities or in the retroperitoneum, but about 12 cases have been reported to arise primarily in the larynx.[54,59,97,120,139,154,157,171,175,188,195,211] The tumour mainly affects men from the fourth to the seventh decades of life. The excised neoplasm may vary considerably, and sometimes a relative pallor may belie its highly vascular nature.

The tumour contains numerous thin-walled vascular channels, lined by apparently normal flattened endothelium, separated by sheets of tumour cells ranging from polyhedral to spindle-shaped, or even stellate, and showing varying degrees of compactness (Figs 15.38, 15.39). Nuclei vary in size and shape, tending to reflect the degree of pleomorphism which may be present, and mitoses may occasionally be seen. Reticulin staining outlines the basal lamina of the vascular channels, thus emphasizing the extravascular location of the tumour cells and thereby helping to distinguish this tumour from angiosarcoma. Areas of poor cellularity and fibrosis may be present. In the more malignant varieties, the tumour may sometimes be misinterpreted as a fibrosarcoma.

There are still no specific markers for haemangiopericytoma. The tumour is usually positive for vimentin and, in a few instances, for actin and S-100 protein.

A consistent aspect revealed by electron microscopy is the demarcation of the relatively normal vascular endothelium from the tumour cells by a basal lamina. Intercellular material is invariably present, either as a basement membrane-like substance surrounding individual cells or forming more diffuse accumulations of more flocculent nature, which may become intermingled with collagen fibrils. Pinocytotic vesicles abound, often alongside the outer cell membrane. The cells exhibit dense bundles of intermediate cytoplasmic filaments and interdigitating cytoplasmic processes. The cells also contain a dense endoplasmic reticulum, many pinocytotic vesicles and myofilaments; they form gap junctions.[71] Long-spaced collagen may be present within the basement membrane-like material.

The tumour should be distinguished from angiosarcoma. The perivascular proliferation of the tumour cells helps to distinguish the two lesions: neoplastic cells of endothelial origin proliferate within the lumen of the vessels in angiosarcoma.

The histological distinction between benign and malignant varieties is not easy. Malignant haemangiopericytoma usually exhibits increased cellularity, mitoses, necrosis and haemorrhage, but neoplasms without these features may also infiltrate locally or metastasize.

The behaviour of laryngeal haemangiopericytoma is difficult to predict and all tumours should be considered as potentially malignant. They may recur locally, but metastasis has been reported in only one case. In 1956, Stout[188] reviewed 197 haemangiopericytomas and noted one in the larynx which had metastasized (the secondary site was not specified).

Optimal management consists of wide surgical excision. Neck dissection does not appear necessary. The neoplasm metastasizes haematogenously rather than via the lymphatic system. Adjuvant radiotherapy does not improve the outcome of surgery.

Malignant nerve sheath tumour

The nomenclature for malignant tumours of nerve sheath origin lacks uniformity, and various terms have been used. These include: malignant neurinoma, neurofibrosarcoma, neurogenic sarcoma, neurogenous sarcoma, malignant neurogenous neoplasm, malignant neurofibroma, malignant spindle cell tumour of Schwann-cell origin, malignant Triton tumour, sarcomatous neurofibroma, 'malignant Schwannoma; however, the term recommended by the WHO[180] is 'malignant nerve sheath tumour' (MNST).

The first well-documented MNST of the larynx was reported by Norris and Peale[146] and occurred in a 59-year-old male. Gorenstein et al[84] reported on 17 cases of laryngeal sarcoma treated at the Mayo Clinic from 1949 to 1974, one of which was described as a neurofibrosarcoma. The same case was recently mentioned by Stanley et al.[187] De Lozier[38] published a case of laryngeal MNST occurring in a 46-year-old male patient. The histological diagnosis was confirmed by Batsakis. Cummings et al[35] reported the malignant transformation of one case of neurofibroma and Schwannoma in the larynx that had been described by Pearlman et al[155] and Stricker,[191] but the photomicrographs are not convincing.[35]

The neoplasm may be pedunculated or infiltrating. The tumour consists of spindle-shaped or ovoid cells having oval and blunted nuclei with finely stippled chromatin. The cells can produce reticulin and collagen. A myxoid pattern is often found (Fig. 15.40). A suggestion of palisading or organoid areas is a specific feature of this lesion. Mitoses are numerous. Cartilaginous, osteoid, lipomatous and rhabdomyomatous tissue, as well as epithelial areas with gland formation and melanin granules, have not so far been observed in laryngeal MNST. The tumour is usually positive for S-100 protein.

Diagnosis can be problematic, particularly when the lesion shows evidence of differentiation towards liposarcoma, chondrosarcoma, osteogenic sarcoma and rhabdomyosarcoma. The presence of nuclear palisading or organoid foci is a typical feature of this neoplasm. Immunohistochemical stains are very useful in contributing towards a correct diagnosis, which can be supported by electron microscopy.

Haematogenous metastases are not uncommon and the prognosis seems poor.

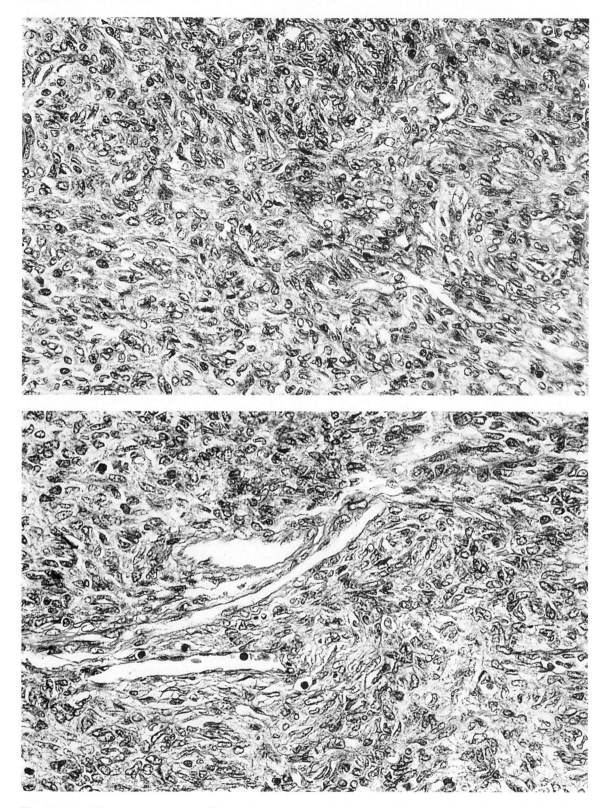

Fig. 15.38 (*top*) Haemangiopericytoma. The neoplasm is composed of round, polyhedral and spindle-shaped cells with hyperchromatic and elongated nuclei. H&E, ×100 OM.

Fig. 15.39 (*bottom*) Same case as in Fig. 15.38. Note perivascular arrangement of the neoplastic cells. H&E, ×100 OM.

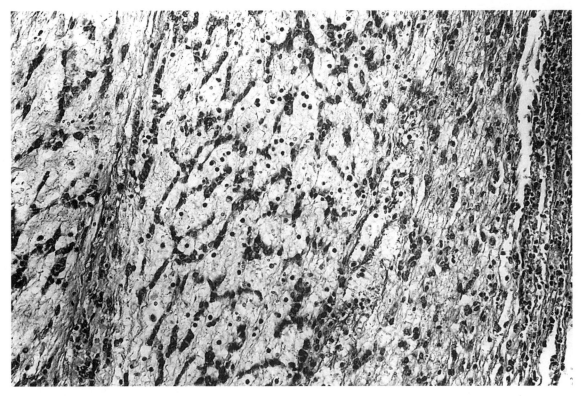

Fig. 15.40 Malignant nerve sheath tumour showing myxoid change. H&E, ×40 OM. (Slide contributed by Dr H. L. DeLozier, Burlington.)

Alveolar soft part sarcoma

This unusual neoplasm has only occasionally been described in the head and neck areas. Michaels[135] described the first case of laryngeal alveolar soft part sarcoma in 1984 (Figs 15.41, 15.42). The lesion involved the supraglottis, with no evidence of lymph node or blood-stream metastases.

The tumour shows an alveolar or organoid pattern and the cells, which contain glycogen, are separated by vascular fibrous septa. Electron microscopy shows that the cells contain crystalline cytoplasmic granules which sometimes have a cross-grid pattern. The tumour is positive for vimentin, desmin, neuron-specific enolase, muscle-specific actin and myosin.[151] Differential diagnosis includes paraganglioma, melanoma, alveolar rhabdomyosarcoma, malignant granular cell tumour and metastatic renal adenocarcinoma.

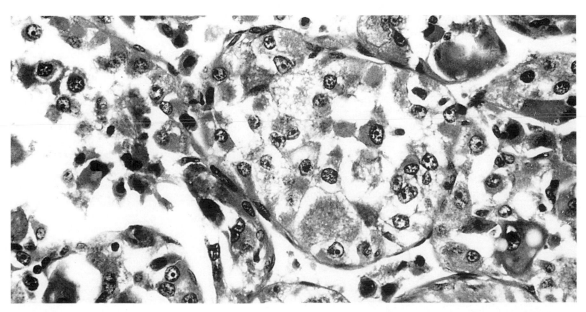

Fig. 15.41 Alveolar soft part sarcoma. Note the organoid pattern. H&E, ×100 OM. (Slide contributed by Professor L. Michaels, London.)

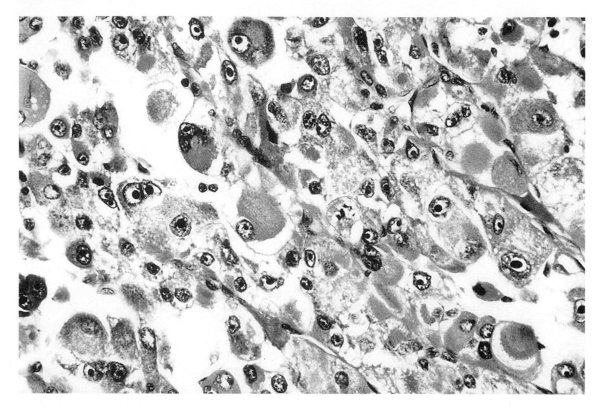

Fig. 15.42   Same case as in Fig. 15.41. The neoplasm is composed of polygonal or rounded cells with a cytoplasm of varying density and vesicular nuclei. H&E, ×100 OM. (Slide contributed by Professor L. Michaels, London.)

Synovial sarcoma

Synovial sarcoma is a malignant soft tissue tumour which occurs primarily in the extremities of young adults. It is no longer considered as a neoplasm derived from synovial lining tissue, but as a lesion developing from a pluripotent mesenchymal stem cell capable of differentiating into cells with epithelial and fibroblast-like features. This tumour is rare in the head and neck region and only about 100 cases have been reported. The most commonly affected site is the pharyngeal area, and the hypopharynx in particular.[150] Involvement of the larynx is usually secondary and the genuinely endolaryngeal localization of this sarcoma is extremely rare. According to Ferlito and Caruso,[62] only seven cases have been reported, one of which is only briefly mentioned[114] and another is reported twice.[77,137] The pathological diagnosis of the latter case was confirmed by the Armed Forces Institute of Pathology. The tumour primarily affects men between the ages of 15 and 30 years. Although few cases have been described, the arytenoid would seem to be the area most frequently involved.

The tumour is typically covered by an intact mucosa and is usually well circumscribed but not encapsulated.

Histologically, one usually sees a biphasic tumour (Fig. 15.43) comprising a fibrosarcomatous component containing glands or gland-like spaces, lined with columnar or cuboidal epithelium. The lumen of these gland-like structures contains PAS diastase resistant material. Myxoid changes and a marked vascularity may be observed. Mitoses are common. The neoplasm may be monophasic. Immunohistochemical staining shows vimentin positivity in the spindle cells and keratin and epithelial membrane antigen positivity in the epithelial component and often in the spindle cells too. The differential diagnosis includes fibrosarcoma, leiomyosarcoma, spindle cell squamous carcinoma, malignant Schwannoma and laryngeal metastases of adenocarcinoma.

Surgery is the treatment of choice. As no lymph node metastases were observed in any of the reported cases of laryngeal synovial sarcoma, neck dissection is not indicated unless there is strong clinical or histological evidence of metastasis. Only one case arising in the hypopharynx developed lymph node metastases.[150]

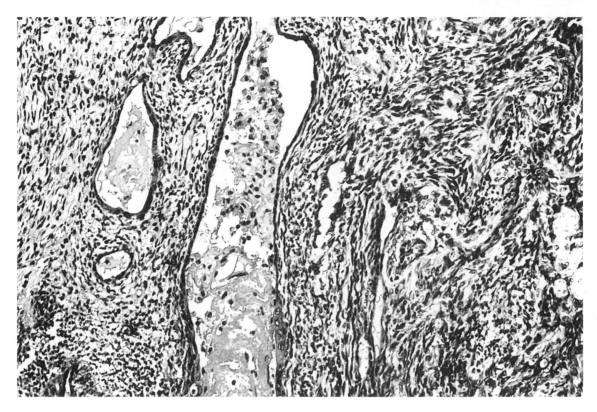

Fig. 15.43   Synovial sarcoma showing biphasic areas. H&E, ×40 OM.

Ewing sarcoma

Abramowsky and Witt[2] described a questionable case of extraskeletal Ewing sarcoma of the larynx in a newborn child (Figs 15.44–15.47). The patient was treated by total laryngectomy at ten days of age and was alive and well two years later.

The histogenesis of this lesion remains unknown, although there is considerable evidence to support its origin from undifferentiated mesenchymal cells.

Malignant granular cell tumour

Malignant variants of granular cell tumours of the larynx are extremely rare. Busanny-Caspari and Hammar[22] reported a case occurring in a 40-year-old man in whom the neoplasm had metastasized to the cervical lymph nodes. The patient died 2 years after diagnosis.

Malignant mesenchymoma

Only one example of malignant mesenchymoma has been reported in the larynx.[108] The tumour exhibited both striated muscle and bone and was positive with PTAH (phosphotungstic acid haematoxylin) and desmin. The tumour appears to arise from pluripotential mesenchymal cells that have undergone divergent differentiation.

Malignant mesenchymoma has not been included among the upper respiratory tract tumours in the WHO classification.[180]

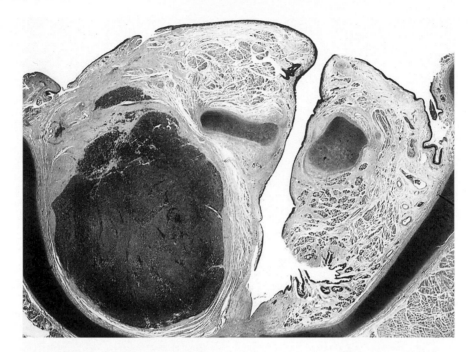

Fig. 15.44 Ewing sarcoma. This transverse section of the larynx taken at the level of the ventricle of the vocal cords shows the circumscribed tumour. The surrounding tissue is compressed and shows a fibrotic reaction to the mass. The arched structure seen inferiorly is the thyroid cartilage. H&E, ×6.5. (Courtesy of Dr. C. Abramowsky, Cleveland, and the editor of *Cancer*.)

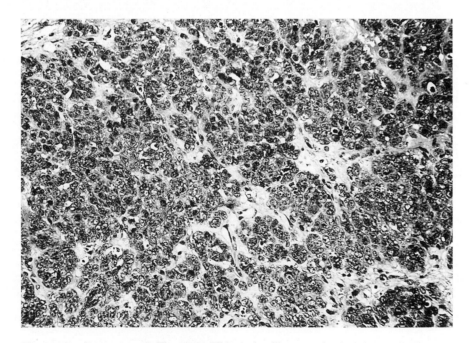

Fig. 15.45 Same case as in Fig. 15.44. This section illustrates the densely populated tumour with the cells variously arranged in cords or sheets. H&E, ×200. (Courtesy of Dr C. Abramowsky, Cleveland, and the editor of *Cancer*.)

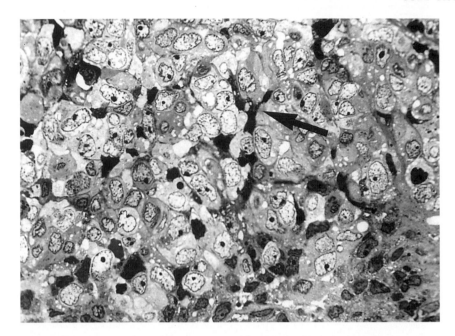

Fig. 15.46   Same case as in Fig. 15.44. A toluidine blue-stained plastic section demonstrates the dual light and dark cell population (arrow) not otherwise differentiated with routine stains. ×600. (Courtesy of Dr C. Abramowsky, Cleveland, and the editor of *Cancer.*)

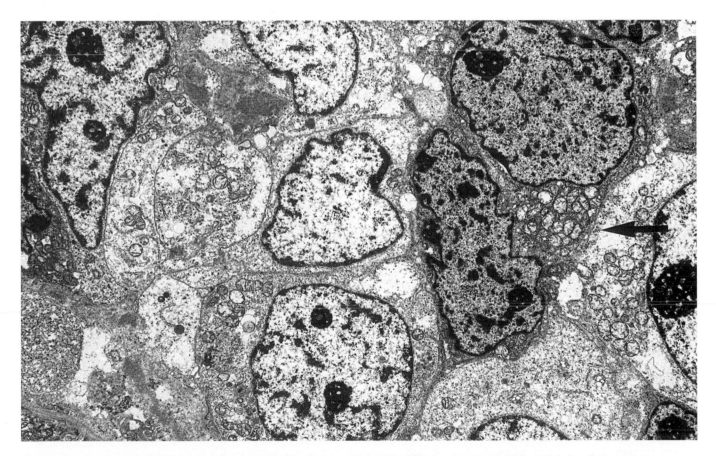

Fig. 15.47   Same case as in Fig. 15.44. The electron micrograph emphasizes the difference between the light and dark cells (arrow). Cytoplasmic glycogen granules are not abundant in this field, but were present in many cells in PAS-stained histological sections. ×6700. (Courtesy of Dr C. Abramowsky, Cleveland, and the editor of *Cancer.*)

REFERENCES

1. Abemayor E, Calcaterra T C 1983 Kaposi's sarcoma and community-acquired immune deficiency syndrome. An update with emphasis on its head and neck manifestations. Arch Otolaryngol 109: 536–542
2. Abramowsky C R, Witt W J 1983 Sarcoma of the larynx in a newborn. Cancer 51: 1726–1730
3. Acheson E D 1985 The acquired immune deficiency syndrome. Health Trends 4: 75–76
4. Alessi D M, Zimmerman M C 1988 Granular cell tumors of the head and neck. Laryngoscope 98: 810–814
5. Allen P W 1972 Nodular fasciitis. Pathology 4: 9–26
6. Allsbrook W C, Harmon J D, Chongchitnant N, Erwin S 1985 Liposarcoma of the larynx. Arch Pathol Lab Med 109:294–296
7. Amendolea L 1968 Leiomiosarcoma della laringe. Valsalva 44: 268–274
8. Azumi N, Ben-Ezra J, Battifora H 1988 Immunophenotypic diagnosis of leiomyosarcomas and rhabdomyosarcomas with monoclonal antibodies to muscle-specific actin and desmin in formalin-fixed tissue. Mod Pathol 1: 469–474
9. Barnes L 1985 Surgical pathology of the head and neck. Marcel Dekker, New York
10. Barnes L, Kanbour A 1988 Malignant fibrous histiocytoma of the head and neck. A report of 12 cases. Arch Otolaryngol Head Neck Surg 114: 1149–1156
11. Bataini J P, Belloir C, Mazabraud A, Pilleron J P, Catigny A, Jaulerry C, Ghossein N A 1988 Desmoid tumors in adults: the role of radiotherapy in their management. Am J Surg 155: 754–760
12. Battifora H A, Elsenstein R, Schild J A 1969 Rhabdomyoma of larynx. Ultrastructural study and comparison with granular cell tumors (myoblastomas). Cancer 23: 183–190
13. Bernáldéz R, Nistal M, Kaiser C, Gavilán J 1991 Malignant fibrous histiocytoma of the larynx. J Laryngol Otol 105: 130–133
14. Bernstein K E, Lattes R 1982 Nodular (pseudosarcomatous) fasciitis: a nonrecurrent lesion; clinicopathologic study of 134 cases. Cancer 49: 1668–1678
15. Bertheau P, Deboise A, De Roquancourt A, Brocheriou C 1991 Léiomyosarcome du larynx. Etude histologique, immunohistochimique et ultrastructurale d'une observation avec revue de la littérature. Ann Pathol 11: 122–127
16. Bianchi C, Muratti G 1975 Rhabdomyoma (adult type) of the larynx. Beitr Pathol 156: 75–79
17. Bisceglia M, Bosman C, Pretto G 1990 Fasciitis-like inflammatory pseudotumour of the larynx. A case report. International Postgraduate Course on Soft Tissue Tumors. Eurograf, Riva del Garda, p 101
18. Blaauwgeers J L G, Troost D, Dingemans K P, Taat C W, van den Tweel J G 1989 Multifocal rhabdomyoma of the neck. Report of a case studied by fine-needle aspiration, light and electron microscopy, histochemistry, and immunohistochemistry. Am J Surg Pathol 13: 791–799
19. Boedts D, Mestagh J 1979 Adult rhabdomyoma of the larynx. Arch Otorhinolaryngol 224: 221–229
20. Bottazzi P, Collini M, Pelizza A 1980 Morbo di Kaposi. Manifestazione secondaria faringo-laringea. Ann Laringol Otol Rinol Faringol 78: 261–268
21. Burke A P, Virmani R 1991 Cardiac rhabdomyoma: a clinicopathologic study. Mod Pathol 4: 70–74
22. Busanny-Caspari von W, Hammar C H 1958 Zur Malignität der sogenannten Myoblastenmyome. Zentralbl Allg Pathol 98: 401–406
23. Canalis R F, Platz C E, Cohn A M 1976 Laryngeal rhabdomyosarcoma. Arch Otolaryngol 102: 104–107
24. Canalis R F, Green M, Konard H R, Hirose F M, Cooper S 1975 Malignant fibrous xanthoma (xanthofibrosarcoma) of the larynx. Arch Otolaryngol 101: 135–137
24a. Carles D, Devars F, Saurel J, Traissac L, Boudard Ph 1992 Leiomyosarcome du larynx: présentation d'un cas. Rev Laryngol 113: 115–117
25. Chang-Lo M 1977 Laryngeal involvement in von Recklinghausen's disease: a case report and review of the literature. Laryngoscope 87: 435–442
26. Chen J M, Novick W H, Logan C A 1991 Leiomyosarcoma of the larynx. J Otolaryngol 20: 345–348
27. Chen K T K, Ballecer R A 1986 Laryngeal myxoma. Am J Otolaryngol 7: 58–59
28. Chen K T K, Weinberg R A 1984 Intramuscular lipoma of the larynx. Am J Otolaryngol 5: 71–72
29. Chizh G I 1976 Leiomyosarcoma of the larynx in an 8-year-old girl. Vestn Otorinolaringol 5: 104–105
30. Claros P, Viscasillas S, Claros A Sr, Claros A Jr 1985 Lymphangioma of the larynx as a cause of progressive dyspnea. Int J Pediatr Otorhinolaryngol 9: 263–268
31. Cohen S R, Thompson J W 1986 Lymphangiomas of the larynx in infants and children. A survey of pediatric lymphangioma. Ann Otol Rhinol Laryngol 95 (suppl 127): 1–20
32. Colev A, Cramer H, Lampe H, McLean C, Slinger R 1989 Malignant fibrous histiocytoma of the larynx: a report of three cases and review of the literature (abstract). Am J Clin Pathol 92: 533
33. Coyas A, Anastassiades O, Kyriakos I 1974 Malignant giant cell tumour of the larynx. J Laryngol Otol 88: 799–803
34. Coyas A, Eliadellis E, Anastassiades O 1983 Kaposi's sarcoma of the larynx. J Laryngol Otol 97: 647–649
35. Cummings C W, Montgomery W W, Balogh K Jr 1969 Neurogenic tumors of the larynx. Ann Otol Rhinol Laryngol 78: 76–95
36. Dahl I, Angervall L, Save-Soderbergh J 1976 Foetal rhabdomyoma. Case report of a patient with two tumours. Acta Pathol Microbiol Scand Sect A 84: 107–112
37. Dehner L P. Enzinger F M, Font R L 1972 Fetal rhabdomyoma. An analysis of nine cases. Cancer 30: 160–166
38. DeLozier H L 1982 Intrinsic malignant schwannoma of the larynx. A case report. Ann Otol Rhinol Laryngol 91: 336–338
39. De Rosa G, Palombini L, D'Angelo 1979 I leiomiomi della laringe. Rassegna della letteratura e presentazione di due casi. Pathologica 70: 209–215
40. De Rosa G, Palombini L, Terracciano L M, D'Angelo L 1990 Primary laryngeal malignant fibrous histiocytoma: a case report. Tumori 76: 403–406
41. De Rosa G, Barra E, Boscaino A, Gentile R, DiPrisco B 1989 Fibromatosis of the larynx in an adult. J Laryngol Otol 103: 1219–1221
42. Diehn K W, Hyams V J, Harris A E 1984 Rhabdomyosarcoma of the larynx: a case report and review of the literature. Laryngoscope 94: 201–205
43. DiNardo L J, Wetmore R F, Potsic W P 1991 Nodular fasciitis of the head and neck in children. Arch Otolaryngol Head Neck Surg 117: 1001–1002
44. Dinsdale R C, Manning S, Brooks D J, Vuitch F 1990 Myxoid laryngeal lipoma in a juvenile. Otolaryngol Head Neck Surg 103: 653–657
45. Diop E M, Sow D, Diop L S 1986 Lipome du larynx. Ann Otolaryngol Chir Cervicofac 103: 207–208
46. Di Sant'Agnese P A, Knowles D M II 1980 Extracardiac rhabdomyoma: a clinicopathologic study and review of the literature. Cancer 46: 780–789
47. Dockerty M B, Parkhill E M, Dahlin D C, Woolner L B, Soule E H, Harrison E G 1968 Tumors of the oral cavity and pharynx. In: Atlas of tumor pathology. Armed Forces Institute of Pathology, Washington DC
48. Dodd-O J M, Wieneke K F, Rosman P 1987 Laryngeal rhabdomyosarcoma. Case report and literature review. Cancer 59: 1012–1018
49. Eagle W W 1965 Lipoma of the larynx and lipoma of the hypopharynx in the same patient. Ann Otol Rhinol Laryngol 74: 851–862

50. El-Serafy S 1971 Rare benign tumours of the larynx. J Laryngol Otol 85: 837–851
51. Enzinger F M, Weiss S W 1988 Soft tissue tumors, 2nd edn. Mosby, St Louis
52. Eusebi V, Ceccarelli C, Daniele E, Collina G, Viale G, Mancini A M 1988 Extracardiac rhabdomyoma: an immunocytochemical study and review of the literature. Appl Pathol 6: 197–207
53. Evans P 1981 Intubation problem in a case of cystic hygroma complicated by a laryngotracheal haemangioma. Anaesthesia 36: 696–698
54. Ey M, Guastella C 1988 Hämangioperizytom des Larynx. Laryngol Rhinol Otol 67: 255–258
55. Feldman B A 1982 Rhabdomyosarcoma of the head and neck. Laryngoscope 92: 424–440
56. Fenoglio J J Jr, McAllister H A Jr, Ferrans V J 1976 Cardiac rhabdomyoma: a clinicopathologic and electron microscopic study. Am J Cardiol 38: 241–251
57. Ferlito A 1978 Histiocytic tumors of the larynx. A clinicopathological study with review of the literature. Cancer 42: 611–622
58. Ferlito A 1978 Primary pleomorphic liposarcoma of the larynx. J Otolaryngol 7: 161–166
59. Ferlito A 1978 Primary malignant haemangiopericytoma of the larynx: a case report with autopsy. J Laryngol Otol 92: 511–519
60. Ferlito A 1985 Soft tissue sarcomas of the larynx. In: Ferlito A (ed) Cancer of the larynx, Vol II. CRC Press, Boca Raton
61. Ferlito A 1990 Laryngeal fibrosarcoma: an over-diagnosed tumor. ORL J Otorhinolaryngol Relat Spec 52: 194–195
62. Ferlito A, Caruso G 1991 Endolaryngeal synovial sarcoma. An update on diagnosis and treatment. ORL J Otorhinolaryngol Relat Spec 53: 116–119
63. Ferlito A, Frugoni P 1975 Rhabdomyoma purum of the larynx. J Laryngol Otol 89: 1131–1141
64. Ferlito A, Caruso G, Nicolai P 1985 Angiosarcoma of the larynx. Case report. Ann Otol Rhinol Laryngol 94: 93–96
65. Ferlito A, Nicolai P, Barion U 1983 Critical comments on laryngeal fibrosarcoma. Acta Otorhinolaryngol Belg 37: 918–925
66. Ferlito A, Nicolai P, Recher G, Narne S 1983 Primary laryngeal malignant fibrous histiocytoma. Review of the literature and report of seven cases. Laryngoscope 93: 1351–1358
67. Ferlito A, Recher G, Polidoro F, Rossi M 1979 Malignant pleomorphic fibrous histiocytoma of the larynx. Further observations. J Laryngol Otol 93: 1021–1029
68. Frank D L 1941 Leiomyosarcoma of the larynx. Arch Otolaryngol 34: 493–500
69. Frankenthaler R, Ayala A G, Hartwick R W, Goepfert H 1990 Fibrosarcoma of the head and neck. Laryngoscope 100: 799–802
70. Frey-Schlottmann M L, Stiens R 1979 Liposarkom im Hypopharynxbereich. Arch Ohr Nas Kehlkopf 223: 419–422
71. Friedmann I, Ferlito A 1988 Granulomas and neoplasms of the larynx. Churchill Livingstone, Edinburgh
72. Frugoni P, Ferlito A 1976 Pleomorphic rhabdomyosarcoma of the larynx. A case report and review of the literature. J Laryngol Otol 90: 687–698
73. Fukuda H, Tsuji D H, Kawasaki Y, Kawaida M, Sakou T 1990 Displacement of the ventricular fold following cordectomy. Auris Nasus Larynx 17: 221–228
74. Fuller A M, van Vliet P D, Lillie J C, Devine K D 1966 Pharyngeal leiomyosarcoma with fever of unknown origin. Arch Otolaryngol 84: 96–98
75. Gadomski S P, Zwillenberg D, Choi H Y 1986 Non-epidermoid carcinoma of the larynx: the Thomas Jefferson University experience. Otolaryngol Head Neck Surg 95: 558–565
76. Garud O, Bostad L, Elverland H H, Mair I W S 1984 Granular cell tumor of the larynx in a 5-year-old child. Ann Otol Rhinol Laryngol 93: 45–47
77. Gatti W M, Strom C G, Orfei E 1975 Synovial sarcoma of the laryngopharynx. Arch Otolaryngol 101: 633–636
78. Gaynor E B, Raghausen U, Weisbrot I M 1984 Primary myxoid liposarcoma of the larynx. Otolaryngol Head Neck Surg 92: 476–480
79. Gertner R, Podoshin L, Fradis M, Misselevitch I, Boss J 1988 Liposarcoma of the larynx. J Laryngol Otol 102: 838–841
80. Glover G W, Park W W 1971 Pharyngeal leiomyosarcoma. J Laryngol Otol 85: 1031–1038
81. Gnepp D R, Chandler W, Hyams V 1984 Primary Kaposi's sarcoma in the head and neck. Ann Intern Med 100: 107–114
82. Godoy J, Jacobs J R, Crissman J 1986 Malignant fibrous histiocytoma of the larynx. J Surg Oncol 31: 62–65
83. Goldofsky E, Hirschfield L S, Abramson A L 1988 An unusual laryngeal lesion in children: granular cell tumor. Int J Pediatr Otorhinolaryngol 15: 263–267
84. Gorenstein A, Neel H B III, Weiland L H, Devine K D 1980 Sarcomas of the larynx. Arch Otolaryngol 106: 8–12
85. Granich M S, Pilch B Z, Nadol J B, Dickersin G R 1983 Fetal rhabdomyoma of the larynx. Arch Otolaryngol 109: 821–826
86. Gridelli C, Palmieri G, Airoma G, Incoronato P, Pepe R, Barra E, Bianco A R 1990 Complete regression of laryngeal involvement by classic Kaposi's sarcoma with low-dose alpha-2b interferon. Tumori 76: 292–293
87. Gross M, Gutjahr P 1988 Therapy of rhabdomyosarcoma of the larynx. Int J Pediatr Otorhinolaryngol 15: 93–97
88. Gryczynski M 1971 Leiomyosarcoma krtani. Otolaryngol Pol 25: 545–548
89. Haerr R W, Turalba C I C, El-Mahdi A M, Brown K L 1987 Alveolar rhabdomyosarcoma of the larynx: case report and literature review. Laryngoscope 97: 339–344
90. Hall-Jones J 1972 Giant cell tumor of the larynx. J Laryngol Otol 86: 371–381
91. Hamper K, Renninghoff J, Schäfer H 1989 Rhabdomyoma of the larynx recurring after 12 years: immunocytochemistry and differential diagnosis. Arch Otorhinolaryngol 246: 222–226
92. Har-El G, Shviro J, Avidor I, Segal K, Sigi J 1985 Laryngeal granular cell tumor in children. Am J Otolaryngol 6: 32–34
93. Harris P F, Maness G M, Ward P H 1967 Leiomyoma of the larynx and trachea. South Med J 60: 1223–1226
94. Havens F Z, Parkhill E M 1941 Tumours of the larynx other than squamous cell epithelioma. Arch Otolaryngol 34: 1113–1122
95. Heffner D K 1984 Problems in pediatric otorhinolaryngic pathology. V. Disease of the larynx and trachea. Int J Pediatr Otorhinolaryngol 7: 203–219
96. Helliwell T R, Sissons M C J, Stoney P J, Ashworth M T 1988 Immunochemistry and electron microscopy of head and neck rhabdomyoma. J Clin Pathol 41: 1058–1063
97. Hertzanu Y, Mendelsohn D B, Kassner G, Hockman M 1982 Haemangiopericytoma of the larynx. Br J Radiol 55: 870–873
98. Hyams V J, Heffner D K 1987 Laryngeal pathology. In: Tucker H M (ed) The larynx. Thieme, New York, pp 33–78
99. Hymes K G, Cheung T, Greene J B, Marcus A, Ballard H 1981 Kaposi's sarcoma in homosexual men — a report of eight cases. Lancet ii: 598–600
100. Iqbal S M, Bhogoliwal S K, Nandi N B 1986 Laryngeal leiomyoma. J Laryngol Otol 100: 723–725
101. Jakobiec F A, Font R L, Tso M O M, Zimmerman L E 1977 Mesectodermal leiomyoma of the ciliary body. A tumor of presumed neural crest origin. Cancer 39: 2102–2113
102. Johnson J T, Poushter D L 1977 Fibrous histiocytoma of the subglottic larynx. Ann Otol Rhinol Laryngol 86: 243–246
103. Jones S R, Myers E N, Barnes E L 1988 Benign neoplasms of the larynx. In: Fried M P (ed) The larynx: a multidisciplinary approach. Brown, Boston
104. Jordan M B, Soames J V 1989 Fibrous histiocytoma of the larynx. J Laryngol Otol 103: 216–218
105. Kapur T R 1968 Recurrent lipomata of the larynx and the pharynx with late malignant change. J Laryngol Otol 82: 761–767
106. Karma P, Hyrynkangas K, Räsänen O 1978 Laryngeal leiomyoma. J Laryngol Otol 92: 411–415
107. Kawabe Y, Kondo T 1967 A laryngeal leiomyosarcoma. Evaluation of the authors' case and observation of the literature. Otolaryngology 39: 427–432
108. Kawashima O, Kamei T, Shimizu Y, Shizuka T, Nakayama M

1990 Malignant mesenchymoma of the larynx. J Laryngol Otol 104: 440–444

109. Kaya S, Saydam L, Ruacan S 1990 Laryngeal leiomyoma. Int J Pediatr Otorhinolaryngol 19: 285–288

110. Keenan J P, Snyder G G III, Toomey J M 1979 Malignant fibrous histiocytoma of the larynx. Otolaryngol Head Neck Surg 87: 599–603

111. Kiel K D, Suit H D 1984 Radiation therapy in the treatment of aggressive fibromatosis (desmoid tumors). Cancer 54: 2051–2055

112. Kinishi M, Amatsu M, Makino K, Yamauchi R, Okada S 1990 Malignant fibrous histiocytoma of the hypopharynx. ORL J Otorhinolaryngol Relat Spec 52: 47–50

113. Klap P, Reizine D, Monteil J P, Despreaux G, Hadjean E, Merland J J, Tran Ba Huy P 1984 Tumeurs et malformations vasculaires du larynx. Aspects angiographiques et indications thérapeutiques. Ann Otolaryngol Chir Cervicofac 101: 579–583

114. Kleinsasser O 1988 Tumors of the larynx and hypopharynx. Thieme, Stuttgart

115. Kleinsasser O, Glanz H 1979 Myogenic tumours of the larynx. Arch Otorhinolaryngol 225: 107–119

116. Kodet R, Fajstavr J, Kabelka Z, Koutecky J, Eckschlager T, Newton W A Jr 1991 Is fetal cellular rhabdomyoma an entity or a differentiated rhabdomyosarcoma? A study of patients with rhabdomyoma of the tongue and sarcoma of the tongue enrolled in the Intergroup Rhabdomyosarcoma Studies I, II, and III. Cancer 67: 2907–2913

117. Konior R J, Holinger L D, Russell E J 1988 Superselective embolization of laryngeal hemangioma. Laryngoscope 98: 830–834

118. Konrad E A, Melster P, Hübner G 1982 Extracardiac rhabdomyoma. Report of different types with light microscopic and ultrastructural studies. Cancer 49: 898–907

119. Krausen A S, Gall A M, Garza R, Spector G J, Ansel D G 1977 Liposarcoma of the larynx: a multicentric or a metastatic malignancy. Laryngoscope 87: 1116–1124

120. Kuzniar A 1971 A case of laryngeal hemangiopericytoma. Otolaryngol Pol 25: 467–468

121. Laurent C, Lindholm C E, Nordlinder H 1985 Benign pedunculated tumours of the hypopharynx. 3 case reports, 1 with late malignant transformation. ORL J Otorhinolaryngol Relat Spec 47: 17–21

122. Lawrence W Jr, Hays D M, Heyn R, Tefft M, Crist W, Beltangady M, Newton W Jr, Wharam M 1987 Lymphatic metastases with childhood rhabdomyosarcoma. A report from the Intergroup Rhabdomyosarcoma Study. Cancer 60: 910–915

123. Lehmann W, Piloux J M, Widmann J J 1981 Larynx. Microlaryngoscopy and histopathology. Inpharzam, Cadempino

124. Löbe L P, Katenkamp D 1984 Malignes fibröses Histiozytom des Larynx. Laryngol Rhinol Otol 63: 257–259

125. Majmudar B, Thomas J, Gorelkin L, Symbas P N 1981 Respiratory obstruction caused by a multicentric granular cell tumor of the laryngotracheobronchial tree. Human Pathol 12: 283–286

126. Majumder N K, Sharma H S, Srinivasan V 1989 Malignant fibrous histiocytoma of the larynx. J Laryngol Otol 103: 219–221

127. Malfatti T 1961 Contributo allo studio del mixoma della laringe. Minerva Otorinolaringol 11: 395–397

128. Manara E 1959 I tumori mesenchimali maligni della laringe. Considerazioni su di un caso di leiomiosarcoma. Otorinolaringol Ital 28: 167–178

129. Mankodi Rc, Shah S S, Kanvinde M S, Joshi J S 1970 Pharyngeal leiomyosarcoma. J Laryngol Otol 84: 327–330

130. Masuda K, Takimoto T, Yoshizaki T, Sakano K, Umeda R 1989 Malignant fibrous histiocytoma arising from vocal cord. ORL J Otorhinolaryngol Relat Spec 51: 365–368

131. McIntosh W A, Kassner G W, Murray J F 1985 Fibromatosis and fibrosarcoma of the larynx and pharynx in an infant. Arch Otolaryngol 111: 478–480

132. McRae R D R, Gatland D J, McNab Jones R F, Khan S 1990 Malignant transformation in a laryngeal hemangioma. Ann Otol Rhinol Laryngol 99: 562–565

133. Meis J M, Mackay B, Goepfert H 1986 Liposarcoma of the larynx. Case report and literature review. Arch Otolaryngol Head Neck Surg 112: 1289–1292

134. Mevio E, Galioto P, Scelsi M, Re P 1990 Neurofibroma of vocal cord: case report. Acta Otorhinolaryngol Belg 44: 447–450

135. Michaels L 1984 Pathology of the larynx. Springer-Verlag, Berlin

136. Miller D, Goodman M, Weber A, Goldstein A 1975 Primary liposarcoma of the larynx. Trans Am Acad Ophthalmol Otolaryngol 80: 444–447

137. Miller L H, Santaella-Latimer L, Miller T 1975 Synovial sarcoma of the larynx. Trans Am Acad Ophthalmol Otolaryngol 80: 448–451

138. Modlin B 1982 Rhabdomyoma of the larynx. Laryngoscope 92: 580–582

139. Moncade J, Demaldent J-E 1979 A propos de deux cas d'hémangiopéricytomes O.R.L. Ann Otolaryngol Chir Cervicofac 96: 789–792

140. Moretti J A, Miller D 1973 Laryngeal involvement in benign symmetric lipomatosis. Arch Otolaryngol 97: 495–496

140a. Mori H, Kumoi T, Hashimoto M, Uematsu K 1992 Leiomyoblastoma of the larynx: report of a case. Head Neck 14: 148–152

141. Mugliston T A H, Sangwan S 1985 Persistent cavernous haemangioma of the larynx — a pregnancy problem. J Laryngol Otol 99: 1309–1311

142. Naito K, Iwata S, Nishimura T, Yagisawa M, Sakurai K 1985 Laryngeal lymphangioma — case report. Auris Nasus Larynx 12: 111–116

143. Narula A, Jefferis A F 1985 Squamous cell carcinoma and liposarcoma of the larynx occurring metachronously. J Laryngol Otol 99: 509–511

144. Neblett L M, Coller F C 1981 Malignant fibrous histiocytoma of the larynx. Am J Otolaryngol 2: 163–166

145. Neivert H, Royer L 1946 Leiomyoma of the larynx. Arch Otolaryngol 44: 214–216

146. Norris C M, Peale A R 1961 Sarcoma of the larynx. Ann Otol Rhinol Laryngol 70: 894–909

147. Nuutinen J, Syrjänen K 1983 Angioleiomyoma of the larynx. Report of a case and review of the literature. Laryngoscope 93: 941–943

148. O'Connor A F F, Freeland A P 1980 Neonatal laryngeal neurofibromatosis. Ear Nose Throat J 59: 174–177

149. Ogura J H, Toomey J M, Setzen M, Sobol S 1980 Malignant fibrous histiocytoma of the head and neck. Laryngoscope 90: 1429–1440

150. Oppedal B R, Royne T, Titterud I 1985 Synovial sarcomas of the neck. A report of two cases. J Laryngol Otol 99: 101–104

151. Ordonez N G, Ro J Y, Mackay B 1989 Alveolar soft part sarcoma. An ultrastructural and immunocytochemical investigation of its histogenesis. Cancer 63: 1721–1736

152. Ortiz C L, Weber A L 1991 Laryngeal lipoma. Ann Otol Rhinol Laryngol 100: 783–784

153. Parham D M, Webber B, Holt H, Williams W K, Maurer H 1991 Immunohistochemical study of childhood rhabdomyosarcomas and related neoplasms. Results of an Intergroup Rhabdomyosarcoma Study Project. Cancer 67: 3072–3080

154. Parke R B, Donovan D T, Schwartz M R, Irani D R 1988 Soft tissue tumors of the larynx. Second International Conference on Head and Neck Cancer, Boston, abstract 357, p 137

155. Pearlman S J, Friedman E A, Appel M 1950 Neurofibroma of the larynx. Arch Otolaryngol 52: 8–14

156. Pennelli N, Mazzilli G 1962 Leiomiosarcoma del laringe. Arch Ital Laringol 70: 343–355

157. Pesavento G, Ferlito A 1982 Haemangiopericytoma of the larynx. A clinico-pathological study with review of the literature. J Laryngol Otol 96: 1065–1073

158. Pownell P H, Brown O E, Argyle J C, Manning S C 1990 Rhabdomyoma of the cricopharyngeus in an infant. Int J Pediatr Otorhinolaryngol 20: 149–158

159. Pratt L W, Goodof I I 1968 Hemangioendotheliosarcoma of the larynx. Arch Otolaryngol 87: 484–489

160. Quesada P, Medina A, Ortiz F 1978 Angioleiomioma de laringe. An Otorrinolaringol Ibero Am 5: 265–270

161. Ramadass I, Balasubramanian V C, Annamala L 1984 Malignant pleomorphic fibrous histiocytoma of the larynx. A case report with a review of the literature. J Laryngol Otol 98: 93–96

162. Raney R B Jr, Crist W M, Maurer H M, Foulkes M A 1983 Prognosis of children with soft tissue sarcoma who relapse after achieving a complete response. A report from the Intergroup Rhabdomyosarcoma Study I. Cancer 52: 44–50

163. Rangdaeng S, Truong L D 1991 Comparative immunohistochemical staining for desmin and muscle-specific actin. A study of 576 cases. Am J Clin Pathol 96: 32–45

164. Reid A P, Hussain S S M, Pahor A L 1987 Lipoma of the larynx. J Laryngol Otol 101: 1308–1311

165. Ribari O, Elemer G, Balint A 1975 Laryngeal giant cell tumour. J Laryngol Otol 89: 857–861

166. Rivas S, Peris J L, Mayayo E, Tortosa V 1982 Histiocytoma fibroso maligno de laringe. Acta Otorrinolaringol Esp 33: 637–640

167. Robb P J, Girling A 1989 Granular cell myoblastoma of the supraglottis. J Laryngol Otol 103: 328–330

167a. Roels H 1992 Histopathology of laryngeal tumours. Acta Otorhinolaryngol Belg 46: 127–139

168. Rolander T, Kim O J, Shumrick D A 1972 Fibrous xanthoma of the larynx. Arch Otolaryngol 96: 168–170

169. Rosenberg H S, Vogler C, Close L G, Warshaw H E 1981 Laryngeal fibromatosis in the neonate. Arch Otolaryngol 107: 513–517

170. Rosenman D, Gertner R, Fradis M, Podoshin L, Misslevitsch A, Boss J H 1986 Rhabdomyoma of the larynx. J Laryngol Otol 100: 607–610

171. Rubin J S, Silver C E 1988 Surgical approach to vascular tumors of the supraglottis. Second International Conference on Head and Neck Cancer, Boston, abstract 285, p 119

172. Saha A M, Mukherjee D, Chatterjee D N, Mukherjee A L, Mondal A 1989 Malignant fibrous histiocytoma of the larynx. J Indian Med Assoc 87: 73–74

173. Schaeffer B T, Som P M, Biller H F, Som M L, Arnold L M 1986 Schwannomas of the larynx: review and computed tomographic scan analysis. Head Neck Surg 8: 469–472

174. Schrader M 1988 Verbesserte Diagnostik des Larynxlipoms durch die Computertomographie. HNO 36: 161–163

175. Schwartz M R, Donovan D T 1987 Hemangiopericytoma of the larynx: a case report and review of the literature. Otolaryngol Head Neck Surg 96: 369–372

176. Scrivner D, Meyers J S 1980 Multifocal recurrent adult rhabdomyoma. Cancer 46: 790–795

177. Sena T, Brady M S, Huvos A G, Spiro R H 1991 Laryngeal myxoma. Arch Otolaryngol Head Neck Surg 117: 430–432

178. Setzen M, Sobol S, Toomey J M 1977 Clinical course of unusual malignant sarcomas of head and neck. Ann Otol Rhinol Laryngol 88: 486–494

179. Shah M C, Lowry L D 1984 Primary liposarcoma of the larynx. Trans Pa Acad Ophthalmol Otolaryngol 37: 49–52

180. Shanmugaratnam K 1991 Histological typing of tumours of the upper respiratory tract and ear. World Health Organization. International histological classification of tumours, 2nd edn. Springer-Verlag, Berlin

181. Shibata K, Komune S 1980 Laryngeal angiomyoma (vascular leiomyoma): clinicopathological findings. Laryngoscope 90: 1880–1886

182. Shikhani A H, Jones M M, Marsh B R, Holliday M J 1986 Infantile subglottic hemangiomas. An update. Ann Otol Rhinol Laryngol 95: 336–347

183. Shin W-Y, Abramson A L 1976 The value of electron microscopy in the diagnosis of fibrosarcoma of the larynx. Trans Am Acad Ophthalmol Otolaryngol 82: 582–587

184. Sidman J, Wood R E, Poole M, Postma D S 1987 Management of plexiform neurofibroma of the larynx. Ann Otol Rhinol Laryngol 96: 53–55

185. Smith N M, Stafford F W 1991 Postcricoid lymphangioma. J Laryngol Otol 105: 220–221

186. Sokolenko S M, Kornilov B E, Averin A A 1984 Leiomyosarcoma of the larynx. Vestn Otorinolaringol 3: 75

187. Stanley R J, Scheithauer B W, Weiland L H, Neel H B III 1987 Neural and neuroendocrine tumors of the larynx. Ann Otol Rhinol Laryngol 96: 630–638

188. Stout A P 1956 Tumors featuring pericytes: glomus tumor and hemangiopericytoma. Lab Invest 5: 217–233

189. Stout A P 1961 Pseudosarcomatous fasciitis in children. Cancer 14: 1216–1222

190. Stout A P, Murray M R 1942 Hemangiopericytoma: a vascular tumor featuring Zimmerman's pericytes. Ann Surg 116: 26–33

191. Stricker F J 1949 Neurinom und Spindelzellsarkom des Kehlkopfes. HNO 1: 554–555

192. Supance J S, Quenelle D J, Crissman J 1980 Endolaryngeal neurofibromas. Otolaryngol Head Neck Surg 88: 74–78

193. Sutow W W, Lindberg R D, Gehan E A, Rogab A H, Raney R B Jr, Ruymann F, Soule E H 1982 Three-year relapse-free survival rates in childhood rhabdomyosarcoma of the head and neck. Report from the Intergroup Rhabdomyosarcoma Study. Cancer 49: 2217–2221

194. Szczudrawa J, Betkowski A 1971 Przyczynek do rzadkich guzow krtani Haemangioleiomyolipoma. Patol Pol 22: 387–389

195. Taguchi K, Yoda M, Maruyama Y 1974 Hemangiopericytoma of the larynx: a case report. Otolaryngology (Tokyo) 46: 21–33

196. Talavera Sanchez J, Segura Coronado E, Sanchez Hidalgo A 1969 Associaciòn laringocele leiomiosarcoma de la cuerda vocal. Acta Otorrinolaringol Esp 20: 74–85

197. Tewary A K, Pahor A L 1991 Leiomyosarcoma of the larynx: emergency laryngectomy. J Laryngol Otol 105: 134–136

198. Thedinger B A, Cheney M L, Montgomery W W, Goodman M 1991 Leiomyosarcoma of the trachea. Case report. Ann Otol Rhinol Laryngol 100: 337–340

199. Thomas R L 1979 Non-epithelial tumours of the larynx. J Laryngol Otol 93: 1131–1141

200. Tobey D N, Wheelis R F, Yarington C T Jr 1979 Electron microscopy in the diagnosis of liposarcoma and fibrosarcoma of the larynx. Ann Otol Rhinol Laryngol 88: 867–871

201. Tommerup B, Mogensen Chr, Nielsen A L 1985 A leiomyosarcoma of the hypopharynx. J Laryngol Otol 99: 605–608

202. Toncini C, Pesce C 1985 Granular cell tumours of the oesophagus and larynx. J Laryngol Otol 99: 1301–1304

203. Triplet I, Vankemmel B, Madelain M 1974 Hémangioendothéliome malin du larynx avec métastases sous-cutanées. Lille Médical 19: 743–745

204. Tse J J, Vander S 1985 The soft tissue myxoma of the head and neck region — report of a case and literature review. Head Neck Surg 7: 479–483

205. Tucker H M 1987 The larynx. Thieme, New York

206. Van Den Eeckhaut J, Fievez CL, Remacle M, Coffyn M-B, Marbaix E 1983 Rhabdomyome adulte du larynx. A propos d'un cas. Ann Otolaryngol Chir Cervicofac 100: 151–153

207. Vanhaudenarde J M, Berrier A, Parent M, Martiat B, Piquet J J 1987 Les Schwannomes isolés du larynx — Etude de 4 cas. Revue de la littérature. Acta Otorhinolaryngol Belg 41: 94–107

208. Velek J P 1976 Liposarcoma of the larynx. Trans Am Acad Ophthalmol Otolaryngol 82: 569–570

209. Volmer J 1985 Malignes fibröses Histiozytom des Larynx. Laryngol Rhinol Otol 64: 579–581

210. von Urfer F 1946 Myxolipom des Kehlkopfes. Pract Otorhinolaryngol 8: 545–550

211. Walike J W, Bailey B J 1971 Head and neck hemangiopericytoma. Arch Otolaryngol 93: 345–353

211a. Weber B-P, Kempf H-G, Kaiserling E 1992 Maligne fibröse Histiozytome in Kopf-Hals-Bereich. Laryngol Rhinol Otol 71: 43–49

211b. Weber R, Kronsbein H 1992 Der Seltene Fall — Neurilemmom der Stimmlippe. Laryngol Rhinol Otol 71: 426–428

212. Weiss A J, Lackman R D 1989 Low-dose chemotherapy of desmoid tumors. Cancer 64: 1192–1194

213. Wenig B M, Weiss S W, Gnepp D R 1990 Laryngeal and hypopharyngeal liposarcoma. A clinicopathologic study of 10 cases with a comparison to soft tissue counterparts. Am J Surg Pathol 14: 134–141

214. Werning J T 1979 Nodular fasciitis of the orofacial region. Oral Surg 48: 441–446

215. Wetmore R F 1987 Fibrous histiocytoma of the larynx in a child. Case report and review. Clin Pediatr 26: 200–202

216. Wharam M D, Beltangady M S, Heyn R M, Lawrence W, Raney R B Jr, Ruymann F B, Soule E H, Tefft M, Maurer H M 1987 Pediatric orofacial and laryngopharyngeal rhabdomyosarcoma. An Intergroup Rhabdomyosarcoma Study Report. Arch Otolaryngol Head Neck Surg 113: 1225–1227

217. Wharam M D Jr, Foulkes M A, Lawrence W Jr, Lindberg R D,

Maurer H M, Newton W A Jr, Ragab A H, Raney R B Jr, Tefft M 1984 Soft tissue sarcoma of the head and neck in childhood: nonorbital and nonparameningeal sites. A report of the Intergroup Rhabdomyosarcoma Study (IRS-1). Cancer 53: 1016–1019

218. Winther L K 1976 Rhabdomyoma of the hypopharynx and larynx. Report of two cases and a review of the literature. J Laryngol Otol 90: 1041–1051

219. Wolfowitz B L, Schmaman A 1973 Smooth-muscle tumours of the upper respiratory tract. S Afr Med J 47: 1189–1191

220. Yankauer S 1924 Angio-sarcoma of the larynx removed by indirect laryngoscopy. Laryngoscope 34: 488

221. Yokoi H, Takasu A, Horibe Y, Takigawa T. Matsunaga H, Nishimura T, Iwata S 1982 Malignant fibrous histiocytoma of the larynx: a case report. J Otolaryngol Jap 85: 70

222. Yokoyama R, Shinohara N, Tsuneyoshi M, Masuda S, Enjoji M 1989 Extra-abdominal desmoid tumors: correlations between histologic features and biologic behavior. Surg Pathol 2: 29–42

223. Zak A, Rowinska E 1988 Coexistence of leiomyosarcoma and carcinoma planoepitheliale of the larynx. Wiad Lek 41: 1387–1389

224. Zakrzewski A 1965 Subglottic lipoma of the larynx. J Laryngol Otol 79: 1039–1048

225. Zarbo R J, Crissman J D, Venkat H, Weiss M A 1986 Spindle cell carcinoma of the upper aerodigestive tract mucosa. An immunohistologic and ultrastructural study of 18 biphasic tumors and comparison with seven monophasic spindle cell tumors. Am J Surg Pathol 10: 741–753

16. Cartilaginous and osteogenic neoplasms

A. Ferlito

Cartilaginous and osteogenic neoplasms of the larynx include chondroma, chondrosarcoma and osteosarcoma. Several neoplasms reported as giant cell tumours of the larynx were in fact cases of malignant fibrous histiocytoma, giant cell variant or aneurysmal bone cyst.

CHONDROMA

Chondromas of the larynx are considered uncommon and occur most frequently in males, usually in middle age. These tumours may be solitary or multiple and can arise from any cartilage of the laryngeal skeleton. The neoplasm resembles the histology of normal cartilage (Fig. 16.1), but increased cellularity may be seen. Diagnosis is made by direct laryngoscopy and biopsy. Traves is credited with the first description of this lesion in the larynx in 1816,[68] and about 250 cases had been reported up to 1981.[3] A congenital chondroma of the larynx has also been reported.[1] A critical review of chondroma cases is virtually impossible, because most reports lack pathological documentation and follow-up data. Accounts of cases in which a diagnosis of primary chondroma was followed by the diagnosis of chondrosarcoma for the recurrent tumour lead us to assume that the incidence of chondroma has always been overestimated.[55] Only two cases of laryngeal chondroma were seen at the Mayo Clinic between 1910 and 1979 among a total of 33 cartilaginous tumours of the larynx.[52] Of 323 cases of benign neoplasms of the larynx reviewed from the pathology files of the Eye and Ear Hospital and Presbyterian University Hospital of Pittsburgh, dating from 1955 to 1984, only two cases were observed.[42] No cases of chondroma were found at the ENT Department of Padua University between 1966 and 1992. A lot of cases reported even in recent years as chondroma are found to be chondrosarcomas when the material is reviewed by experts.[66]

In the past, chondroma of the larynx has also been confused with chondrometaplasia. The differential clinical and pathological appearances between the two lesions are presented in Table 16.1. Chondrometaplasia is characterized by fibroblastic proliferation with myxoid changes in the stroma and the appearance of lacunae, simulating hyaline cartilage. Elastic stains demonstrate excessive elastic deposits in the cartilaginous areas as observed in normal elastic cartilage. The extent of metaplastic change may vary from focal areas to concentric nodules of elastic cartilage. Cartilaginous changes in vocal cord nodules represent metaplasia rather than neoplasia and should be considered as a variant in vocal cord nodules exposed to excessive trauma or irradiation.[17,38] In a study of 205 unselected human larynxes removed at autopsy, foci of fibroelastic cartilage of metaplastic origin were found in about 1–2% of the organs examined. The age of subjects ranged from 14 to 98 years. A focus of metaplastic fibroelastic cartilage was also found in both the vestibular folds of an orangutan (*Pongo pygmaeus*).[35] In a review of 377 vocal cord nodules resected at the Massachusetts Eye and Ear Infirmary over a two-year period, 34 nodules were found to contain elastic cartilage.[8]

Nodules of elastic cartilage are quite commonly found in the false cord and true cord.[48]

Table 16.1 The differential diagnosis of chondrometaplasia and chondroma of the larynx[1]

	Chondrometaplasia	Chondroma
Symptoms	Hoarseness (possibly asymptomatic)	Obstruction of the airway or swelling of the neck
Gross presentation	Small nodule less than 1 cm in diameter	Multilobular tumour
Site of lesion	Ventricular fold and vocal cord	Cricoid and thyroid cartilages
Type of cartilage	Elastic	Hyaline (usually)

[1]From Ferlito and Recher.[20]

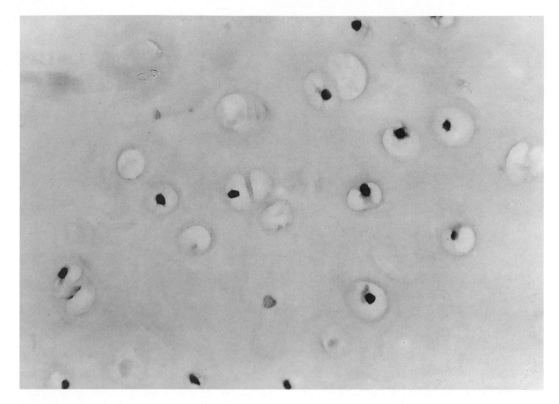

Fig. 16.1 Chondroma of the larynx. The cellularity of this chondroma approaches that of normal cartilage. H&E, ×400. (Courtesy of Dr L. Barnes, Pittsburgh.)

The treatment of chondroma is surgical[14] and a conservative approach should be used wherever possible.

CHONDROSARCOMA

Introduction

Chondrosarcomas are slow-growing tumours rarely encountered in the head and neck, where the larynx is one of the most frequently affected sites.

These neoplasms account for approximately 20% of all bone tumours in the body as a whole.

Terminology

New[54] first used the term 'chondrosarcoma of the larynx' in 1935. Various terms have since been applied to this neoplastic lesion, such as non-calcifying chondrosarcoma, malignant chondroma, dedifferentiated chondrosarcoma, chondrosarcoma which malignant mesenchymal component, extraskeletal chondrosarcoma, extra-osseous chondrosarcoma.

Definition

Chondrosarcoma is a malignant tumour characterized by the formation of cartilage by the tumour cells.

Incidence

Chondrosarcoma (and not fibrosarcoma, as was commonly thought in the past) must be considered the most frequent sarcoma of the larynx.[19,21] In a review by Nicolai et al,[55] approximately 200 cases of this malignant tumour were collected from the world literature. Several more cases have since been reported.[4a,5a,6a,7,14a,27,36,49,51,58a,61,64a,66a,72] Two cases have been reported in association with prior radiation treatment.[26,27]

Clinical features

This neoplasm is most frequent in patients between the age of 50 and 70, but it may also occur in young people.[72] The male-to-female ratio is 3:1. The most common site of origin is the cricoid cartilage (75%), especially the posterior lamina (Fig. 16.2). However, there are also reports of its onset in the thyroid cartilage, arytenoid cartilages, epiglottis and accessory cartilages. Observation of some chondrosarcoma cases originating from the epiglottis (Figs 16.3–16.5)[22,29,40,43,58,72] disproves the commonly held notion that this tumour occurs only in hyaline and not in elastic cartilage.[62] Chondrosarcoma may also involve the hyoid bone,[13,23,30,33a] but this is not anatomically a part of the larynx.

Symptoms consist of progressive hoarseness, dyspnoea and dysphagia, varying according to tumour location.

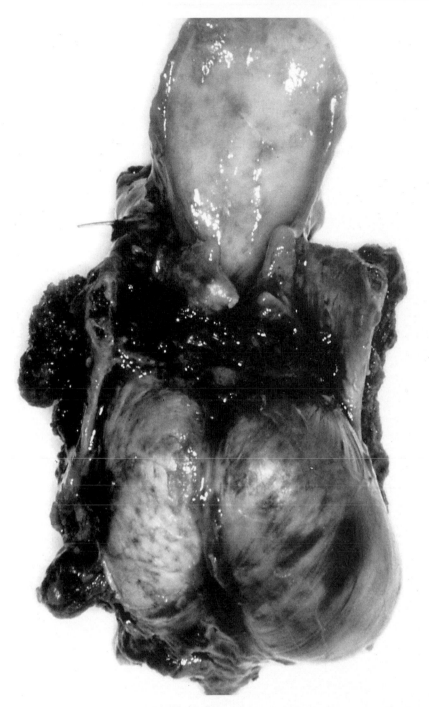

Fig. 16.2 Front view of a surgical specimen of a laryngeal chondrosarcoma showing lobulated aspect.

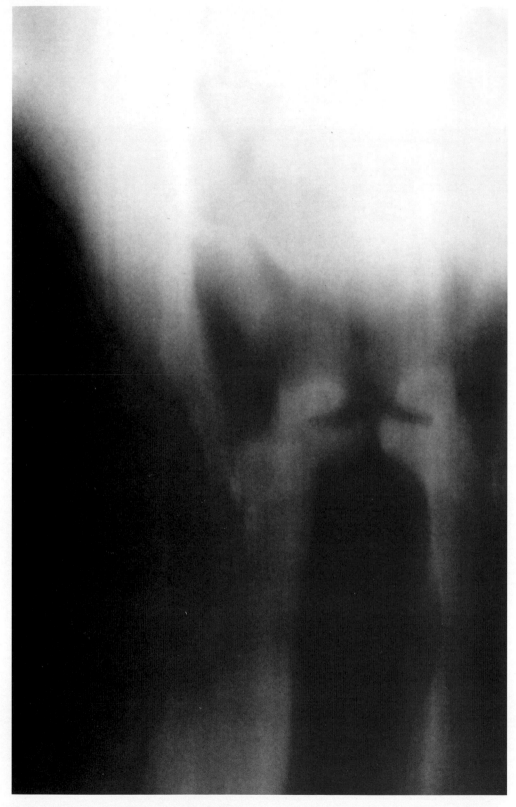

Fig. 16.3 Tomogram of the larynx, showing a large mass at the level of the epiglottis, with normal true and false vocal cords. (Courtesy of Dr D.G. John, Cardiff, and the editor of *Journal of Laryngology and Otology*.)

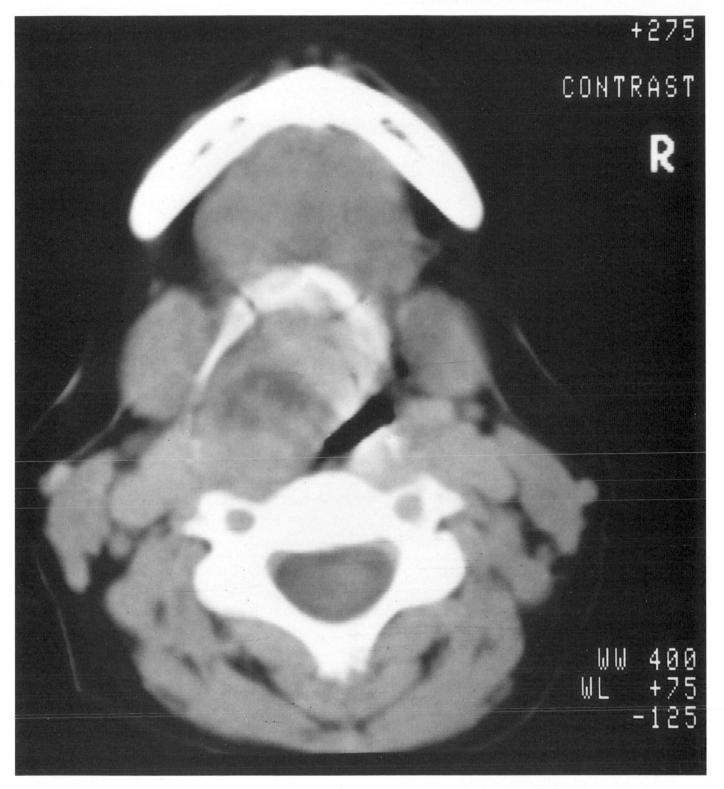

Fig. 16.4 CT scan showing horizontal section at the level of the hyoid bone. A large mass is seen in the area of the epiglottis, which, on the left, extends as far as the lateral pharyngeal wall and which severely narrows the airway. (Courtesy of Dr D. G. John, Cardiff, and the editor of *Journal of Laryngology and Otology*.)

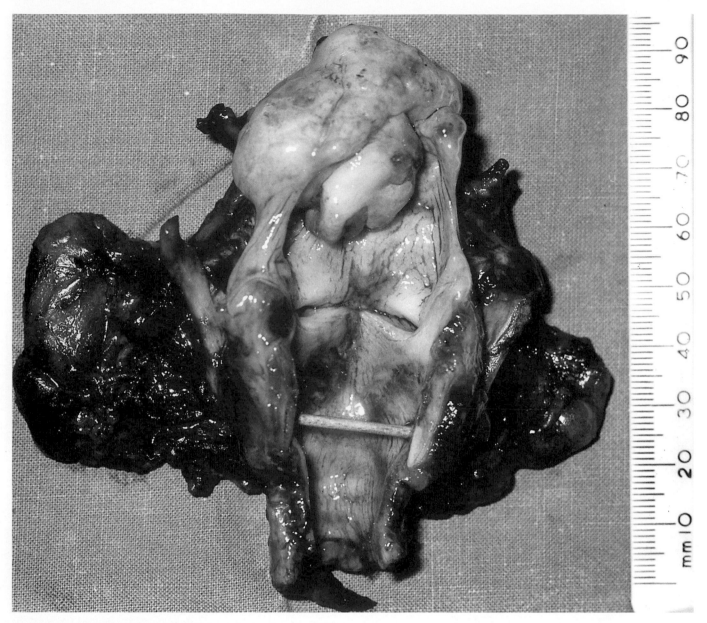

Fig. 16.5 Laryngectomy specimen opened posteriorly, with large epiglottic tumour. (Courtesy of Dr D. G. John, Cardiff, and the editor of *Journal of Laryngology and Otology*.)

Dyspnoea will predominate if the neoplasm extends anteriorly into the lumen of the airway. If it develops posteriorly into the pharynx, dysphagia will result. As the neoplasm is usually slow-growing, the patient may adapt to progressive narrowing of the airway until an episode of acute inspiratory dyspnoea leads to emergency tracheostomy.[44] When the neoplasm originates from the thyroid cartilage, the major complaint may be the presence of a hard lump in the neck produced by the tumour mass. As found in some cases reported in the literature,[32,47,55] the first clinical sign may be vocal cord paralysis, apparently unassociated with other laryngeal or non-laryngeal lesions and thus labelled as idiopathic. Vocal cord paralysis is almost exclusively an early sign of cricoid chondro-

sarcoma and may be related to involvement of the recurrent nerve or fixation of the cricoarytenoid joint.

On routine radiographs of the neck, the neoplasm usually appears as a mass with variable patterns of calcification.[61]

Computed tomography with contrast medium is very useful for demonstrating the extent of the lesion (Figs 16.6, 16.7) and for leading to the diagnosis of a cartilaginous tumour. A lesion with calcified areas, extensively involving one or more cartilages and moderately enhancing after injection of intravenous contrast medium, is a typical CT finding for laryngeal cartilaginous tumour.[51] However, there are no reliable radiographic criteria to enable differentiation between chondrosarcoma and chondroma.

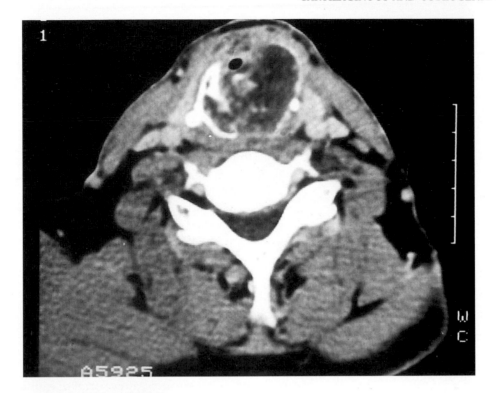

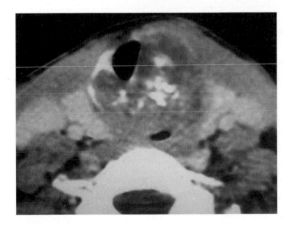

Fig. 16.6 (*top*) Axial computed tomogram showing a large, hypodense lesion arising from cricoid cartilage and severely narrowing airway.

Fig. 16.7 (*bottom*) Axial computed tomogram demonstrating a massive lesion stemming from cricoid cartilage with multiple foci of coarse calcification.

According to recent reports, magnetic resonance imaging (Fig. 16.8) can also demonstrate the lesion within the larynx and has the additional advantage of superior contrast resolution of the neoplasm and paralaryngeal tissues.[36,49,55,64a]

Pathology

Gross pathology

The tumour presents as a lobulated submucosal, rounded or oval mass covered by intact laryngeal mucosa. The neoplasm may be uniformly hard or may have soft and even cystic areas of degeneration (Fig. 16.9). Even in the more advanced stages, the tumour tends to develop within the cartilage (Fig. 16.10) and only rarely, or in the case of recurrence, extends beyond the external perichondrium, invading the surrounding tissues.[2,26]

Histopathology

Chondrosarcomas must be distinguished as low-grade (grade I), medium-grade (grade II) and high-grade (grade III).

The histological pattern of low-grade chondrosarcoma is similar to that of benign chondroma. The neoplasm is composed of abundant basophilic and metachromatic cartilaginous matrices in which the cells show small, densely staining nuclei. Binucleated and occasionally even multinucleated cells may be found (Fig. 16.11) Features of nuclear irregularity and the prominence of nucleoli are also indicative of malignancy. Mitoses are usually absent. Calcification and bone formation are frequent. In the larynx the tumour is usually well differentiated.[23]

Medium-grade chondrosarcoma shows an increased cellularity, particularly at the periphery of the lobules. The nucleus–cytoplasm ratio of the chondrocytes is low (i.e. cytoplasm is abundant with respect to nucleus size). Plump binucleated cells are also seen. Mitoses, if any, are scarce.

High-grade chondrosarcoma shows pronounced cellularity, and plump binucleated and multinucleated cells are often seen. The chondrocytes have large nuclei with nucleoli and delicate chromatin, and the nucleus–cytoplasm ratio is relatively high. Mitoses are frequently seen.[18]

A particular variant, called dedifferentiated chondrosarcoma, has also been reported in the larynx.[5,5a,11a,22,32,41,49a,71,71a] This term indicates a neoplasm in which a spindle cell component is associated with cartilaginous proliferation (Figs 16.12–16.14).

Another morphological variant of chondrosarcoma occasionally found in the larynx is myxoid chondrosarcoma.[21] The tumour is composed of rounded or elongated cells arranged in nests or ribbons embedded in basophilic homogeneous myxoid material.

Immunocytochemistry

Chondrosarcomas show positive staining for S-100 protein (Fig. 16.15) and vimentin.[5a,55] The dedifferentiated and myxoid chondrosarcomas are also positive for S-100 protein.[5,5a,72]

Electron microscopy

The tumour shows malignant chondrocytes, mostly round, with short processes and scalloping of the membrane. Nuclei are indented or very irregular and have dispersed chromatin, occasionally with large nucleoli. Cytoplasm is abundant and contains numerous short, branching segments of rough endoplasmic reticulum, often distended (Fig. 16.16), with variable amounts of flocculent material. The Golgi apparatus is prominent, and small clusters of glycogen and a few lipid droplets are also observed. The matrix is composed of fine elements and small proteoglycan granules. (Fig. 16.17) Binucleated cells are often present.[15,22]

Diagnosis and differential diagnosis

It is not always easy to obtain an adequate biopsy sample from laryngeal cartilaginous tumours because of their submucosal location and consistency. It is advisable to take the biopsy sample under general anaesthesia and it often proves necessary to perform a preliminary tracheotomy to obtain easier access to the lesion. Laryngeal chondrosarcomas often present areas with different degrees of differentiation, so that only a generous biopsy sample provides a reliable definition of the tumour's nature and microscopic features. A correct diagnosis has also been obtained from a needle biopsy under CT scan guidance.

The distinction between benign and malignant varieties of cartilaginous neoplasms of the larynx is often difficult. Cases reported in the literature as benign chondromas, which were actually laryngeal chondrosarcomas, are not uncommon—and correct diagnosis could not be established until recurrence or metastases developed. In addition, according to Thomas[67] there is no evidence of the transformation of chondroma into chondrosarcoma.

To establish the diagnosis between benign and malignant lesions, attention should be concentrated more on the cells than on the intercellular substance. In well-differentiated examples, malignancy is to be suspected in the presence of: many cells with plump nuclei; more than occasional cells with two such nuclei; giant cartilage cells with large, single or multiple nuclei or with irregular clumps of chromatin. Nuclear irregularity and the prominence of nucleoli are additional features suggestive of malignancy. Mitoses are usually scanty. Lobularity is often also a microscopic feature, the periphery of lobules often showing high cellularity and cytological irregularities.[25]

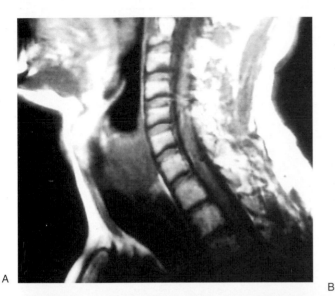

A

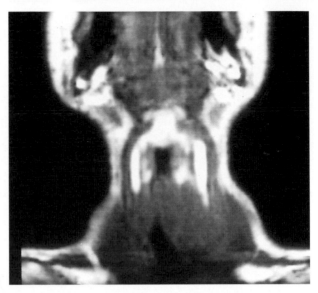

B

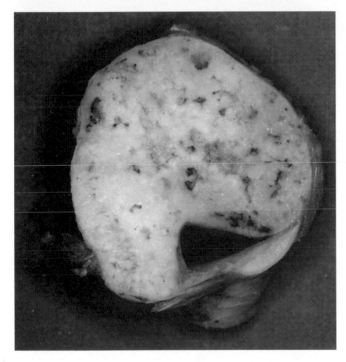

Fig. 16.8   A. (*top, left*) T1-weighted magnetic resonance images. Note posterior extension of tumour, extensive destruction of cricoid cartilage, and partial involvement of both thyroid cartilage and first tracheal ring. Sagittal plane. B. (*top, right*) Coronal plane.

Fig. 16.9 (*bottom*) Cross section of the specimen of tumour shown in Fig. 16.2.

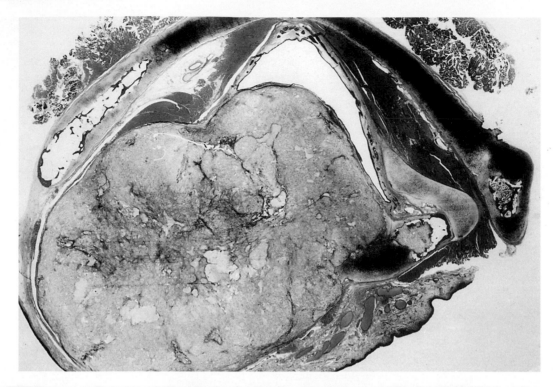

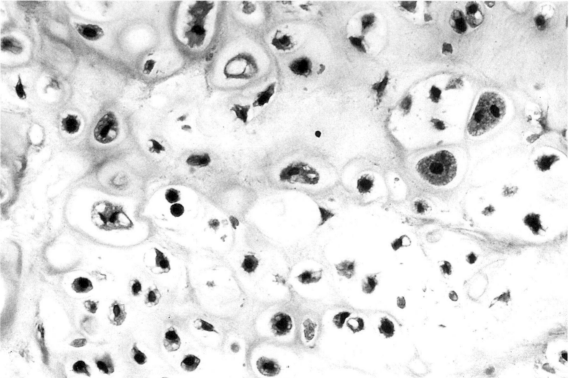

Fig. 16.10 (*top*) Cross section through a total laryngectomy specimen made on the level of the upper portion of the cricoid. A large, expansile cartilaginous lesion — still limited by external perichondrium — is visible.

Fig. 16.11 (*bottom*) Low-grade chondrosarcoma. Lacunae contain plump irregular cells which are occasionally binucleated. H&E, ×100 OM.

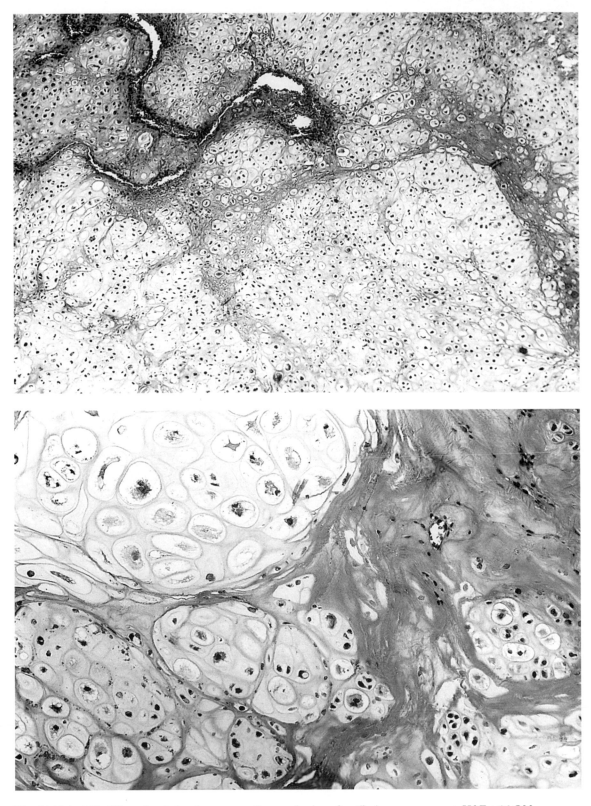

Fig. 16.12 (*top*) Dedifferentiated chondrosarcoma. Panoramic view of cartilaginous component. H&E, ×16 OM.

Fig. 16.13 (*bottom*) The tumour shows lobulated cartilaginous tissues. H&E, ×100 OM.

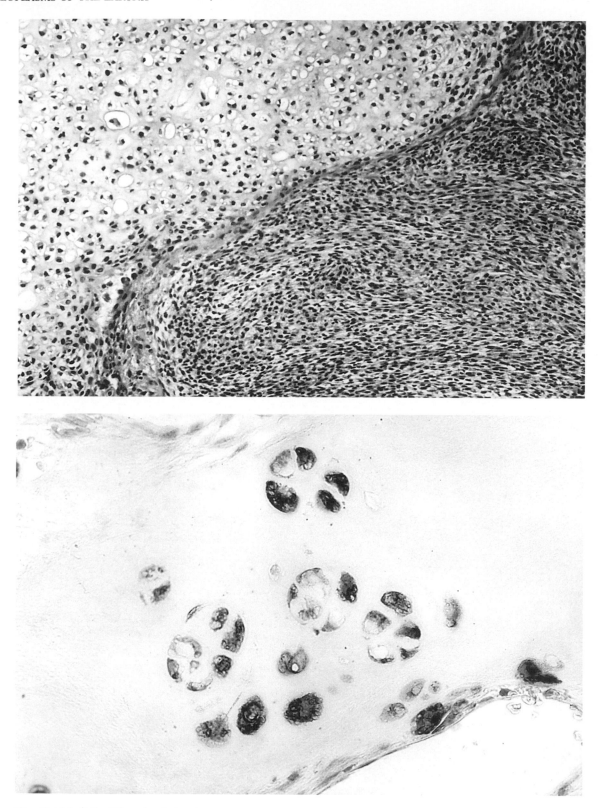

Fig. 16.14 (*top*) Dedifferentiated chondrosarcoma. Note the association of cartilaginous and spindle cell components. H&E, ×40 OM.

Fig. 16.15 (*bottom*) Diffuse positivity for S-100 protein is present. Immunoperoxidase, ×100 OM.

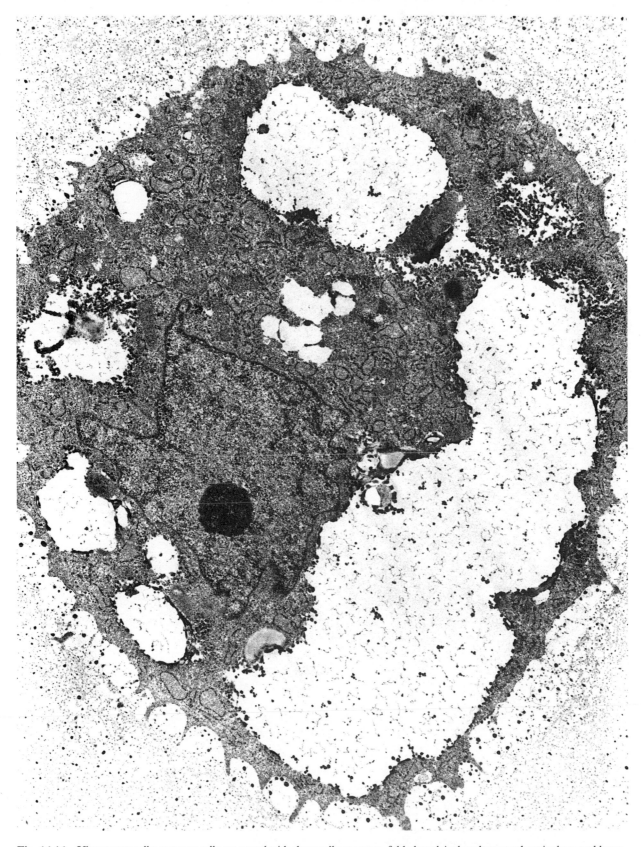

Fig. 16.16   Ultrastructurally, tumour cells are round with short cell processes, folded nuclei, abundant rough reticulum and large pools of intracytoplasmic proteoglycans. ×4000 OM.

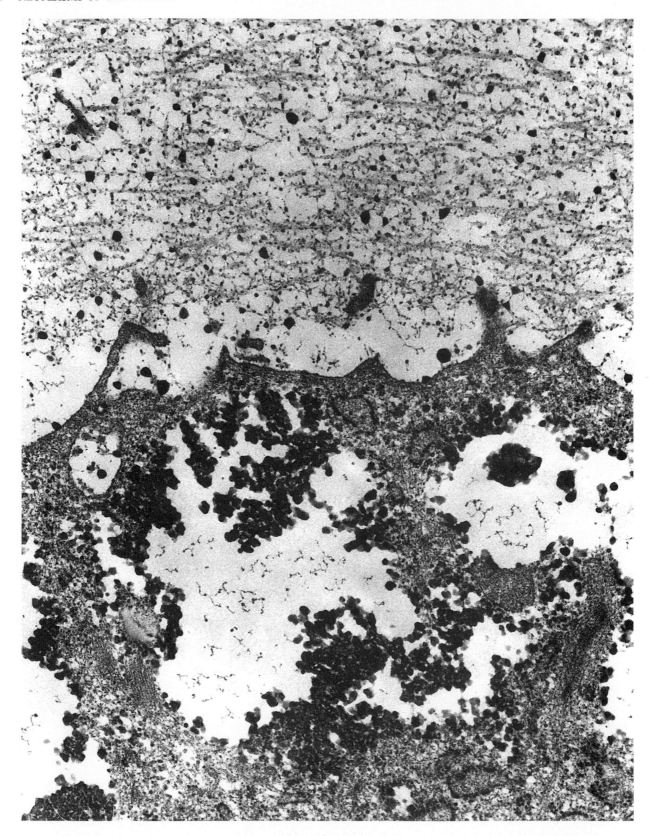

Fig. 16.17 At higher magnification the matrix is composed of fibrils and proteoglycan granules. ×10 000 OM.

Photometric investigation of the DNA content of cells may provide an aid in the differential diagnosis of chondroma and highly differentiated chondrosarcoma.[34] The differential diagnosis of chondroblastic osteosarcoma may be assisted by examining the alkaline phosphatase in smears or cryostat sections. All osteosarcomas (whether osteoblastic, chondroblastic, fibroblastic or anaplastic) produce abundant alkaline phosphatase, whereas this enzyme is not found in high-grade chondrosarcomas.[60] Areas of calcification and non-neoplastic bone may be present in chondrosarcoma but, unlike osteosarcoma, bone formation by the tumour cells is not seen.

Differential diagnosis must also be made with respect to fibrosarcoma, myxoid liposarcoma, embryonal rhabdomyosarcoma, spindle cell squamous carcinoma with cartilaginous metaplasia and chondrometaplasia.[20]

Spread

Chondrosarcoma of the larynx is primarily a local invader but lymphogenous and haematogenous metastases (Figs 16.18, 16.19) have been observed in 19 cases (see Table 16.2). The lungs and lymph nodes are most frequently involved. Other metastases have occurred in the kidney, spleen and cervical spine.[22]

Therapy

Surgical excision is commonly regarded as the treatment of choice for this tumour. Radiotherapy does not seem to play an important role, though it has been used in the past for recurrent tumours unsuitable for surgical treatment.[2,6] Conservative surgical techniques may certainly be considered the mainstay for treating laryngeal chondrosarcoma, but must be strictly applied to ensure that the tumour is radically removed, with a wide margin of normal tissue, and that the external perichondrium is resected on a level with the lesion.[55] The majority of recurrences observed in the past were probably related to piecemeal excisions sparing the external perichondrium. Supraglottic laryngectomy is indicated only when the lesion is restricted to the supraglottic region.[22,40]

The problem becomes more complex when dealing with cricoid lesions, because this cartilage is considered the keystone in maintaining an adequate laryngeal airway. When the lesion is limited in size and involves less than half of the cricoid, conservative removal through a laryngofissure can be used. Different techniques have been described to reconstruct the laryngeal lumen and to prevent stenosis.[4,9] Neis et al[53] have reported using a rib graft after removing more than half of the cricoid for a grade I chondrosarcoma. Although the results of these reconstruction techniques seem encouraging, the number of cases is so limited that no conclusions can be drawn as yet.[55]

Considering that cervical lymph node metastases are rare, neck dissection must be reserved for cases in which the clinical picture or imaging techniques suggest lymph node involvement.

Chemotherapy has not proved to be effective for chondrosarcoma of the larynx.

Prognosis

Chondrosarcomas range from locally aggressive non-metastasizing neoplasms which occasionally invade the thyroid gland[59] to high-grade malignancies which metastasize via the blood stream to the lungs.[25]

A statistically significant evaluation of prognostic determinants and different surgical techniques (conservative versus radical) is hindered by the fact that the data in the literature do not allow for a comparative analysis between sufficiently homogeneous groups of patients.[55] Lavertu and Tucker[46] compared the results of conservative and radical operations in a total of 46 patients suffering from laryngeal chondrosarcoma and concluded that the difference, in terms of cure rate, was not significant (77% versus 86%). However, the groups of patients used for comparison varied as to the lesion's site, extent and differentiation and the duration of follow-up.

Generally speaking, the clinical course of this neoplasm depends on the tumour's degree of differentiation and extent, as well as on the adequacy of primary treatment. Grade I chondrosarcomas usually show a local malignancy with a minimal propensity for metastasizing. Metastases are more frequent in grade II and even more so in grade III.

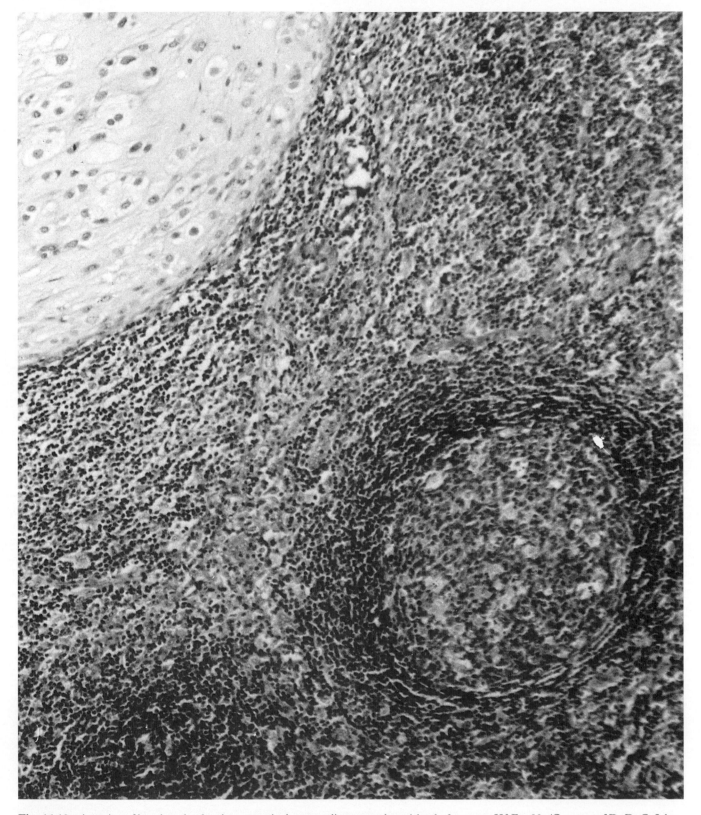

Fig. 16.18   A section of lymph node, showing a germinal centre adjacent to a large island of tumour. H&E, ×80. (Courtesy of Dr D. G. John, Cardiff, and the editor of *Journal of Laryngology and Otology*.)

Table 16.2 Summary of 19 reported cases of metastasizing laryngeal chondrosarcoma

Reference	Age (Years)/sex	Site	Treatment	Metastases	Follow-up
1. Ungerecht[69]	62/M	Cricoid, lateral trachea	Laryngofissure; laryngectomy for recurrence after 7 months	Lungs	Died of metastases 28 months after surgery
2. Frenzel[24]				Cervical lymph node	
3. Sirota[63]	65/M	Cricoid	Total laryngectomy	Cervical lymph nodes, lungs, renal artery tumour embolus	Died of metastases 18 months after surgery
4. Bronzini[6]	72/M	Corniculate	Total laryngectomy and radiotherapy, left radical neck dissection and radiotherapy after 7 months	Cervical lymph node, widespread	
5. Ghalib et al[26]	74/F	Cricoid	Total thyroidectomy with excision of a soft tissue mass on the left side of the neck	Lungs	Died of respiratory failure on the third postoperative day
6. Al-Saleem et al[2]	70/F	Cricoid	Several endoscopic resections; total laryngectomy 1 month after the last resection; radiotherapy for nodal metastasis	Cervical lymph node	Died 8 months after total laryngectomy
7. Huizenga and Balogh[37]	68/M	Cricoid	Laryngofissure; total laryngectomy after 5 years; excision after 3 years; radiotherapy after 9 years	Lung, kidney, and neck	Died 30 years after diagnosis for recurrence
8. Hyams and Rabuzzi[38]	71/F	Cricoid	Local resection; tracheotomy for recurrence after 23 years; radiotherapy	Subcutaneous nodules	
9. Hellquist et al[34]	65/F	Cricoid	Tracheotomy; total laryngectomy after 1 month	Lungs, spleen	Died of metastases 42 months after laryngectomy
10. Harwood et al[33]	75/M		Excision; palliative radiotherapy to lung metastases	Lungs	
11. Neel and Unni[52]			Total laryngectomy; cervical spine surgery after 8 years for metastasis	Cervical spine	Alive and well 10 years after total laryngectomy
12. Ferlito et al[22]	74/M	Thyroid	Total laryngectomy	Lungs	Died 30 months after total laryngectomy for local recurrence and metastases
13. Escher et al[16]	53/M	Cricoid	Laryngofissure; multiple resections for recurrence (4.5; 5; 6 years), total laryngectomy (1 year)	Lungs	Alive with disease 11.5 years after the first treatment with lung metastases and stomal recurrence
14. Gray et al[29]		Epiglottis		Lungs	Fulminating fatal outcome
15. Kasanzew et al[43]	46/F	Epiglottis	Total laryngectomy and removal of deep cervical nodes adjacent to the larynx on both sites; left radical neck dissection	Two paralaryngeal nodes	Alive and well 6 months after neck dissection
16. Hakky et al[32]	56/M	Cricoid	Total laryngectomy with removal of regional lymph nodes	Cervical lymph nodes	Alive and well 3 years after surgical treatment
17. Jacobs et al[40]	52/M	Epiglottis	Supraglottic laryngectomy and right modified neck dissection; segmental lobectomy (3 years)	Cervical lymph node, lung (3 years)	
18. Glaubiger et al[27]	57/M	Thyroid	Total laryngectomy, partial pharyngectomy, total thyroidectomy, left modified radical neck dissection, right radical neck dissection	Cervical and mediastinal lymph nodes	
19. Brandwein et al[5a]	69/M	Cricoid	Partial laryngectomy, endoscopic laser treatments, total laryngectomy, tracheal resection, radiotherapy	Cervical lymph nodes	Died 18 years after diagnosis for a cerebral vascular accident

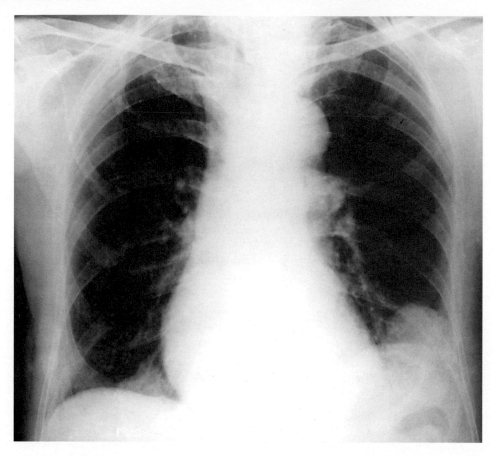

Fig. 16.19 Chest radiograph showing bilateral pulmonary metastases.

OSTEOSARCOMA

Although the commonest primary malignant neoplasm of the bony skeleton, osteosarcoma is one of the rarest mesenchymal malignant neoplasms of the larynx. It was first described by Jackson and Jackson in 1942.[39] There have been only 13 cases reported in the literature.[11,12,28, 31,39,45,50,56,57,58a,64,65,70]

Clinical data indicate that this neoplasm occurs in men in their sixth or seventh decades, and that the lesion is not directly correlated with tobacco exposure.

Macroscopically (Figs 16.20, 16.21), the neoplasm is mainly polypoid or exophitic in appearance.

Microscopy shows that the tumour is composed of frankly malignant, spindle-shaped mesenchymal cells, associated with osteoid and immature neoplastic bone formation (Figs 16.22, 16.23). The nuclei show considerable hyperchromasia or pleomorphism and mitoses may be numerous. Atypical and bizarre giant cells and multinucleated osteoclast-like cells (Fig. 16.24) have been described.[12] Venous invasions may be identified

(Fig. 16.25). Histologically, the extraskeletal osteogenic sarcomas may be divided into the following categories: osteoblastic, fibroblastic, chondroblastic, osteoclastic and telengietasic.

Immunohistochemical studies have shown that the neoplasm was positive for vimentin and negative for desmin, S-100 protein, cytokeratin and epithelial membrane antigen.[56,70]

Electron microscopy showed cells resembling osteoblasts with pleomorphic nuclei and nucleoli of variable size within the abundant cytoplasm containing numerous dilated cisternae of rough endoplasmic reticulum.[12,56,65] The cells were enveloped by interlacing collagen fibres. Osteoblastic elements predominated but cartilaginous and fibrous tissue could be found. According to the predominant component—osseous, stromal or cartilaginous—the tumour may be distinguished as osteoblastic, fibroblastic or chondroblastic.

The *diagnosis* of osteosarcoma depends on the identification of osteoid production by malignant cells.[10] The demonstration of alkaline phosphatase is helpful in making the diagnosis. The case described by van Laer et

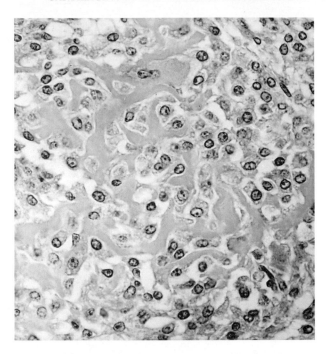

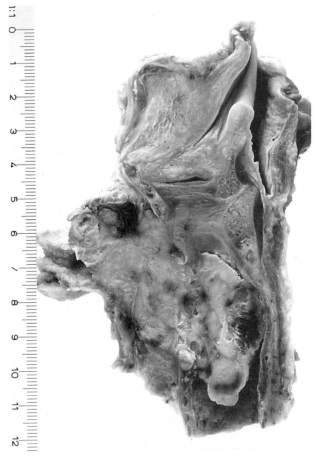

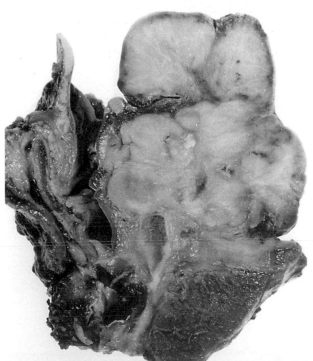

Fig. 16.20 (*top, left*) Sagittal section of an osteosarcoma of the larynx. (Courtesy of Dr W. Remagen, Basel.)

Fig. 16.21 (*bottom*) Sagittal section of tumour, showing airway narrowing with intact mucosa. (Courtesy of Professor P. M. Stell, Liverpool, and the editor of *Annals of Otology, Rhinology and Laryngology*.)

Fig. 16.22 (*top, right*) Focus of lace-like osteoid production by malignant cells. H&E, ×600 OM. (Courtesy of Professor P. M. Stell, Liverpool and the editor of *Annals of Otology, Rhinology and Laryngology*.)

al[70] probably arose from dedifferentiation of a low-grade chondrosarcoma of the cricoid cartilage. The case mentioned by Laskin et al[45] was a post-radiation sarcoma in a patient treated for squamous cell carcinoma of the larynx. Radiotherapy is a known predisposing agent for osteogenic sarcoma of the head. In the cases reported by Morley et al[50] and Pinsolle et al[56], the tumours were suggested to have arisen from the soft tissues of the larynx.

The *differential diagnosis* includes spindle cell squamous carcinoma with osteoid differentiation, chondrosarcoma, malignant fibrous histiocytoma, fibrosarcoma, and myositis ossificans affecting the larynx.[21,25,70]

Osteosarcoma is typically a highly malignant neoplasm that metastasizes early; it also has a marked tendency to recur.[50,56,70] There are reports of metastases to regional lymph nodes[50] and lungs.[12,31]

The majority of patients in the case reports died within a few months. Surgery is the treatment of choice, and chemotherapy might improve the prognosis for patients with disseminated lesions.[70]

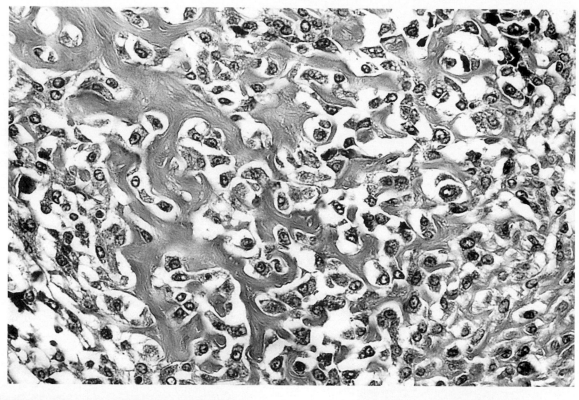

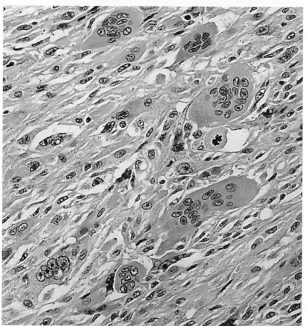

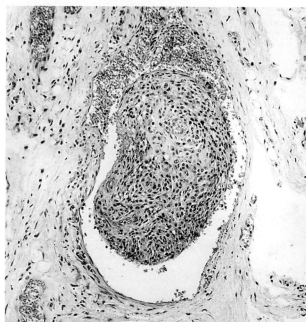

Fig. 16.23 (*top*) Another area of the osteosarcoma with the presence of osteoid material. H&E, ×100 OM. (Slide contributed by Dr T. R. Helliwell, Liverpool.)

Fig. 16.24 (*bottom, left*) Osteoclast-like giant cells in osteosarcoma. H&E, ×375 OM. (Courtesy of Professor P. M. Stell, Liverpool and the editor of *Annals of Otology, Rhinology and Laryngology*.)

Fig. 16.25 (*bottom, right*) Mass of osteosarcoma in vein in perilaryngeal tissue. H&E, ×150 OM. (Courtesy of Professor P. M. Stell, Liverpool and the editor of *Annals of Otology, Rhinology and Laryngology*.)

REFERENCES

1. Adler D, Maier H, Paul K 1985 Kongenitales Chondrom des Larynx. Laryngol Rhinol Otol 64: 459–460
2. Al-Saleem T, Tucker G F Jr, Peale A R, Norris C M 1970 Cartilaginous tumors of the larynx. Clinical-pathologic study of ten cases. Ann Otol Rhinol Laryngol 79: 33–41
3. Barsocchini L M, McCoy G 1968 Cartilaginous tumors of the larynx: a review of the literature and report of four cases. Ann Otol Rhinol Laryngol 77: 146–153
4. Benali B 1981 Chondrome du larynx. Acta Otorhinolaryngol Belg 35: 115–130
4a. Bernal-Sprekelsen M, Storkel S 1990 Chondrosarcoma of the larynx and laryngectomy. Report of two cases. Acta Otorrinolaringol Esp 41: 253–256
5. Bleiweiss I J, Kaneko M 1988 Chondrosarcoma of the larynx with additional malignant mesenchymal component (dedifferentiated chondrosarcoma). Am J Surg Pathol 12: 314–320
5a. Brandwein M, Moore S, Som P, Biller H 1992 Laryngeal chondrosarcoma: a clinicopathologic study of 11 cases, including two 'dedifferentiated' chondrosarcomas. Laryngoscope 102: 858–867
6. Bronzini E 1959 Condrosarcoma della laringe. Ann Laringol Otol Rinol Faringol 58: 497–509
6a. Burggraaff B A, Weinstein G S 1992 Chondrosarcoma of the larynx. Ann Otol Rhinol Laryngol 101: 183–184
7. Burkey B B, Hoffman H T, Baker S R, Thornton A F, McClatchey K D 1990 Chondrosarcoma of the head and neck. Laryngoscope 100: 1301–1305
8. Burtner D, Goodman M, Montgomery W 1972 Elastic cartilaginous metaplasia of vocal cord nodules. Ann Otol Rhinol Laryngol 81: 844–847
9. Cantrell R W, Reibel J F, Jahrsdoerfer R A, Johns M E 1980 Conservative surgical treatment of chondrosarcoma of the larynx. Ann Otol Rhinol Laryngol 89: 567–571
10. Chung A B, Enzinger F M 1987 Extraskeletal osteosarcoma. Cancer 60: 1132–1142
11. Clerf L H 1946 Sarcoma of the larynx: report of eight cases. Arch Otolaryngol 44: 517–524
11a. Dahlin D C, Unni K K 1986 Bone tumors: general aspects and data on 8542 cases, 4th edn. Thomas, Springfield
12. Dahm L J, Schaefer S D, Carder H M, Vellios F 1978 Osteosarcoma of the soft tissue of the larynx. Report of a case with light and electron microscopic studies. Cancer 42: 2343–2351
13. Dalla Palma P, Piazza M 1983 Peripheral chondrosarcoma of the hyoid bone. Report of a case. Appl Pathol 1: 333–338
14. Damiani K K, Tucker H T 1981 Chondroma of the larynx. Surgical technique. Arch Otolaryngol 107: 399–402
14a. Dekker P J, Andrew A C 1992 Laryngeal chondrosarcoma — an unusual presentation. J Laryngol Otol 106: 450–452
15. Erlandson R A, Huvos A G 1974 Chondrosarcoma: a light and electron microscopic study. Cancer 34: 1642–1652
16. Escher A, Escher F, Zimmermann A 1984 Zur Klinik und Pathologie chondromatoser Tumoren des Larynx. HNO 32: 269–285
17. Fechner R E 1984 Chondrometaplasia of the larynx. Arch Otolaryngol 110: 554–556
18. Ferlito A 1985 Soft tissue sarcomas of the larynx. In: Ferlito A (ed) Cancer of the larynx, Vol II. CRC Press, Boca Raton
19. Ferlito A 1990 Laryngeal fibrosarcoma: an over-diagnosed tumor. ORL J Otorhinolaryngol Relat Spec 52: 194–195
20. Ferlito A, Recher G 1985 Chondrometaplasia of the larynx. ORL J Otorhinolaryngol Relat Spec 47: 174–177
21. Ferlito A, Barion U, Nicolai P 1983 Myositis ossificans of the head and neck. Review of the literature and report of a case. Arch Otorhinolaryngol 237: 103–113
22. Ferlito A, Nicolai P, Montaguti A, Cecchetto A, Pennelli N 1984 Chondrosarcoma of the larynx: review of the literature and report of three cases. Am J Otolaryngol 5: 350–359
23. Finn D G, Goepfert H, Batsakis J G 1984 Chondrosarcoma of the head and neck. Laryngoscope 94: 1539–1544
24. Frenzel H. Quoted by Singh J, Black M J, Fried I 1980 Cartilaginous tumors of the larynx: a review of literature and two case experiences. Laryngoscope 90: 1872–1879
25. Friedmann I, Ferlito A 1988 Granulomas and neoplasms of the larynx. Churchill Livingstone, Edinburgh
26. Ghalib S H, Warner E D, DeGowin E L 1969 Laryngeal chondrosarcoma after thyroid irradiation. JAMA 210: 1762–1763
27. Glaubiger D L, Casler J D, Garrett W L, Yuo H S, Lillis-Hearne P K 1991 Chondrosarcoma of the larynx after radiation treatment for vocal cord cancer. Cancer 68: 1828–1831
28. Gorenstein A, Neel H B III, Weiland L H, Devine K D 1980 Sarcomas of the larynx. Arch Otolaryngol 106: 8–12
29. Gray S D, Blanke S B, Babin R W, Robinson R A 1984 Chondrosarcoma of the epiglottis with pulmonary metastases. Abstract, Scientific Poster. Presented at the Annual Meeting of the American Academy of Otolaryngology–Head and Neck Surgery, Inc, Las Vegas
30. Greer J A, Devine K D, Dahlin D C 1977 Gardner's syndrome and chondrosarcoma of the hyoid bone. Arch Otolaryngol 103: 425–427
31. Haar J G, Chaudhry A P, Karanjia M D, Milley P S 1978 Chondroblastic osteosarcoma of the larynx. Arch Otolaryngol 104: 477–481
32. Hakky M, Kolbusz R, Reyes C V 1989 Chondrosarcoma of the larynx. Ear Nose Throat J 68: 60–62
33. Harwood A R, Krajbich J I, Fornasier V L 1980 Radiotherapy of chondrosarcoma of bone. Cancer 45: 2769–2777
33a. Hasan S, Kannan V, Shenoy A M, Nanjundappa, Naresh K N 1992 Chondrosarcoma of the hyoid. J Laryngol Otol 106: 273–276
34. Hellquist H, Olofsson J, Gröntoft O 1979 Chondrosarcoma of the larynx. J Laryngol Otol 93: 1037–1047
35. Hill M J, Taylor C L, Scott G B D 1980 Chondromatous metaplasia in the human larynx. Histopathology 4: 205–214
36. Horowitz D R, Perusek M C, Nguyen V D 1991 A rare cause of laryngeal distress: chondrosarcoma of the larynx. Comput Med Imag Graph 15: 67–71
37. Huizenga C, Balogh K 1970 Cartilaginous tumors of the larynx: a clinicopathologic study of 10 new cases and a review of the literature. Cancer 26: 201–210
38. Hyams V J, Rabuzzi D D 1970 Cartilaginous tumors of the larynx. Laryngoscope 80: 755–767
39. Jackson C, Jackson Cl 1942 Diseases and injuries of the larynx. Macmillan, New York
40. Jacobs R D, Stayboldt C, Harris J P 1989 Chondrosarcoma of the epiglottis with regional and distant metastasis. Laryngoscope 99: 861–864
41. Johnson S, Tetu B, Ayala A G, Chawla S P 1986 Chondrosarcoma with additional mesenchymal component (dedifferentiated chondrosarcoma). I. A clinicopathological study of 26 cases. Cancer 58: 278–286
42. Jones S R, Myers E N, Barnes E L 1988 Benign neoplasms of the larynx. In: Fried M P (ed) The larynx: a multidisciplinary approach. Brown, Boston
43. Kasanzew M, John D G, Newman P, Lesser T J H, Thomas P L 1988 Chondrosarcoma of the epiglottis. J Laryngol Otol 102: 374–377
44. Kramer D S, Brown G P, Schuller D E 1983 Proximal airway obstruction presenting as dyspnea. A case of chondrosarcoma of the larynx. Postgrad Med 5: 133–135
45. Laskin W B, Silverman T A, Enzinger F M 1988 Postradiation soft tissue sarcomas. An analysis of 53 cases. Cancer 62: 2330–2340
46. Lavertu P, Tucker H M 1984 Chondrosarcoma of the larynx. Case report and management philosophy. Ann Otol Rhinol Laryngol 93: 452–456
47. Leonetti J P, Collins S L, Jablokow V, Lewy R 1987 Laryngeal chondrosarcoma as a late-appearing cause of 'idiopathic' vocal cord paralysis. Otolaryngol Head Neck Surg 97: 391–395
48. Michaels L 1984 Pathology of the larynx. Springer-Verlag, Berlin
49. Mishell J H, Schild J A, Mafee M F 1990 Chondrosarcoma of the larynx. Diagnosis with magnetic resonance imaging and computed tomography. Arch Otolaryngol Head Neck Surg 116: 1338–1341
49a. Mitschke H 1975 Chondrome des Kehlkopfes und ihre Behandlung. Wien Med Wochenschr 125: 153–155
50. Morley A R, Cameron D S, Watson A J 1973 Osteosarcoma of the larynx. J Laryngol Otol 87: 997–1005

51. Munoz A, Penarrocha L, Gallego F, Olmedilla G, Poch-Broto J 1990 Laryngeal chondrosarcoma: CT findings in three patients. AJR 154: 997–998
52. Neel H B III, Unni K K 1982 Cartilaginous tumors of the larynx: a series of 33 patients. Otolaryngol Head Neck Surg 90: 201–207
53. Neis P R, McMahon M F, Norris C W 1989 Cartilaginous tumors of the trachea and larynx. Ann Otol Rhinol Laryngol 98: 31–36
54. New G B 1935 Sarcoma of the larynx: report of two cases. Arch Otolaryngol 21: 648–652
55. Nicolai P, Ferlito A, Sasaki C T, Kirchner J A 1990 Laryngeal chondrosarcoma: incidence, pathology, biological behavior, and treatment. Ann Otol Rhinol Laryngol 99: 515–523
56. Pinsolle J, Lecluse I, Demeaux H, Laur P, Rivel J, Siberchicot F 1990 Osteosarcoma of the soft tissue of the larynx: report of a case with electron microscopic studies. Otolaryngol Head Neck Surg 102: 276–280
57. Remagen W, Löhr J, von Westernhagen B 1983 Osteosarkom des Kehlkopfes. HNO 31: 366–368
58. Réthi A Quoted by Bronzini E 1959 Condrosarcoma della laringe. Ann Laringol Otol Rinol Faringol 58: 497–509
58a.Roels H 1992 Histopathology of laryngeal tumours. Acta Otorhinolaryngol Belg 46: 127–139
59. Ross D E 1971 Chondrosarcoma of the larynx invading the thyroid gland. Laryngoscope 81: 379–386
60. Sanerkin N G 1980 Definitions of osteosarcoma, chondrosarcoma, and fibrosarcoma of bone. Cancer 46: 178–185
61. Shankar L, Hawke M 1991 The C T appearance of cricoid chondrosarcoma. J Otolaryngol 20: 297–298
62. Shearer J E, Goldberg A L, Lupetin A L, Rothfus W E 1988 Chondrosarcoma of the larynx. Report of a case with characteristic computed tomography findings. J Comput Tomogr 12: 292–294
63. Sirota H H Quoted by Hyams V J, Rabuzzi D D 1970 Cartilaginous tumors of the larynx. Laryngoscope 80: 755–767
64. Sprinkle P M, Allen M S, Brookshire P F 1966 Osteosarcoma of the larynx (a true primary sarcoma of the larynx). Laryngoscope 76: 325–333
64a.Stiglbaner R, Steurer M, Schimmerl S, Kramer J 1992 MRI of cartilaginous tumours of the larynx. Clin Radiol 46: 23–27
65. Suchatlampong V, Sriumpai S, Khawcharoenporn V 1981 Osteosarcoma of the larynx. The first case report in Thailand with ultrastructural study. J Med Assoc Thai 64: 301–307
66. Thomas R L 1979 Non-epithelial tumours of the larynx. J Laryngol Otol 93: 1131–1141
66a.Timon C I, Gullane P J, Van Nostrand A W P, O'Dwyer T 1992 Chondrosarcoma of the larynx: a histo-radiologic analysis. J Otolaryngol 21: 358–363
67. Tiwari R M, Snow G B, Balm A J M, Vos W, Bosma A 1987 Cartilagenous tumours of the larynx. J Laryngol Otol 101: 266–275
68. Traves F 1816 A case of ossification and bony growth of the cartilages of the larynx. Med Chir Trans 7: 150
69. Ungerecht K 1951 Multiple Chondrome und Chondrosarkome des Larynx under der Trachea mit chondromyxosarkomatösen Rezidiven. Arch Ohrenheilk 160: 158–169
70. van Laer C G, Helliwell T R, Atkinson M W A, Stell P M 1989 Osteosarcoma of the larynx. Ann Otol Rhinol Laryngol 98: 971–974
71. Wick M R, Abenoza P, Manivel J C 1988 Diagnostic immunopathology. In: Gnepp D R (ed) Pathology of the head and neck. Churchill Livingstone, New York
71a.Varletzides E, Theodosiou A 1977 Chondrosarcoma of the larynx of unusual size. Panminerva Med 19: 279–285
72. Wilkinson A H III, Beckford N S, Babin R W, Parham D M 1991 Extraskeletal myxoid chondrosarcoma of the epiglottis: case report and review of the literature. Otolaryngol Head Neck Surg 104: 257–260

17. Haemopoietic neoplasms

K. A. MacLennan, J. B. Schofield

INTRODUCTION

Haemopoietic neoplasms of the larynx are uncommon either as primary tumours or in association with disseminated disease. Despite their relative rarity, a wide variety of disease entities have been described in the larynx; these include the acute and chronic leukaemias, the non-Hodgkin's lymphomas and — very rarely — Hodgkin's disease. Because of their rarity, the natural history of haemopoietic neoplasms affecting the larynx is poorly documented, and this problem is compounded by a degree of terminological confusion which perpetually surrounds these tumours. In this short review we will attempt to document what little is known about the pathology and behaviour of haemopoietic neoplasms in this anatomical location.

NON-HODGKIN'S LYMPHOMA OF THE LARYNX

Non-Hodgkin's lymphomas present with extra-nodal disease in approximately a quarter of cases; common sites include the gastrointestinal tract, skin, testis and the head and neck region, where salivary gland, thyroid, nasopharynx and tonsil are all frequent sites of disease.[32,76]

The classification of the non-Hodgkin's lymphomas remains controversial, with major differences in the diagnostic criteria and terminology employed between American and European workers. Many European (and some American) workers have adopted the cytological approach to lymphoma classification espoused by Lennert and co-workers[53,54] and embodied in the updated Kiel classification[80] (Table 17.1). Many American authors use the working formulation[85] which, although never intended to be a classification, has, by common usage, become one (Table 17.2).

These terminological difficulties become magnified when we consider the extranodal lymphomas whose histological appearance and natural history are divergent from node based lymphoproliferative disease.[45] These pathological and clinical differences have led to the recognition of a distinctive type of lymphoma which has been termed

Table 17.1 Updated Kiel classification of malignant lymphomas[80]

Low grade	*Low grade*
*Lymphocytic — chronic lymphocytic and prolymphocytic leukaemia; hairy-cell leukaemia	Lymphocytic — chronic lymphocytic and prolymphocytic leukaemia
	Small, cerebriform cell-mycosis fungoides, Sézary's syndrome
Lymphoplasmacytic/cytoid (LP immunocytoma)	Lymphoepithelioid (Lennert's lymphoma)
Plasmacytic	Angioimmunoblastic (AILD, LgX)
*Centroblastic/centrocytic	
— follicular ± diffuse	
— diffuse	
	T zone
	Pleomorphic, small cell (HTLV-I ±)
High grade	*High grade*
Centroblastic	Pleomorphic, medium and large cell (HTLV-I ±)
*Immunoblastic	Immunoblastic (HTLV-I ±)
*Large cell anaplastic (Ki-1 +)	Large cell anaplastic (Ki-1 +)
Burkitt lymphoma	••
*Lymphoblastic	Lymphoblastic
Rare types	*Rare types*

*Indicates some degree of correspondence, either in morphology or in functional expression, between categories in two columns.

malignant lymphoma of mucosa associated lymphoid tissue (MALT[45]). In some extranodal sites, such as the stomach, MALT lymphoma has been associated with a favourable clinical course.[14,56]

The larynx appears to be a rare site of extranodal lymphoma, and this group of tumours accounts for less than 1% of all neoplasms at this site.[4] The majority of laryngeal lymphomas reported in the literature are of B cell lineage, with only a small minority possessing a T cell phenotype.[63]

B CELL LYMPHOMA OF THE LARYNX

In common with the majority of extranodal lymphomas (other than cutaneous lymphoma) most laryngeal lymphomas have morphological features of, or have been phenotyped as, B cell neoplasms.

Table 17.2 A working formulation of non-Hodgkin's lymphomas for clinical usage[85]

Low grade
A. Malignant lymphoma
    Small lymphocytic
        consistent with CLL
        plasmacytoid
B. Malignant lymphoma, follicular
    Predominantly small cleaved cell
        diffuse areas
        sclerosis
C. Malignant lymphoma, follicular
    Mixed, small cleaved and large cell
        diffuse areas
        sclerosis

Intermediate grade
D. Malignant lymphoma, follicular
    Predominantly large cell
        diffuse areas
        sclerosis
E. Malignant lymphoma, diffuse
    Small cleaved cell
        sclerosis
F. Malignant lymphoma, diffuse
    Mixed, small and large cell
        sclerosis
        epithelioid cell component
G. Malignant lymphoma, diffuse
    Large cell
        cleaved cell
        non-cleaved cell
        sclerosis

High grade
H. Malignant lymphoma
    Large cell, immunoblastic
        plasmacytoid
        clear cell
        polymorphous
        epithelioid component
I. Malignant lymphoma
    Lymphoblastic
        convoluted cell
        non-convoluted cell
J. Malignant lymphoma
    Small non-cleaved cell
        Burkitt's
        follicular areas

Miscellaneous
    Composite
    Mycosis fungoides
    Histiocytic
    Extramedullary plamacytoma
    Unclassified
    Other

Primary laryngeal lymphomas probably arise from specialized, submucosal aggregates of lymphoid cells which are predominantly of B cell lineage and are closely related to the bronchial lymphoid tissue (Bienenstock et al.[6-8]) Malignant lymphomas arising from mucosa associated lymphoid tissue (MALT) have distinctive characteristics which have been described by Isaacson and his co-workers (for a review see reference[45]). Indeed, it would now appear that many of the lesions previously regarded as pseudolymphomas of the larynx are probably low-grade lymphomas of the MALT type.[21,22,28]

Laryngeal lymphomas also share certain patterns of clinical behaviour in common with other extranodal lymphomas. They have a tendency to remain localized, and when they disseminate they preferentially involve other extranodal sites such as the gastrointestinal tract or respiratory system.

Twenty-seven cases of localized laryngeal lymphoma have been documented in the literature.[4,10,12,13,15,19-23, 27,38,40,52,55,63,71,81,83,87] Age at presentation ranges from 4 to 81 years (mean age 55 years); 12 males and 15 females have been reported. These patients have presented with symptoms indistinguishable from those of other laryngeal tumours — such as hoarseness, cough, stridor, dysphonia, dysphagia and weight loss.

The majority of stage Ie laryngeal lymphomas present in the supraglottic or glottic region with a particular tendency to involve the aryepiglottic folds; four cases have been recorded in the subglottis.[19,55,81,83] The majority are macroscopically described as polypoid, smooth surfaced, non-ulcerated lesions which may attain a considerable size before clinical presentation (Fig. 17.1).[63]

Histological features

The literature regarding histological subtyping of laryngeal lymphomas is confusing as various classifications have been applied which are not readily translated into modern lymphoma terminology. With some certainty we can say that seven of the reported cases are large cell lymphomas: two reticulum cell sarcomas,[39,87] one histiocytic lymphoma,[12] three centroblastic lymphomas and one immunoblastic lymphoma,[63] and that this subtype probably represents the largest single well-defined group. Other histological subtypes described include poorly differentiated lymphocytic lymphoma (two cases[27,83]), lymphosarcoma (eight cases[13,19,20,23,52,55,71]), lymphoblastic lymphoma (six cases[4,10,15,19,40,87]), one case of non-Hodgkin's lymphoma of intermediate cell type[81] and one case of low-grade lymphoma of MALT.[19]

In the four cases that one of the authors (KAM) had the opportunity to review histologically, the tumours appeared identical to node based, large cell lymphoma (Figs 17.2, 17.3).[63]

Treatment and prognosis

Primary laryngeal lymphoma responds well to radiotherapy, and this has been recommended as the treatment of choice for stage Ie disease.[63] However, as the number of patients treated is rather small, and their management by no means uniform, it is difficult to provide firm guidelines.

Disseminated lymphoma involving the larynx has been recorded[5,27,62] and is associated with a poor prognosis.

T CELL LYMPHOMA OF THE LARYNX

Introduction

T cell lymphoma is a relatively rare occurrence in the head and neck. In a recent study of 114 cases of extranodal

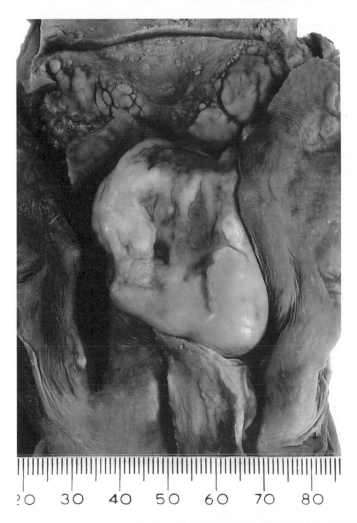

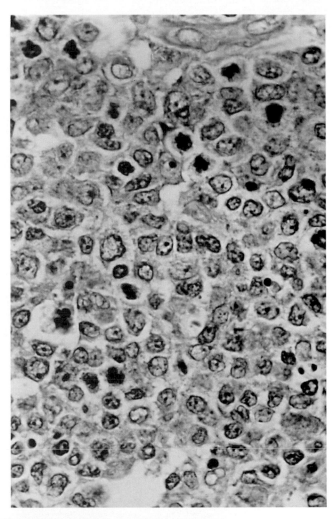

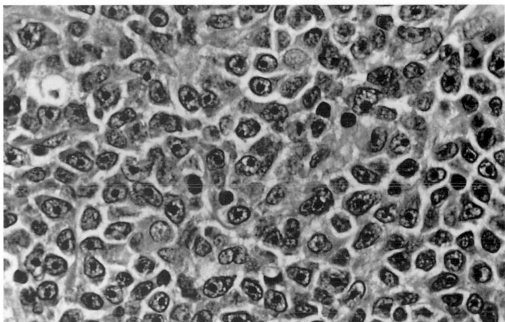

Fig. 17.1 (*top, left*) Autopsy specimen of the larynx showing a polypoid lesion.

Fig. 17.2 (*top, right*) Laryngeal biopsy specimen showing a diffuse, large, noncleaved follicle centre cell lymphoma (centroblastic). H&E, ×400 OM.

Fig. 17.3 (*bottom*) Laryngeal biopsy specimen showing a diffuse infiltrate of immunoblastic sarcoma. H&E, ×600 OM.

lymphoma in this anatomical region, only 11% showed a T cell immunophenotype. These 13 cases (from an area of Japan not endemic for adult T cell leukaemia/lymphoma) involved nasopharynx (four cases), nasal cavity (three cases), palatine tonsil (five cases) and oral cavity (one case).[79] In addition, the head and neck region is the site of a number of destructive, usually midline lesions, which are variously termed lethal midline reticulosis, lymphomatoid granulomatosis, polymorphic reticulosis, and are also known by other names. Many of these lesions have eventually been shown to be T cell lymphomas. However, these lesions rarely involve the larynx.[4] Nakashima et al[64] reported the case of a 28-year-old female who presented with hoarseness, dyspnoea and fever. On laryngeal fibrescopy, a left glottic mass and swelling of the right vocal cord were seen. Biopsy showed the subepithelial tissues to be extensively infiltrated by atypical pleomorphic lymphoid cells, but there was no involvement of the overlying squamous epithelium; no vasculitis or granulomata were present. On the basis of these findings the patient was treated with external beam radiotherapy (40 Gy in 20 days), but she deteriorated and died five weeks later. At autopsy the tumour was found to involve both vocal cords and extended into the subglottic region; additionally, lymphoma was present in tongue, pharynx and lung. Within the larynx there was extensive infiltration of the intrinsic musculature, and an angiocentric pattern in some areas. Epitheliotropic lesions are not mentioned. Immunohistochemistry performed on post mortem tissues confirmed the T cell nature of the proliferation.

Primary T cell lymphoma

Primary T cell lymphoma of the larynx is extremely rare, with only three convincing reports in the English language literature. Laryngeal involvement occurs in a pattern analogous to cutaneous T cell lymphoma (also known as mycosis fungoides), with definite 'epitheliotropic' characteristics. Similar lesions may be seen in the oral mucosa, tongue and soft palate.[17,48] This contrasts with lymphoid sites in the head and neck region, e.g. tonsil and Waldeyer's ring, where node based peripheral, and, less commonly, central (thymic, lymphoblastic) T cell lymphomas are more frequent.

Mycosis fungoides limited to the larynx was first reported by Hood et al.[41] The patient described in their paper was an 80-year-old female who initially presented with hoarseness and was found to have an ulcerated tumour involving the epiglottis and extending to the aryepiglottic fold. There was no evidence of disease outside the larynx or of any past history of cutaneous disease. The biopsy appearances were misinterpreted as an undifferentiated small cell tumour, and the patient was treated with radiotherapy; two years later the patient

relapsed with widespread cutaneous plaques and nodules showing the typical histological appearance of mycosis fungoides. The patient died 4 years after the onset of disease. At autopsy the larynx was found to be extensively infiltrated by tumour which was confined by the laryngeal cartilages; there was widespread visceral involvement. Microscopically there was extensive subepithelial infiltration of the larynx by pleomorphic and atypical lymphoid cells, some with hyperconvoluted (so-called 'cerebriform') nuclear characteristics, and focal infiltration of the squamous epithelium with formation of lymphoid (Pautrier's type) microabscesses.

Agarwal et al[1] reported a further case of mycosis fungoides limited to the larynx. The patient was a 55-year-old male with a ten-week history of dysphagia and alteration of voice. Indirect laryngoscopy showed a diffuse swelling involving the right arytenoid cartilage, the right false cord and extending to the aryepiglottic fold and laryngeal surface of the epiglottis. No other clinical abnormalities were noted and the skin appeared normal. Biopsy showed focal ulceration of the squamous epithelium and a lymphomatous infiltrate containing cerebriform cells typical of mycosis fungoides. The patient apparently refused treatment and was lost to follow-up.

Secondary involvement by T cell lymphoma

'Secondary' laryngeal involvement appears to be exceptionally rare in cases of disseminated node based or extranodal T cell lymphoma. It has been described in a case of the HTLV1 related adult T cell leukaemia lymphoma (ATLL). Inagi et al[44] reported the case of a 51-year-old male with 'smouldering' ATLL who developed hoarseness and was found to have a deposit of T cell lymphoma in the left vocal cord. The patient was alive 6 years after initial diagnosis.

Although lymphoblastic lymphoma and, occasionally, immunoblastic lymphoma, may be associated with a T-cell immunophenotype, to our knowledge their localization in the larynx has not been reported.

Ferlito and Recher[29] report the case of a 74-year-old male with a six-year history of cutaneous T cell lymphoma who presented with laryngeal involvement as the first manifestation of visceral disease. A further case of upper aero-digestive tract involvement by mycosis fungoides was reported by Strahan and Calcaterra.[82] Autopsy studies in mycosis fungoides have shown that although laryngeal involvement may occur, this is not a common feature.[25,73]

The association of coeliac disease with non-Hodgkin's lymphoma of the gastrointestinal tract is well recognised.[84] However, Seddon et al[78] reported the case of a 46-year-old male with a history of coeliac disease who presented with upper airway obstruction and was found to have a large cell lymphoma of T-cell immuno-phenotype, apparently arising in the upper trachea. The patient was treated with combination chemotherapy and was alive and well 7 years after diagnosis.

Histological features

A diagnosis of T cell lymphoma may be suspected in many cases on morphological grounds. There are two principal diagnostic problems: firstly, the separation of T cell lymphoma from B cell lymphoma, and secondly, the differentiation between early forms of T cell lymphoma and their non-neoplastic mimics. The cyto-logical features of neoplastic T cells are characteristic in some cases, in particular when hyperchromatic 'cerebri-form' (convoluted and multiply cleaved) nuclei are present as in mycosis fungoides. The presence of these cells, which are often seen in aggregates within the overlying squamous mucosa (Pautrier's microabscesses) is diagnostic of T cell lymphoma. Other diagnostic clues seen in some forms of T cell lymphoma are the presence of abundant clear cytoplasm in the neoplastic lymphoid cells, vascular proliferation with particularly prominent endothelial cells (so-called high endothelial venules), infiltration of vessel walls by lymphoid cells, and an associated eosinophil granulocyte infiltration.

Confirmation of the diagnosis of T cell lymphoma may be achieved by immunophenotyping. Positive staining for T cell restricted antigens on frozen section or, more recently, on conventionally fixed and processed material, using antibodies such as UCHL 1 (CD 45 R0[67]) and polyclonal CD 3[58] enables the pathologist to establish the T cell lineage of the tumour. Aberrant expression or loss of T cell epitopes is often seen in T cell neoplasms, and may be useful in diagnosis.[70] It is important to be aware that a number of B cell lymphomas contain many T cells and that these may predominate (so-called T-cell-rich B-cell lymphoma[66,72]) causing diagnostic confusion. Finally, the use of molecular biological techniques to detect rearrange-ment of the T cell receptor gene can confirm the presence of a neoplastic T-cell clone in many cases.[49]

Treatment and prognosis

Because of the very small number of cases recorded, optimal treatment for this condition is unknown. The prognosis appears to be extremely poor.

PLASMACYTOMA OF THE LARYNX

Introduction

Plasmacytoma is a neoplastic clonal proliferation of the B lymphoid immunoglobulin producing cell, the plasma cell. The clonal nature of the expansion can be confirmed by detection of excess production of one of the two immunoglobulin light chains, kappa or lambda (light chain restriction), and many of these tumours are associated with amyloid deposition of AL (light chain) type. Most cases of plasma cell neoplasia involve the bone marrow and are multifocal; this variant is termed multiple myeloma and is associated with raised serum immuno-globulin levels and a monoclonal band on serum electro-phoresis. Less frequently, plasma cell neoplasms present as a single localized tumour involving either bone (plasmacytoma) or non-osseous tissue (extramedullary plasmacytoma). Localized lesions may respond well to radiotherapy, but subsequent development of dissemi-nated disease (multiple myeloma) may occur. It is important to distinguish these neoplastic processes from the reactive 'plasma cell granuloma', nodular amyloidosis, and the extremely rare, probably benign, mucocutaneous plasmacytosis.

Plasma cell neoplasms in the larynx are rare. At this site, solitary extramedullary plasmacytoma is more common than involvement by multiple myeloma, but it is mandatory to screen the patient for evidence of dissemi-nated disease at the time of presentation as the therapy required is more intensive and the prognosis worse in multiple myeloma. Solitary lesions often respond well to radiotherapy and/or surgery; some present with multiple myeloma after a variable time period.

Extramedullary plasmacytoma accounts for less than 5% of plasma cell neoplasms, but over 80% of these occur in the head and neck region; nevertheless, this lesion accounts for less than 1%,[89] and probably nearer 0.05%[36] of all head and neck malignancies. Between 4.5 and 18% of all extramedullary plasmacytomas involve the larynx;[37,51] of the approximately 350 recorded head and neck cases in the literature, there are over 80 examples of laryngeal plasmacytoma. Between 10 and 20% of the lesions will manifest multiple lesions.[51] The peak inci-dence is in the 50- to 70-year-old age group (but rare cases have been reported in children), and males are more commonly affected, the male-to-female ratio vary-ing between 2:1 and 4:1 in different series.

Clinical presentation of plasmacytoma of the larynx is usually with hoarseness, change in voice or dysphagia, which has generally been present for several months and, in some cases, for years. Rarely, patients may first present with acute laryngeal obstruction[37] or metastasis to cervical lymph nodes.[30]

The largest published series is that of Pahor[68] who reviewed details of 31 cases of laryngeal plasmacytoma in the medical literature and found a male-to-female ratio of 2.3:1; 74% of the cases presented between the ages of 30 and 69. The sites of tumour involvement were epiglottis (six cases), true vocal cord (five cases), false vocal cord (five cases), ventricle (six cases), aryepiglottic fold (four cases), arytenoid (three cases), subglottis (three cases) and anterior commissure (two cases). Twelve of the cases (38%) had involvement of other sites in the aerodigestive tract, one case had a lymph node metastasis, and in one case there was a single bony tumour.

Hyams et al[43] studied 53 patients referred to the Armed Forces Institute of Pathology (AFIP), Washington, with a diagnosis of extramedullary plasmacytoma of the upper respiratory tract; nine of these (17%) involved the larynx. Other sites of involvement in this series were sinonasal cavity (28 cases, 52%), nasopharynx (10 cases, 19%), pharynx (3 cases, 6%) and tonsil (3 cases, 6%). Of the laryngeal tumours, three involved the ventricular fold, one the true vocal cord, three the supraglottis, and two the epiglottis. Age at presentation varied widely but centred in the 40–80-year age group, and the male-to-female ratio was approximately 3:1. The tumour was polypoid in 20% of cases, but the remainder were mucosa-covered rubbery grey to red sessile masses. Kost[51] extensively reviewed the literature and added four further cases. The patients were all male and were aged 35 to 76 years. Two cases were supraglottic, one was glottic and one was glottic/subglottic.

Although laryngeal involvement by plasmacytoma is usually extramedullary, laryngeal disease may be seen in multiple myeloma.[2,24,35,46]

Extramedullary plasmacytoma has occasionally been reported in the upper trachea and at the carina.[16,50]

Histological features

Microscopically, these tumours are characterized by large sheets of uniform cells replacing the infiltrated tissue, without other inflammatory cells being present (cf. plasma cell granuloma). Many of the tumour cells are indistinguishable from normal plasma cells, with typical eccentric nucleus containing five to eight masses of condensed chromatin, giving the so-called cartwheel pattern. The cytoplasm is non-granular and contains a prominent paranuclear area of pallor (hof) corresponding to the large amount of Golgi apparatus. Plasmablastic forms can usually be found but meticulous search is often required as they may be present in only very small numbers; these cells are less well differentiated than the mature plasma cells with larger nuclei, less marked chromatin clumping, and often a central nucleolus.

The presence of numerous plasmablastic forms or many mitotic figures (these are not seen in reactive plasma cell populations) correlates with a more aggressive pattern of behaviour. In the AFIP study,[43] cases of tumours with mean nuclear diameter less than 6μm had no evidence of metastasis or local recurrence 1 year after treatment. The presence of multinucleated forms was not of prognostic value.

Russell bodies (eosinophilic spheroidal bodies 50–150 μm in diameter, corresponding to cytoplasmic immuno-globulin) may be present, but these are more often seen in reactive plasma cell infiltrates (only 7 of the 53 AFIP cases contained Russell bodies).[43] It is of interest to note that Russell bodies and amyloid were not found in the same tumours.

Marked amyloid deposition is seen in more than 20% of tumours but was not associated with altered prognosis.[59] However, amyloid deposition may be so marked as to simulate nodular amyloidosis and produce a diagnostic problem. In such cases, careful scrutiny of the plasma cell component, combined with immunohistochemical demonstration of immunoglobulin light chain restriction, helps the pathologist to reach an accurate diagnosis. Raised serum immunoglobulins were not seen in the AFIP cases,[43] whereas in the study of Wiltshaw,[90] about 10% of cases showed this phenomenon in the late stages of the disease when associated with a large tumour bulk.

Differential diagnosis

Diagnosis of this condition may in some cases be difficult and is not infrequently delayed. This is probably due to a combination of factors, including the relative rarity of the lesion, its non-specific gross appearance, and the difficulty of histological diagnosis. Initial biopsies in this condition may be mistaken for a chronic inflammatory process, either unspecified or 'plasma cell granuloma', because of the excess of morphologically normal plasma cells. The absence of other inflammatory cells should alert the pathologist to the possibility of the diagnosis of plasmacytoma. Some cases are almost indistinguishable, on morphology alone, from nodular amyloidosis, and immuno-histochemistry is helpful in establishing a diagnosis of plasmacytoma. Tumours with gross plasmablastic features may resemble large cell lymphoma, but these are unusual at this site. Immunhistochemistry and electron microscopy may be of assistance in this situation.

Treatment and prognosis

Prognosis in cases of extramedullary plasmacytoma is substantially better than in cases of multiple myeloma. In particular, extramedullary plasmacytoma in the head and neck region is associated with a better prognosis than is plasmacytoma at other sites, possibly because the tumours present when still relatively small, and well localized. Regional lymph node involvement is seen in 14 to 26% of cases, but it does not appear to affect prognosis.[51] Recurrence usually occurs within 24 months but may occur as late as 10 years after treatment. Some authors have found an increased risk of dissemination in those cases with local recurrence. Dissemination to bone or soft tissues occurs in 17 to 35% of cases and is usually seen within 24 months of diagnosis, but, as with local recurrence, this may occur years later.

The prognostic value of nuclear size has already been mentioned. A mean nuclear diameter of greater than 6 µm (which correlates with the presence of plasmablastic forms) is associated with a more aggressive course.[43] However, other morphological features, such as the presence of amyloid or multinucleated cells, does not appear to be significant.

Woodruff et al[91] proposed a clinical staging system (stage 1: tumour confined to primary site; stage 2: tumour involvement of draining lymph nodes; stage 3: metastatic tumour spread). However, in the recent review by Kost,[51] lymph node metastases were found in up to 25% of cases and did not affect prognosis. On the other hand, subsequent systemic dissemination, seen in 17–35% of cases, did significantly shorten survival.

In general, these tumours are radiosensitive, and treatment of the plasmacytoma of the larynx is usually by radiotherapy, sometimes in combination with conservative surgery; chemotherapy is indicated only in patients with disseminated disease (multiple myeloma). Although radiotherapy plays an important role in treatment, the optimal dosage regime is not known. Reviewing groups of extramedullary plasmacytomas, Harwood et al recommended a dose of 3500 cGy in 3 weeks,[39] but Gaffney et al suggested 4000 cGy in 3–4 weeks.[34] Mill and Griffith[61] proposed 5500–6000 rads in 6–7 weeks. Kost[51] highlighted the fact that higher doses of radiotherapy carry significant morbidity (one of the patients received 7000 rads and developed radionecrosis of the larynx requiring laryngectomy).

Chemotherapy is reserved for cases with locally advanced, recurrent or disseminated disease. The favoured agents are similar to those used to treat multiple myeloma, namely melphalan and cyclophosphamide. In cases of disseminated disease, complete remission was seen in 55% and partial remission in 33%, with remission lasting from 1 to 122 months.[34]

Overall 5-year survival for extramedullary plasmacytoma is approximately 50%,[34,89] but the well-recognised risk of late recurrence or dissemination makes long term follow-up essential.

LEUKAEMIC AND MAST CELL INFILTRATES OF THE LARYNX

Although extramedullary manifestations of leukaemia are not uncommon (principally involving the skin, gums, tonsils and central nervous system),[3] leukaemic infiltrations of the larynx are extremely rare. In a series of 61 cases of granulocytic sarcoma (chloroma, soft tissue acute myeloid leukaemia), involvement of the upper respiratory tract was seen in only one case (nasopharynx), and laryngeal disease was not seen.[65] Of a further series of

eight cases in which extensive immunohistochemistry was performed,[33] two cases had nasopharyngeal disease and one additional case had pharyngeal involvement.

Granulocytic sarcoma of the human larynx appears to have been reported only rarely. Ti et al[86] reviewed the literature and found only 10 cases of leukaemia with significant laryngeal involvement. They described a 68-year-old woman presenting with stridor due to laryngeal involvement by previously undiagnosed acute myeloid leukaemia. The patient died despite corticosteroid treatment, and at autopsy there was widespread leukaemic infiltration (liver, spleen, lymph nodes, bone marrow, kidneys, adrenals, gastrointestinal tract, larynx and trachea). The epiglottis, glosso-epiglottic and aryepiglottic folds and vocal cords were thickened, and there was an ulcerated greenish mass in the glottis below the tracheostomy side. Histologically there was massive, diffuse infiltration of the larynx and trachea by acute myeloid leukaemia, with mucosal ulceration.

Schilling et al[77] reported three patients with laryngeal involvement by chronic myeloid leukaemia and one with acute myeloid leukaemia, all of whom died before therapy could be started. A further three cases of acute leukaemic infiltration of the larynx were reported by Jones and Shalom,[47] all of whom died of rapidly progressive disease. Marks[57] reported a case of laryngeal acute myeloid leukaemia which responded initially to radiotherapy, but the patient died of disease within 2 months, and Warthin[88] reported a similar case in which sudden death was due to acute laryngeal obstruction.

Fergusson et al[26] describe a 69-year-old man presenting with right-sided throat pain and odynophagia. Chronic granulocytic leukaemia (CGL) had been diagnosed 3 years previously, with blast transformation treated with hydroxyurea and prednisolone 6 months prior to ENT presentation. An ulcerated area on the right side of the epiglottis was found on indirect laryngoscopy; it was biopsied and showed extensive infiltration of the laryngeal tissues by granulocytic sarcoma composed of sheets of blast cells. The patient was treated with local radiotherapy with apparent complete tumour resolution, but he died 6 months later.

Laryngeal infiltration by chronic myelomonocytic leukaemia was reported by Brito-Babapulle et al.[11] The patient was a 71-year-old woman presenting with a two-week history of dyspnoea, one week's stridor and 3 days dysphagia and dysphonia. The lesion was a large, smooth mass below the larynx causing partial obstruction. The patient was leukaemic (WBC $89.9 \times 10^9/\ell$) with 30% blasts and dysplastic features, indicating CMML. Several biopsies were performed, showing ulceration of the surface epithelium and a diffuse infiltration of the subepithelial tissues by polymorphous monocytic and myeloid cells, including blast cells and mature neutrophils. The patient had a good response to Mitoxantrone (laryngoscopy 3 weeks later showed disappearance of the lesion) but relapsed with cutaneous lesions and peripheral blood recurrence 1 year later. Interestingly, the larynx was not involved at relapse; the patient was refractory to further treatment, and died.

Mast cell sarcoma has been reported on only one occasion in the larynx.[42] The patient was a 71-year-old woman who presented with hoarseness and was found to have a laryngeal mass. The initial biopsy was diagnosed as Wegener's granulomatosis but subsequent excision established the diagnosis as mast cell sarcoma. There was no evidence of cutaneous mastocytosis. Further tumours appeared on her back and arm, which showed similar histological features. She subsequently developed nodules in the breasts, submandibular and axillary lymph nodes, followed by recurrence of her laryngeal tumour. She was treated with bleomycin and local radiotherapy to the larynx and skin lesions, with some improvement, but within 8 months there was recurrence which again responded to combined chemotherapy and radiotherapy. However, 5 months later there was further recurrence and the patient died with a haemorrhagic diathesis and circulatory failure. The histological appearances seen in several biopsies were initially similar; in the larynx, the subepithelial tissues were diffusely infiltrated by medium-sized cells with smooth, focally clefted nuclei with only mild nuclear pleomorphism; the cytoplasm was eosinophilic and contained numerous granules. The granules showed metachromatic staining with toluidine blue, and were strongly positive with the chloroacetate esterase procedure, confirming the mast cell nature of the tumour. In later biopsies, a much more pleomorphic population of highly mitotically active cells was present and metachromatic granules were scanty, suggesting tumour dedifferentiation. Electron microscopy confirmed the presence of typical electron-dense granules in the cytoplasm in the earlier biopsies.

SINUS HISTIOCYTOSIS WITH MASSIVE LYMPHADENOPATHY

Sinus histiocytosis with massive lymphadenopathy (SHML; Rosai–Dorfman disease) is a rare proliferative disease of histiocytes. It is probably not neoplastic and is regarded as an idiopathic histiocytosis.[74,75] Although not a true neoplasm, the disease may cause large tumourous masses at any nodal or extranodal site in the body. SHML is diagnosed by its characteristic histological appearances, the pathognomonic cell being a large histiocyte with a vesicular nucleus containing a prominent nucleolus which is often central; there is abundant cytoplasm which often contains phagocytosed lymphocytes and inflammatory cells. These histiocytes infiltrate tissues as swathes, and aggregates of cells and are usually associated with a heavy, predominantly chronic, inflammatory cell infiltrate; foci of necrosis may occur. The head and neck region is commonly affected; cervical lymph nodes are the most frequently involved lymph node region (87.3%[31]). The nasal cavity, paranasal sinuses, orbit, salivary gland and oral cavity are the commoner sites of extranodal disease in the head and neck.[31]

Seven cases of laryngeal involvement by SHML have been described in the literature.[9,18,21,31,60,69] All regions of the larynx may be affected, but there appears to be a predominance of glottic disease; the lesions are described as smooth-surfaced and sessile or polypoid. The majority of patients have nodal as well as additional extranodal sites of SHML, and these frequently include the nose and paranasal sinuses.[31] The clinical course of SHML is unpredictable, with some cases undergoing spontaneous regression and others having persistent or progressive disease which may prove fatal. There have been too few cases of laryngeal SHML to be able to draw firm conclusions about prognosis, but two-thirds of patients appear to have persistent disease.[31]

REFERENCES

1. Agarwal M K, Gupta S, Gupta O P 1982 Mycosis fungoides of the larynx. Asian Med J 25: 180–184
2. Agarwal M K, Samant H C, Gupta O P, Khanna S 1981 Multiple myeloma invading the larynx. Ear Nose Throat J 60: 395–397
3. Amromin G D 1968 The pathology of leukaemia. Harper & Row, New York
4. Anderson H A, Maisell R H, Cantrell R W 1976 Isolated laryngeal lymphoma. Laryngoscope 86: 1251–1257
5. Babitt D C, Yarington C T, Yonkers A J 1973 Malignant lymphoma of the larynx. J Laryngol Otol 87: 807–810
6. Bienenstock J, Befus A D 1980 Mucosal immunology. Immunology 41: 249–270
7. Bienenstock J, Johnston N, Perey D Y E 1973 Bronchial lymphoid tissue: I. Morphologic characteristics. Lab Invest 28: 686–692
8. Bienenstock J, Johnston N, Perey D Y E 1973 Bronchial lymphoid tissue: II. Functional characteristics. Lab Invest 28: 693–698
9. Biller H F, Pilch B Z 1981 A 51 year old man with upper airway obstruction and lymphadenopathy. New Engl J Med 305: 1572–1580
10. Boutens F, Cuvelier C 1981 Non-Hodgkin's lymphoma presenting as a solitary laryngeal tumour. J Belge Radiol 64: 357–359
11. Brito-Babapulle F, Lord J A D, Babatis C, Whitmore D N 1989 Laryngeal infiltration in chronic myelomonocytic leukaemia. Clin Lab Haemat 11: 403–406
12. Chen K T K 1984 Localised laryngeal lymphoma. J Surg Oncol 26: 208–209
13. Clerf L H 1946 Sarcoma of the larynx. Arch Otolaryngol 44: 517–524
14. Cogliatti S B, Hansmann M L, Schumacher U, Eckert F, Schmidt U, Lennert K 1990 Primary gastric lymphoma. Clinical and prognostic features of 145 cases. Abstract 75, Fourth International Conference on Malignant Lymphoma, Lugano
15. Cohen S R, Landing B H, Feig S, Byrne W J, Isaacs H 1978 Primary lymphosarcoma of the larynx in a child. Ann Otol Rhinol Laryngol 52 (suppl): 20–24
16. Cohen S R, Landing BH, Isaacs H, King K K, Hanson V 1978 Solitary plasmacytoma of the larynx and upper trachea associated

with systemic lupus erythematosus. Ann Otol Rhinol Laryngol Suppl 52: 11–14

17. Cohn A M, Park J K, Rappaport H 1971 Mycosis fungoides with involvement of the oral cavity. Arch Otolaryngol 93: 330–333

18. Courteney-Harris R G, Goddard M J 1992 Sinus histiocytosis with massive lymphadenopathy (Rosai–Dorfman disease): a rare cause of subglottic narrowing. J Laryngol Otol 106: 61–62

19. DeSanto L W, Weiland L H 1970 Malignant lymphoma of the larynx. Laryngoscope 80: 966–978

20. Dickson R 1971 Lymphoma of the larynx. Laryngoscope 81: 578–585

21. Diebold J, Audouin J, Viry B, Ghandour C, Betti P, D'Ornano G 1990 Primary lymphoplasmacytic lymphoma of the larynx: a rare localization of MALT-type lymphoma. Ann Otol Rhinol Laryngol 99: 577–580

22. Dindzans L J, Irvine B W H, Hayden R E 1984 An unusual case of airway obstruction. J Otolaryngol 13: 252–254

23. Dogra T S 1972 Lymphosarcoma of the larynx. J Laryngol Otol 86: 535–541

24. East D 1978 Laryngeal involvement in multiple myeloma. J Laryngol Otol 92: 61–65

25. Epstein E H, Levin F L, Croft J D, Lutzner M A 1972 Mycosis fungoides: survival prognostic features, response to therapy, and autopsy findings. Medicine 51: 61–72

26. Ferguson J L, Maragos N E, Weiland L H 1987 Granulocytic sarcoma (chloroma) of the epiglottis. Otolaryngol Head Neck Surg 6: 588–590

27. Ferlito A, Carbone A, Volpe R 1981 Diagnosis and assessment of non-Hodgkin's malignant lymphoma of the larynx. ORL J Otorhinolaryngol Relat Spec 43: 61–78

28. Ferlito A, Doglioni C, Bontempini L, Arrigoni A 1984 Metachronous coexistence of laryngeal pseudolymphoma and squamous cell carcinoma. ORL J Otorhinolaryngol Relat Spec 46: 202–209

29. Ferlito, Recher G 1986 Laryngeal involvement by mycosis fungoides. Ann Otol Rhinol Laryngol 95: 275–277

30. Fishkin B G, Speigelberg H L 1976 Cervical lymph node metastasis as the first manifestation of localised extramedullary plasmacytoma. Cancer 38: 1641–1644

31. Foucar E, Rosai J, Dorfman R F 1990 Sinus histiocytosis with massive lymphadenopathy (Rosai–Dorfman disease): review of the entity. Sem Diagn Pathol 7:19–73

32. Freeman C, Berg J W, Cutler S J 1972 Occurrence and prognosis of extranodal lymphomas. Cancer 29: 252–260

33. Furebring-Freden M, Martinsson U, Sundstrom C 1990 Myelosarcoma without acute leukaemia: immunohistochemical and clinico-pathologic characterization of eight cases. Histopathology 16: 243–250

34. Gaffney C C, Dawes P J D K, Jackson D 1987 Plasmacytoma of the head and neck. Clin Radiol 38: 385–388

35. Georghiou P A, Hogg M L 1988 Immunoglobulin A myeloma presenting with laryngeal obstruction. Med J Aust 149: 447–449

36. Gorenstein A G, Neel H B III, Devine K D, Weiland L H 1977 Solitary extramedullary plasmacytoma of the larynx. Arch Otolaryngol 103: 159–161

37. Gormley P K, Primrose W J, Bharucha H 1985 Subglottic plasmacytoma of the larynx: an acute presentation. J Laryngol Otol 99: 925–929

38. Gregor R T 1981 Laryngeal malignant lymphoma: an entity? J Laryngol Otol 95: 81–94

39. Harwood AR, Knowling M A, Bersagel D E 1965 Radiotherapy of extramedullary plasmacytoma of the head and neck. Clin Radiol 16: 395–399

40. Holmes G W, Schulz M D 1946 Radiation treatment of localised malignant lymphoma. New Eng J Med 235: 789–790

41. Hood A F, Mark G J, Hunt J V 1979 Laryngeal mycosis fungoides. Cancer 43: 1527–1532

42. Horny H P, Parwaresch M R, Kaiserling E, Muller K, Olbermann M, Mainzer K, Lennert K 1986 Mast cell sarcoma of the larynx. J Clin Pathol 39: 596–602

43. Hyams V J, Batsakis J G, Michaels L 1988 Lymphoreticular tissue neoplasia. In: Atlas of tumour pathology. 2nd series, fascicle 25. Armed Forces Institute of Pathology, Washington DC

44. Inagi K, Tabahashi H, Okamoto M, Yao K, Furukawa K 1989 A case of adult T cell leukaemia with a laryngeal tumor. J Otolaryngol Jpn 92: 46–50

45. Isaacson P G, Spencer J 1988 Malignant lymphoma of mucosa-associated lymphoid tissue. In: Habeshaw J A, Lauder I (eds) Malignant lymphomas. Churchill Livingstone, Edinburgh, pp 179–200

46. Jones N S, Kenyon G S, Mahy N 1987 Multiple myeloma in bony metaplasia of the cricoid cartilage (a rare cause of laryngeal obstruction). J Laryngol Otol 101: 1301–1305

47. Jones R V, Shalom A S 1968 Laryngeal involvement in acute leukaemia. J Laryngol Otol 82: 123–128

48. Karcher D S, Perry D J, Hurwitz M A, Detrick-Hooks B 1982 T cell lymphoma occurring in the oropharynx. Cancer 50: 1155–1159

49. Knowles D M 1989 Immunophenotypic and antigen receptor gene rearrangement analysis in T cell neoplasia. Am J Pathol 134: 761–785

50. Kober S J 1979 Solitary plasmacytoma of the carina. Thorax 34: 567–568

51. Kost K M 1990 Plasmacytomas of the larynx. J Otolaryngol 19: 141–146

52. Lachmann J 1951 Sarcoma of the larynx. Arch Otolaryngol 53: 299–307

53. Lennert K, Stein H, Kaiserling E 1975 Cytologic and functional criteria for the classification of malignant lymphomata. Br J Cancer 31 (suppl II) 29–43

54. Lennert K (in collaboration with Mohri N, Stein H, Kaiserling E, Muller-Hermelink H K) 1978 Malignant lymphomas other than Hodgkin's disease. Histology, cytology, ultrastructure and immunology. Springer-Verlag, Berlin

55. Mackenty J E 1934 Malignant disease of the larynx. Arch Otolaryngol 20: 297–328

56. MacLennan K A, Bennett M H, Morton J, Leyland M J, MacLennan S, Vaughan Hudson B, Vaughan Hudson G 1990 The prognostic significance of histological pattern in primary gastric lymphoma: an analysis of 80 patients. Abstract 76, 4th International Conference on Malignant Lymphoma, Lugano

57. Marks M M 1953 Monocytic leukaemia — oral and anorectal involvement. J Int Coll Surg 20: 750–752

58. Mason D Y, Krissansen G W, Davey F R, Crumpton M J, Gatter K C 1988 Antisera against epitopes resistant to denaturation on T 3 (CD 3) antigen can detect reactive and neoplastic T cells in paraffin embedded tissue biopsy specimens. J Clin Pathol 41: 121–127

59. Michaels L, Hyams V J 1979 Amyloid in localised deposits and plasmacytomas of the respiratory tract. J Pathol 128: 29–38

60. Miettinen M, Paljakka P, Haveri P et al 1987 Sinus histiocytosis with massive lymphadenopathy: a nodal and extranodal proliferation of S 100 positive histiocytes? Am J Clin Pathol 88: 270–277

61. Mill W B, Griffith R 1980 The role of radiation therapy in the management of plasma cell tumours. Cancer 45: 647–652

62. Mora E, Sertoli M R, Campara E, Parodi G 1981 Epiglottic non-Hodgkin's lymphoma: case report. Tumori 67: 507–510

63. Morgan K, MacLennan K A, Narula A, Bradley P J, Morgan D A L 1989 Non-Hodgkin's lymphoma of the larynx (stage 1E). Cancer 64: 1123–1127

64. Nakashima T, Inamitsu M, Uemura T, Sugimoto T 1989 Immunopathology of polymorphic reticulosis of the larynx. J Laryngol Otol 103: 955–960

65. Neiman R S, Barcos M, Berard C, Bonner H, Mann R, Rydell R E, Bennett J M 1981 Granulocytic sarcoma: a clinicopathologic study of 61 biopsied cases. Cancer 48: 1426–1437

66. Ng C S, Chan J K C, Hui P K, Lau W H 1989 Large B-cell lymphomas with a high content of reactive T cells. Hum Pathol 20: 1145–1154

67. Norton A J, Isaacson P G 1989 Lymphoma phenotyping in formalin-fixed and paraffin wax-embedded tissue: II. Profiles of reactivity in the various tumour types. Histopathology 14: 557–579

68. Pahor A L 1978 Plasmacytoma of the larynx. J Laryngol Otol 92: 223–232

69. Penneys N S, Ahn Y S, McKinney E C, McCleod T, Byrne G, Byrnes J, Nadji M 1982 Sinus histiocytosis with massive lymphadenopathy. A case with unusual skin involvement and a therapeutic response to vinblastine-loaded platelets. Cancer 49: 1994–1998

70. Picker L J, Weiss L M, Medeiros L J et al 1987 Immunophenotypic criteria for the diagnosis of non-Hodgkin's lymphoma. Am J Pathol 128: 181–201

71. Podoshin L, Fradis M, Schalit M 1971 Lymphosarcoma of the larynx. J Laryngol Otol 82: 1063–1068

72. Ramsey A D, Smith W J, Isaacson P G 1988 T-cell-rich B-cell lymphoma. Am J Surg Pathol 12: 433–443

73. Rappaport H, Thomas L B 1974 Mycosis fungoides: the pattern of extracutaneous involvement. Cancer 34: 1199–1229

74. Rosai J, Dorfman R F 1969 Sinus histiocytosis with massive lymphadenopathy: a newly recognised benign clinicopathological entity. Arch Pathol 87: 63–70

75. Rosai J, Dorfman R F 1972 Sinus histiocytosis with massive lymphadenopathy: a pseudolymphomatous benign disorder. Analysis of 34 cases. Cancer 30: 1174–1188

76. Rudders R A, Ross M E, DeLellis R A 1978 Primary extra-nodal lymphoma: response to treatment and factors influencing prognosis. Cancer 42: 406–416

77. Schilling B B, Abell M R, Work W P 1967 Leukaemic involvement of larynx. Arch Otolaryngol 85; 658–665

78. Seddon D J, Chung K F, Paradinas F J, Newlands E S, Snashall P D 1989 Long-term survival after treatment of disseminated T cell lymphoma presenting with tracheal obstruction in a patient with coeliac disease. Thorax 44: 519–520

79. Shima N, Kobashi Y, Tsutsui K et al 1990 Extranodal non-Hodgkin's lymphoma of the head and neck. A clinicopathologic study in the Kyoto-Nara area of Japan. Cancer 66: 1190–1197

80. Stansfeld A G, Diebold J, Kapanci Y, Kelenyi G, Lennert K, Misoluzewska O, Noel H, Rilke F, Sundstrom C, Van Unnik J A, Wright D H 1988 Updated Kiel classification for lymphomas. Lancet i: 292–293

81. Stepnick D, Sawyer R 1989 Isolated subglottic lymphomas. Otolaryngol Head Neck Surg 101: 578–580

82. Strahan R W, Calcaterra T C 1971 Otolaryngologic aspects of mycosis fungoides. Laryngoscope 81: 1912–1916

83. Swerdlow J B, Merl S A, Davey F R, Gacek R R, Gottlieb A J 1984 Non-Hodgkin's lymphoma limited to the larynx. Cancer 53: 2546–2549

84. Swinson C M, Slavin G, Coles E C, Booth C C 1983 Coeliac disease and malignancy. Lancet i: 111

85. The Non-Hodgkin's Lymphoma Pathologic Classification Project 1982 National Cancer Institute sponsored study of classifications of non-Hodgkin's lymphomas: summary and description of a working formulation for clinical usage. Cancer 49: 2112–2135

86. Ti M, Villafuerte R, Chase P H, Dosik H 1974 Acute leukaemia presenting as laryngeal obstruction. Cancer 34: 427–430

87. Wang C C 1972 Malignant lymphoma of the larynx. Laryngoscope 82: 97–100

88. Warthin A S 1909 Death due to leukaemic infiltration of the larynx. International Clinic Series 4: 280–295

89. Webb H E, Harrison E, Masson J K, Remine W H 1962 Solitary extramedullary plasmacytoma (myeloma) of the upper part of the respiratory tract and oropharynx. Cancer 15: 1142–1155

90. Wiltshaw E 1976 The natural history of extramedullary plasmacytoma and its relation to solitary myeloma of bone and myelomatosis. Medicine 55: 217–238

91. Woodruff R K, Whittle J M, Malpas J S 1979 Solitary plasmacytoma. Cancer 43: 2340–2343

18. Blastoma, hamartoma and teratoma

A. Ferlito

BLASTOMA

The term 'pulmonary blastoma' was coined by Spencer in 1961,[20] replacing the earlier name of 'embryoma of the lung'.[3] Spencer[20] considered pulmonary blastomas as deriving from a primitive totipotential blastoma cell capable of differentiating into epithelium and mesenchyme and in many ways similar to Wilm's tumour of the kidney. The embryological basis of this concept is no longer acceptable and the histogenesis of the neoplasm is uncertain.

Eble et al[9] first reported a blastoma of the pyriform sinus in 1985; it was described as a neoplasm morphologically similar to pulmonary blastoma. The case was also reviewed by John G. Batsakis. Considering that the lesion is unique, it is preferable to give the pathological findings in the author's own words:[9]

Grossly, the neoplasm formed an exophytic mass in the right pyriform fossa (Fig. 18.1). It was polypoid, 33 × 17 × 16 mm, and had a base approximately 15 mm wide on the lateral wall of the pyriform fossa. The surface of the neoplasm was lobulated and rough. Before fixation, the surface was brown and mottled with congestion and hemorrhage, but did not appear ulcerated. Its cut surface was a homogeneous gray-tan with neither grossly obvious necrosis nor cysts. . . . Light microscopy showed the

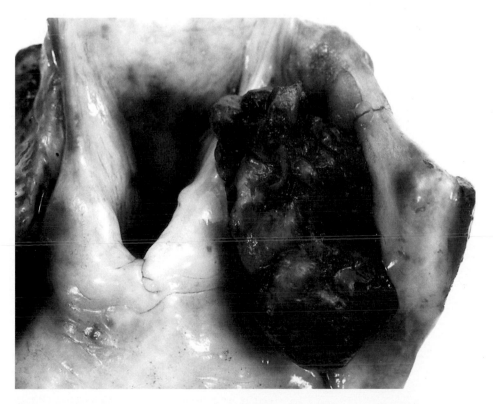

Fig. 18.1 External appearance of blastoma in the right pyriform fossa. (Courtesy of Dr J. N. Eble, Indianapolis, and the editor of *American Journal of Clinical Pathology*.)

surface of the neoplasm to be multilobular (Fig. 18.2) with foci of adherent exudate and debris. Some lobules had small areas of necrosis and hemorrhage near the surface. The neoplasm consisted of a mixture of blastematous, mesenchymal and epithelial components, in which transitions from one to another occurred abruptly and frequently (Fig. 18.3). The blastematous component predominated and consisted of cells with small round-to-oval nuclei with thick nuclear membranes and frequently with small nucleoli. The cytoplasm was pale, sparse and wispy, with ill-defined borders. These cells were arranged haphazardly in sheets, often forming nodules, some of which contained a central blood vessel (Fig. 18.4). In a few foci, the blastematous cells had more abundant cytoplasm and more hyperchromatic nuclei than elsewhere. The mesenchymal component consisted, in part, of stellate and spindle cells arranged in a faintly basophilic matrix (Figs 18.5, 18.6) which stained weakly with Alcian blue at pH 2.5, and moderately with Alcian blue at pH 4.0. Sections stained with periodic acid–Schiff (PAS) showed that this matrix was PAS-negative. In other parts of the tumour the stroma consisted of spindle cells with wispy, faintly eosinophilic cytoplasm. These were areas in which the stroma was intimately mixed with cords of epithelial cells (Fig. 18.7). There was moderate nuclear pleomorphism. Multinuclear forms were not present. Epithelial elements were scattered throughout the neoplasm and were varied in their morphological features. Glandular structures with well-formed lumens lined by low columnar epithelium and well-differentiated squamous elements were found within the lesion. Squamous differentiation was most apparent at the surface at the base of the lesion. The predominant epithelial component consisted of cords of polygonal cells that interlaced in a complex pattern against a background of spindle-cell stroma. Islands of epithelial cells were found scattered in the sheets of blastema and the transition from blastema to epithelium or stroma was seen throughout the lesion. Mitotic figures were found in stroma, epithelium and blastema. Thin sections showed nests and cords of epithelial cells that varied from spindle to cuboidal. These nests were surrounded by incomplete basal lamina. Cytoplasm was moderate in quantity and contained rough endoplasmic reticulum, Golgi structures, round and oval mitochondria, bundles of tonofilaments and a few lysosomes. Cells were connected by desmosomes. Some epithelial cells lined central areas that resembled small, glandular structures by light microscopy. The cells lining these areas had pseudopodia and surface specialization resembling microvilli, but microvillous, microfilamentous cores and tripartite junctions were lacking. A few glycogen lakes were seen.

Blastematous elements consisted of cells that were irregularly shaped and connected by desmosomes. They had moderate quantities of cytoplasm that contained rough endoplasmic reticulum, oval and round mitochondria, Golgi structures and a few lysosomes. They also contained prominent glycogen lakes. Nuclei were irregularly shaped and contained moderately granular chromatin. Mesenchymal elements included poorly differentiated mesenchymal cells, immature fibroblasts and cells resembling myofibroblasts.

Differential diagnosis must be made from spindle cell squamous carcinoma, teratocarcinoma[9] and laryngeal carcinoma with multidirectional differentiation[8]. Glandular structures are absent in spindle cell squamous carcinoma but present in laryngeal blastoma. There is no blastematous component in teratocarcinoma, which, conversely, contains organoid structures not found in blastoma.[9]

The blastematous component was not found in the case of laryngeal carcinoma with multidirectional differentiation recently reported by Doglioni et al[8] in which the presence of areas of carcinoma in situ and microinvasive squamous cell carcinoma also go against the diagnosis of blastoma. Immunocytochemical studies must be used to make a correct diagnosis of unusual tumours.

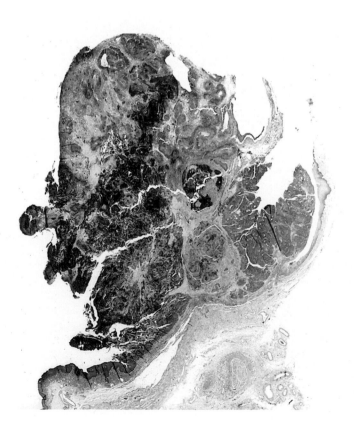

Fig. 18.2 (*left*) Whole-mount section showing lobular architecture, broad base and varied tissue types of laryngeal blastoma. H&E, ×1. (Courtesy of Dr J. N. Eble, Indianapolis, and the editor of *American Journal of Clinical Pathology.*)

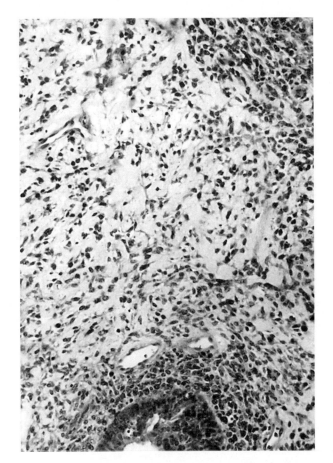 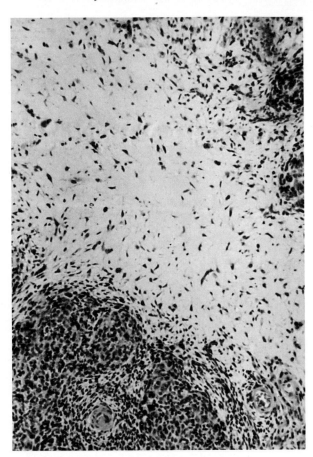

Fig. 18.3 (*left*) A glandular epithelial element surrounded by a cuff of blastema (lower) with an abrupt transition to stellate and spindle-cell mesenchyme. The edge of another nodule of blastema is shown in the upper right. H&E, ×6. (Courtesy of Dr J. N. Eble, Indianapolis, and the editor of *American Journal of Clinical Pathology*.)

Fig. 18.4 (*right*) A nodule of blastema with a central blood vessel (lower left). Stellate mesenchymal cells in the myxoid matrix. H&E, ×63. (Courtesy of Dr J. N. Eble, Indianapolis, and the editor of *American Journal of Clinical Pathology*.)

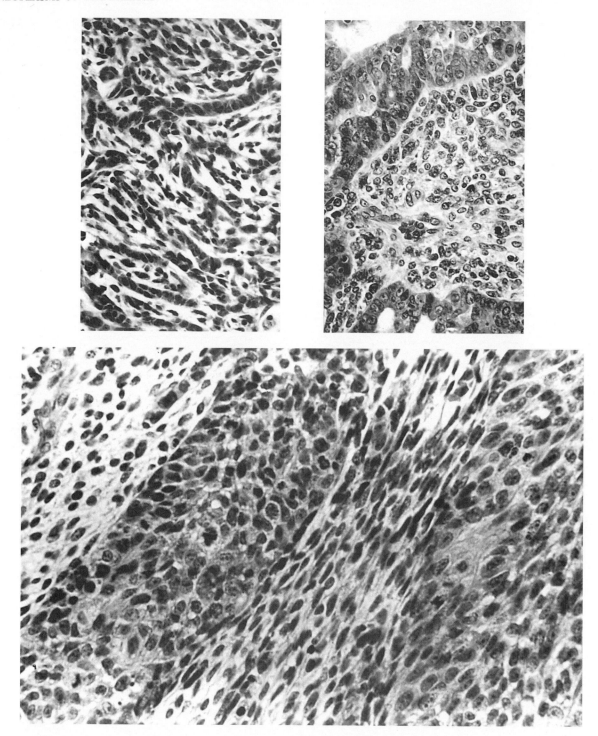

Fig. 18.5 (*top, left*) Admixture of interlacing cords of epithelial cells with mesenchymal spindle cells. H&E, ×250. (Courtesy of Dr J. N. Eble, Indianapolis, and the editor of *American Journal of Clinical Pathology*.)

Fig. 18.6 (*top, right*) Glandular structures with well-formed lumens arising in a background of blastema. H&E, ×250. (Courtesy of Dr J. N. Eble, Indianapolis, and the editor of *American Journal of Clinical Pathology*.)

Fig. 18.7 (*bottom*) Transitions of blastema to epithelium to spindle-cell stroma to epithelium. Note mitotic figures in the epithelial compartments. H&E ×250. (Courtesy of Dr J. N. Eble, Indianapolis, and the editor of *American Journal of Clinical Pathology*.)

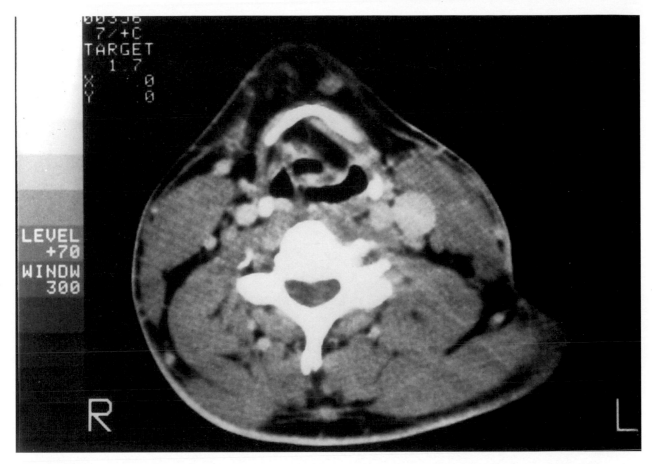

Fig. 18.8   Pre-operative CT scan reveals complete distortion of the supraglottic larynx by hamartoma. (Courtesy of Dr S. M. Archer, Lexington, and the editor of *International Journal of Pediatric Otorhinolaryngology.*)

HAMARTOMA

The term 'hamartoma' derives from the Greek word 'hamartanein' which means 'to go wrong', and Albrecht[1] introduced this term in 1904 to distinguish tumour-like malformations from true neoplasms. Hamartoma designates an excessive focal overgrowth of normal cells and tissue indigenous to its site of origin. The lesion is not a neoplasm but a development anomaly. In other words, it represents a simple exaggeration of a normal physiological process.[4]

A hamartoma may occur in any organ, but it often involves the spleen, liver and lungs. Hamartomas of the larynx are rare, and only a few cases have been reported.[2,17,19–23] Archer et al[2] described two cases (Figs 18.8–18.12) requiring partial laryngectomy. The lesion has also been found in the hypopharynx.[18] Cohen[6] reported two cases of hamartoma associated with posterior clefts and causing severe episodes of airway obstruction. Meyer-Breiting and Burkhardt[16] observed a hamartomatous laryngeal polyp with Cowden's disease in a 49-year-old female patient.

Posterior cleft larynx associated with hamartoma is a rare malformation complex well documented in the literature.[6,13,14]

The preponderant tissue further defines the lesion as cartilaginous hamartoma, myxochondromatous hamartoma, neuromyomatous hamartoma, mesenchymal hamartoma, epithelial hamartoma, glandular hamartoma, etc.

Diagnosis may be problematic and must differentiate from choristoma, teratoma and rhabdomyoma, among others. Choristoma (or heterotopia) is characterized by the presence of mature tissue elements not normally occurring in the locations where they are found. Teratoma usually shows multiple mature and immature tissues, mainly of neural type, resembling neuroblasts. Hamartoma contains an admixture of adipose and fibrous tissue in addition to skeletal muscle cells which allows it to be distinguished from rhabdomyoma. Differential diagnosis also concerns mixed tumour, chondroma and chondrometaplasia.

Management should consist of conservative excision. Recurrences are usually associated with incomplete removal.

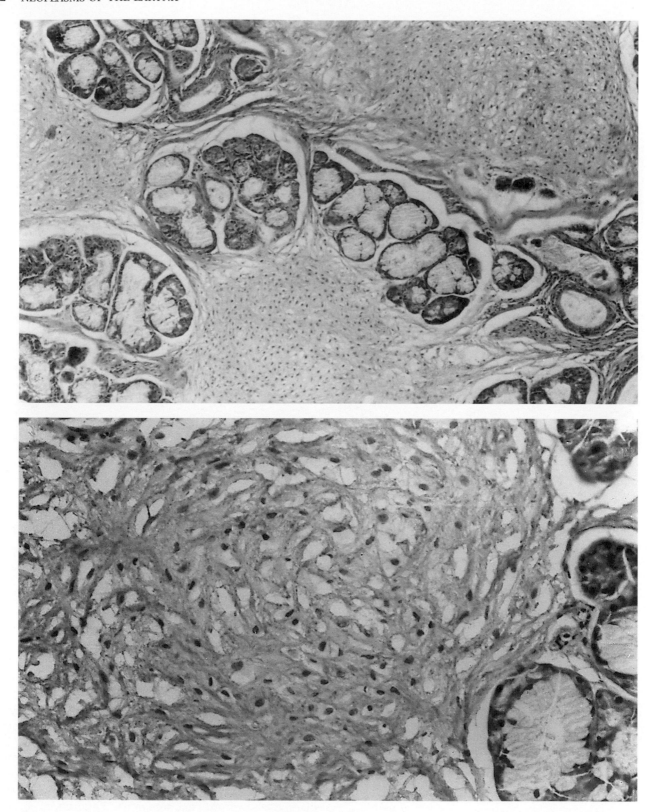

Fig. 18.9 (*top*), **18.10** (*bottom*) Myxochondromatous hamartoma of the larynx. Multifocal nodules of benign cartilage and a myxoid matrix are seen in the low- and high-power photomicrographs. Note the fat, skeletal muscle and nerve around the chondromatous matrix. (Courtesy of Dr S. M. Archer, Lexington, and the editor of *International Journal of Pediatric Otorhinolaryngology*.)

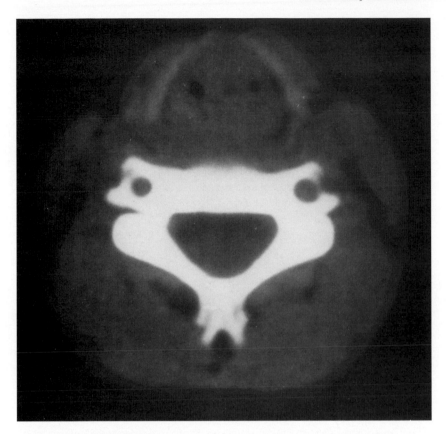

Fig. 18.11   Pre-operative CT scan showing the infiltrative nature of a laryngeal hamartoma. (Courtesy of Dr S. M. Archer, Lexington, and the editor of *International Journal of Pediatric Otorhinolaryngology*.)

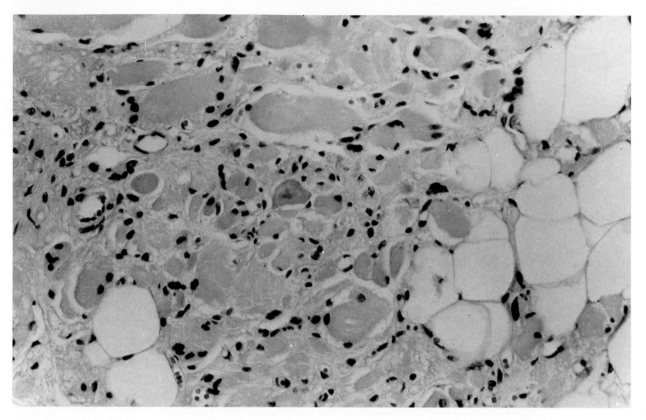

Fig. 18.12   The microscopic appearance of a laryngeal hamartoma is that of a non-encapsulated tumour mass composed of poorly organized skeletal muscle and neural elements and interspersed with fat cells. (Courtesy of Dr S. M. Archer, Lexington, and the editor of *International Journal of Pediatric Otorhinolaryngology*.)

TERATOMA

Teratomas are rare lesions containing multiple tissues in varying amounts, involving all three, or at least two, basic germ cell layers (ectoderm, mesoderm and endoderm) in various degrees of maturation.[12] They are therefore distinguished as mature (entirely composed of well-differentiated tissues) and immature (with some tissues of immature or embryonic appearance) and occur prevalently in the sacrococcygeal region, ovaries, mediastinum and retroperitoneum.

Only approximately 10% of teratomas occur in the head and neck areas, the neck and nasopharynx being the most common sites.[4] These lesions are very rare in the larynx, and only a few cases have been reported.[7,10,11,15]

In 1987, Cannon et al[5] described one case of immature teratoma of the larynx occurring in a 32-year-old woman complaining of hoarseness of 3 months' duration. The lesion involved the true vocal cord and was completely excised. The patient is currently well 5 years later. The teratoma was composed of primitive cells, with uniform nuclei and scant cytoplasm. There was an irregular distribution of melanin containing cells recapitulating the retinal anlage (Figs 18.13, 18.14); there was also a mucoid matrix and the cells resembled fetal cartilage (Fig. 18.15). Part of the surface of the lesion was covered by a flattened epithelial lining (Fig. 18.16) The absence of mitoses and necrosis suggested a benign lesion.[5] The treatment of choice is surgery, and the biological behaviour is usually benign.

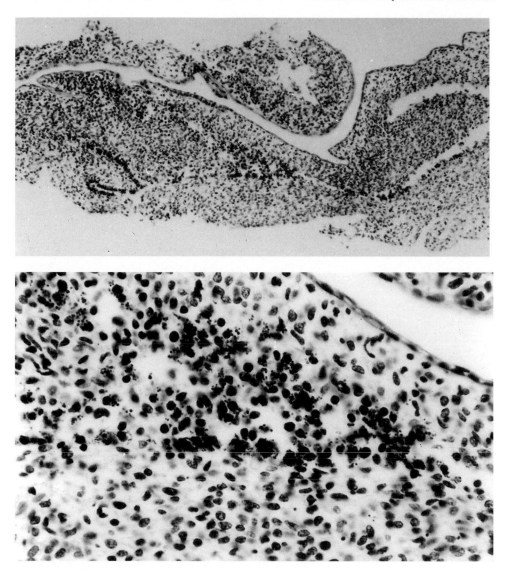

Fig. 18.13 (*top*) Immature teratoma of the larynx. A portion of the tumour consists of immature cells. An irregularly shaped, but well-delineated line of pigmented cells recapitulates retina. H&E, ×20 OM. (Courtesy of Dr R. E. Fechner, Virginia, and the editor of *Otolaryngology, Head and Neck Surgery*.)

Fig. 18.14 (*bottom*) The melanin-containing cells are seen at higher power. H&E, ×200 OM. (Courtesy of Dr R. E. Fechner, Virginia, and the editor of *Otolaryngology, Head and Neck Surgery*.)

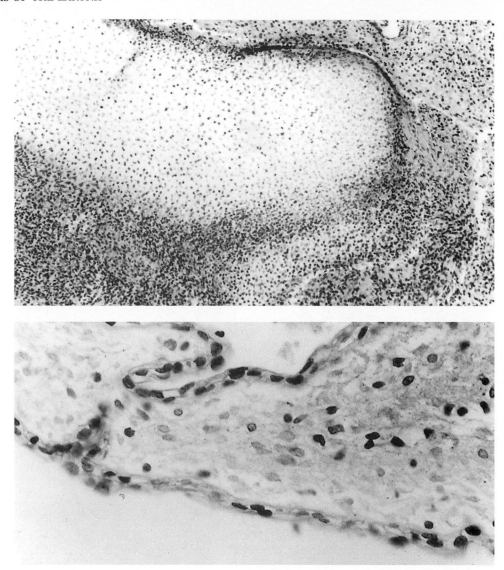

Fig. 18.15 (*top*) Part of the tumour has a dense zone of undifferentiated mesenchymal cells that are condensed around stroma, with the appearance of immature cartilage. H&E, ×100. OM. (Courtesy of Dr R. E. Fechner, Virginia, and the editor of *Otolaryngology, Head and Neck Surgery*.)

Fig. 18.16 (*bottom*) A flattened epithelial lining, without distinguishing features, covers much of the lesion. H&E, ×200. (Courtesy of Dr R. E. Fechner, Virginia, and the editor of *Otolaryngology, Head and Neck Surgery*.)

REFERENCES

1. Albrecht E 1904 Uber Hamartome. Verh Dtsch Ges Pathol 7: 153–157
2. Archer S M, Crockett D M, McGill T J I 1988 Hamartoma of the larynx: report of two cases and review of the literature. Int J Pediatr Otorhinolaryngol 16: 237–243
3. Barnard W G 1952 Embryoma of lung. Thorax 7: 299–301
4. Batsakis J G 1979 Tumors of the head and neck, 2nd edn. Williams & Wilkins, Baltimore
5. Cannon C R, Johns M E, Fechner R E 1987 Immature teratoma of the larynx. Otolaryngol Head Neck Surg 96: 366–368
6. Cohen S R 1984 Posterior cleft larynx associated with hamartoma. Ann Otol Rhinol Laryngol 93: 443–446
7. Chumakov F I, Voinova V G 1973 Unusual case of teratoma of the larynx: Vestn Otorinolaringol 73: 92–94
8. Doglioni C, Ferlito A, Chiamenti C, Viale G, Rosai J 1990 Laryngeal carcinoma showing multidirectional epithelial, neuroendocrine and sarcomatous differentiation. ORL J Otorhinolaryngol Relat Spec 52: 316–326
9. Eble J N, Hull M T, Bojrab D 1985 Laryngeal blastoma. A light and electron microscopic study of a novel entity analogous to pulmonary blastoma. Am J Clin Pathol 84: 378–385
10. Fleischer K 1956 Drei seltene Kehlkopftumoren. Speicheldrüsenmischtumor–Teratom–Granuloblastom. Laryngol Rhinol Otol 35: 346–354
11. Fournie R, Benkiran D, Carresse J, Tahiri M 1965 A propos d'un cas de tératome foetoide anisopage endocymiens inclus de la région latero-laryngée. J Fr Otorhinolaryngol 14: 893–903
12. Gonzales-Crussi F 1982 Extragonadal teratomas. In: Atlas of tumor pathology, 2nd series, fasc 18. Armed Forces Institute of Pathology, Washington DC
13. Holinger L D, Tansek K M, Tuker G F 1985 Cleft larynx with airway obstruction. Ann Otol Rhinol Laryngol 94: 622–626
14. Lyons T J, Variend S 1958 Posterior cleft larynx associated with hamartoma: a case report and literature review. J Laryngol Otol 102: 471–472
15. Johnson L F, Strong M S 1953 Teratoma of the larynx. Arch Otolaryngol 58: 435–441
16. Meyer-Breiting E, Burkhardt A 1988 Tumours of the larynx. Springer-Verlag, Berlin
17. Mozota Ortiz J R, Medina Sola J J, Munilla Moneo L, Aguado Martinez F, Arruti Gonzales I, Alfaro Garcia J, Hueto Prado J 1988 Laryngeal hamartoma. Report of a case. Acta Otorrinolaringol Esp 39: 45–47
18. Patterson H C, Dickerson G R, Pilch B Z, Bentkover S H 1981 Hamartoma of the hypopharynx. Arch Otolaryngol 107: 767–772
19. Smith H W 1959 Skeletal muscle rhabdomyoma of the larynx: report of a case. Laryngoscope 69: 1528–1536
20. Spencer H 1961 Pulmonary blastomas. J Pathol Bacteriol 82: 161–165
21. Weinberger J, Kassim O, Birt B D 1985 Hamartoma of the larynx. J Otolaryngol 14: 305–308
22. Wilhelm H J, Dietz R, Schoendorf J 1980 Diagnosis and treatment of rare tumours in the laryngeal-pharyngeal area. Laryngol Rhinol Otol 59: 137–143
23. Zapf B, Lehmann W B, Snyder G G 1981 Hamartoma of the larynx: an unusual cause for stridor in an infant. Otolaryngol Head Neck Surg 89: 797–799

19. Secondary neoplasms

A. Ferlito

INTRODUCTION

Laryngeal involvement in the course of systemic malignant neoplasms (such as in acute and chronic leukaemias and lymphomas) and infiltration of the larynx by neoplasms arising in contiguous structures (e.g. thyroid gland, trachea, tongue base, hypopharynx and cervical oesophagus) should not be considered as metastases.

INCIDENCE

While metastatic tumours to the lung represent the most frequent pulmonary neoplasms, metastatic neoplasms to the larynx are considered rare. The comparative paucity of metastatic tumours in the larynx may be explained by its terminal position in the lymphatic and vascular system.[34] The first documented case of secondary cancer of the larynx was reported by Eppinger in 1880[20] and concerned a skin melanoma metastatic to the left ventricular band. Several reviews of the literature on the subject have been published.[4,25,26,35,37,87] Taking into account other and more recently published cases,[17,28,38,43,61,70,73,79,80] the total number of secondary laryngeal tumours reported to date amounts to 134.[1-90] The essential data are summarized in Table 19.1.

In a series of more than 4000 malignant neoplasms of the larynx observed at the ENT Department of Padua University from 1966 to 1992, there were only eight cases of metastases (six from skin melanoma and two from renal adenocarcinoma).

The increasing number of reports may reflect a true increase in the incidence of the disease, a longer survival due to improved local control of the primary neoplasm, or a more careful evaluation of the larynx.

SITES OF PRIMARY LESION

The primary sources of metastatic tumour, in order of frequency, are: skin (melanoma, Figs 19.1–19.6), kidney (Figs 19.7–19.11), breast, lung, prostate, colon (Fig. 19.12), stomach and ovary. Occasional cases of metastases from the pancreas, testis, uterine cervix, bone, nasopharynx, nose, trachea, oesophagus, gall bladder, liver, adrenal gland, etc. have also been reported. There was one case in which nasal melanoma metastasized to subglottic and tracheal areas.[8] One amelanotic melanoma of the eye metastasized to the supraglottic region.[75] Only six cases have been reported of mesenchymal tumours causing laryngeal metastases.[3,4,12,50,71,88]

CLINICAL FEATURES

Men are most frequently affected, but the male-to-female ratio is less than 2:1. The age range is 24 to 83 years.

The most common sites are the supraglottic and the subglottic regions, in that order, because of their abundant vascularity. The vocal cord is seldom involved,[38,70] though multiple laryngeal metastases may occur. Being composed of elastic cartilage, the epiglottis is the laryngeal cartilage offering least resistance to metastatic spread. Ossified cartilages are more easily invaded by metastatic tumours because they have a direct blood supply. The perichondrium acts as a barrier against metastatic spread.

Glanz and Kleinsasser[37] divided laryngeal metastases into two groups: (i) those metastasizing to soft tissues, mainly to the vestibular and aryepiglottic folds and sometimes to the vocal cords or epiglottis—such as melanoma and renal adenocarcinoma; (ii) those which tend to spread to the marrow spaces in the ossified cricoid and thyroid cartilages and occasionally even in the arytenoid cartilages—such as lung and breast carcinomas.

Symptoms of metastatic tumours to the larynx are comparable with those of primary tumours and vary according to the site affected. Haemoptysis is an important symptom of laryngeal metastasis from renal adenocarcinoma because of the abundant vascularization of the tumour. Some of the cases reported were asymptomatic, and the laryngeal involvement was an autopsy finding.[2,18,32,54] In other cases,[7,27,37,49,75]

Table 19.1   Reported cases of laryngeal metastases with regard to primary tumour

Primary tumour	Histological type	Number of cases	(%)
Skin	Melanoma	46	34.32
Nasal mucosa	Melanoma	1	0.74
Eye	Melanoma	1	0.74
Kidney	Adenocarcinoma (20) Sarcoma (1)	21	15.67
Breast	Carcinoma	13	9.70
Lung	Carcinoma (6) Adenocarcinoma (2) Small cell carcinoma (3)	11	8.20
Prostate	Carcinoma (8) Small cell carcinoma (1)	9	6.71
Colon	Adenocarcinoma	6	4.47
Stomach	Adenocarcinoma (2) Leiomyosarcoma (1)	3	2.23
Ovary	Cystadenocarcinoma (1) Mesonephroid carcinoma (1) Anaplastic carcinoma (1)	3	2.23
Pancreas	Adenocarcinoma (1) Pleomorphic carcinoma (1)	2	1.49
Testis	Seminoma	2	1.49
Uterine cervix	Carcinoma	2	1.49
Bone	Giant cell tumour (1) Unspecified (1)	2	1.49
Nasopharynx	Carcinoma	2	1.49
Nose	Esthesioneuroblastoma	1	0.74
Trachea	Small cell carcinoma	1	0.74
Oesophagus	Carcinoma	1	0.74
Gall bladder	Carcinoma	1	0.74
Liver	Carcinoma	1	0.74
Adrenal gland	Sympathicoblastoma	1	0.74
Scalp/face	Angiosarcoma	1	0.74
Jaw	Sarcoma	1	0.74
Mediastinum	Sarcoma	1	0.74
Retroperitoneum	Sarcoma	1	0.74
TOTAL		134	

however, the larynx was the first location producing symptoms reported by the patient and led to the discovery of the primary neoplasm, which otherwise might have gone undetected.

PRIMARY OR METASTATIC GROWTH?

The question of whether a given neoplasm in the larynx is primary or metastatic arises particularly in patients with a solitary nodule. Clear cell carcinoma in the larynx may be metastatic from clear cell renal adenocarcinoma, which is more common than primary laryngeal clear cell carcinoma.[67] Stains for glycogen and lipids are usually positive in renal adenocarcinoma cells. A marked vascularity is

another histological feature that may characterize a metastasis from kidney tumour.[26] An intravenous pyelogram and renal arteriogram should be performed in all patients before diagnosing primary clear cell carcinoma of the larynx in order to exclude a primary kidney tumour.

Histochemical stains with periodic acid–Schiff, Best's carmine, oil red O and Sudan black may be used to establish a correct diagnosis. Although primary malignant melanoma of the larynx may occur, a melanoma presenting in the larynx is more likely to be secondary than primary—even if there is no detectable primary skin tumour. Some melanomas may be self-eliminating, but the clinical disappearance of the primary neoplasm does not prevent the onset of distant metastases.

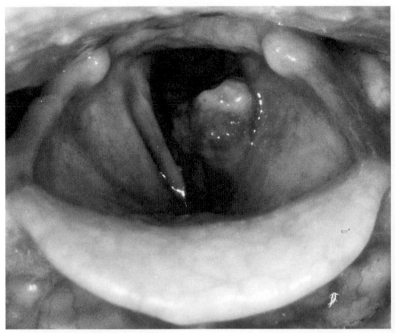

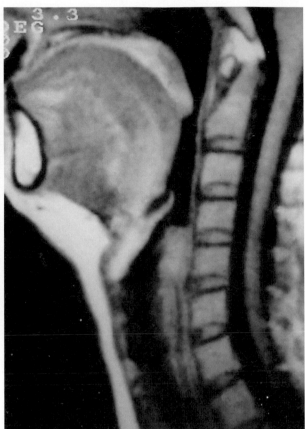

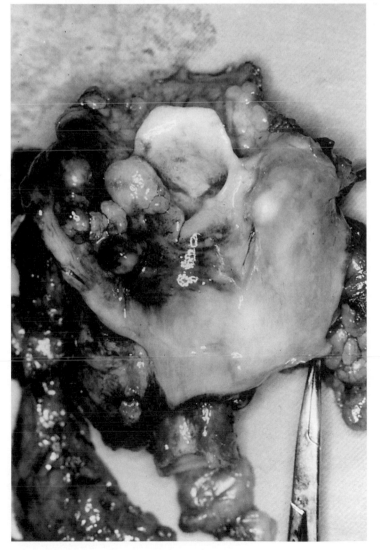

Fig. 19.1 (*top left*) Telescopic view of a metastasis of a malignant melanoma involving the left laryngeal ventricle. (Courtesy of Professor J. Olofsson, Bergen.)

Fig. 19.2 (*bottom left*) Total pharyngolaryngectomy specimen showing extensive metastatic melanoma occupying the left side of the larynx and hypopharynx from a 36-year-old woman. The primary tumour had been resected from her back 7 years before. (Courtesy of Dr Miyata, Kochi, and the editor of *The Larynx Japan*.)

Fig. 19.3 (*top right*) Sagittal T2-weighted magnetic resonance imaging scan showing a large tumour. Same case as in Fig. 19.2. (Courtesy of Dr Miyata, Kochi, and the editor of *The Larynx Japan*.)

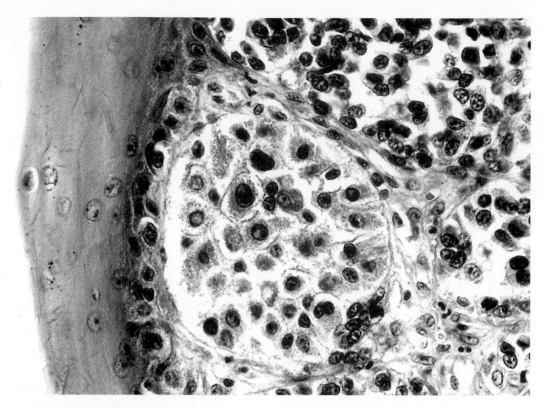

Fig. 19.4   Histological appearance of laryngeal metastasis from melanoma. Same case as in Figs 19.2 and 19.3. H&E, ×100 OM. (Slide contributed by Dr Miyata, Kochi.)

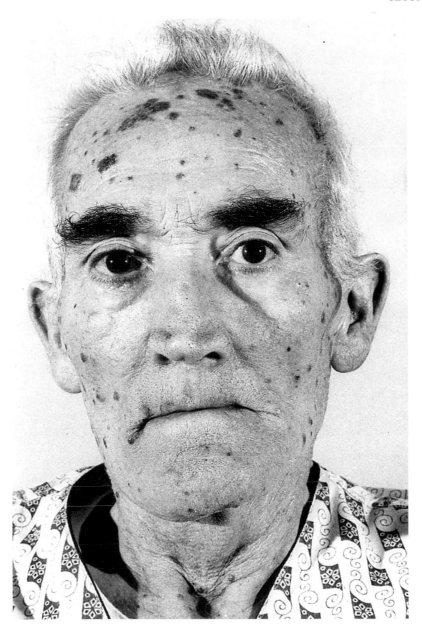

Fig. 19.5   Diffuse facial metastases of primary melanoma of the right leg.

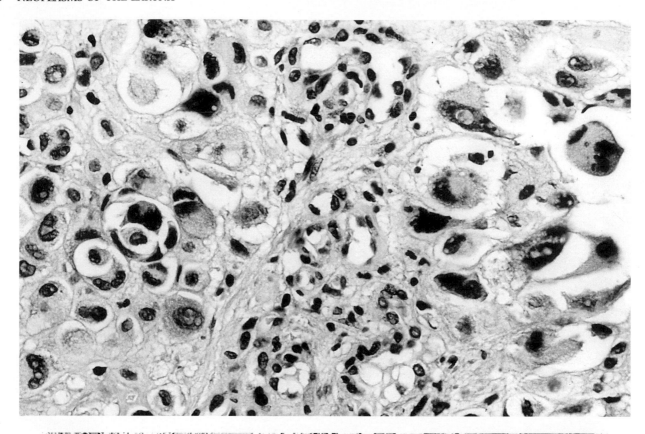

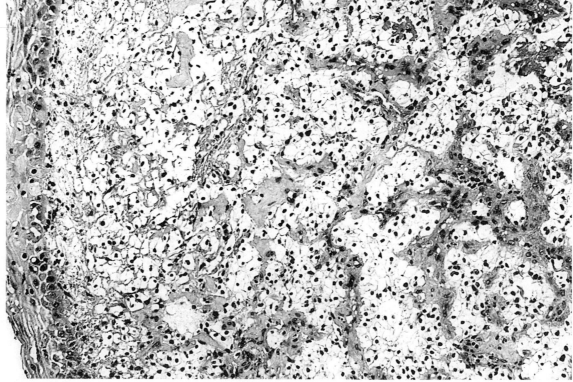

Fig. 19.6 (*top*) Same case as in Fig. 19.5. Great cellular pleomorphism is present. H&E, ×100 OM.

Fig. 19.7 (*bottom*) Metastatic renal adenocarcinoma of the larynx. Note the intact squamous epithelium. H&E, ×40 OM.

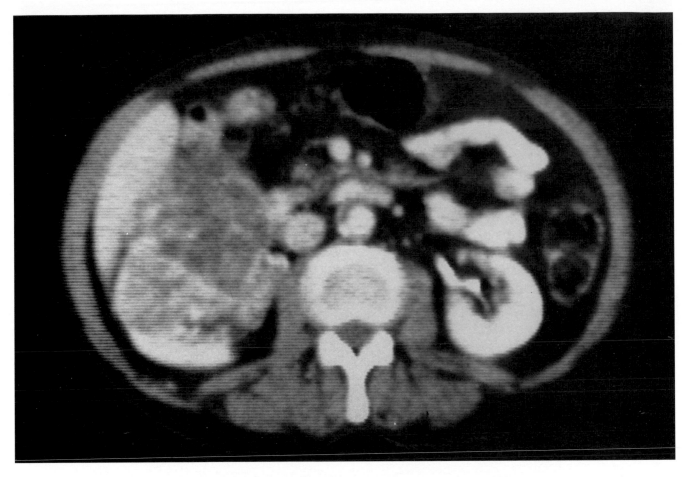

Fig. 19.8   CT scan showing a large mass in the right kidney.

Before a diagnosis of primary laryngeal carcinoma can be made in patients with a previous malignant cancer, the two neoplasms should be compared and their clinical features evaluated. Special studies, including histochemistry, immunocytochemistry and electron microscopy may prove useful.

PATHOGENESIS

The simplest and perhaps most common mechanism of metastatic spread is through the systemic circulation (Fig. 19.13): inferior vena cava, right heart, lungs, left heart, aorta, external carotid artery, upper thyroid artery, upper laryngeal artery. However, spread may also take place via the retrograde circulation of the paravertebral venous plexus and thoracic duct, and these must be considered in obscure cases of laryngeal metastases with no pulmonary involvement.

THERAPY

It is justified to treat a secondary tumour of the larynx only if it is a single metastasis; the type of treatment depends on the biological behaviour of the primary neoplasm and the laryngeal symptoms, taking into account the patient's quality of life. The options are partial or total laryngectomy, or radiotherapy and/or chemotherapy.

PROGNOSIS

The prognosis in patients with secondary laryngeal tumours is naturally very poor, but there are some well-documented instances of prolonged survival.[14,28,37,52,75] Maung et al[52] reported a case of metastatic renal adenocarcinoma to the larynx with no evidence of residual or recurrent tumour two years after hemilaryngectomy and 17 years after nefrectomy. Chamberlain[14] described a patient with metastasis to the larynx from a skin melanoma who was still alive and recurrence-free 6 years after radiotherapy. One patient[37] with an isolated metastasis from a seminoma to the epiglottis was alive and well after 14 years (H. Glanz, oral communication, 1986). There have been no reports of spontaneous regression.

It is important to perform routine indirect laryngoscopy in neoplastic patients, particularly those 'at risk' with malignant melanoma of the skin or renal adenocarcinoma. As Freeland et al[32] pointed out, this is a simple test which should be part of standard 'metastatic' screening procedures for all cancer patients, especially if a curative treatment of the primary lesion is planned.

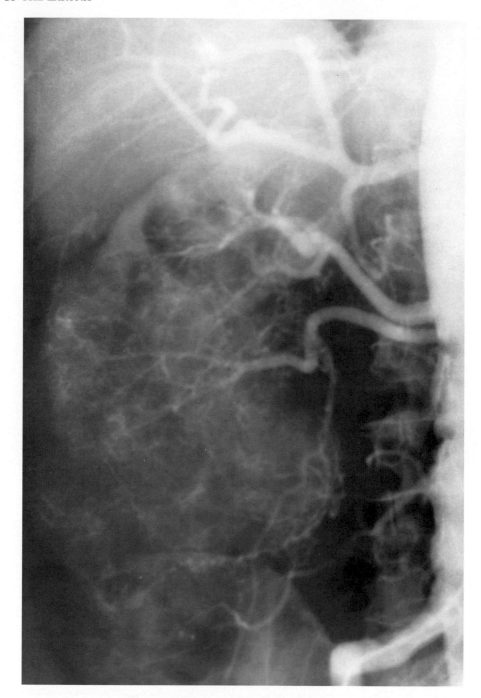

Fig. 19.9 Angiography showing abnormality of the distribution of the renal vessels.

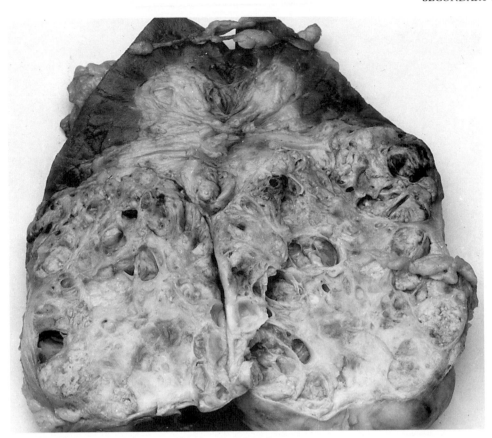

Fig. 19.10   Gross appearance of the renal adenocarcinoma occupying the lower two-thirds of the kidney.

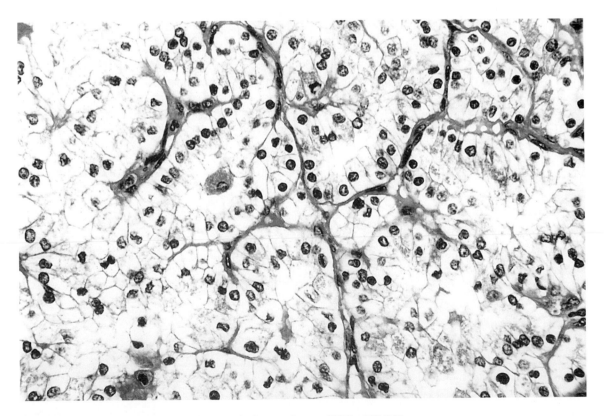

Fig. 19.11   Microscopical features of the renal adenocarcinoma. H&E, ×100 OM.

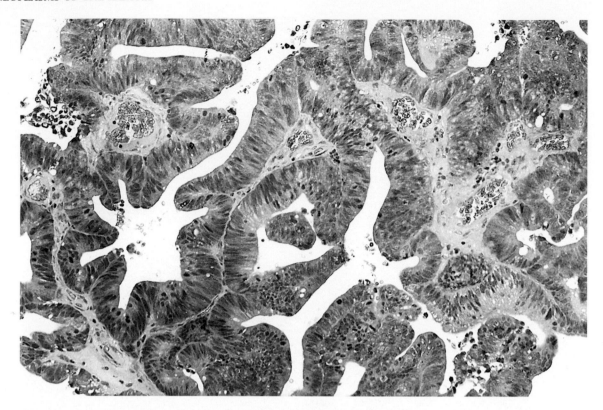

Fig. 19.12   Histology of metastasis to the larynx from a colonic adenocarcinoma. H&E, ×100 OM. (Slide contributed by Dr O. Cavicchi, Bologna.)

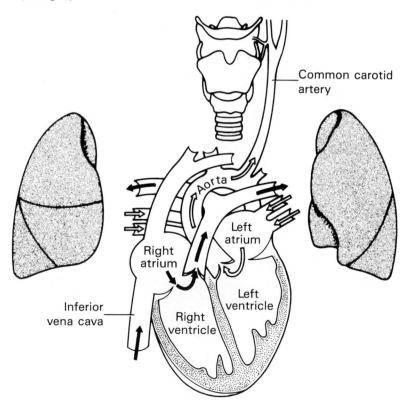

Fig. 19.13   Diagram illustrating the most common mechanism of metastatic spread through the systemic circulation.

REFERENCES

1. Abemayor E, Cochran A J, Calcaterra T C 1983 Metastatic cancer to the larynx: diagnosis and management. Cancer 52: 1944–1948
2. Auriol M. Chomette G, Abelanet R 1959 Métastases laryngées des tumeurs malignes (à propos de quelques observations). Gaz Med 66: 233–239
3. Bardach J, Korzon T. Quoted by Stankiewicz C, Mostowski L 1979 Przerzut raka jasnokomórkowego nerki do krtani. Otolaryngol Pol 33: 543–545
4. Batsakis J G, Luna M A, Byers R M 1985 Metastases to the larynx. Head Neck Surg 7: 458–460
5. Batsakis J G, Regezi J A, Solomon A R, Rice D H 1982 The pathology of head and neck tumors: mucosal melanomas, part 13. Head Neck Surg 4: 404–418
6. Bauer J , Fuchs G 1961 Lokalization und Therapie der Melanome im Ohren-Nasen-Hals-Bereich. Krebsarzt 16: 411–424
7. Bergstedt M, Herberts G 1962 Hypernephrometastasis in the larynx: Radical extirpation before diagnosis of primary tumour. Acta Otolaryngol 54: 95–98
8. Blatchford S J, Koopmann C F Jr, Coulthard S W 1986 Mucosal melanoma of the head and neck. Laryngoscope 96: 929–934
9. Bolla A, Cabassa N, Scolari R 1968 Metastasi solitaria alla laringe da microcitoma polmonare. Arch Ital Otol 79: 74–82
10. Bolognesi C, Caliceti G 1960 Seminoma metastatico della laringe. Otorinolaringol Ital 29: 15–25
11. Bolognesi C, Nucci C 1963 Metastasi laringea da neoplasia della mammella. Otorinolaringol Ital 32: 280–290
12. Caboche H, Paisseau. Quoted by Bolognesi C, Nucci C 1963 Metastasi laringea da neoplasia della mammella. Otorinolaringol Ital 32: 280–290
13. Cavicchi O, Farneti G, Occhiuzzi L, Sorrenti G 1990 Laryngeal metastasis from colonic adenocarcinoma. J Laryngol Otol 104: 730–732
14. Chamberlain D 1966 Malignant melanoma metastatic to the larynx. Arch Otolaryngol 83: 231–232
15. Chapuis (1896) Quoted by Ellis M, Winston P 1957 Secondary carcinoma of the larynx. J Laryngol Otol 71: 16–24
16. Coakley J F, Ranson D L 1984 Metastasis to the larynx from a prostatic carcinoma: a case report. J Laryngol Otol 98: 839–842
17. Cullen J R 1990 Ovarian carcinoma metastatic to the larynx. J Laryngol Otol 104: 48–49
18. Ehrlich A 1954 Tumor involving the laryngeal cartilages. Arch Otolaryngol 59: 178–185
19. Ellis M, Winston P 1957 Secondary carcinoma of the larynx. J Laryngol Otol 71: 16–24
20. Eppinger H 1880 Pathologische Anatomie der Larynx und der Trachea. In: Klebs E (ed) Handbuch der pathologischen Anatomie. Hirschwald Publisher, Berlin
21. Eschwege F, Cachin Y, Micheau C 1975 Treatment of adenocarcinoma of the larynx. Can J Otolaryngol 4: 291–292
22. Faaborg-Andersen K 1953 Melanoma malignum laryngis. Acta Otolaryngol 43: 539–531
23. Fabbi F 1948 Metastasi laringea di simpaticoblastoma primitivo della surrenale destra: sindrome della coda equina da metastasi midollare. Otorinolaringol Ital 17: 75–94
24. Ferlito A 1985 Secondary tumours of the larynx. In: Ferlito A (ed) Cancer of the larynx, vol II. C R C Press, Boca Raton
25. Ferlito A, Caruso G 1984 Secondary malignant melanoma of the larynx. Report of two cases and review of 79 laryngeal secondary cases. ORL J Otorhinolaryngol Relat Spec 46: 117–133
26. Ferlito A, Caruso G, Recher G 1988 Secondary laryngeal tumors Report of seven cases with review of the literature. Arch Otolaryngol Head Neck Surg 114: 635–639
27. Ferlito A, Pesavento G, Meli S, Recher G, Visonà A 1987 Metastasis to the larynx revealing a renal cell carcinoma. J Laryngol Otol 101: 843–850
28. Fiaoni M, Colonna A, Leonardi M Jr, Passamonti G L 1989 Metastasi laringea solitaria di carcinoma a piccole cellule polmonari 'cosidetto microcitoma'. Descrizione di un caso clinico. Valsalva 65: 203–209

29. Field J A 1966 Renal carcinoma metastasis to the larynx. Laryngoscope 76: 99–101
30. Fisher G E, Odess J S 1951 Metastatic malignant melanoma of the larynx. Arch Otolaryngol Head Neck Surg 54: 639–642
31. Franzoni M 1964 I melanomi metastatici della laringe. Boll Mal Orecchio Gola Naso 82: 113–129
32. Freeland A P, van Nostrand A W P, Jahn A F 1979 Metastases to the larynx. J Otolaryngol 8: 448–456
33. Freire F, Câmara J, Paiva L 1958 Sòbre un caso de carcinoma metastatico a carcinoma broncogenico. Rev Paul Med 52: 59–64
34. Friedmann I, Ferlito A 1988 Granulomas and neoplasms of the larynx. Churchill Livingstone, Edinburgh
35. Friedmann I. Osborn D A 1965 Metastatic tumours in the ear, nose and throat region. J Laryngol Otol 79: 576–591
36. Gadomski S P, Zwillemberg D, Choi H Y 1986 Non-epidermoid carcinoma of the larynx: The Thomas Jefferson University experience. Otolaryngol Head Neck Surg 95: 558–565
37. Glanz H, Kleinsasser O 1978 Metastasen im Kehlkopf. HNO 26: 163–167
38. Grignon D J, Ayala A G, Ro J Y, Chong C 1990 Carcinoma of prostate metastasizing to vocal cord. Urology 36: 85–88
39. Hajek M 1927 Bronchuskarzinom mit Larynx-metastasen. Monatsschr Ohrenheilkd 62: 125
40. Henderson L T, Robbins K T, Weitzner S 1986 Upper aerodigestive tract metastases in disseminated malignant melanoma. Arch Otolaryngol Head Neck Surg 112: 659–663
41. Hessan H, Strauss M, Sharkey F E 1986 Urogenital tract carcinoma metastatic to the head and neck. Laryngoscope 96: 1352–1356
42. Hofer G 1921 Schilddrüsenmetastasen eines Magenkarzinoms mit Einwachsen in den Kehlkopf. Monatsschr Ohrenheilkd 56: 220
43. Ikeda M, Takahashi H, Karaho T, Kitahara S, Inouye T 1991 Amelanotic melanoma metastatic to the epiglottis. J Laryngol Otol 105: 776–779
44. Kubo R, Ono M 1968 Case of malignant femoral melanoma with metastasis. J Otolaryngol Jpn 71: 165–178
45. Kyriakos M, Berlin B D, DeSchryver-Kecskemeti K 1978 Oat cell carcinoma of the larynx. Arch Otolaryngol 104: 168–176
46. Landgraf 1888 Ein Fall von secundärem (infectiösem) Carcinom des Larynx. Charite Ann 13: 258–260
47. Levine H L, Applebaum E L 1976 Metastatic adenocarcinoma to the larynx: report of a case. Trans Am Acad Ophthalmol Otolaryngol 82: 536–541
48. Levine H L, Tubbs R 1986 Nonsquamous neoplasms of the larynx. Otolaryngol Clin North Am 19: 475–488
49. Loughead J R 1952 Malignant melanoma of the larynx. Ann Otol Rhinol Laryngol 61: 154–158
50. Maddox J C, Evans H L 1981 Angiosarcoma of skin and soft tissue: A study of 44 cases. Cancer 49: 1907–1921
51. Massei F Quoted by Franzoni M 1964 I melanomi metastatici della laringe. Boll Mal Orecchio Gola Naso 82: 113–129
52. Maung R, Burke R C, Hwang W S 1987 Metastatic renal carcinoma to larynx. J Otolaryngol 16: 16–18
53. Maxwell J H 1942 Metastatic hypernephroma of the larynx. Mich Univ Hosp Bull 8: 29–30
54. Mazzarella L A, Pina L H, Wolff D 1966 Asymptomatic metastasis to the larynx. Laryngoscope 76: 1547–1554
55. Menzel K M 1912 Ein malignes Hypernephrom im Larynx: Ein Unikum. Arch Laryngol Rhinol 26: 265–269
56. Miyamoto R, Helmus C 1973 Hypernephroma metastatic to the head and neck. Laryngoscope 83: 898–905
57. Miyata T, Kishimoto S, Katto Y, Masuda T 1989 Metastatic malignant melanoma involving the larynx and hypopharynx. Report of a case. Larynx Jpn 1: 146–149
58. Morgan A H, Norris J W, Hicks J N 1985 Palliative laser surgery for melanoma metastatic to the larynx: report of two cases. Laryngoscope 95: 794–797
59. Motloch E 1927 Melanosarcommetastase in Schilddrüse und Larynx (Präparat). Monatsschr Ohrenheilkd 61: 853–854

60. Mullin W V, Langsten F V 1930 Malignant tumor of breast with metastasis to opposite side of larynx and contralateral vocal cord paralysis. Ann Otol Rhinol Laryngol 39: 125–127

61. Nambu T, Shinohara M, Takada A, Susuki K, Koyama Y, Irie G 1990 Ca case of icteric hepatoma with laryngeal metastasis and coexisting pancreatic cancer. Gan No Rinsho 36: 515–520

62. Neumann H Quoted by Ellis M, Winston P 1957 Secondary carcinoma of the larynx. J Laryngol Otol 71: 16–24

63. Nguyen C H, Weitzner S 1983 Metastatic carcinoma of breast in the hypopharynx. South Med J 73: 1590–1591

64. Oku T, Hasegawa M, Watanabe I, Nasu M, Aoki N 1980 Pancreatic cancer with metastasis to the larynx. J Laryngol Otol 94: 1205–1209

65. Oppikofer E 1932 Die Hypernephronmetastasen in den oberen Luftwegen und im Gehörorgan. Arch Ohrenheilkd 129: 271–292

66. Palacios E J, Hanchey C C, White H J 1970 Renal cell carcinoma metastatic to the larynx: Case report. J Arkansas Med Soc 66: 484–485

67. Pesavento G, Ferlito A, Recher G 1980 Primary clear cell carcinoma of the larynx. J Clin Pathol 33: 1160–1164

68. Quinn F B Jr, McCabe B F 1957 Laryngeal metastases from malignant tumors in distant organs. Ann Otol Rhinol Laryngol 66: 139–143

69. Rachel T, Reinfuss M 1974 Nerwiak wechowy z przerzutem do krtani. Otolaryngol Pol 4: 487–489

70. Radici M, Croce A, Leante M, Bicciolo G 1988 Metastasi alla laringe da neoplasie primitive sistemiche. Revisione critica. Valsalva 63: 105–110

71. Rebattu J, Martin H, Takizawa 1950 Sarcome laryngé (métastatique d'une tumeur rénale) à localization bilatérale et symétrique. Lyon Med 184: 267–269

72. Ritchie W W, Messmer J M, Whitley D P, Gopelrund D R 1985 Uterine carcinoma metastatic to the larynx. Laryngoscope 95: 97–98

73. Robin P E, Olofsson J 1987 Tumours of the larynx. In: Stell P M (ed) Scott-Brown's otolaryngology — laryngology, 5th edn. Butterworths, London

74. Schmorl G 1908 Ueber Krebsmetastasen im Knochensystem. Verh Dtsch Ges Pathol 12: 89–95

75. Shaheen O H 1960 A case of metastatic amelanotic melanoma of the larynx. J Laryngol Otol 74: 182–187

76. Snow G B, Esch E P, van der Slooten E A 1978 Mucosal melanomas of the head and neck. Head Neck Surg 1: 24–30

77. Stankiewicz C, Mostowski L 1979 Przerzut raka jasnokomórkowego nerki do krtani. Otolaryngol Pol 8: 448–456

78. Stepanov W M, Bénimecki J S, Makarowa L A. Quoted by Coyas A, Anastassiades O Th, Kyriakos I 1974 Malignant giant cell tumour of the larynx. J Laryngol Otol 88: 799–803

79. Szmeja Z, Obrebowski A, Lukaszewski B 1986 A case of metastasis of breast cancer to the larynx. Otolaryngol Pol 40: 212–216

80. Szmeja Z, Kruk-Zagajewska A, Salwa-Zurawska W, Muszynski M 1987 Metastases of renal adenocarcinoma to the larynx and paranasal sinuses. Otolaryngol Pol 41: 221–227

81. Tamura H. Nakamoto M 1956 Ein Fall von Grawitztumor mit Metastasen in Kehlkopf. Monatsschr Ohrenheilkd 90: 354–357

82. Teoh T B 1957 Epidermoid carcinoma of the nasopharynx among Chinese: a study of 31 necropsies. J Pathol 73: 451–465

83. Tolstov U P, Saburov P A 1977 Metastatic melanoma of the larynx. Vestn Otorinolaringol 2: 99–100

84. Turner A L 1924 Metastatic malignant tumor of the larynx secondary to adenocarcinoma of the right kidney. J Laryngol Otol 39: 181–194

85. Walter H E 1948 Krebsmetastasen. Schwabe, Basel

86. Wanamaker J R, Good T L, Kraus D H, Eliachar I, Lavertu P 1991 Unusual manifestations of metastatic breast carcinoma to the head and neck. Am Laryngol Rhinol Otol Soc, abstract

87. Whicker J H, Carder G A, Devine K D 1972 Metastasis to the larynx: Report of a case and review of the literature. Arch Otolaryngol 96: 182–184

88. Willis R A 1952 The spread of tumours in the human body, 2nd edn. Butterworths, Stoneham, Mass

89. Yeatman T J, Seagle M B, Cassisi N J 1986 A rare manifestation of metastatic adenocarcinoma. Laryngoscope 96: 692–694

90. Zuchowska-Vogelgesang B, Sokolowski S, Skolyszewski J 1976 Przypadek przerzutu do krtani plaskonablonkowego raka oskrzela. Otolaryngol Pol 6: 621–623

20. Clinical manifestations and diagnostic procedures

J. Olofsson

CLINICAL MANIFESTATIONS OF TUMOURS OF THE LARYNX

The symptomatology of tumours arising within the larynx varies with the location and size of the tumour. The symptoms certainly vary if the tumour arises from the mucosa or submucosally from neurogenic tissue, vessels, salivary glands or the laryngeal framework.

Location

Glottic tumours are characterized by hoarseness as the earliest and most prominent symptom. Dyspnoea and stridor may occur in larger tumours.

Supraglottic tumours are characterized by being fairly large when diagnosed. Cough and irritation in the throat may be early symptoms, and dysphagia is another symptom that may be seen in both ulcerated and exophytic lesions. Exophytic tumours overhanging the laryngeal inlet may cause inspiratory stridor.

When dealing with squamous cell carcinomas, nodal metastases — micro or macro — occur in about 30% of patients with a primary squamous cell carcinoma of the supraglottis at the time of diagnosis.

Subglottic tumours give symptoms late and are often advanced when diagnosed. Slowly-increasing stridor is not a seldom initial symptom. In invasive squamous cell carcinomas the tumour often grows circumferentially. When the vocal cords are involved hoarseness may occur. Thus, this symptom is often late in primary subglottic tumours.

Various symptoms

Haemoptysis may occur in richly vascularized tumours of the larynx or in thyroid carcinomas invading the larynx and trachea. Haemoptysis is otherwise not a frequent symptom in primary laryngeal tumours.

Swelling of the neck may occur e.g. in a primary cartilaginous tumour of the thyroid cartilage.

Nodal metastases occur (see above) in about 30% of supraglottic carcinomas and may be the initial symptom of these carcinomas or of a carcinoma arising in the pyriform sinus.

Subglottic primary carcinomas are rare and they make up less than 5% of all laryngeal carcinomas. Nevertheless, they have a high incidence of nodal metastases, especially paratracheally and to the lower part of the neck.

DIAGNOSTIC PROCEDURES

Examination and diagnosis

Diagnosis may be based on: (i) history; (ii) examination of the larynx; (iii) examination of the neck; (iv) general examination of the patient; (v) radiology; (vi) clinical investigations; and (vii) histological examination.

The clinical examination of laryngeal lesions comprises external inspection and palpation of the larynx to rule out any growth through the laryngeal framework, or spread outside the larynx.

Mirror laryngoscopy is still perhaps the most common mode of inspection; this is supplemented — and in certain departments entirely replaced — by the use of telescopes. The 70° telescope in particular provides better visualization of the laryngeal surface of the epiglottis and the anterior commissure region. Biopsy specimens can be removed by indirect techniques, at least when dealing with larger tumours (Fig. 20.1).

Fibre laryngoscopic examination provides a good complement in the diagnostic armamentarium, especially in individuals difficult to inspect with other techniques. Many of the patients who nowadays can be examined by fibrescopes previously had to be examined under general anaesthesia. Examination using the thin, specially designed fibrelaryngoscopes without suction channels can be performed without problems using only Xylocain jelly on the scope for an easier passage through the nose. At the same time, a careful inspection can be performed of the nasopharynx and pharynx. For removal of biopsy specimens from visible lesions a larger fibrescope with a suction and biopsy channel can be used. In these instances I usually prefer the fibrebronchoscopes or, if possible, anaesthetization of the patient for a microlaryngoscopy.

Stroboscopy

The word stroboscopy is derived from the Greek words strobos (to rotate) and scopos (target).

In stroboscopy an optical illusion is produced that arises from the persistence of vision. Admission of light to the retina leaves a positive after-image which lasts for 0.2 seconds. The sequence of pictures presented at intervals shorter than 0.2 seconds will thus appear as a continuously moving picture. A life-like impression of movements is obtained, but it really represents only fragments of the complete movement (Prytz, brochure B & K).[30]

In principle there are two vibratory movements of the vocal folds: the transverse movement of the muscular 'body' and the vertical travelling wave movement of the mucosal 'cover'. While the muscle is still vibrating in the upper portion of the vocal fold edge in the laterally directed opening phase, a narrow mucosal edge occurs in the subglottis or at the lower vocal cord edge, initiating the closing phase and producing a double contour of the vocal cord edge (Fig. 20.2).

There are at least three major clinical implications.[24]

Phonatory function

The size of the mucosal waves and vibratory amplitudes are closely correlated, increasing with falling pitch and rising intensity. Disturbances may be normalized following successful voice therapy if the patient is capable of using his/her new voice during examination.

Adhesions and invasive processes

The most common cause of adhesion of the mucosa to the underlying 'body' is previous surgery, when deeper submucous loose tissue covering the vocal ligament has been included in the removal of a benign process such as polyps, nodules, Reinke's oedema, etc.

An epithelialization, directly of the ligament or on the muscular layer of the vocal folds without intervening soft tissue, impedes the normal vibratory pattern and causes hoarseness. No mucosal wave can be seen. Unnecessary adhesions should be avoided by the laryngologist, especially when performing 'phono surgery'; such adhesions have a status comparable to that of an adhesive eardrum following ear surgery. Following surgery to the vocal folds, return of the glottic wave within 7 to 10 days is a sign of uncomplicated recovery.

Localized lesions may cause the disappearance of the mucosal wave. The most important cause is invasive

squamous cell carcinoma. Stroboscopy is an important tool to follow patients with 'chronic laryngitis', keratosis and erythroplasia. As long as the mucosa is freely mobile there is at least no invasiveness, and removal of a biopsy specimen for histopathological examination may not always be necessary.

After irradiation treatment of glottic carcinomas, a mucosal wave remains in about half of the patients. The disappearance of this wave indicates a recurrence, and microlaryngoscopy and removal of a biopsy specimen have to be performed. If the loss of mucosal wave is limited, the laryngologist gets a good indication of where to excise the mucosa.

Vocal fold pareses

The loss of mucosal waves in a paretic vocal fold is well described. A remaining mucosal wave in a laryngeal paresis indicates re-innervation of the vocal fold.[31]

Fex[9] found that if the EMG showed denervation there was a complete loss of mucosal waves. A return of mucosal waves was always combined with signs of re-innervation in the EMG. Thus, stroboscopic examination is an aid in foretelling the prognosis e.g. in vocal cord paresis following thyroid surgery.

An immobile vocal cord with normal mucosal waves may indicate a crico-arytenoid ankylosis and rule out a recurrant palsy.

Microlaryngoscopy

A direct laryngoscopy should nowadays be performed using the operating microscope—microlaryngoscopy—a technique introduced by Kleinsasser[25] in the 1960s. The microlaryngoscopic examination is a major advantage in the diagnosis and endoscopic surgery for laryngeal lesions. The possibilities of removing representative biopsy specimens have been greatly improved, and it has facilitated a photographic documentation (Figs 20.3–20.5).

The value of microlaryngoscopy is reflected in the increased number of premalignant lesions being diagnosed.[17,19] The microlaryngoscopic appearance of premalignant lesions varies from leukoplakia to erythroplasia and is often a mixture of both.

The combination of videolaryngostroboscopic examination and microlaryngoscopy makes possible a more precise and less traumatic excision. For those of us who have experienced the older, monocular non-magnified way of performing excisions in the larynx — or who have had to go back to this modality in the rare patient who is not amenable to microlaryngoscopy—the great advantages of microlaryngoscopy are obvious.

The microlaryngoscopic examination should never overlook lesions that may be located around the larynx proper, i.e. in the valleculae, pyriform sinuses, post-

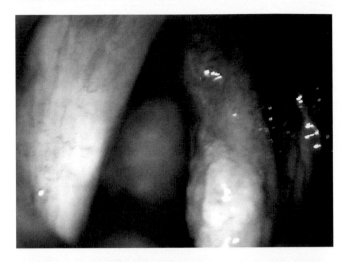

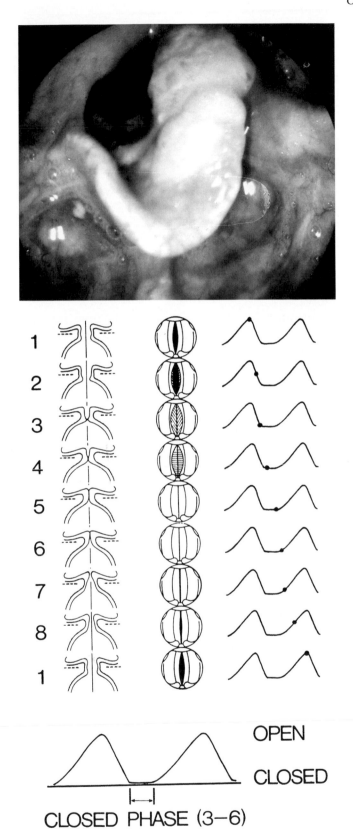

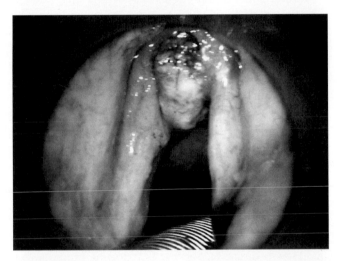

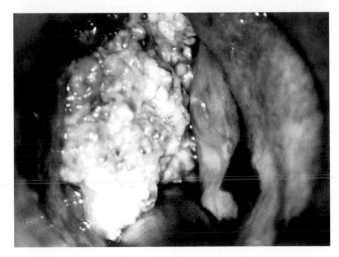

OPEN

CLOSED

CLOSED PHASE (3–6)

Fig. 20.3 (*top right*) Microlaryngoscopy. Carcinoma of the full length of the right vocal cord.

Fig. 20.4 (*middle right*) Microlaryngoscopy. Carcinoma involving the anterior commissure.

Fig. 20.5 (*bottom right*) Verrucous carcinoma of the left vocal cord with supra- and subglottic extension.

Fig. 20.1 (*top left*) Telescopic view showing an exophytic supraglottic carcinoma.

Fig. 20.2 (*bottom left*) Stroboscopy. Schematic presentation of the vocal fold with vibratory pattern during phonation in normal chest register. Frontal sections (*left*), laryngoscopic view (*middle*) and area function of the glottis (*right*). (Reprinted by permission from *Journal of Otolaryngology* 14: 151–157, 1987[24])

cricoid region or in the posterior commissure behind the intubation tube.

The microlaryngoscopic examination may be supplemented by the use of 90° optical instruments for inspection of the posterior surface of the epiglottis, the lower margin of an exophytic supraglottic neoplasm or the undersurface of the vocal cords and the anterior commissure area. This might be the only way to exactly assess the subglottic extent of a glottic carcinoma, if not using a fibrescope.

Toluidine blue staining

Toluidine blue, an acidophilic, metachromatic dye belonging to the thiazine group, selectively stains acid tissue components (sulphate, carboxylate and phosphate radicals) such as DNA and RNA. Shedd et al,[32,33] Myers,[29] and Iwano et al[20] stated that toluidine blue was useful in diagnosing and delineating dysplastic and neoplastic oral epithelium. They had no false-negative findings, but encountered a few false-positive ones due to inflammation or trapping of dye in fissures and small crypts.[32,33] There was a risk that heavily keratinized tumours and submucosally located carcinomas may not stain.[6,32,33,37] Despite these problems, toluidine blue has been recommended as an aid in obtaining a 'positive' biopsy specimen.[37]

Tarkkanen et al[38] found toluidine blue to be a valuable asset in the diagnosis of bronchial carcinoma. They found it useful in respiratory epithelium, although most authors have reported less satisfactory results as the goblet cells give false-positive responses. Staining of mucin was less regular and less intense than staining of nucleic acids.

Our own results using toluidine blue in the microlaryngoscopic diagnosis of glottic lesions showed that the toluidine blue test was sensitive—as indicated by the proportion of positive reactions among the malignant lesions: 91% (135/148). There was no difference in sensitivity for patients who had received or had not received radiotherapy. Eleven of the 13 false-negative staining reactions were ascribed to the presence of clinically evident keratosis.

The specificity of the toluidine blue staining reaction, as indicated by the number of negative staining reactions in the benign group of lesions, was only 52% (64/124). The specificity was significantly lower (P < 0.01) for previously irradiated lesions—33% (14/43)—than for the non-irradiated group—62% (50/81). This difference may be due to intraepithelial oedema, with consequent widening of the intercellular spaces, or post-irradiation inflammation.

Toluidine blue staining is easy to perform, but care has to be taken not to traumatize the vocal cords as abrasions and bleeding may interfere with the assessment of the staining. The sensitivity of the staining is sufficiently high, but the specificity is low.

Toluidine blue offers, especially to the less experienced microlaryngoscopist, an improved chance of obtaining representative biopsy specimens. Toluidine blue staining is by no means an alternative to histological examination, but it should be considered as a diagnostic complement that provides a better chance of obtaining representative biopsy specimens.[26]

Smear cytology

The role of smear cytology in the diagnosis of laryngeal lesions has been debated in the literature. Früwald[13] considered smear cytology to be of no value as a screening procedure of laryngeal lesions due to the high frequency of false-negative results in malignancy (low sensitivity). Conversely, several authors[10,11,40,41] have reported cytology most useful as a complement in laryngeal diagnosis.

In a prospective study, samples were taken from the vocal cords in 540 patients of whom 111 had received irradiation treatment for laryngeal malignancies.[28] Most of the specimens were taken with both a wooden pin and a brush. All specimens obtained were immediately fixed in 95% alcohol.

The smears were stained according to Papanicolau and classified into four stages: benign, including mild atypia (non-malignant changes), moderate atypia, severe atypia or CIS, and invasive carcinoma. It is important to notice that the classification used for cervical cytological smears cannot be directly transferred into the larynx with a well-differentiated, often keratinized vocal cord epithelium, but must be upgraded considerably. Smears with moderate atypia are considered control patients, and biopsy specimens should be removed or excisions performed, at least from visible lesions.

In 3.7% (20/540), insufficient material was obtained, and these cases were discarded. Of the remaining 520 cases, cytology could prove carcinoma in 137/147 histologically verified cases, i.e., a sensitivity of 93%. In severe dysplasia—CIS—the sensitivity was 83% (59/71), and for moderate dysplasia it was 45% (17/38).

The specificity of the cytological technique, i.e., proportion of negative smears in the histologically benign group, was 80% (210/264). Forty-eight of the 59 specimens (49 patients) with a false-positive cytological evaluation, out of a total of 264 cases showing normal histology or hyperplasia, keratosis or mild dysplasia, were cytologically classified as moderate atypia. Interestingly, two of these patients later developed invasive carcinoma: one severe dysplasia and one moderate dysplasia.

Laryngeal smear cytology can by no means supersede the histological examination, which definitely has to provide the final diagnosis on which the treatment decision has to be based. Smear cytology may, however, have a role — especially in diffuse lesions and as a part of screening procedures for high-risk patients (Fig. 20.6).

Scanning electron microscopy (SEM)

Do ultrastructural surface studies have any diagnostic importance? In normal squamous cell epithelium at low magnification the picture is uniform with a mosaic of polygonal cells of similar size and shape and with sharp and slightly elevated borders.[27] An increasing irregularity is observed in dysplasia, giving the surface a cobble-stone appearance. A highly disorganized pattern is seen in carcinoma in situ. The cells are rounded and swollen, and they protrude with ill-defined intercellular junctions. In invasive carcinoma the picture varies with degree of differentiation.

SEM has been shown to be more sensitive than light microscopy for revealing delicate surface changes which may be benign, premalignant or malignant.

However, SEM does not allow any prognostic predictions.[7,23] It may, however, be possible to combine SEM with functional surface labelling techniques.[7,22] Statistical, quantitative and form-analytic definitions should be applied to obtain any significance in clinical work.

Photometry

The squamous cell lesion is the pathological entity whose evaluation involves the largest number of subjective components.[2] The nomenclature has been poorly defined and inconsistently applied. It is therefore all the more important for the laryngologist to be thoroughly familiar with the terminology of the pathologist.

To obtain a more objective classification of squamous cell lesions, photometric determination of DNA content and nuclear size may be performed directly on histological section using scanning cytophotometric methods.[14,16,19] No abnormalities could be disclosed in the size and DNA content of the nuclei in normal, keratotic epithelia, and only a slight increase was noticed in the value in hyperplastic epithelia. However, except for a few nuclei, the tetraploid value was not reached. This was consistent with the findings in other proliferative tissue, such as the chondroma.[18] The photometric patterns of severe dysplasia and carcinoma in situ differed distinctly from normal: they resembled that of invasive carcinoma (Figs 20.7, 20.8).[19]

A milestone was set when, in 1983, Hedley and coworkers[15] described their method of obtaining isolated nuclei on formalin-fixed, paraffin-embedded tumours, enabling the retrospective study of groups of patients with known clinical outcome. There was, however, no significant difference in DNA values between small glottic carcinomas that recurred after a full course of radiotherapy and those that did not.[12]

Morphometry

Laryngeal biopsies of squamous cell lesions, with or without dysplasia, can be graded by means of morphometry[21] and using a number of non-correlated nuclear parameters preselected with linear discriminant analysis and tested for their prognostic significance in follow-up studies. In the progressive group, 73% of the biopsies were morphometrically classified as prognostically unfavourable. The following parameters were measured:

1. The mean nuclear contour index in the basal layer
2. The mean nuclear area in the superficial layer
3. The standard deviation of the nuclear area in the basal layer
4. The total number of nuclei per (arbitrary) unit area in the basal layer
5. Nuclear crowding in the superficial layer.

For a valuable morphometrical classification of lesions of individual patients our results up to now are still insufficient. Morphometrical classification probabilities may, however, be improved when the numbers of untreated patients with squamous cell hyperplasia with atypia do increase.[21]

Radiological examinations

The purpose of the radiographic examination is to determine the superficial spread of the tumour and the extent of its infiltration of deep structures. Nowadays, computed tomography and magnetic resonance imaging have replaced plain films, tomography, laryngography and xerography.

Conventional tomography gives only inferior data regarding submucosal margins of the tumour. CT is superior in assessing cartilage destruction and distortion and in demonstrating tumour spread outside the larynx.[5,34]

There are a number of reports stating that CT is more accurate than contrast laryngography in identifying and delineating areas of tumour involvement.

Deep invasion, such as pre-epiglottic space invasion, invasion of the paraglottic space and the subglottis, is more accurately assessed by CT. CT has the additional advantage of visualizing the laryngeal cartilages. CT thus complements the laryngoscopic examination more than other radiological examinations, and it provides information about the depth of tumours and of cartilage involvement and spread outside the laryngeal framework. CT assists in clarifying suspected pathology beneath the laryngeal mucosa. In addition, it gives information regarding lymph node metastases that may not be diagnosed by palpation.

Magnetic resonance imaging (MRI) seems to be superior to CT in demonstrating invasion of the laryngeal cartilages, and Castelijns et al[5] recommend it for radiological examination of laryngeal tumours. These authors even conclude that MR imaging should be included in the diagnostic work-up of all patients with laryngeal cancer who have not been treated previously — but with

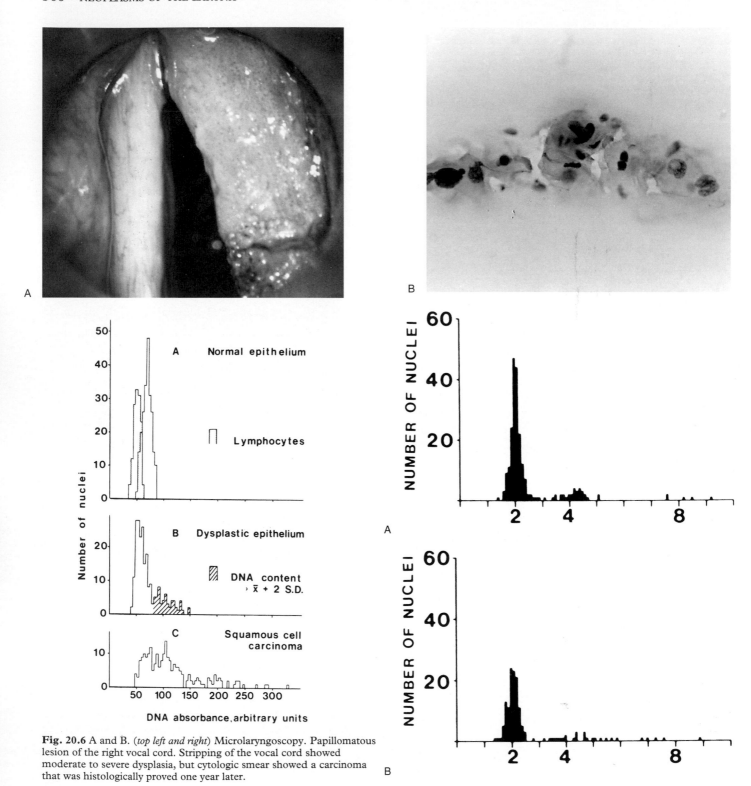

A

B

A

B

Fig. 20.6 A and B. (*top left and right*) Microlaryngoscopy. Papillomatous lesion of the right vocal cord. Stripping of the vocal cord showed moderate to severe dysplasia, but cytologic smear showed a carcinoma that was histologically proved one year later.

Fig. 20.7 (*bottom left*) DNA histogram of a normal laryngeal epithelium (A); dysplastic epithelium (B); squamous cell carcinoma (C). (Reprinted with permission from *Acta Oto-Laryngologica 86: 473–479, 1978.*[14])

Fig. 20.8 A and B. (*Middle and bottom right*) Cytofluorometry of cytologic smears. A. A lesion with moderate dysplasia showing a DNA histogram with hypertetraploid cells (above 5c). This patient later developed an invasive squamous cell carcinoma. B. Severe dysplasia with hypertetraploid cells in the DNA histogram. This patient later developed a microinvasive carcinoma. The presence of hypertetraploid cells may have prognostic significance. (Olofsson J et al 1985 In: Myers E (ed) New dimensions in oto-rhino-laryngology/head & neck surgery. Elsevier, Amsterdam, pp 663–664)

the exception of those with a small tumour such as a glottic T1 lesion. If MR imaging fails — due to metallic implants in the area of interest, a pacemaker, surgical clips, or movement artefacts — CT may still play a role.

MR imaging appears to be less effective in patients suspected of having a recurrent residual tumour after radiotherapy. It seems to be difficult to make a distinction between cancer, oedema and post-irradiation fibrosis.

Neck nodes

Neck nodes should be assessed by palpation and by fine-needle aspiration cytology of any palpable, suspected nodes. However, nodes containing smaller deposits may be missed. On the other hand, not all enlarged nodes contain metastatic deposits.

There is a large inter-observer variation in the assessment of cervical lymph nodes. The overall error in assessing the presence or absence of cervical lymph node metastasis lies between 20 and 30%.[1]

Do we reach a better assessment using imaging techniques? Most experience has been achieved by CT. Central necrosis and size, particularly minimum axial diameter, seem to be the most useful radiological criteria for nodal metastases.[4] Several studies have proven CT and MRI superior to palpation in demonstrating cervical lymph node metastases.[4,8,35,36]

Fine-needle aspiration cytology guided by ultrasound (USgFNAC) seems, however, to be the most valuable technique in establishing metastases in cervical lymph nodes.[3]

SUMMARY

Indirect and direct laryngoscopy, with the use of telescopic, fibrescopic, stroboscopic and microlaryngoscopic techniques, provides the basis for laryngoscopic diagnosis. Toluidine blue staining may guide the removal of adequate biopsies in squamous cell lesions. Cytological smears may be useful in screening procedures.

Histological examination is still the basis for an accurate diagnosis. Light microscopy may be complemented by immunochemistry for the diagnosis of more unusual neoplasms. Cytophotometry and morphometry may add information in squamous cell premalignant and malignant lesions and in e. g. chondrogenic tumours.

Radiological examinations are a prerequisite for classification of laryngeal carcinomas according to the rules for classification.[39] Computed tomography and MR imaging are the preferred examination techniques which enable delineation of deep tumour extent, cartilage invasion and spread of tumour outside the laryngeal framework. These techniques can thereby guide us in selecting an optimal treatment modality both from the functional point of view and for cure.

Ultrasound-guided fine-needle aspiration cytology (USg FNAC) seems to be the most reliable examination method (and better than CT and MR) for assessing the cervical lymph nodes.

REFERENCES

1. Ali S, Tiwari R M, Snow G B 1985 False-positive and false-negative neck nodes. Head Neck Surg 8: 78–82
2. Batsakis J G 1974 In: Miller A H, Batsakis J G Premalignant laryngeal lesions, carcinoma in situ, superficial carcinoma — definition and management. Can J Otolaryngol 3: 515
3. van den Brekel M W M, Castelijns J A, Stel H V et al 1991 Occult metastatic neck disease: detection with US and US-guided fine-needle aspiration cytology. Radiology 180: 457–461
4. van den Brekel M W M, Stel H V, Castelijns J A et al 1990 Cervical lymph node metastasis: assessment of radiologic criteria. Radiology 177: 379–384
5. Castelijns J A, Snow G B, Valk J, Gerritsen G J, Hanafee W N 1991 M R imaging of laryngeal cancer. Kluwer Academic Publishers, Dordrecht
6. Chüden H 1969 Krebsdiagnostik im Bereich der Mundhöhle mit einem Farbtest. Med Welt 35: 1871–1872
7. Davina J H M, Stadhouders A M, Lamers G E M, van Haelst U J G M, Kenemans P 1981 Ectocervical cell surface properties related to the location in the epithelium. Nijmegen, The Netherlands: Human reproduction in three dimensions, International SEM Symposium, abstract 1
8. Feinmesser R, Freeman J L, Noyek A M, Birt B D 1987 Metastatic neck disease: a clinical/radiographic/pathologic correlative study. Arch Otolaryngol Head Neck Surg 113: 1307–1310
9. Fex S 1970 Judging the movements of vocal cords in larynx paralysis. Acta Otolaryngol 263: 82–83
10. Franz B 1978 Unsere bisherigen Erfahrungen über den Stellenwert der Kehlkopfzytologie. Arch Oto-Rhino-Laryngol 219: 378–379
11. Franz B, Wetzel M 1980 Zytologie des frühinvasiven Larynxkarzinoms. Laryngol Rhinol Otol 59: 401–405
12. Franzén G, Olofsson J, Klintenberg C, Brunk U 1987 Prognostic value of malignancy grading and DNA measurements in small glottic carcinomas. ORL J Otorhinolaryngol Relat Spec 49: 73–80
13. Früwald H 1979 Zum Wert der Larynxzytologie als Screening-Untersuchung. Laryngol Rhinol Otol 58: 698–699
14. Gröntoft O, Hellquist H, Olofsson J, Nordström G 1978 The DNA content and nuclear size in normal, dysplastic and carcinomatous laryngeal epithelium. A spectrophotometric study. Acta Otolaryngol 86: 473–479
15. Hedley D W, Friedlander M L, Taylor I W, Rugg C A, Musgrove E A 1983 Method for analysis of cellular DNA content of paraffin-embedded pathological material using flow cytometry. J Histochem Cytochem 31: 1333–1335
16. Hellquist H, Olofsson J 1981 Photometric evaluation of laryngeal epithelium exhibiting hyperplasia, keratosis and moderate dysplasia. Acta Otolaryngol 92:157–165
17. Hellquist H, Lundgren J, Olofsson J 1982 Hyperplasia, keratosis, dysplasia and carcinoma in situ of the vocal cords — a follow-up study. Clin Otolaryngol 7: 11–27
18. Hellquist H, Olofsson J, Gröntoft O 1979 Chondrosarcoma of the larynx. J Laryngol Otol 93: 1037–1047
19. Hellquist H, Olofsson J, Gröntoft O 1981 Carcinoma in situ and severe dysplasia of the vocal cords. A clinico-pathological and photometric investigation. Acta Otolaryngol 92: 543–555
20. Iwano T, Yanagizawa I, Iwayanagi T 1965 An in vivo staining test using toluidine blue for oral cytodiagnosis. Shikwa Gaku 65: 66–69

21. Kalter P O, Delemarre J F M, Alons C L, Meijer C J L M, Snow G B 1986 The prognostic significance of morphometry for squamous cell hyperplasia of the laryngeal epithelium. Acta Otolaryngol 102: 124–130

23. Kenemans P, Davina J H M, de Haan R W et al 1981 Cell surface morphology in epithelial malignancy and its precursor lesions. Scan Electron Microsc (part III) 23–36

24. Kitzing P 1985 Stroboscopy — a pertinent laryngological examination. J Otolaryngol 14: 151–157

25. Kleinsasser O 1968 Mikrolaryngoscopie und endolaryngeale Mikrochirurgie Technik und typische Befunde. F K Schattauer, Stuttgart

26. Lundgren J, Olofsson J, Hellquist H 1979 Toluidine blue. An aid in the microlaryngoscopic diagnosis of glottic lesions? Arch Otolaryngol 105: 169–174

27. Lundgren J, Olofsson J, Hellquist H, Gröntoft L 1983 Scanning electron microscopy of vocal cord hyperplasia, keratosis, papillomatosis, dysplasia and carcinoma. Acta Otolaryngol 96: 315–327

28. Lundgren J, Olofsson J, Hellquist H, Strandh J 1982 The role of smear cytology in laryngeal diagnosis. J Otolaryngol 11: 371–378

29. Myers E N 1970 The toluidine blue test in lesions of the oral cavity. CA 20: 134–139

30. Prytz S 1985 Laryngostroboscopy, Brüel & Kjær, Nærum, Denmark, pp 1–12

31. Schönhärl E 1960 Die Stroboskopie in der praktischen Laryngologie. Georg Thieme Verlag, Stuttgart

32. Shedd D P, Hukill P B, Bahn S 1965 In vivo staining properties of oral cancer. Am J Surg 110: 631–634

33. Shedd D P, Hukill P B, Bahn S, Ferraro R H 1967 Further appraisal of in vivo staining properties of oral cancer. Arch Surg 95: 16–22

34. Sökjer H, Olofsson J 1981 Computed tomography in carcinoma of the larynx and pyriform sinus. Clin Otolaryngol 6: 335–343

35. Stern W B R, Silver C E, Zeifer B A, Persky M S, Heller K S 1990 Computed tomography of the clinically negative neck. Head Neck 12: 109–113

36. Stevens M H, Harnsberger H R, Mancuso A A, Davis R K, Johnson L P, Parkin J L 1985 Computed tomography of cervical lymph nodes: staging and management of head and neck cancer. Arch Otolaryngol 111: 735–739

37. Strong M S, Vaughan C W, Incze J S 1968 Toluidine blue in the management of carcinoma of the oral cavity. Arch Otolaryngol 87:527–531

38. Tarkkanen J, Paavolainen M, Saksela E 1972 Toluidine blue staining in the endoscopic diagnosis of carcinoma of the bronchus. Ann Clin Res 4:7–9

39. UICC (Union Internationale Contre le Cancer). 1987 TNM classification of malignant tumours. Hermanek P, Sobin L H (eds). Springer, Berlin

40. Wetzel M, Franz B 1979 Larynxdysplasien und zytologische Befunde. Arch Oto-Rhino-Laryngol 223: 415–416

41. Wetzel M, Franz B, Neumann O G 1978 Vergleichende Wertung verschiedener, in der HNO-Praxis durchführbarer diagnostischer Methoden bei der laryngologischen Krebsfrüherkennung. Arch Oto-Rhino-Laryngol 219: 380.

21. Documentation

E. Yanagisawa

INTRODUCTION

In the early and mid-19th century, Bozzini (1806), Babington (1829), Avery (1840) and Desormeaux (1853) attempted to examine the larynx using various devices. In 1854, Manuel Garcia, a Spanish-born singing teacher practising in London, observed the movements of his own vocal cords with a dental mirror and a hand-held mirror with which he reflected the sunlight into his open mouth.[16] This marked the birth of indirect laryngoscopy. In the summer of 1857, Garcia's method was tried by Professor Ludwig Turck of Vienna who had to abandon it during the winter because of insufficient sunlight for illumination. In the November of 1857, Professor Johann Nepomuk Czermak of Budapest borrowed Turck's mirror and substituted artificial illumination for sunlight.[11] Czermak attempted to photograph the larynx but was not successful. Morell MacKenzie (1865) of London, a skillful laryngologist and teacher, redesigned the laryngeal mirror and popularized indirect laryngoscopy.[29,34,47,54,56]

In 1882, Thomas French of New York described the first successful technique for photographing the larynx using a box camera to which a laryngeal mirror was attached. He used sunlight as a light source via a sunlight concentrator (Fig. 21.1A).[14] In 1884, French published a paper entitled 'On a Perfected Method of Photographing the Larynx',[15] producing the first publishable black-and-white photographs of the larynx. These pictures were of amazingly good quality (Fig. 21.1B).

Since French's successful documentation, many different methods of photographic documentation of the larynx have been described. They include: (i) indirect laryngoscopic photography,[13,39] (ii) direct laryngoscopic photography,[13,22–24,40] (iii) fibrescopic photography,[9,12,19,25,41,43–45,55–58,60,61,63,65–67,70] (iv) telescopic photography,[1–8,10,17,18,28,33,35–37,46,49,53,56,58–61,63,66–68,70] and (v) microscopic photography.[1,26,27,30–32,38,39,42,48,51,69] Among these contributions, the following are worthy of special mention.

In 1941, P. Holinger, J. D. Brubaker and J. E. Brubaker collaborated to produce several models of the Brubaker–Holinger endoscopic camera which were designed primarily for open-tube endoscopic photography of the larynx, bronchi and oesophagus.[22,24] These cameras used an open-tube system with a proximal illumination and optical system. Colour photographs of the larynx taken by Paul Holinger were of exceptionally high quality. Clarity of the details was excellent. His laryngeal colour pictures have been used widely in otolaryngological and other medical texts throughout the world.[22–24] The Holinger–Brubaker camera is no longer available.

In 1953, the Zeiss operating microscope was developed and used for otological surgery. Oscar Kleinsasser of Cologne adapted the binocular Zeiss microscope to direct laryngoscopy (the birth of microlaryngoscopy), using a 400 mm objective lens.[30–32] He employed general endotracheal anaesthesia along with wider-diameter laryngoscopes and a chest holder. Using a single lens reflex (SLR) camera attached to the photoadapter via a beam splitter, Kleinsasser was able to obtain 'perfectly clear pictures of the internal larynx.'. His unexcelled microlaryngoscopic photographs of laryngeal disorders were shown in his classic book, *Microlaryngoscopy and Endolaryngeal Microsurgery* (1968).[31]

In 1954, Yutaka Tachiki, a professor of otolaryngology at Tohoku University, Japan, demonstrated the first successful television recording of the larynx, using a 'tele-endoscope' attached to a large television camera.[50] He emphasized the advantages of simultaneous viewing by many others, even at a distance, and simultaneous voice recording. He predicted that televised video recording would become a most useful method of laryngeal documentation in the future.

In 1968, Sawashima and Hirose of Tokyo introduced flexible fibrescopic laryngoscopy to laryngology.[41] Since then, the flexible fibrescope has been widely used for evaluation and documentation of the function and pathology of the larynx. One of the most significant advances in endoscopic documentation was the development of the modern telescopes with the Hopkins rod lens system (Karl Storz), the Lumina optic system (Richard Wolf) and the full lumen system (Nagashima). Paul Ward, George Berci,

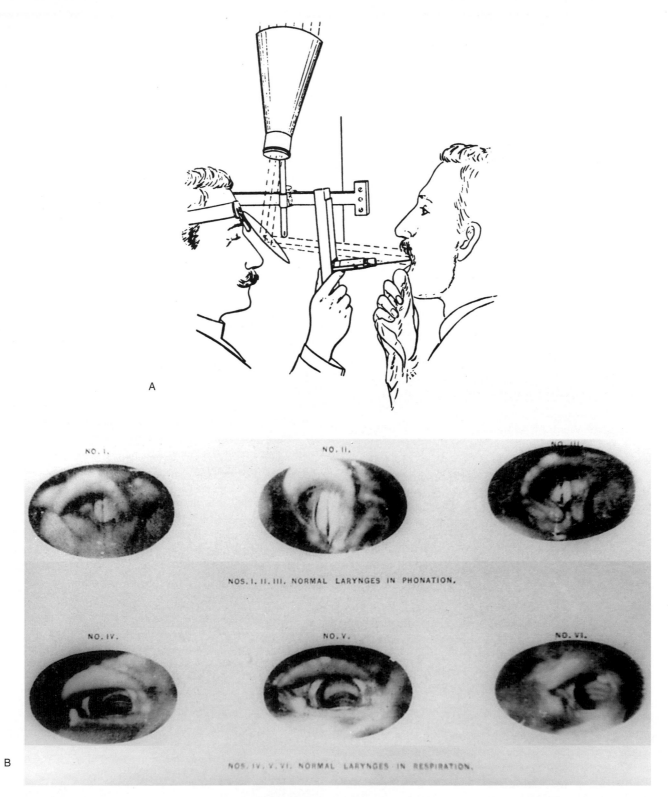

Fig. 21.1 A. (*top*) Dr French's method of laryngeal photography in 1882, using a sunlight concentrator as a light source, a camera with a throat mirror attached and a perforated forehead reflector. B. (*bottom*) Photographs taken by Dr French using his method.

Bruce Benjamin and others have set the high standard for the newer generation of telescopic documentation.[4,5,6-8,46,53,56,68] The optics of these newer systems are such that light transmission and magnification are significantly increased, thereby providing a brighter and more easily perceived image and an improved resolution of depth. Telescopic documentation with a still or video camera produces large, clear images of the larynx. Koichi Yamashita, a skilful endoscopist, pioneer of modern VTR (video-tape recorded) endoscopy, set the high standard of video-endoscopic documentation.[55,56,58] His ENT video images of superb quality are illustrated in his recent textbook entitled, *Diagnostic and Therapeutic ENT Endoscopy* (in Japanese) (1988) which concisely describes the historical development, current techniques and clinical application of VTR endoscopy.[56] More than three decades after Tachiki's discovery, thanks to remarkable advances in video and optical technology, videoendoscopy of the larynx has been widely adapted and has become a useful addition to the daily practice of laryngology. Many have advocated the use of television (video tape) for laryngeal documentation.[9,21,25,28,33,43,44,48,51,55,56,58-60,64-68,70,72] In 1990, Kantor, Berci, Partlow et al[28] introduced a completely new approach to microlaryngeal surgery and its documentation, using a specially designed 'video-microlaryngoscope' with a built-in rigid telescope and an attached camera. In this method, surgery is performed and recorded while observing the laryngeal images on the television screen.

Laryngeal documentation can be accomplished by different modalities: (i) still photography, (ii) videography, and (iii) cinematography. Although still photography of the larynx is still a valuable method of laryngeal documentation today, videography is increasingly gaining favour. Cinematography has the advantage of producing excellent quality pictures in motion and has been used widely until recently as an important and effective means of documentation and presentation.[6,13,19,20,23,24,31,52] Sixteen-millimetre colour movies have been shown to large audiences without the need for multiple television monitors. However, because of the cost of films, time-consuming film development and editing, and the availability of newer generation video projectors for large screens, cinematography is infrequently used today and is being replaced by videography.

In this chapter, various techniques of still photography and videography of the larynx, personally used by the author, will be described.

STILL PHOTOGRAPHY OF THE LARYNX

The larynx has traditionally been documented by still photography for many years. Still photography is a convenient and effective way of documenting the larynx and is still the method of choice for many laryngologists, particularly those who have no easy access to videographic or cinematographic equipment.

Still photography of the larynx can be accomplished with a 35 mm SLR camera (Fig. 21.2A) by means of a laryngeal mirror, a laryngoscope, a flexible fibrescope, a rigid telescope or an operative microscope. Other cameras specially designed for endoscopes can also be used. One of the distinct advantages of still photography is that colour slides and/or prints for presentation and publication can easily be made.

Still photography in the office

Indirect still laryngoscopic photography

During indirect laryngoscopy, the larynx can be photographed using a laryngeal mirror, a 35 mm SLR camera and a fibreoptic headlight as a light source. In this method, the patient sits facing the examiner. While the examiner exposes the laryngeal image, an assistant photographs the laryngeal image on the mirror using a 35 mm SLR camera with a 100 mm telephoto lens with a ring light and ASA 400 or faster Ektachrome colour film. The use of a tripod is recommended. A special close-up macrolens with a ring light, such as the Nikon Medical close-up lens, is useful. This is a relatively inexpensive method, but focusing of the laryngeal image on the mirror through the viewfinder of the camera is difficult, because of motion. Besides the examiner, an experienced photographer should be present. Results are unpredictable and poor in the author's hand. (The success rate is approximately 20%.)

Fibrescopic still laryngeal photography

Fibrescopic still laryngeal photography in the office can be accomplished with a flexible fibrescope such as Olympus ENF-P2 (3.4 mm) or P3 (3.4 mm), Machida 4L (4 mm) or 3L (3.3 mm), Pentax FNL-10S (3.5 mm) or Olympus ENF-L (4.4 mm).[43,44,65]

The following equipment is recommended for this procedure: (i) the Olympus OM2 35 mm SLR camera with an autowinder, clear-glass focusing screen 1–9, and 2× teleconverter (Fig. 21.2A), (ii) ENF-P2 or P3 fibrescope (the author's choice) (Fig. 21.2B), (iii) Olympus SMR endoscopic coupler (Fig. 21.2A), (iv) Karl Storz xenon cold-light source 487C or 615, (v) Ektachrome ASA 400 or 800 daylight film. The camera is set on automatic mode with the appropriate ASA setting.

The flexible fibrescope is connected to the 2× teleconverter attached to the SLR camera using the Olympus SMR endoscopic coupler. Instead of the SMR coupler, the 100 mm macrolens with the Karl Storz quick-connect adapter may also be used. The examiner may perform the

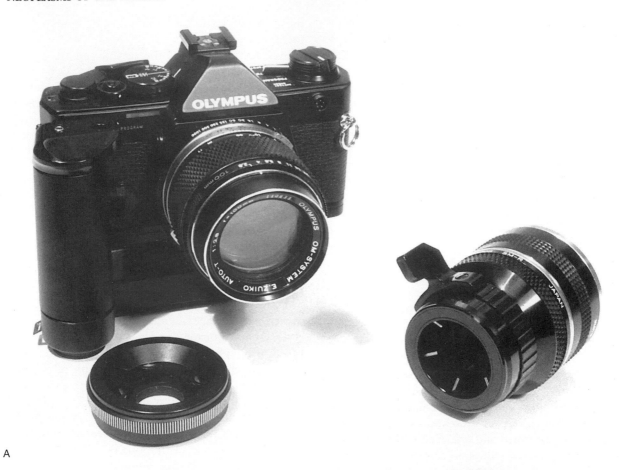

A

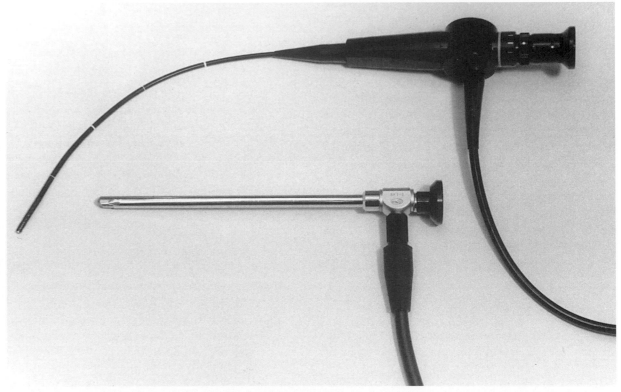

B

Fig. 21.2   A. (*top*) Single-lens-reflex (SLR) camera system for still photography: (*top left*) Olympus OM-2 35 mm SLR camera with an autowinder and 100 mm macrolens; (*bottom left*) Karl Storz quick-connect adapter; (*right*) Olympus SMR coupler to which a 2× extender is attached. B. (*bottom*) Endoscopes: (*top*) Olympus ENF-P3 flexible fibrescope; (*bottom*) Nagashima SFT-1 rigid telescope.

procedure in either a sitting or standing position (Fig. 21.3A). The nose is sprayed with 3% Ephedrine to shrink hypertrophied turbinates and lightly anaesthetized with 4% Xylocaine spray. The laryngeal image is centred and focused in the viewfinder of the camera, and the pictures are taken both on respiration and phonation. The clearest pictures are obtained on inspiration immediately after phonating 'ee'. A series of pictures is taken using the autowinder. The exposure is bracketed using the exposure compensation dial of the camera. Because the size of the laryngeal image is small and a large amount of the field is unlit, most automatic cameras adjust to the darkness of the image and overcompensate, thus producing a washed-out laryngeal image. Accordingly, the best picture is taken when the compensation dial is set at −1 or −2 (underexposure). The xenon light source is set at the high filming mode during the photography. When the xenon light source is not available, faster films, such as ASA 800, are needed. The success rate in the author's hand is approximately 50%. Fibrescopic pictures appear grainy (Fig. 21.3Ba,b) and it may be difficult to identify small lesions.

Telescopic still laryngeal photography

Telescopic laryngeal photography can be accomplished using a rigid right-angled telescope (Fig. 21.4A). The equipment used includes: (i) Olympus 35 mm SLR OM2 camera system as described for fibrescopic photography; (ii) a telescope, such as the Nagashima SFT-1 (70°) (the new SFT-1 with an 'Olympus-type' eyepiece) (Fig. 21.2B), Karl Storz right-angled telescope 8702D (90°), Stuckrad magnifying telescope (Wolf), or the newer Karl Storz 70° rigid telescope 8706 CL; (iii) a xenon light source (Karl Storz 487C, 610, 615C); (iv) ASA 400 or 800 Ektachrome daylight film. The advantage of using a xenon light source over an electronic unit is that there is no warm-up period required between the exposures. The patient often cannot tolerate repeated or prolonged exposures. The technique of telescopic still photography is shown in Fig. 21.4A. By having the patient say 'ee', the larynx is fully exposed in most cases. Pictures are taken during respiration and phonation. A series of pictures is taken using the autowinder of the camera. Exposures are bracketed using the automatic compensation dial at +1, 0, −1 and −2. The success rate with this method is 70–80%. Telescopic still photography gives the clearest laryngeal images taken in the office (Fig. 21.4Ba,b,c).[59, 62,66,70]

Microscopic still laryngeal photography

Microscopic photography can be performed in the office during indirect laryngoscopy. The larynx is exposed using the laryngeal mirror and the Zeiss operating microscope to which the 35 mm SLR camera is attached via the photoadapter. The wall-mounted microscope is easier to manipulate than the floor-based microscope. It is important for the microscope to be fixed during exposure to prevent blurred images due to movement.

The following equipment is recommended (i) the Zeiss operating microscope with a straightforward eyepiece and 250 or 300 mm objective lens; (ii) a 35 mm SLR camera; (iii) a photoadapter; and (iv) Ektachrome ASA 160 film pushed to ASA 320.

Some have good results with this method, but the success rate is approximately 30% in the author's hand. The poor percentage of this technique is due to difficulty in exposing and focusing the larynx using the operating microscope.

Still photography in the operating room

Direct laryngoscopic photography

The larynx can be photographed directly through the laryngoscope at the time of laryngoscopy using a 35 mm SLR camera with a telephoto lens (Fig. 21.5A). For this purpose, the SLR camera with a 100 to 200 mm telephoto lens is placed on the tripod. The larynx is centred and focused through the viewfinder of the camera and pictures are taken. When using the Dedo or Ossoff photographic laryngoscope with two large fibreoptic light cables attached, there is an adequate amount of light at the larynx. Ektachrome Tungsten ASA 160 film is used and pushed to ASA 320 when developed. This technique is inexpensive and produces quite satisfactory pictures (Fig. 21.5B). However, it is inconvenient and time-consuming since both the camera and the tripod have to be re-adjusted and re-positioned each time the surgeon finds an interesting and worthwhile lesion to be photographed. The surgery has to be interrupted. The success rate is 70–80%.

Another method of direct laryngoscopic photography is by an aperture-preferred automatic 35 mm SLR camera with a 50 mm macrolens (Fig. 21.6A). For this technique, 35 mm SLR cameras such as the Nikon FE or the Olympus OM 2 are excellent. The camera is hand-held. The larynx is focused through the laryngoscope and photographed. The photographed image on the finished slide is small but quite recognizable (Fig. 21.6). This photograph can be cropped and enlarged. Ektachrome Tungsten ASA 160 film is used and pushed to ASA 320. This is the simplest method of laryngeal photography.

Telescopic laryngeal photography

Telescopic laryngeal photography in the operating room can be accomplished by passing a straightforward telescope

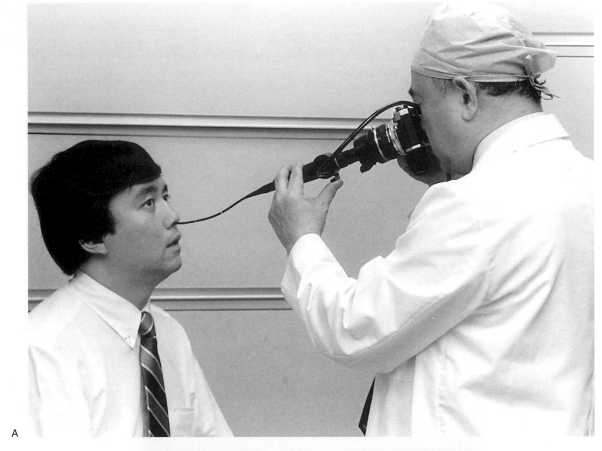

A

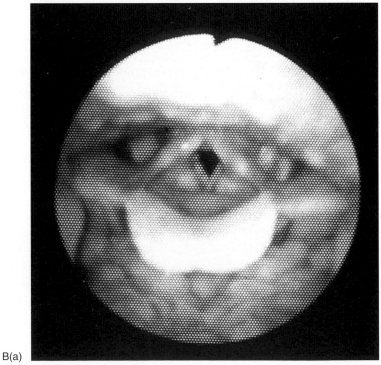

B(a)

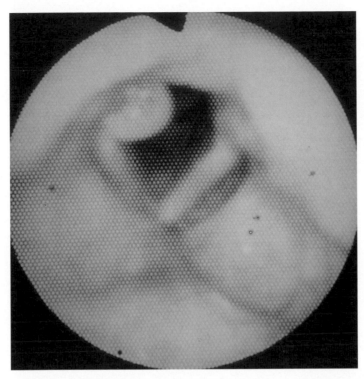

B(b)

Fig. 21.3 A. (*opposite page, top*) Method for fibrescopic still laryngeal photography in the office. B. Still photographs taken with this method: (a) (*opposite page, bottom*) normal larynx and hypopharynx; (b) (*above*) post-intubation granuloma.

into the laryngoscope (Fig. 21.7A).[4,5] For this purpose, the author uses the Hopkins 0° straightforward telescope 8700A with a xenon light source. The telescope is attached to the Olympus OM2 camera with a 100 mm macrolens, a Karl Storz quick-connect adapter, a 1-9 focusing screen and an autowinder. Ektachrome daylight ASA 400 film is used. A xenon light source such as the Karl Storz 487C, 615 is used.

Although photography with this method is time-consuming and the telescope may be expensive, this telescopic system produces excellent pictures of the larynx (Fig. 21.7B). The success rate is very high (90% or better).

Microscopic laryngeal photography

Microscopic laryngeal photography can be accomplished by utilizing the optical system of an operating microscope. It can be done with or without the use of a photoadapter.[27,30,31,38,66,69] Photographs of acceptable quality and of various magnification may be obtained.

Microlaryngoscopic photography using a 35 mm SLR camera with a photoadapter. When a special photoadapter (Zeiss, Designs for Vision, etc.) is attached to the beam splitter of the operating microscope and the laryngoscope is suspended with a laryngoscope holder, the larynx can be photographed with relative ease (Fig. 21.8A). It is important to obtain an accurate axial alignment of the

optical system of the microscope and the lumen of the laryngoscope.

The equipment recommended includes: (i) Zeiss operating microscope; (ii) a beam splitter; (iii) a photoadapter; (iv) an adapter ring for a 35 mm SLR camera; and (v) an automatic 35 mm SLR camera. High-speed Ektachrome Tungsten ASA 160 film was used and pushed to 320 when developed.

One of the major advantages of microscopic photography with the use of a photoadapter is that the surgeon can be the photographer. While performing the operation, he can photograph the larynx at any time without depending on his assistant. Other advantages are: (i) the surgery is minimally interrupted because the operator is the photographer; (ii) the larynx can be photographed at different magnifications (6×, 10×, 25× and 40×); (iii) copying and enlargement of the slides is not necessary when pictures are taken at higher magnification (Fig. 21.8B); and (iv) TV and movie documentation can be conveniently and simultaneously done when used with a Telestill photoadapter.

Some of the disadvantages are: (i) photoadapter and beam splitter are expensive; (ii) the depth of field is very shallow, particularly at high magnification; and (iii) it requires bright illumination. With the use of a photographic laryngoscope, such as Dedo or Ossoff (Pilling), there is adequate light for satisfactory photography.

The success rate is approximately 70%.

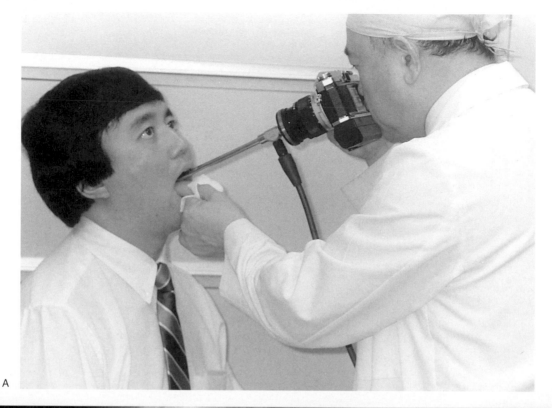

A

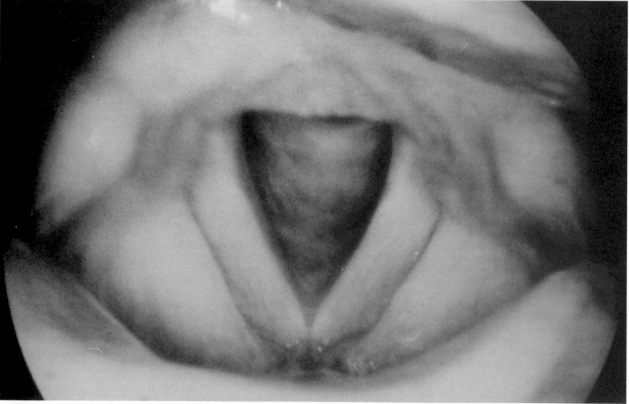

B(a)

Fig. 21.4 A. (*top*) Method for telescopic still laryngeal photography in the office. B. Photographs taken with this method: (a) (*bottom*) normal larynx on respiration; (b) (*opposite page, top*) bilateral post-intubation granulomas; (c) (*opposite page, bottom*) extensive supraglottic carcinoma.

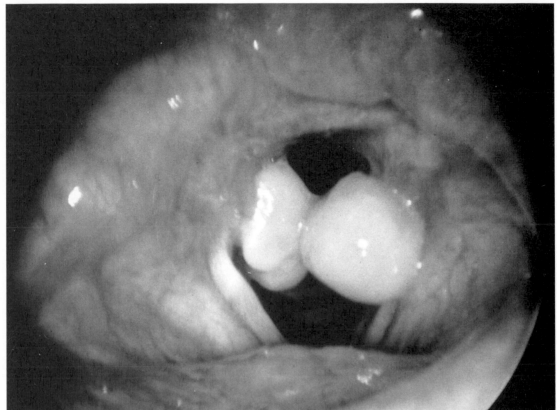

B(b)

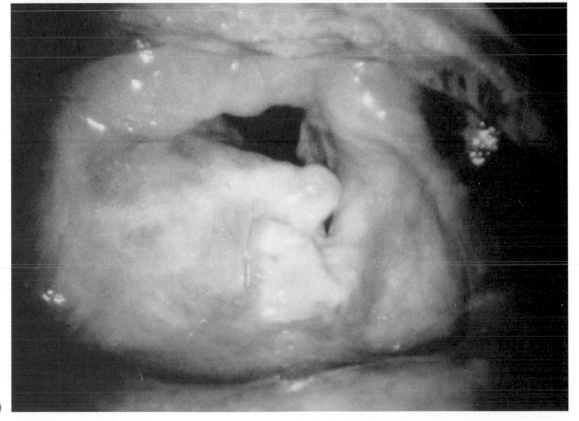

B(c)

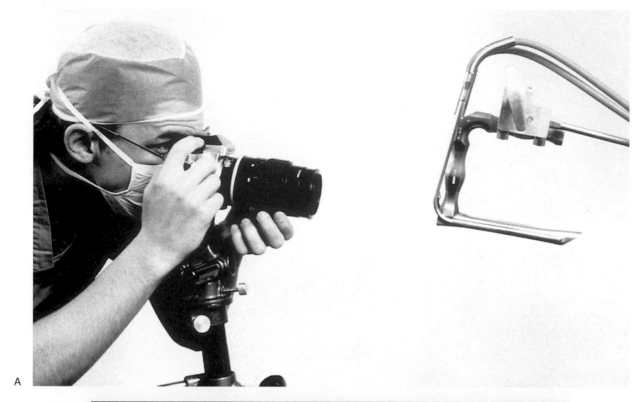

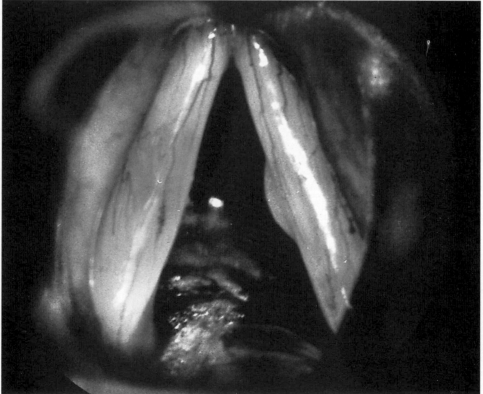

Fig. 21.5   A. (*top*) Method for direct laryngoscopic photography in the operating room using an SLR camera with a 100 mm telephoto lens mounted on the tripod. B. (*bottom*) Photograph taken with this method showing early Reinke's oedema on the left and a small polyp on the right.

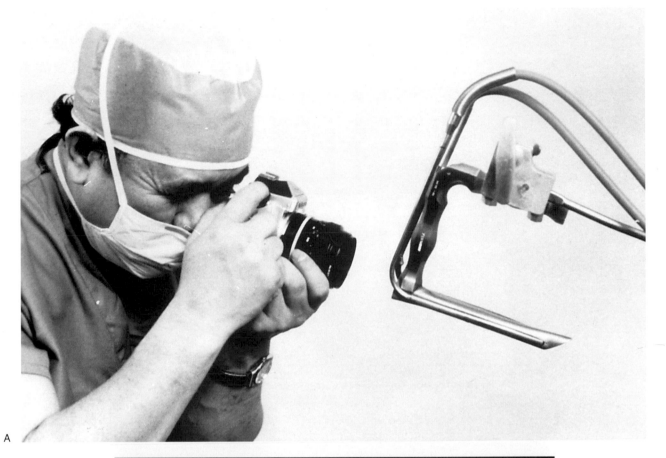

A

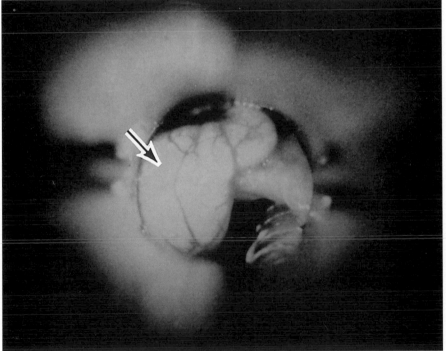

B

Fig. 21.6   A. (*top*) Method for direct laryngoscopic photography using an SLR camera with a 50 mm macrolens. B. (*bottom*) Photograph taken with this technique showing a pedunculated vallecular cyst (arrow) overlying the top of the epiglottis.

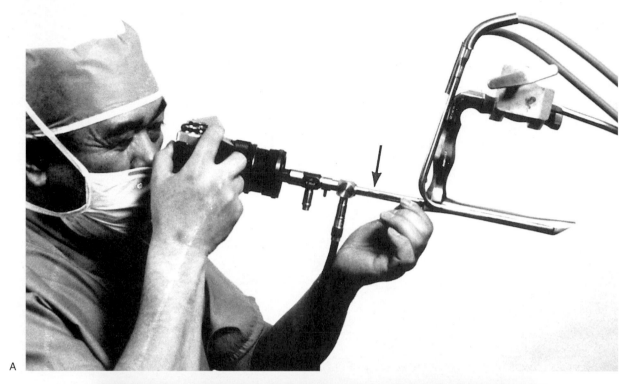

A

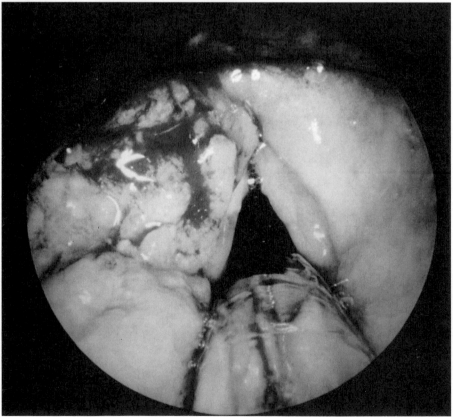

B

Fig. 21.7   A. (*top*) Method for telescopic still photography in the operating room using the Hopkins 8700A telescope (arrow) attached to the SLR camera lens inserted into the laryngoscope. B. (*bottom*) Photograph taken with this method showing transglottic carcinoma on the left.

Microlaryngoscopic photography using the SLR camera without a photoadapter ('microscopic macrolens technique').[66,69] This is a simple method of laryngeal photography through the eyepiece of the operating microscope using the 35 mm SLR camera with a macrolens (Fig. 21.9A).

The equipment used includes: (i) a Zeiss operating microscope; (ii) an 'aperture-preferred' automatic 35 mm SLR camera, such as the Nikon FE, Pentax ME, Olympus OM2, etc.; (iii) a 50 mm macrolens; and (iv) a Dedo or Ossoff photographic laryngoscope. Ektachrome Tungsten ASA 160 film is used and pushed to 320.

In this technique, the camera is set at infinity with the lens wide open (usually at f3.5). The eyepiece of the microscope is set at 0. The larynx is focused via the microscope first. The microscope knob is tightened. The macrolens of the camera is placed on the eyepiece of the microscope (Fig. 21.9A). The larynx is now focused through the eyepiece of the camera and the pictures are taken. Photographs taken by this technique are of surprisingly good quality and are ready for use in teaching without cropping or enlargement (Fig. 21.9B). Some of the disadvantages are: (i) it is sometimes difficult to hold the camera still on the eyepiece of the camera; (ii) the surgery is interrupted because the picture has to be taken by either an assistant or the surgeon himself. The success of this technique depends on illumination, critical focusing, and stability of the patient, microscope and camera. The macrolens technique is simple, and it is the least expensive method of microscopic laryngeal photography. The success rate is 70–80%.

VIDEOGRAPHY OF THE LARYNX

Videographic documentation of the larynx can be accomplished using a flexible fibrescope, a rigid telescope, or an operating microscope. Due to the availability of compact light-sensitive CCD video cameras, xenon light sources and vastly improved optical and endoscopic equipment, videographic documentation of the larynx has become an accepted method of effective laryngeal documentation. Excellent laryngeal images can be easily recorded and hard copies of these images can be instantaneously obtained with a newer colour video printer.[35,66]

Videography of the larynx in the office

Fibrescopic videolaryngoscopy[61,65,66,70]

Fibrescopic videolaryngoscopy is of great value in evaluating and documenting the physiological functions and pathological conditions of the larynx. It permits simultaneous voice and video recording.

The following equipment is used: (i) a flexible fibrescope; (ii) a colour video camera; (iii) a video camera adapter; (iv) a light source (a xenon light source is preferable);

(v) a video recorder (3/4", 1/2", 8 mm); and (vi) a colour monitor. Fibrescopes, such as the Olympus ENF-P2 or P3, Machida ENT4L or 3L, and Pentax FNL 10S or 15S, can be used. The Olympus ENF-P3 is the author's choice. There are many fine-quality miniature CCD video cameras available for fibrescopic video laryngoscopy; they include: (i) Karl Storz Mini 9000 CCD (17 lux), 9050B, 90820E and Supercam 9060B (7 lux) (Fig. 21.10A); (ii) Olympus OTV-S2; (iii) Toshiba CCD distributed by Nagashima CCD (10 lux); (iv) Elmo EC-202 CCD (10 lux) (Figs 21.10A, B; 21.11); Elmo EC (Olympus) 102 CCD (15 lux) (Fig. 21.10B), and Elmo MN401 (10 lux); (v) Jedmed Micro CCD (8 lux); (vi) Storz ENT 62 CCD (7 lux); and (vii) Wolf CCD (10 lux). Most of these cameras are equipped with C-mount couplers and require special adapters for the endoscopes (Fig. 21.10A,B). The cost of these cameras ranges from US$3500 to US$10 000. More recently, high-resolution three-chip CCD mini cameras (Sony DXC-750, approximately US$18 000) have been introduced. While these cameras are compact and convenient, the cost of the camera is often prohibitive to many otolaryngologists. Yanagisawa et al advocated the use of reasonably priced home video cameras for endoscopic videolaryngoscopy and obtained excellent results.[61,65–68,70] Home video cameras used include: (i) JVC GX NBU (10 lux, US$800) (Fig. 21.11, no longer available); (ii) Olympus Movie 8 VX801-62 (7 lux, approximately US$1500) (Fig. 21.11); (iii) Ricoh R620 CCD (4 lux, approximately US$1500) (Fig. 21.22); and (iv) Ricoh R66 (4 lux). These home video cameras have a macrozooming device but the lens is not detachable. With the use of a Karl Storz quick-connect adapter, however, a fibrescope can be easily attached to the front of the lens (Fig. 21.12A). These cameras can be used with endoscopes, but cannot be used with the operating microscope. The adaptability of these video cameras to endoscopic adapters should be checked prior to purchase. If the video camera is ultra light-sensitive, a standard light source such as the Pilling 2× luminator suffices. It has a built-in adapter for most other endoscopes available today. If illumination is not sufficient, the xenon light source is recommended. The examiner performs the procedure as described for still fibrescopic laryngeal photography. The larynx is centred on the screen and the patient is ready for video taping (Fig. 21.12A). The larynx is examined and videotaped on respiration, phonation, effort closure and swallowing. Laryngeal pathology can be easily detected and documented (Fig. 21.12Ba,b,c).

One of the most significant advantages of fibrescopic video laryngoscopy is the ease of the examination. Other advantages are: (i) it is a quick and comfortable way of examining the larynx; (ii) children and adults with gag reflex can be effectively examined; (iii) it is valuable for voice analysis and for the study of the physiological function of the larynx; and (iv) it allows the examination of subglottic

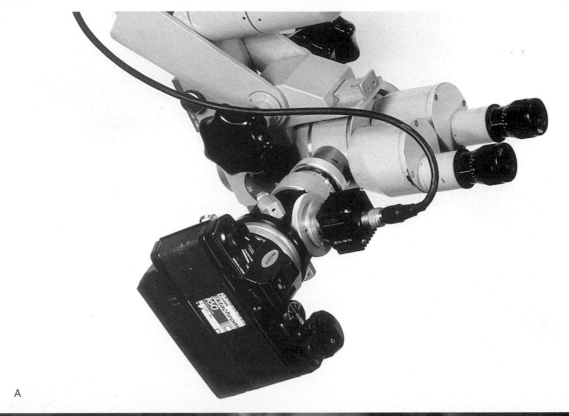

A

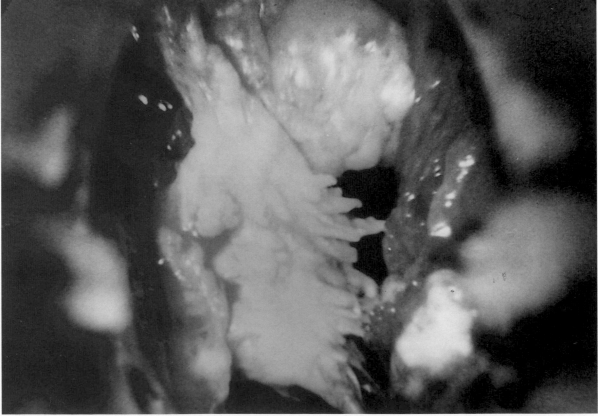

B

Fig. 21.8   A. (*top*) Method for microlaryngoscopic still photography using a photoadapter. The SLR camera with the autowinder attached is connected to the Zeiss operating microscope via a photoadapter. B. (*bottom*) Photograph taken with this method showing extensive verrucous carcinoma of the larynx.

and tracheal lesions. Some of the disadvantages are: (i) it provides a smaller, less clear, more distorted picture of the larynx than does telescopic examination; (ii) it requires more illumination due to the small diameter of the scope, and documentation may not be easy; (iii) it requires a light-sensitive camera (low lux); and (iv) it often produces Moiré effect (multiple abnormal colour strips) on the television screen interfering with detailed interpretation. The success rate is 95%, including young children and infants.

Telescopic videolaryngoscopy[61,66,70]

Telescopic videolaryngoscopy using a rigid telescope and a video camera in the office is an effective method of documenting the normal physiology and pathology of the larynx (Fig. 21.13A, Ba,b,c). It is particularly important for precise evaluation of structural changes of the larynx.

Equipment used for telescopic videolaryngoscopy is essentially the same as for fibrescopic videolaryngoscopy except for the use of the rigid telescope. There are several excellent right-angled telescopes especially designed for laryngeal examination; they are: (i) Berci–Ward Karl Storz 3702D; (ii) Karl Storz 8704D; (iii) Karl Storz 8706CL; (iv) Wolf Stuckrad; and (v) Nagashima SFT-1 (Fig. 21.2B). The prism angle of the Nagashima SFT-1 and Karl Storz 8706CL telescopes is 70°—permitting excellent visualization of anterior and posterior commissures of the larynx and being particularly useful for laryngostroboscopy. These telescopes are connected to a miniature CCD camera via a specific adapter, or to the front of the home video camera via the Karl Storz quick-connect adapter (Fig. 21.2A).

After the soft palate and posterior half of the tongue have been topically anaesthetized using 4% Xylocaine solution, the examiner inserts the telescope into the mouth with one hand while holding the patient's tongue with the other hand (Fig. 21.13A). Prior to the procedure, the tip of the telescope is dipped into warm water and dried to prevent fogging of the lens during the examination. When the desired image appears on the monitor screen, the video recording is begun.

Some of the advantages of telescopic videolaryngoscopy are: (i) it provides a wide-angle view and large clear images; (ii) a close-up view of telescopic examination is of great value for detecting early lesions; and (iii) it allows easy videographic documentation. The telescope produces a much brighter and clearer stroboscopic image since the diameter of the telescope is generally larger than that of a fibrescope and, therefore, the telescope transmits more light. The disadvantages of telescopic videolaryngoscopy are: (i) children and some adults with hyperactive

gag reflex may not be able to tolerate the procedure; (ii) fogging of the telescope lens during the procedure is common; (iii) the voice is distorted; and (iv) normal speech is impossible.

The author prefers telescopic documentation to fibrescopic documentation since the former gives clearer, sharper and larger images of the larynx (Fig. 21.13Ba, b,c), which is so essential for accurate diagnosis. The success rate is 90% in the author's hand.

Microscopic videolaryngoscopy

Microscopic videolaryngoscopy in the office can be done during indirect laryngoscopy in the same way as described for microscopic still photography, except that the video camera is attached to the Zeiss operating microscope via a photoadapter instead of a 35 mm SLR camera (Fig. 21.14).

Because of technical difficulty, time- and cost-ineffectiveness and the availability of simpler and more effective endoscopic techniques, microscopic videolaryngoscopy is no longer performed by the author in the office.

Videography in the operating room

Telescopic videolaryngoscopy

Telescopic videolaryngoscopy in the operating room can be accomplished by using the straightforward Hopkins rigid telescope 8700A and video camera along with a xenon light source (Fig. 21.15A). For use in the operating room, a miniature CCD camera is more useful and convenient than a home video camera. The telescope is attached to the miniature CCD camera and passed into the laryngoscope which is suspended using the laryngoscope holder. When the laryngeal image is centred on the TV monitor, video taping is begun. One of the disadvantages of this method is that the procedure has to be interrupted for video documentation. The images obtained through this method are superb (Fig. 21.15B). They can be video-printed using a colour video printer at the time of, or after, the procedure.

Telescopic video documentation of a subglottic lesion is possible with a Hopkins 4 mm 70° telescope (Karl Storz 7200C) via a tracheostomy opening.

Microscopic videolaryngoscopy[66]

Microscopic videolaryngoscopy using the operating microscope and colour video camera is the most effective and convenient method of teaching and documenting microsurgery of the larynx (Fig. 21.16A, Ba, b, c).

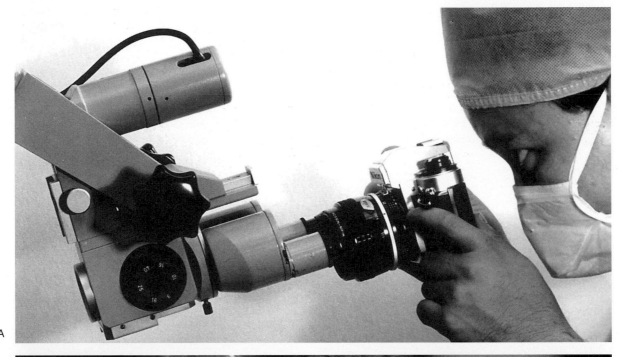

A

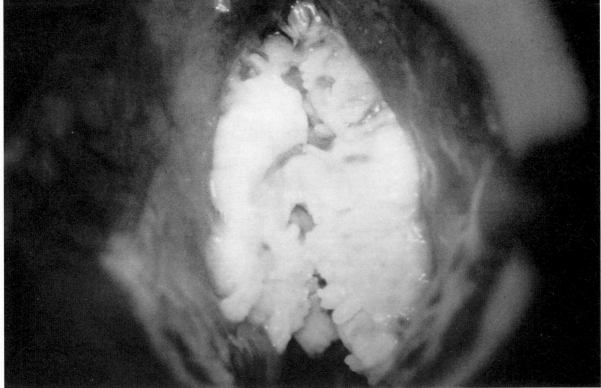

B

Fig. 21.9 A. Method for microscopic still photography without photoadapter ('microscopic macrolens technique'). The macrolens of the hand-held camera is placed over the eyepiece of the microscope. B. Photograph taken with this method showing extensive verrucous carcinoma of the larynx.

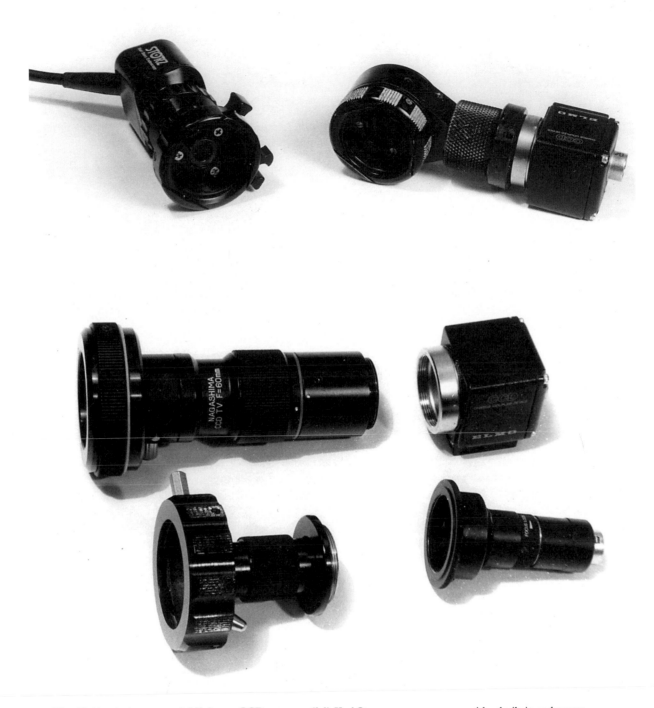

Fig. 21.10 A. (*upper group*) Miniature CCD cameras: (*left*) Karl Storz supercam camera with a built-in endoscope adapter; (*right*) Elmo EC202 CCD camera with Karl Storz beam splitter adapter. B. (*lower group*) Video adapters: Nagashima videoadapter (*top, left*) for C-mount miniature CCD camera, Elmo EC-202 (*top, right*), Olympus videoadapter (*bottom, left*) for C-mount miniature camera, Elmo EC-102 (Olympus) (*bottom, right*).

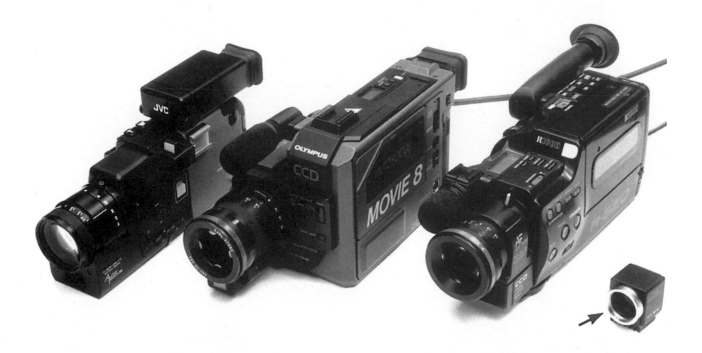

Fig. 21.11 Home video cameras: JVC GX-N8U (*left*); Olympus CCD Movie 8 camera (*middle*); Ricoh 620 CCD (*right*) compared with miniature CCD camera Elmo EC-202 (*arrow*).

The equipment used includes: (i) a laryngoscope especially designed for photographic documentation (Dedo, Ossoff); (ii) a light source such as the Pilling Illuminator 2×; (iii) a Zeiss operating microscope with a straight eyepiece and 400 mm objective lens; (iv) a beam splitter; (v) a photoadapter such as the Zeiss video adapter or the Telestill photoadapter; (vi) a video camera, either the miniature CCD camera or pick-up tube camera; (vii) a video recorder; and (viii) a colour TV monitor. Some of the newer CCD miniature cameras (such as Storz CCM-1, Elmo EC202 (Fig. 21.16A), Elmo MN 401E, CN401E) can be conveniently and effectively used with the microscope. Because of the small size and the light weight of the camera, the microscope can be easily manipulated, thus making it easy to operate and document the microlaryngeal surgery at the same time. Heavier and more expensive three-tube cameras such as Hitachi-DK5050 (Fig. 21.16A) or Ikegami ITC-350 M produce exceptionally high-quality video images (Fig. 21.16Ba,b,c). Since the three-tube camera is no longer available, those who desire top-quality high-resolution laryngeal pictures may have to resort to newer three-chip video cameras, such as the Sony DXC-750 (approximately US$16 000) and Hitachi three-chip CCD camera.

Some of the advantages of microscopic videography of the larynx are: (i) it can document either a part or the entire microsurgery procedure with minimal interference to surgery; (ii) live viewing by an unlimited audience is possible; (iii) equipment, although expensive, is already available in most medical centres, and the system is familiar to most surgeons; (iv) higher magnifications can be easily and quickly obtained, producing very sharp images at the plane of focus, allowing visualization and precise operation of a minute lesion; (v) microlaryngoscopes are available for both paediatric and adult patients; (vi) televized microscopic laryngoscopy is an excellent method of teaching; and (vii) instant colour video print-outs can be obtained for documentation and patient's record using a video printer. Some of the disadvantages are: (i) it provides a shallower depth of field; (ii) the microscope is placed between the surgeon and the patient, making instrumentation more difficult; (iii) a light-sensitive miniature video camera and light source are needed; (iv) the surgery may have to be carried out through one eyepiece due to a small proximal opening of the laryngoscope; and (v) refocusing at different magnifications is necessary.

Kantor–Berci telescopic video microlaryngoscopy[28]

In 1990 Kantor, Berci, Partlow et al introduced a new approach to microlaryngeal surgery and its documentation using a specially designed 'video-microlaryngoscope' with a built-in rigid telescope and an attached video camera (Fig. 21.17A). The ability to perform surgery of the larynx by viewing the high-resolution TV image and simultaneously video-documenting the surgery was demonstrated. This technique was recommended by Kantor, Berci, Partlow et al over the standard microscopic technique for its increased visibility with greater depth of view, unimpeded access to instrument, instant documentation and superior teaching value.

Recommended equipment includes: (i) Kantor–Berci video microlaryngoscope (Karl Storz 8590 VJ) with straightforward telescope (Karl Storz 8575A) and Lewy laryngoscope holder; (ii) Karl Storz supercam micro CCD video camera (9050B) (which has a built-in adapter for a telescope); (iii) xenon light source (Karl Storz 615); (iv) large, high-resolution TV monitor and recorder; and (v) colour video printer (Sony UP-5000). Some of the advantages of Kantor–Berci telescopic video microlaryngoscopy are: (i) it gives a clear sharp image, (ii) it has an excellent depth of field; (iii) no microscope is interposed between the surgeon and the patient; (iv) the image can be seen with both eyes; and (v) it provides superior documentation. The disadvantages are (i) the equipment is costly; (ii) special equipment such as angled forceps are needed; (iii) it requires a dedicated video camera; (iv) refocusing is necessary (supercam camera) when the zoom lens is used; (v) there is some image distortion; and (vi) there is no paediatric laryngoscope available.

The author tried this new technique as well as the standard microscopic technique at the same setting on a series of patients. The Kantor–Berci system provides superior visualization of the anterior larynx with an exceptional depth of field (Fig. 21.17B). It is a most effective method of documentation of microsurgery of the larynx. The standard microscopic technique has the advantage of visualizing and documenting at various magnifications allowing precise diagnosis and surgical procedure. The microscopic system provides better depth of field than generally expected.

VIDEO IMAGE TRANSFER TO SLIDE AND PRINT

Video images can be transferred to slides and prints with relative ease. When it becomes necessary to produce slides for presentation, the author photographs the laryngeal image on the monitor using daylight Ektachrome ASA 400 colour film (Fig. 21.18).[66,71] To photograph the TV images, the standard 35 mm SLR camera equipped with a 50 mm macrolens and an orange-coloured filter (Kodak CC40R or Tiffen CC40) is used. The camera is placed on the tripod. The laryngeal image on the TV is focused through the eyepiece of the camera. The photographs are taken with the shutter speed of half a second or slower (otherwise, there will be streaks across the picture). The exposure is bracketed using the f stops. The use of ASA 400 colour Ektachrome film is recommended. Another way of producing colour slides for presentation is to copy the colour video print-outs using colour slide films.

To produce a black-and-white print for publication or documentation, the same technique described above is used utilizing ASA 400 Tri-X film.[60,62,66] Photographs shown in Figures 21.12Ba, b, c, and 21.13Ba,b,c were photographed from the television screen using ASA400 Tri-X black-and-white film. It is recommended that, during photography, the room be made dark to prevent reflection on the surface of the TV screen, which may show on the finished picture. For obtaining black-and-white prints, the author has also been photographing video print-outs using ASA 400 Tri-X film (Fig. 21.19). Photographs shown in Figures 21.15B, 21.16Ba,b,c, and 21.17B were photographed from colour prints produced by Sony UP5000 video printer, using ASA400 Tri-X black-and-white film.

More recently, the author has been using the Sony UP-5000 colour video printer (Fig. 21.20A).[35,66] This unit, although expensive (US$7000), produces a superb colour print of the video images of high resolution. A print costs approximately US$1.25. The image can be produced in single or multiple images (4 or 9). A newer, affordable colour video printer, the Sony CVPG500 (Fig. 21.20B) (approximately US$1500), produces quite acceptable colour video printouts.[35,66]

SUMMARY AND CONCLUSION

Laryngeal documentation can be effectively accomplished either by means of still photography or videography.

Flexible fibrescopic still photography provides inferior photographic images because of graininess caused by the multiple fibres in the cable. Telescopic still photography provides superior laryngeal images of excellent depth and resolution. Microscopic still photography can be done with or without the use of a photoadapter, providing excellent magnified views of the laryngeal pathology.

Fibrescopic videolaryngoscopy is a simple, fast and effective method of laryngeal evaluation and documentation. Telescopic videolaryngoscopy, on the other hand, provides superior images of anatomical and pathological changes of the laryngeal structures. Microscopic videolaryngoscopy is the most effective method of documenting and teaching the microsurgery of the larynx. Video printouts of laryngeal images on the TV screen can be easily and instantaneously made for recording the initial pathology and the results of treatment. As a permanent record, they are valuable for patient management and teaching.

Although still photography is a valuable method of laryngeal documentation today, videography is increasingly gaining favour. Because of its simplicity, reproducibility, time/cost effectiveness and capacity to produce instantaneous high-quality hard copies while recording laryngeal images and voice, videography may some day replace still photography of the larynx.

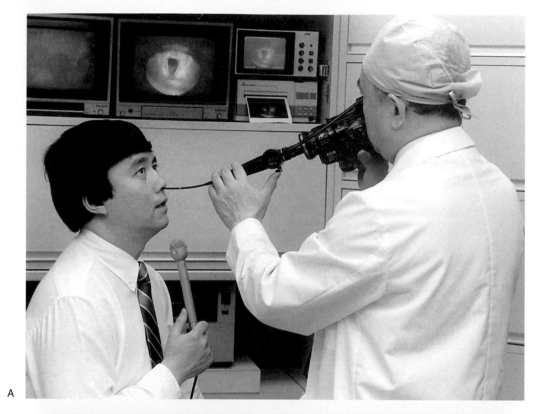

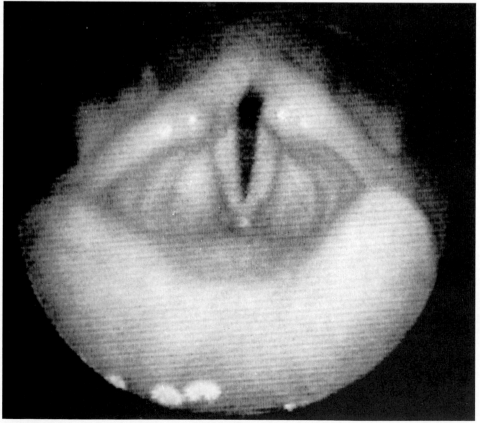

Fig. 21.12 A. (*top*) Method of flexible fibrescopic videolaryngoscopy in the office using a home video colour camera. B. Video photographs taken with this method: (a) (*bottom*) normal larynx upon respiration; (b) (*opposite page, top*) laryngocele; and (c) (*opposite page, bottom*) sessile laryngeal polyp.

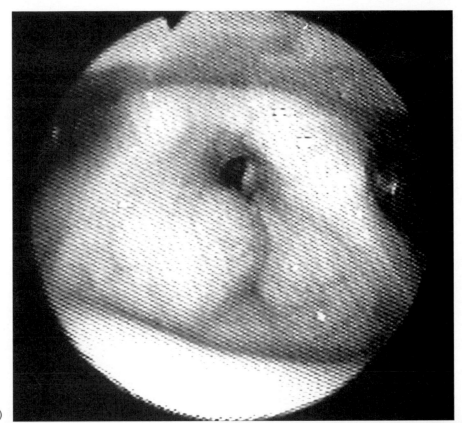

B(b)

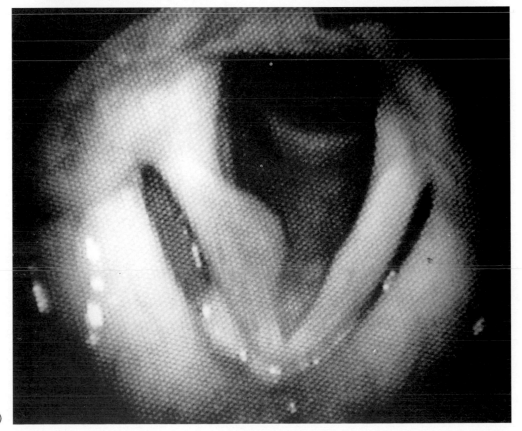

B(c)

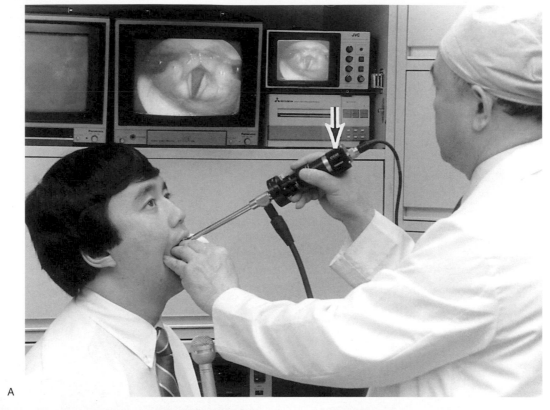

A

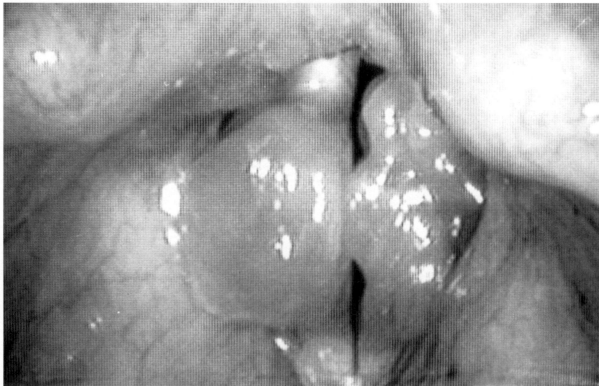

B(a)

Fig. 21.13   A. (*top*) Method for telescopic videolaryngoscopy in the office using the miniature CCD video camera (Elmo EC202) (arrow) and Nagashima SFT-1 telescope. B. Photographs taken with this method: (a) (*bottom*) bilateral laryngeal polyps; (b) (*opposite page, top*) bilateral extensive Reinke's oedema; (c) (*opposite page, bottom*) laryngeal papillomas.

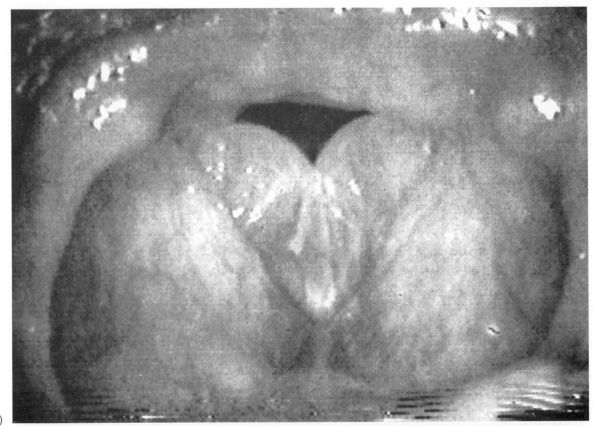

B(b)

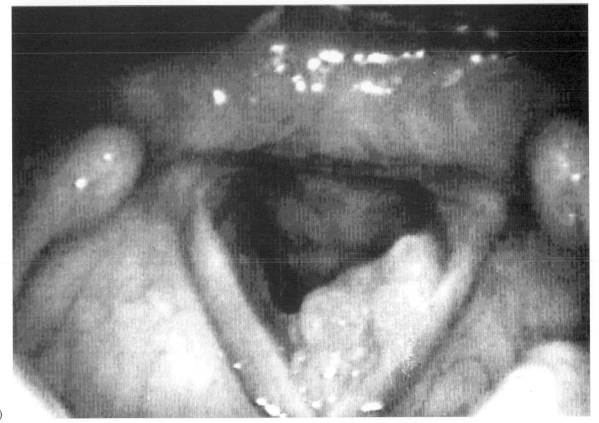

B(c)

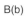

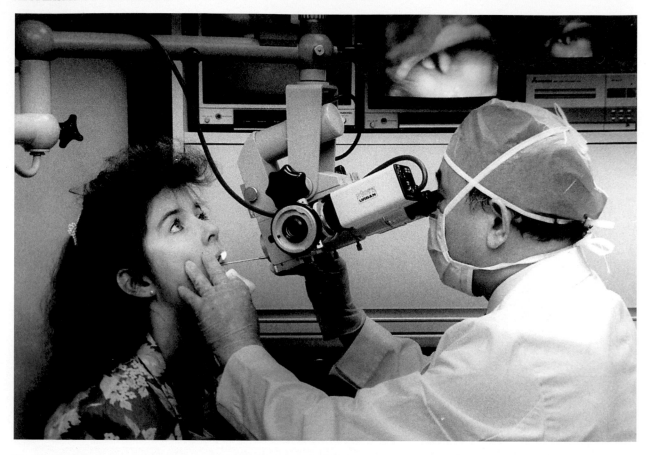

Fig. 21.14 Microscopic videolaryngoscopy in the office using the Zeiss operating microscope and medium size CCD colour video camera.

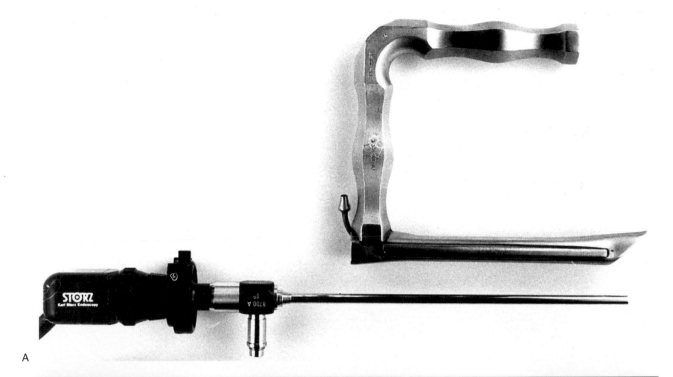

A

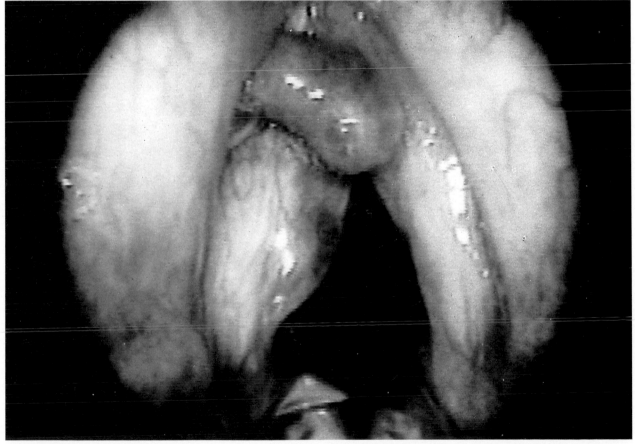

B

Fig. 21.15   Telescopic videolaryngoscopy in the operating room. A. (*top*) Dedo laryngoscope (*top*) and the Karl Storz supercam CCD miniature camera attached to the 8700A 0° telescope. B. (*bottom*) Photograph taken with this method showing multiple laryngeal polyps.

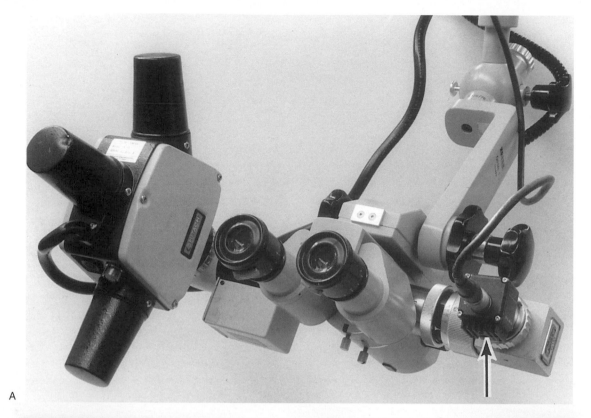

A

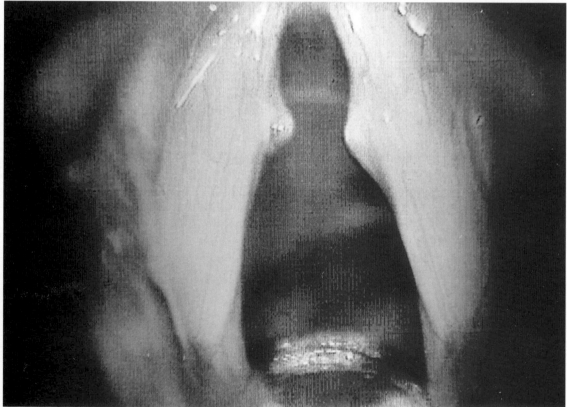

B(a)

Fig. 21.16 A. (*top*) Technique for microscopic videography with Hitachi three-tube camera on the left side of a beam-splitter and Elmo 202 mini-CCD camera attached to the Zeiss photo adapter on the right (*arrow*). B. Photographs taken with this technique: (a) (*bottom*) laryngeal nodules; (b) (*opposite page, top*) multiple obstructive laryngeal polyps; (c) (*opposite page, bottom*) extensive laryngeal carcinoma.

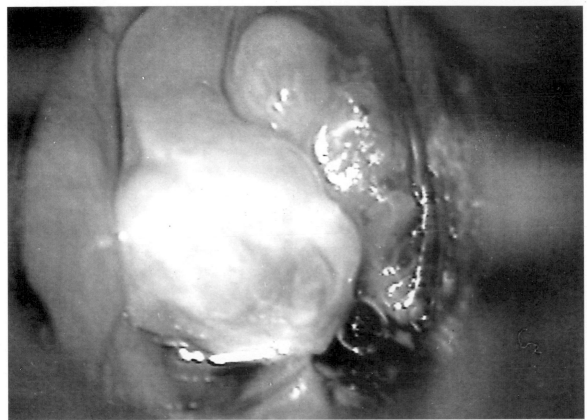

B(b)

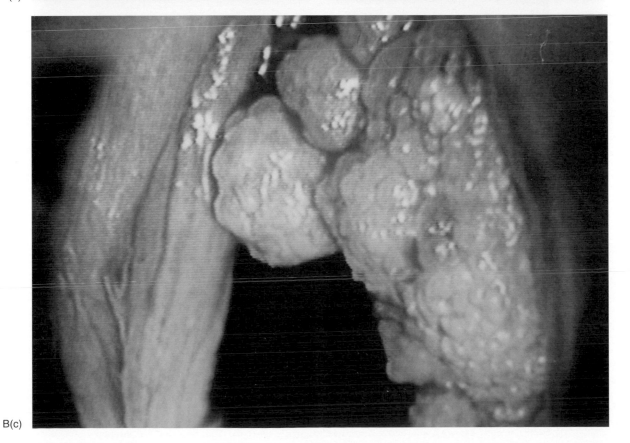

B(c)

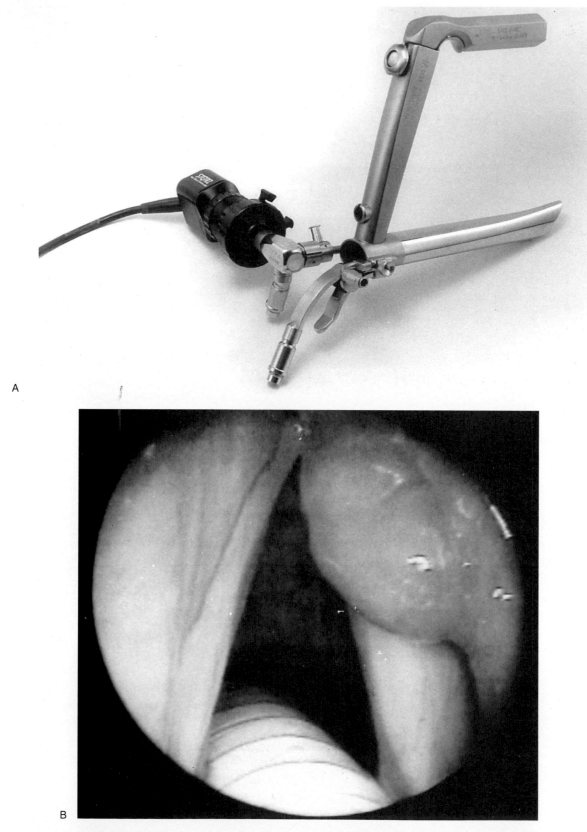

Fig. 21.17   A. (*top*) Kantor–Berci's video microlaryngoscopic technique. Karl Storz supercam CCD miniature camera is attached to the specially designed telescope (Karl Storz 8575A) inserted into the left side of the Kantor–Berci video microlaryngoscope (Karl Storz 8590BJ). B. (*bottom*) Photograph taken with this technique showing false cord polyp.

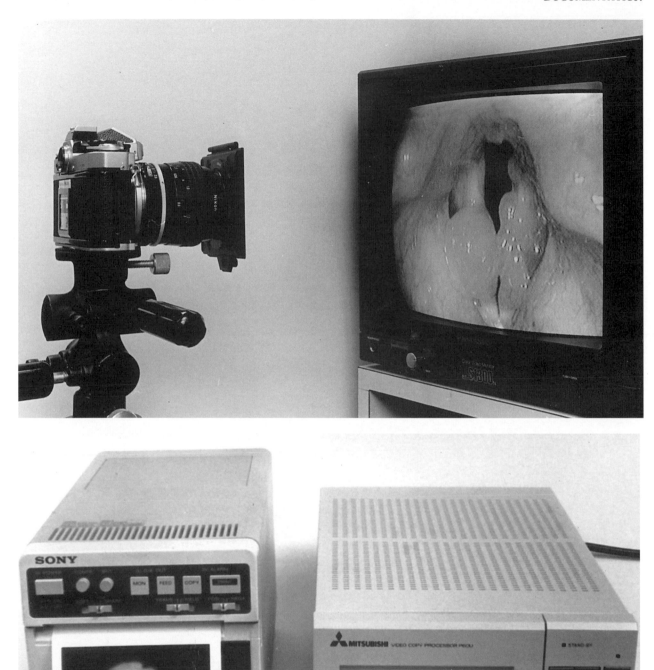

Fig. 21.18 (*top*) Technique for photographing the video images on the TV monitor showing the Nikon 35 mm SLR camera mounted on the tripod. A special filter (Kodak CC40R or Tiffen CC40R) is used.

Fig. 21.19 (*bottom*) Black and white video printers: (*left*) Sony UP811 video printer; (*right*) Mitsubishi P60U video printer.

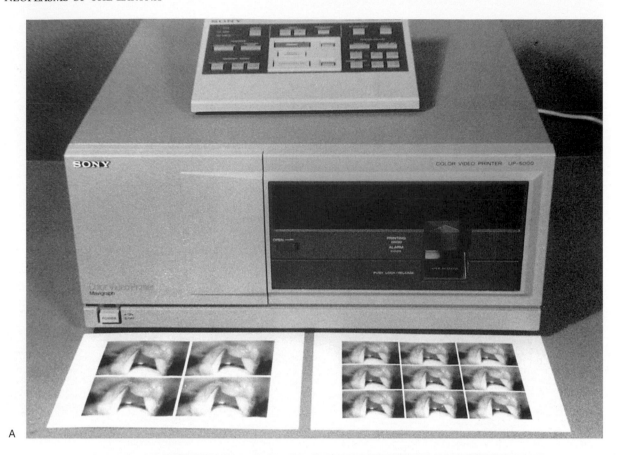

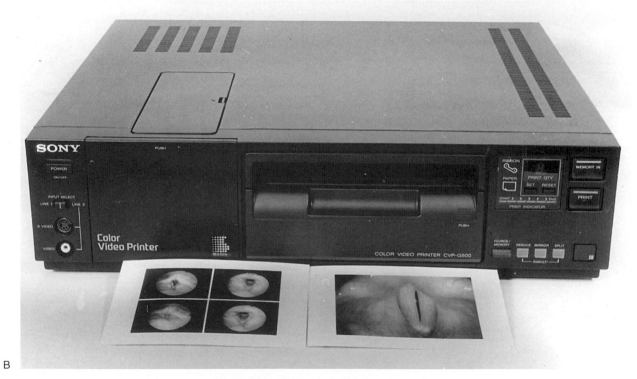

Fig. 21.20 Colour video printers. A. (*top*) Sony UP 5000 colour video printer. B. (*bottom*) Sony CVP G500 colour video printer.

REFERENCES

1. Alberti P W 1975 Still photography of the larynx — an overview. Can J Otolaryngol 4: 759–765
2. Albrecht R 1956 Zur Photographie des Kehlkopfes. HNO 5: 196–199
3. Andrews A H 1962 Laryngeal telescope. Trans Am Acad Ophthalmol Otolaryngol 66: 268
4. Benjamin B 1984 Technique of laryngeal photography. Ann Otol Rhinol Laryngol; 93(suppl 109)
5. Benjamin B 1990 Diagnostic laryngology — adults and children. Saunders, Philadelphia
6. Berci G 1976 Endoscopy. Appleton-Century-Crofts, New York
7. Berci G, Caldwell F H 1963 A device to facilitate photography during indirect laryngoscopy. Med Biol Illus 13: 169–176.
8. Berci G, Calcaterra T, Ward P H 1975 Advances in endoscopic techniques for examination of the larynx and nasopharynx. Can J Otolaryngol 4: 786–792
9. Brewer D W, McCall G 1974 Visible laryngeal changes during voice study. Ann Otol Rhinol Laryngol 83: 423–427
10. Clement P A R 1985 Endoscopy in otolaryngology. In: Clement PAR (ed) Recent advances in ENT-endoscopy. Scientific Society for Medical Information, Brussels pp 11–14
11. Czermak J 1858 Uber den Kehlkopfspiegel. Wien Med Wschr 8: 196–198
12. Davidson T M, Bone R C, Nahum A M 1974 Flexible fiberoptic laryngobronchoscopy. Laryngoscope 84: 1876–1882
13. Ferguson G B, Crowder W J 1970 A simple method of laryngeal and other cavity photography. Arch Otolaryngol 92: 201–203
14. French T R 1882 On photographing the larynx. Trans Am Laryngol 4: 32–35
15. French T R 1884 On a perfected method of photographing the larynx. N Y Med J 4: 655–656
16. Garcia M 1855 Observations on the human voice. Proc R Soc Lond 7: 399–420
17. Gould W J 1973 The Gould laryngoscope. Trans Am Acad Ophthalmol Otolaryngol 77: 139–141
18. Hahn C, Kitzing P 1978 Indirect endoscopic photography of the larynx — a comparison between two newly constructed laryngoscopes. J Audiov Media Med 1: 121–130
19. Hirano M 1981 Clinical examination of voice. Springer, Wien
20. Hirano M, Yoshida Y, Matsushima H, Nakajima T 1974 An apparatus for ultra-high-speed cinematography of the vocal cords. Ann Otol Rhinol Laryngol: 83 1–7
21. Hirose H, Kiritani S, Imagawa H 1988 High-speed digital image analysis of laryngeal behavior in running speech. In: Fujimura O (ed) Vocal fold physiology, Vol 2. Raven Press, New York, pp 335–345
22. Holinger P H 1942 Photography of the larynx, trachea, bronchi and esophagus. Trans Am Acad Ophthalmol Otolaryngol 46: 153–156
23. Holinger P H, Tardy M E 1986 Photography in otorhinolaryngology and bronchoesophagology. In: English G M (ed) Otolaryngology, Vol 5. Lippincott, Philadelphia, Chapter 22
24. Holinger P H, Brubaker J D, Brubaker J E 1975 Open tube, proximal illumination mirror and direct laryngeal photography. Can J Otolaryngol 4: 781–785
25. Inoue T 1983 Examination of child larynx by flexible fiberoptic laryngoscope. Int J Pediatr Otorhinolaryngol 5: 317–323
26. Jako G J 1970 Laryngoscope for microscopic observation, surgery and photography. Arch Otolaryngol 91: 196–199
27. Jako G J, Strong S 1972 Laryngeal photography. Arch Otolaryngol 96: 268–271
28. Kantor E, Berci G, Partlow E, Paz-Partlow M 1991 A completely new approach to microlaryngeal surgery. Laryngoscope 101: 678–679
29. Karmody C 1988 The history of laryngology. In: Fried M P (ed) The larynx — a multidisciplinary approach. Little Brown, Boston, pp 3–13
30. Kleinsasser O 1963 Entwicklung und Methoden der Kehlkopffotografie. (Mit Beschreibung eines neuen einfachen Fotolaryngoskopes). HNO 11: 171–176
31. Kleinsasser O 1968 Microlaryngoscopy and endolaryngeal microsurgery. Saunders, Philadelphia
32. Kleinsasser O 1988 Tumors of the larynx and hypopharynx. Thieme, New York, pp 124–130
33. Konrad H R et al 1981 Use of video tape in diagnosis and treatment of cancer of larynx. Ann Otol Rhinol Laryngol 90: 398–400
34. Mackenzie M 1871 The use of the laryngoscope. Hardwicke, London
35. Mambrino L, Yanagisawa E, Yanagisawa K, Gallo O 1991 Endoscopic ENT photography: a comparison of pictures by standard color films and newer color video printers. Laryngoscope 101: 1229–1232
36. Muller-Hermann F, Pedersen P 1984 Modern endoscopic and microscopic photography in otolaryngology. Ann Otol Rhinol Laryngol 93: 399
37. Oeken F W, Brandt R H 1967 Lupenkontrolle endolaryngealer Operationen. Modifikation der Schwenklupenhalterung nach Brunings. HNO 15: 210–211
38. Olofsson J, Ohlsson T 1975 Techniques in microlaryngoscopic photography. Can J Otolaryngol 4: 770–780
39. Padovan I F, Christman N T, Hamilton L H, Darling R J 1973 Indirect microlaryngoscopy. Laryngoscope 83: 2035–2041
40. Rosnagle R, Smith H W 1972 Hand-held fundus camera for endoscopic photography. Trans Am Acad Ophthalmol Otolaryngol 76: 1024–1025
41. Sawashima M, Hirose H 1968 New laryngoscopic technique by use of fiber optics. J Acoust Soc Am 43: 168–169
42. Scalo A N, Shipman W F, Tabb H G 1960 Microscopic suspension laryngoscopy. Ann Otol Rhinol Laryngol 69: 1134–1138
43. Selkin S G 1983 'How I do it: head and neck and plastic surgery.' A targeted problem and its solution. Flexible fiberoptics for laryngeal photography. Laryngoscope 93: 657–658
44. Selkin S G 1983 The otolaryngologist and flexible fiberoptics: photographic considerations. J Otolaryngol 12: 223–227
45. Silberman H D, Wilf H, Tucker J A 1976 Flexible fiberoptic nasopharyngolaryngoscope. Ann Otol Rhinol Laryngol 85: 640–645
46. Steiner W, Jaumann M P 1978 Moderne otorhinolaryngologische Endoskopie beim Kind. Padiat Prax 20: 429–435
47. Stevenson R S, Guthrie D A 1949 A history of oto-laryngology. ES Livingstone, Edinburgh, p 98
48. Strong M S 1975 Laryngeal photography. Can J Otolaryngol 4: 766–769
49. Stuckrad Hv, Lakatos I 1975 Uber ein neues Lupenlaryngoskop (Epipharyngoskop). Laryngol Rhinol Otol 54: 336–340
50. Tachiki Y 1956 Laryngeal examination. Kanehara Shuppan, Tokyo
51. Tardy M E, Tenta L T 1970 Laryngeal photography and television. Otolaryngol Clin North Am 3: 483–492
52. von Leden H 1960 Laryngeal physiology. Cinematographic observations. J Laryngol Otol 74: 705–712
53. Ward P H, Berci G, Calcaterra T C 1974 Advances in endoscopic examination of the respiratory system. Ann Otol Rhinol Laryngol 83: 754–760
54. Willemot J 1985 The birth of otolaryngologic endoscopy. In: Clement PAR (ed) Recent advances in ENT-endoscopy. Scientific Society for Medical Information, Brussels; pp 25–31
55. Yamashita K 1983 Endonasal flexible fiberoptic endoscopy. Rhinology 21: 233–237
56. Yamashita K 1988 Diagnostic and therapeutic ENT endoscopy. Medical View, Tokyo
57. Yamashita K, Mertens J, Rudert H 1984 Die flexible Fiberendoskopie in der HNO-Heilkunde. HNO 32: 378–384
58. Yamashita K, Oku T, Tanaka H, Sato K 1977 VTR endoscopy. J Otolaryngol Jpn 80: 1208–1209
59. Yanagisawa E 1982 Office telescopic photography of the larynx. Ann Otol Rhinol Laryngol 91: 354–358
60. Yanagisawa E 1984 Videolaryngoscopy using a low cost home video system color camera. J Biolog Photogr 52: 9–14
61. Yanagisawa E. Videolaryngoscopy 1986 In: Lee K J, Stewart C H (eds) Ambulatory surgery and office procedures in head and neck surgery. Grune & Stratton, Orlando; Chapter 6

62. Yanagisawa E, Carlson R D 1985 Videophotolaryngography using a new low cost video printer. Ann Otol Rhinol Laryngol 94: 584–587

63. Yanagisawa E, Carlson R D 1989 Physical diagnosis of the hypopharynx and the larynx with and without imaging. In: Lee K J (ed) Textbook of otolaryngology and head and neck surgery. Elsevier, New York; Chapter 37

64. Yanagisawa E, Walker R 1986 Instantaneous 'video photography' with a low-cost black-and-white video printer: its value in otolaryngology and head and neck surgery. Otolaryngol Head Neck Surg 95: 230–233

65. Yanagisawa E, Yamashita K 1986 Fiberoptic nasopharyngo-laryngoscopy. In: Lee K J, Stewart C H (eds) Ambulatory surgery and office procedures in head and neck surgery. Grune & Stratton, Orlando; pp 31–40

66. Yanagisawa E, Yanagisawa R 1991 Laryngeal photography. Otolaryngol Clin North Am 24: 999–1022

67. Yanagisawa E, Carlson R D, Strothers G 1985 Videography of the larynx — fiberscope or telescope? In: Clement PAR (ed) Recent advances in ENT-endoscopy. Scientific Society for Medical Information, Brussels, pp 175–183

68. Yanagisawa E, Casuccio J R, Suzuki M 1981 Video laryngoscopy using a rigid telescope and video home system color camera. A useful office procedure. Ann Otol Rhinol Laryngol 90: 346–350

69. Yanagisawa E, Eibling D E, Suzuki M 1980 A simple method of laryngeal photography through the operating microscope. 'Macrolens technique'. Ann Otol Rhinol Laryngol 89: 547–550

70. Yanagisawa E, Owens T W, Strothers G, Honda K 1983 Videolaryngoscopy — a comparison of fiberscopic and telescopic documentation. Ann Otol Rhinol Laryngol 92: 430–436

71. Yanagisawa K, Shi J, Yanagisawa E 1987 Color photography of video images of otolaryngological structures using a 35 mm SLR camera. Laryngoscope 97: 992–993

72. Yoshida Y, Hirano M, Nakajima T 1979 A videotape recording system for laryngostroboscopy. J Jpn Bronchoesophagol Soc 30: 1–5.

22. Diagnostic imaging*

M. S. Mendelsohn, H. S. Shulman, A. M. Noyek

INTRODUCTION

Contemporary radiological imaging provides a high level of sophistication in the analysis of laryngeal tumours. In particular, the development of computerized tomography (CT) and magnetic resonance imaging (MR) provides information unobtainable by clinical assessment. Evaluation of the role of MR in the analysis of laryngeal tumours was begun in the 1980s and still continues. We have now reached a stage where meaningful comparison of the indications and limitations of these two techniques is possible.

Imaging confirms the clinical findings and permits evaluation of areas not accessible by clinical means. It is non-invasive and displays the larynx in a resting state free from encumbrances such as endotracheal tubes. The films are a permanent record which permit comprehensive evaluation, quantification and display to the patient and to all team members involved.

The increased complexity and power of contemporary imaging techniques highlight the need for close cooperation with the laryngeal radiologist. Although in practice the laryngologist orders the test, it is the radiologist who best understands the benefits and limitations of each procedure. The radiologist can manipulate the test protocol to display the specific information requested by the laryngologist. This cooperation ensures optimal imaging in a cost-effective and time-efficient way.

THE ROLE OF IMAGING

Laryngeal imaging complements the clinical process by answering specific questions which affect management. Imaging techniques may provide information for diagnosis, staging, assessment of the airway or assessment of metastatic disease.

* Supported by the Saul A. Silverman Family Foundation and the Latner Family Trust (Dynacare), Toronto, Canada as a Canada-International Scientific Exchange Program in Otolaryngology (CISEPO II) Project.

Every patient with a laryngeal cancer needs a chest X-ray. This may be the only radiological investigation required. Many small tumours are adequately assessed clinically. Even some large tumours have a clear management course, not affected by greater analysis of tumour extent. In these cases radiological investigation is not mandatory, but it is often undertaken for teaching purposes or to verify the surgeon's assessment. These indications must be balanced against increasing costs of medical investigation.

Diagnosis

Most laryngeal tumours arise from the mucosal surface. They can usually be diagnosed at endoscopy. However, diagnosis of early recurrent disease can be a frustrating and difficult process. Recurrences after surgery or radiotherapy often present submucosally and are thereby hidden.[12] Early detection of recurrent disease is critical, and usually this diagnosis requires a strong index of suspicion and sometimes repeated 'blind' biopsies. Radiological imaging can demonstrate changes in the deeper tissues suggestive of recurrence which can serve to guide biopsy.

Unusual soft tissue tumours often arise submucosally. Laryngeal imaging can differentiate solid masses from laryngocoeles and cysts. Vascular lesions, such as haemangiomas and glomus tumours enhance with intravenous contrast. The radiological appearance of cartilaginous tumours is diagnostic, although the differentiation between chondroma and chondrosarcoma is usually not possible. The red blood cell scan can suggest the diagnosis of cavernous haemangioma, which may obviate injudicious biopsy and airway haemorrhage.[8]

Laryngocoeles may be an accompaniment of laryngeal cancers.[2] Their preoperative diagnosis and assessment hinges upon laryngeal imaging. The presence of a laryngocoele and spread of cancer within it has important management considerations, especially in relation to conservation laryngectomy.[4]

Radiological imaging provides a non-invasive means of tumour identification in the paediatric age group. Tumours, such as haemangiomas, papillomas and rhabdomyosarcomas need to be excluded in cases of hoarseness or progressive stridor. Office assessment may be very limited. However, radiological evidence of a tumour is an indication for direct laryngoscopy.

Invasion

Radiology provides a non-invasive means of mapping extension of tumour into submucosal tissues. Important areas of assessment include the pre-epiglottic space, paraglottic space, laryngeal framework and extralaryngeal tissues. These areas are difficult to assess clinically yet their involvement is an integral part of assessing T stage and consequent management.

Pre-epiglottic space invasion by a supraglottic lesion transforms it to a T3 tumour. This factor makes cure with radiotherapy less likely.[9,20] Framework invasion or extralaryngeal spread, such as tongue base invasion, transforms a lesion to T4. Radiotherapy is less likely to effect a cure in these lesions.[9] Involvement of the carotid vessels, prevertebral tissues or skull base may have important management implications.

Assessment of invasion is difficult after any previous therapy. The differentiation between fibrosis, oedema, radionecrosis and recurrent tumour may require repeated biopsy. Radiology may be used to follow changes over time or demonstrate a deep mass.

Airway assessment

Radiology plays a key role in defining the airway in patients with respiratory compromise. It may be impossible to determine clinically the pattern of airway invasion by the tumour. Exophytic tumour may obstruct the airway at any level, precluding a view beyond the upper margin. The normal anatomy may be distorted and destroyed.

Laryngeal imaging can map out the dimensions of the airway at each level and in different plans. This provides the surgeon and anaesthetist with a guide to the safety of intubation. When the patient needs a tracheostomy under local anaesthetic, imaging provides a view of cancer spread at the subglottis and trachea, guiding placement of the tracheostoma.

Metastatic disease

Much of the controversy in elective neck management relates to the difficulty in determining the true incidence of occult disease. Improved detection of small nodal masses promises significantly to affect guidelines for management of the neck. Radiological imaging can upstage the N0 neck. MR and CT are more sensitive than clinical examination in detecting nodal masses.[7,10,14] Ultrasound-guided fine-needle biopsy can provide a tissue diagnosis of small neck nodes.[19] Imaging may be particularly helpful in the patient with the short fat neck or one who has had previous neck treatment.

Subglottic spread of disease is associated with spread to the prelaryngeal (Delphian), paratracheal and pretracheal nodes. Radiological imaging can evaluate the paratracheal, pretracheal and mediastinal nodes in a non-invasive fashion.

Tumour volume

Tumour volume has been identified as a prognostic factor in radiotherapy for laryngeal tumours.[11] Radiological imaging is the only diagnostic test which can estimate tumour volume. Three-dimensional reconstruction may one day be a standard part of the imaging process.[21]

PLAIN X-RAYS

The chest film is used as a screen for lung spread and may show bony metastases. It may indicate cardiac and pulmonary disease. The chest film is always a routine part of the work-up for any patient with laryngeal cancer, and may be the only radiological investigation required.

The plain lateral soft tissue examination of the neck is a low-cost screening modality in benign disease. Its role in the evaluation of tumours is mainly in the paediatric age group. It permits a view of the air–mucosa interface. Imaging of the supraglottis shows excellent detail of the vallecula, epiglottis, aryepiglottic folds and arytenoid eminences (Fig. 22.1). Imaging of the glottis is hampered by the overlapping thyroid cartilages; in children, they have neither calcified nor ossified — providing an improved view compared to that in adults. The ventricles are seen as a well-demarcated shadow. The subglottis and trachea are also well seen.

Paediatric airway tumours are uncommon. Those most commonly detected are papilloma, subglottic haemangioma and rhabdomyosarcoma. Diagnosis of a mass will ultimately lead to endoscopy to establish a specific diagnosis.

The high kV filtered anteroposterior view complements the lateral soft tissue radiograph as a screening test in the paediatric age group. The technique can be utilized to display the glottis without the shadow of the cervical spine, which normally obscures conventional radiographs. It is cheaper, faster and uses less radiation than tomography. In older children and adults it can be combined with functional manoeuvres such as inspiration, phonation and Valsalva to improve the visibility of the air–soft tissue interface.

XERORADIOGRAPHY

This process provides greater edge enhancement than the plain lateral airways view. Any structure with a sharply defined edge is seen with particular clarity. It can be utilized when the plain lateral airways film is inadequate. It has been replaced by CT and MR scans in the evaluation of adult tumours.

Xeroradiography utilizes a normal X-ray source which impinges on a charged plate. A blue powder adheres to

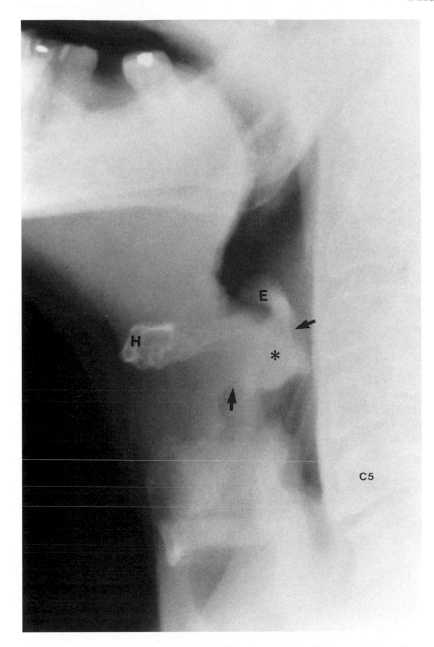

Fig. 22.1 Lateral soft tissue of the neck. When appropriate soft tissue technique is used, there is good visualization of the soft tissue structures of the neck. A supraglottic tumour of the larynx arising from the laryngeal surface of the epiglottis is well demonstrated (*). Its superior and inferior margins are fairly well delineated (arrows). E = epiglottis; H = hyoid bone; C5 = 5th cervical vertebral body. (Courtesy of A. M. Noyek, D. Fliss and H. Shulman.[18])

this plate, and this powder is then transferred to paper by contact, and sealed. Despite its improved resolution, the popularity of the technique suffers from the disadvantage of a four-fold increase in radiation dosage and the high cost of leasing arrangements.

CORONAL (AP) TOMOGRAPHY

Coronal tomography has a role in displaying the airway and in providing a functional assessment of the larynx. It provides superb displays of the airway profile from the laryngeal vestibule through to the trachea. The coronal format provides a more direct and continuous airway demonstration than do axial CT scans—which are tangential to the plane of the airway. It is the technique of choice in the patient who cannot tolerate CT or MR due to claustrophobia or an inability to lie down.

The tomogram provides best imaging of structures which lie at right-angles to the coronal plane. It displays the epiglottis, the false and true cords, the ventricle and the subglottis. The images can be modified by the use of physiological manoeuvres. Tomography during phonation can provide functional assessment of vocal cord mobility. The ventricle is best assessed during modified Valsalva and reverse phonation.

The limited grey scale and soft tissue resolution capability of tomography has been outpaced by CT scan and MR. Using tomography, a lesion must be 3–4 mm in size to be adequately assessed, even with a 0.5 cm examination technique.

CT SCAN AND MR

CT scan and MR are the current benchmarks of laryngeal imaging. They have application in assessment of tumour invasion, airway involvement, metastatic spread, estimation of tumour volume and in tumour diagnosis (Table 22.1). Whether CT or MR imaging is better for laryngeal evaluation depends upon the specific information required for each case. Understanding the benefits and limitations of each technique by close liaison with a laryngeal radiologist can maximize the diagnostic yield.

Both CT and MR provide high-resolution images of the deep laryngeal anatomy and the airway (Figs 22.2, 22.3). The paraglottic and paralaryngeal spaces are synonymous, with the former term used by surgeons, and the latter a radiological finding. This deep anatomy cannot be effectively evaluated by clinical inspection. The

Table 22.1   Clinical indications for CT scan or MR

Evaluation
  of invasion when considering conservation laryngeal surgery or radiotherapy
  of extralaryngeal spread
  of cervical, paratracheal or mediastinal nodes
  of the airway in a patient with airway symptoms
  of the submucosal mass
Calculation of tumour volume

ability to image in different planes confers a significant advantage to MR. This benefit is greatest in evaluation of laryngeal tumour invasion and in imaging of the airway.

Assessment of invasion

Paraglottic (paralaryngeal) and pre-epiglottic spaces

These regions lie deep to the laryngeal mucosal surface and therefore cannot be accurately assessed clinically. These spaces are clinically important because they serve as a highway for deep tumour spread without disturbance of the overlying laryngeal mucosa. These spaces are contiguous. Once a tumour invades them it can become transglottic (Figs 22.4, 22.5). A tumour invading the pre-epiglottic space can escape the larynx into the tongue base. A tumour invading the paraglottic space can escape through the cricothyroid membrane (Fig. 22.6). Since

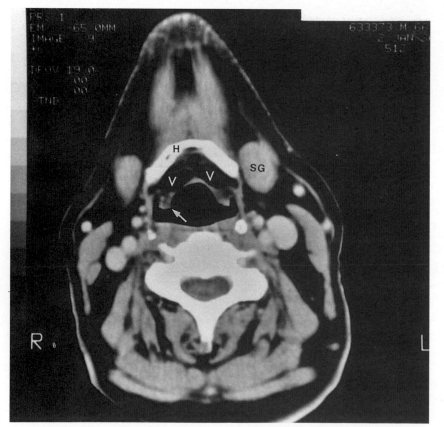

Fig. 22.2   Normal CT. A. (*left*) Just below the base of the tongue, we can identify the valleculae (V), hyoid bone (H), submandibular gland (SG) and the superior aspect of the aryepiglottic fold (arrow). B. (*opposite page, top*) 5 mm caudad to (A), fat in the pre-epiglottic space (pes) can be seen extending laterally as the paralaryngeal fat (PL) into the aryepiglottic fold. E = epiglottis. C. (*opposite page, bottom*) 5 mm caudad to (B), the level is between the hyoid and thyroid cartilages — a site for potential spread of tumour through the larynx into the neck. aef = aryepiglottic fold; ic = internal carotid artery; ihs = infrahyoid strap muscles; JV = jugular vein; PL = paralaryngeal fat. D. (*page 406*) 5 mm caudad to (C). The posterior portion of the image is at the true cord level, but the anterior aspect is slightly cephalad to the anterior commissure. A = arytenoid; Cr = cricoid; V = true cord; JV = jugular vein; SM = sternomastoid muscle E. (*page 406, bottom*) 5 mm caudad to (D). The subglottis is characterized by an oval airway which merges caudally into the round tracheal airway. T = thyroid gland; Tr = tracheal airway (Courtesy of A. M. Noyek, D. Fliss and H. Shulman.[18])

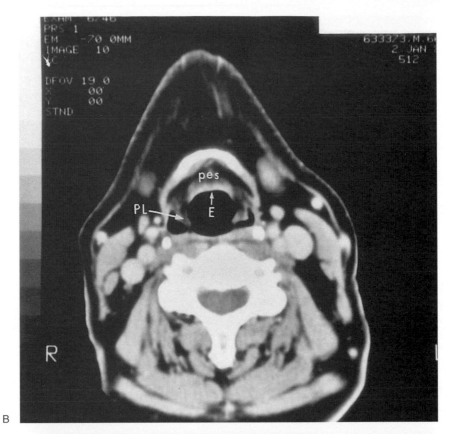

B

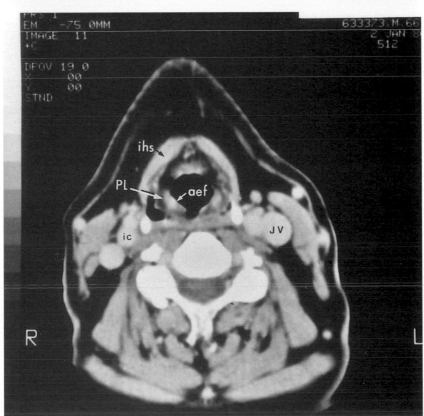

C

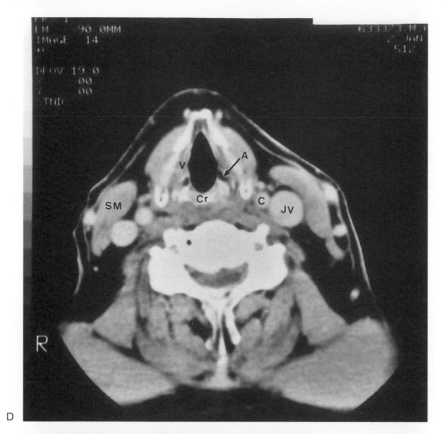

D

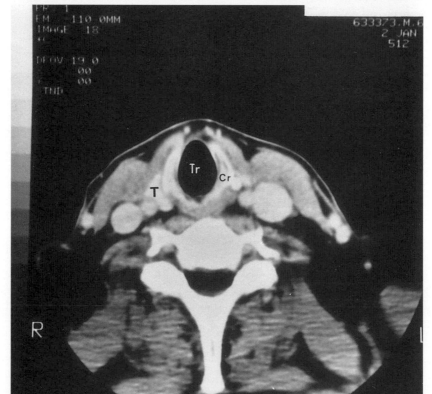

E

deep invasion can occur without disturbing the overlying laryngeal mucosa, diagnosis requires a high level of clinical suspicion. The diagnosis is made by directed deep biopsy or radiological imaging study.

The paraglottic and pre-epiglottic spaces are well displayed in both CT and MR as areas of fat density (Figs 22.2, 22.3). The paraglottic space lies medial to the perichondrium of the thyroid cartilage and lateral to the quadrangular membrane, ventricle and conus elasticus. Posteriorly is the piriform fossa, and the pre-epiglottic space lies above. The pre-epiglottic space is a horseshoe-shaped area lying anterior to the epiglottis and posterior to the thyroid cartilage perichondrium and thyrohyoid membrane. The vallecula lies above, and the petiole of the epiglottis is below (Fig. 22.3). The hyoepiglottic ligament is a longitudinal thickening above, and should not be confused with invading tumour.

The paired paraglottic spaces communicate with the pre-epiglottic space above. This communication may allow for the spread of invading tumour. Cancer invasion into the deeper spaces is well seen by both CT and MR (Figs 22.4, 22.5, 22.7). Well-defined tumour margins suggest a pushing edge, whereas poorly defined margins suggest infiltration. Once the cancer has invaded the paraglottic or pre-epiglottic spaces it can become transglottic, invade the thyroid cartilage, or escape the larynx (Figs 22.7, 22.8).

The ventricle is the key landmark used to define the suitability of conservation laryngeal surgery. It represents an embryological dividing line that serves to localize the spread of disease to either the supraglottis above, or the glottis below. Transglottic tumours, that is, those which cross the ventricle, are not suitable for supraglottic or vertical hemilaryngectomy.

Invasion into the pre-epiglottic and paraglottic space can be determined with either CT or MR. However, the coronal MR view will permit more accurate determination of the level of deep invasion with respect to the ventricle. The ventricle can be identified as a longitudinal furrow between the false and true cords (Fig. 22.4). Laterally, the fat of the paraglottic space lies above the thyroarytenoid muscle. The extent of paraglottic invasion cannot be clinically assessed.

CT scanning is restricted to the axial plane. Coronal reconstructions provide limited resolution of fine detail. Using the CT scan, a normal cut through the ventricle does suggest that the tumour has not crossed the ventricle. However, it is not always possible to align the plane of the image with the plane of the ventricle. This generates a slightly slanted image, so that the ventricle may be seen in more than one cut. Due to the small size of the ventricle, and computer averaging techniques, the ventricle may not be seen at all. In the axial projection, the ventricular level is estimated by the distance above the vocal cord and a change in density from fat to the thyroarytenoid muscle.

Glottis

Glottic lesions often present early. Hypertrophic surface lesions of the mucosa may represent dysplasia, carcinoma in situ or microinvasive cancer. These tumours require excision biopsy and do not need laryngeal imaging.

Imaging may be useful in the assessment of any invasive glottic lesion. Direct invasion into the thyroarytenoid muscle may cause impaired vocal mobility. Once the tumour has invaded the paraglottic space it can pass superiorly to become transglottic or inferiorly to escape the larynx through the cricothyroid membrane (Fig. 22.6). This infiltration may not be clinically seen, but it is well displayed by imaging. It may be critical when deciding on the possibility of vertical hemilaryngectomy, as discussed in the section on paraglottic space.

The anterior commissure is an important area for assessment. There should be minimal thickness between the mucosa and the thyroid cartilage as the mucosa and Broyle's ligament are applied directly upon the internal thyroid perichondrium at this point (Fig. 22.9). Anterior commissure tumour may follow Broyle's ligament into the thyroid cartilage.

Vocal cord fixation denotes a T3 lesion (Fig. 22.10). Imaging can help identify the cause of fixation: thyroarytenoid muscle invasion, cricoarytenoid joint invasion, invasion in the region of the recurrent laryngeal nerve or a bulky tumour. There is often more than one reason for a fixed cord.[14,15]

Supraglottis

CT and MR play a valuable role in the assessment of invasion by supraglottic cancers. The extent and patterns of deep tumour invasion are critical when considering conservation surgery or radiotherapy (Figs 22.10–22.12).

Deep invasion by tumours of the false cords and ventricles occurs into the paraglottic space. Anterior lesions pass through the epiglottis into the pre-epiglottic space. Invasive supraglottic cancers can quickly become transglottic by inferior spread within the paraglottic space without disturbing the mucosa of the ventricle (Fig. 22.4). They may invade the thyroid cartilage, or escape the larynx into the tongue base.

Anterior lesions can pass through foramina in the epiglottic cartilage directly into the pre-epiglottic space. The epiglottis rarely mineralizes, so that differentiation between cartilage and tumour invasion is more readily seen with MR utilizing multiple pulse sequences than with CT. From the pre-epiglottic space, tumours can readily advance into the tongue base without ulceration of the vallecular mucosa. This diagnosis requires a high level of clinical suspicion. Although both CT and MR can display the pre-epiglottic space, tongue base invasion is best imaged with MR. Invasion into these regions reduces radiocurability.[9] Mucosal extensions of supraglottic lesions

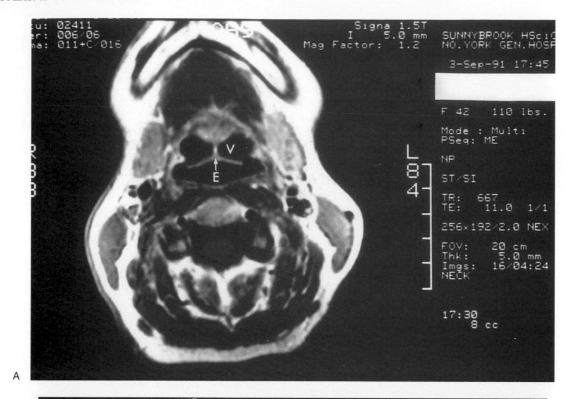

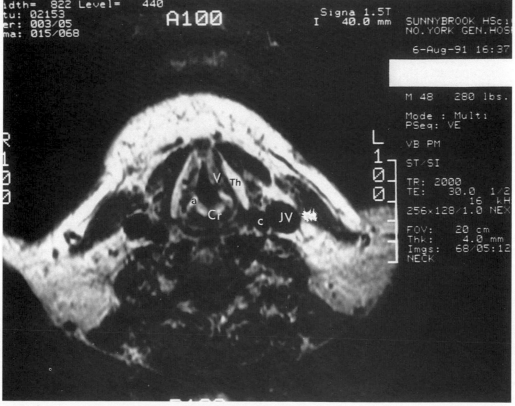

Fig. 22.3 Normal MR. A. (*top*) T1-weighted image obtained below the base of the tongue. The paired valleculae (V) are separated by the median glossoepiglottic fold and are just anterior to the epiglottis (E). B. (*bottom*) First sequence T2-weighted image (the fat is still bright) at the true cord level. a = arytenoid; c = common carotid artery; Cr = cricoid cartilage; JV = jugular vein; Th = medulla of thyroid cartilage; v = vocal cord. C. (*opposite page, top*) T1-weighted image of subglottis. Cr = fat in marrow of cricoid medulla. Arrow = cricothyroid joint. D. (*opposite page, bottom*) T-1 weighted image of the upper trachea. The airway is now round, except for the posterior indentation by the oesophagus (E). C = common carotid artery; J = internal jugular vein; Th = thyroid gland. E. (*page 410, top*) Sagittal T-1 weighted image near the midline. C = cricoid (marrow fat); P = pre-epiglottic space; short arrow = free margin of epiglottis; long arrow = petiole. (Courtesy of A. M. Noyek, D. Fliss and H. Shulman.[18])

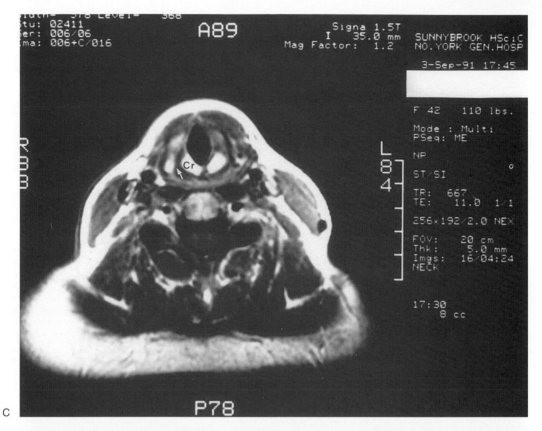

C

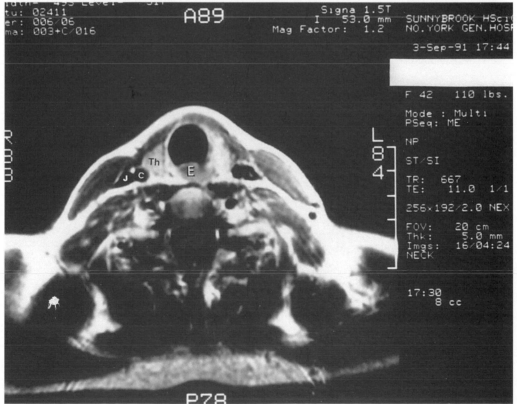

D

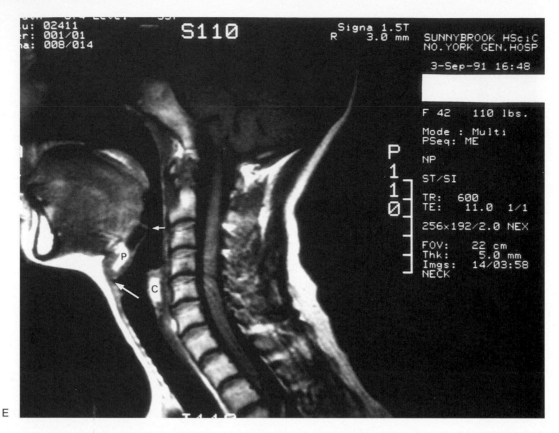

into the ventricle, piriform fossa (Fig. 22.13) or post-cricoid area are well seen at endoscopy.

Subglottis

Subglottic spread along the mucosa can be well assessed at endoscopy. However, submucosal spread in the para-glottic space deep to the conus elasticus can be clinically unsuspected. Either CT or MR can image the subglottis effectively. Any soft tissue thickness at the level of the cricoid ring is abnormal (Fig. 22.14).

The level of subglottic spread is critical when planning conservation surgery. Most authors state that subglottic extension more than 1 cm anteriorly or 5 mm posteriorly contraindicates vertical hemilaryngectomy.[13] These measures are approximate, allowing for the sloping anatomy of the average cricoid ring. Beyond these limits, the tumour is likely to escape through the cricothyroid membrane, and may invade the thyroid and cricoid cartilages.[12] Radio-logical imaging provides a direct correlation of the extent of tumour spread with the level of the cricoid cartilage. The MR has a significant advantage over CT in the ability to compare directly the level of deep subglottic spread in relation to the cricoid cartilage in the coronal and sagittal planes. The cricoid cartilage is well seen on the CT scan, but extrapolation of tumour level is somewhat indirect due to the sloping superior surface of the cricoid cartilage and computer averaging.

Cartilage invasion

Invasion of the laryngeal cartilaginous framework trans-forms laryngeal tumours to a T4 stage. This militates against either conservation therapy or primary radio-therapy. Imaging of framework destruction is most reliable in patients with ossified laryngeal cartilages. Ossification of the thyroid cartilage starts from posteroinferiorly, is frequently patchy and asymmetric. Evaluation of invasion of ossified cartilage is reliable with either MR or CT (Figs 22.6, 22.8, 22.9).

Invasion of non-mineralized cartilage is more difficult. Cartilage and tumour have a similar density on CT scanning, making CT scan determination of invasion un-reliable. Using multiple pulse sequences, MR has been reported to provide greater discrimination between tumour and cartilage.[3]

In either method, the most reliable sign of framework invasion is demonstration of tumour external to the outer surface of the thyroid cartilage.[6] In this situation, MR may overstate the extent of tumour spread due to enhance-ment of oedema.

Piriform fossa

Piriform fossa tumours generally present late. Either CT or MR can detect the extent of local invasion into the paraglottic space, the prevertebral fascia or the carotid

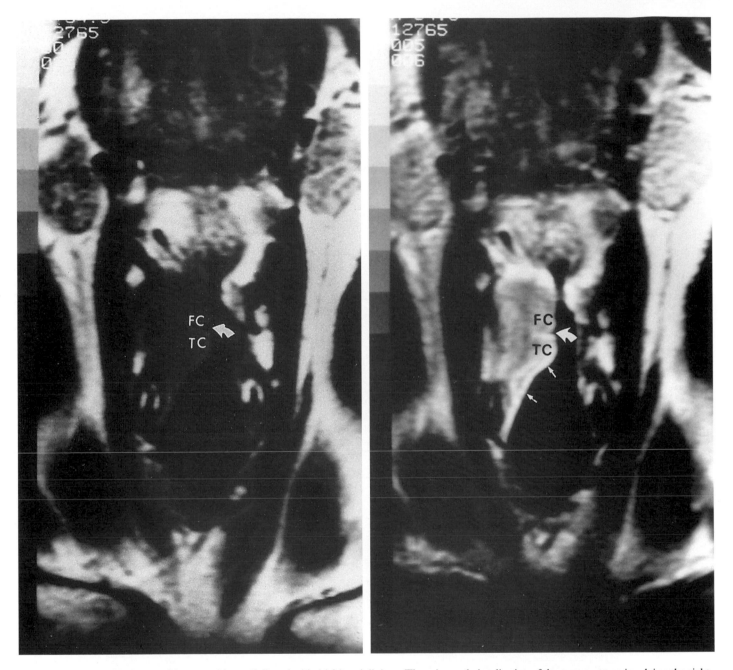

Fig. 22.4 T1-weighted coronal images without (*left*) and with (*right*) gadolinium. There is good visualization of the tumour mass involving the right false cord (FC), right true cord (TC) and subglottis. The abnormal tissue is enhanced with gadolinium, particularly the subglottic mucosa (short arrows). Curved arrow = ventricle. (Courtesy of A. M. Noyek, D. Fliss and H. Shulman.[18])

sheath (Fig. 22.15). The extent of mucosal spread has a large bearing on extent of resection and type of reconstruction. Involvement of the piriform apex, mucosal extension around the pharynx, into the oesophagus or into the supraglottis or postcricoid region is best assessed at endoscopy. Imaging may suggest areas of submucosal spread. Submucosal tongue base extension of piriform fossa tumours can be clinically deceptive. It denotes a T4 lesion, and alters the surgical approach. Tongue base invasion is best evaluated with MR.[14]

Diagnosis

CT and MR play a role in the diagnosis of submucosal tumours. A bulge in the laryngeal wall may be related to a cyst, laryngocoele or non-squamous tumour. The CT and MR can both determine the location and consistency of the lesion. The coronal views of the MR can give improved localization of the lesion relative to the ventricle when this is relevant. CT with contrast may demonstrate vascular enhancement in lesions such as haemangioma and glomus tumours. CT demonstrates chondroma and chondro-

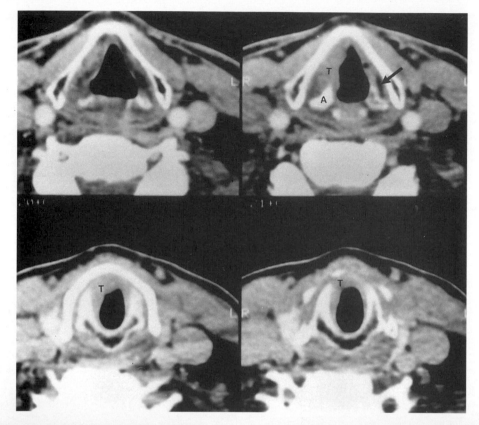

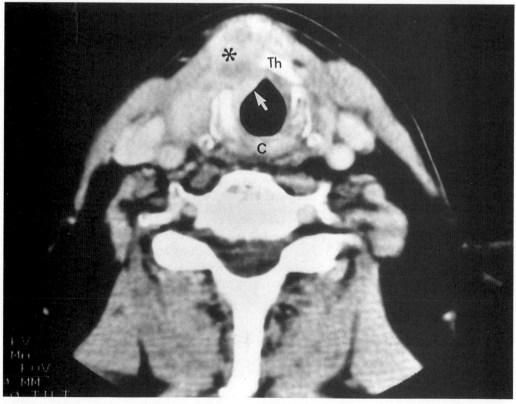

sarcoma more readily than MR due to the superior display of calcification. Ultimate diagnosis and evaluation of differentiation depends upon biopsy.

The diagnosis of recurrent disease continues to tax the surgeon. Recurrences after radiotherapy are frequently submucosal, and can be confused with oedema, fibrosis and radionecrosis. These conditions may coexist. Acute post-radiotherapy oedema usually reaches its maximum at 2–5 weeks after therapy, and should slowly subside. On the other hand, recurrent tumour shows progressive enlargement. Focal oedema is more suspicious than generalized laryngeal oedema. A suspicious lesion requires biopsy, which may be guided by the presence of a mass seen on CT or MR. Biopsy may be unreliable due to a heavy fibrous or inflammatory component, and the frequent presence of tumour nests instead of a discrete solid mass. Rideout[16] has listed six signs which suggest a recurrence: (i) an increasing localized soft tissue mass on serial examination; (ii) progressive loss of the subglottic angle; (iii) erosion or ulceration of mucosal structures that were previously known to be intact; (iv) alteration of vocal cord mobility; (v) change in cartilage structure or composition; (vi) persistent mass 3 to 4 months after treatment. To this list, we would add a seventh: increased vascularity. Our experience has demonstrated that lesions which demonstrate increased vascularity after IV contrast on CT scanning are highly suspicious for tumour. This vascularity is a useful target to guide biopsy.

Radionecrosis is related to entry of infection through the disrupted mucosa, combined with localized vascular impairment. It most commonly affects the epiglottis or arytenoid cartilages, but any cartilage may be involved. The thyroid and cricoid cartilages may disintegrate, collapse inward or even fracture. There is an inflammatory soft tissue reaction, and there may be functional impairment of vocal cord mobility and even airway collapse. Imaging can monitor these changes but is not tissue specific.

Airway

Tumour growth can prevent safe clinical visualization of the airway. In this situation, the surgeon and the anaesthetist need to know the shape and calibre of the airway, and the extent of subglottic or tracheal spread. This information serves as a guide to whether the patient can be intubated and the safe level for a tracheostomy.

The decision as to the safety of the radiological examination in a patient with airway distress is paramount.

This requires close liaison between the surgical and radiological teams. The patient who has significant airway distress, or who cannot tolerate lying down, is not a candidate for preoperative imaging with CT or MR. Some patients become claustrophobic during imaging, especially in the MR machine, which can precipitate an emergency.

Both CT and MR are excellent techniques to demonstrate the airway. Provided the patient can cooperate, MR can provide the best airway assessment due to the multiplanar imaging capabilities. The coronal and sagittal MR images provide a more direct and continuous display of the laryngotracheal airway than does the axial CT views (Figs 22.3–22.5). However, in the patient with even mild respiratory distress who cannot lie still, or who keeps swallowing secretions, the MR images will be unsatisfactory. In these patients CT will be more reliable and faster.

Clinical impression and experience are critical factors in the assessment of the obstructed airway. Some obstructive supraglottic tumours arise from a small base. The patient can be easily intubated allowing the polypoid tumour to be debulked by laser. Some obstructive tumours are rock solid, creating a corkscrew airway which will defy intubation. Imaging techniques cannot determine the compressibility, mobility or pedicle size of laryngeal tumours.

Regional spread

CT and MR play a role in evaluating the extent of large nodal masses and the presence of occult disease (Fig. 22.12). These techniques offer particular benefit in patients who are difficult to examine. This includes patients with a short fat neck, or patients whose neck tissues were woody following previous treatment.

Imaging may reveal that a large nodal mass involves the carotid artery or extends up to the base of the skull. These are ominous signs. The surgeon may need to consider a larger resection, the need for vascular assessment or an alternative treatment plan.

Radiological imaging may suggest the presence of occult nodal disease, thus upstaging the neck. Radiological investigation has a higher clinical accuracy than physical examination alone.[7] CT can reliably detect occult nodes greater than 6 mm in diameter.[14] CT is probably superior to MR for evaluation of the neck because of an increased ability to demonstrate metastatic foci in small nodes and to detect early extracapsular spread.[14] MR can more readily differentiate between nodes and tortuous blood

Fig. 22.5 (*opposite page, top*) Carcinoma of the larynx, extending from the right false cord into the subglottis. There is irregular thickening of the right true cord with an indistinct paralaryngeal fat stripe (compare with normal on left). The increased density of the arytenoid may be a reaction to the adjacent tumour. In the subglottis, tumour is seen mainly on the right side, but it does cross the midline. A = arytenoid; arrow = paralaryngeal fat; T = tumour. (Courtesy of A. M. Noyek, D. Fliss and H. Shulman.[18])

Fig. 22.6 (*opposite page, bottom*) Subglottic extension of tumour. Laryngeal tumour in this patient has extended into the subglottis (arrow). The inferior aspect of the right thyroid ala has been destroyed by tumour which has extended into the neck and is characterized by mixed areas of high and low density. Th = thyroid cartilage; C = cricoid; * = tumour. (Courtesy of A. M. Noyek, D. Fliss and H. Shulman.[18])

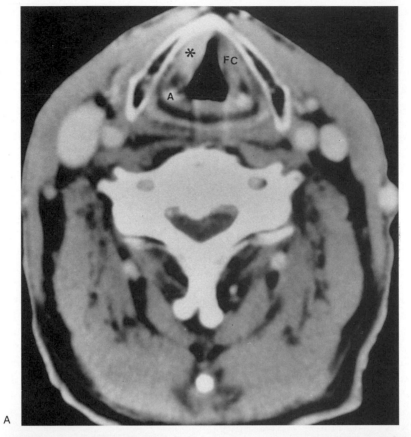

A

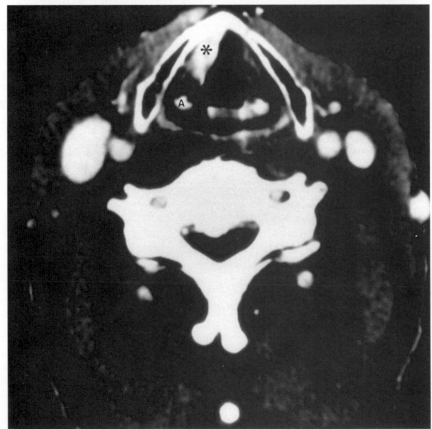

B

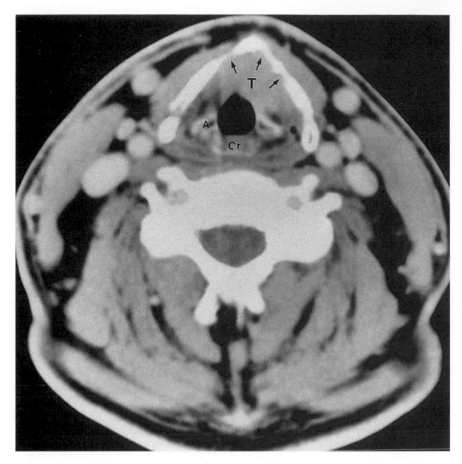

Fig. 22.7 A. (*opposite page, top*) Carcinoma of the right false cord. There is little change in size or contour of the right false cord but the tumour (⋆) is associated with sufficiently increased vascularity to result in 'enhancement' of the soft tissue. FC = left false cord; A = arytenoid cartilage. B. (*opposite page, bottom*) The same image, viewed at a narrower setting, exaggerates the difference in density between the tumour and the surrounding soft tissue. A = arytenoid cartilage. (Courtesy of A. M. Noyek, D. Fliss and H. Shulman.[18])

Fig. 22.8 (*above*) Carcinoma of the larynx involving the anterior one-third of the left true cord and extending across the anterior commissure to involve the right true cord. Thyroid cartilage involvement is seen as irregular scalloping (arrows) along the posterior margin of the cartilage adjacent to the tumour. A = arytenoid; Cr = cricoid; T = tumour. (Courtesy of A. M. Noyek, D. Fliss and H. Shulman.[18])

vessels, which usually have a signal void.[17] However, radiological investigation does not always accurately correlate with the final pathology specimen. CT and MR may undercall, or less commonly overcall, the number of involved nodes.[7]

Occult disease is most common with piriform fossa (35%), supraglottic (20%) and subglottic lesions.[5] All laryngeal lesions can spread to the jugular chain, whereas anterior commissure and subglottic lesions may involve the prelaryngeal (Delphian), pretracheal and paratracheal nodes. Patients with a significant subglottic or tracheal component should undergo imaging of the thoracic inlet and mediastinum.

Radiological diagnostic criteria are based on size and morphology. Nodes 15 mm or larger are highly likely to be malignant.[7] Malignant involvement of nodes less than 15 mm is less certain. A study of 35 patients who received neck dissection for a variety of head and neck primary tumours revealed that each node identified in the neck dissection specimen which was less than 15 mm has a 2.4% chance of malignancy.[7] Ultrasound-guided fine-needle biopsy may have a greater sensitivity and specificity than MR. A positive aspirate is highly specific, but a negative needle result does not exclude malignancy.[19] There is currently no technique which can reliably diagnose the presence of micrometastases.

Morphological criteria include irregular contour, rim enhancement, multiple or matted nodes, central necrosis and obliteration of surrounding fat and tissue planes. Although these factors are highly sensitive for malignant invasion, they are generally seen on the larger nodes which are positive on the basis of the size criteria.

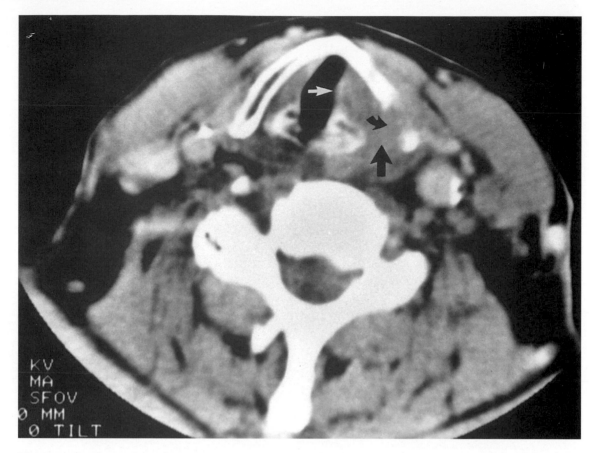

Fig. 22.9 Carcinoma of the left true vocal cord. The left true cord is increased in size and has a slightly lobulated medial margin (white arrow). The tumour has extended posteriorly, widening the cricothyroid joint (straight black arrow) and is invading the adjacent thyroid cartilage (curved arrow). (Courtesy of A. M. Noyek, D. Fliss and H. Shulman.[18])

Tumour volume

There is some evidence that tumour volume is a prognostic factor for laryngeal carcinoma.[11] Gilbert et al found that tumour volume was of greater significance than age, sex or T and N categories in predicting the outcome of radiotherapy. The accuracy of the volume calculations is dependent upon the number of cuts through the tumour. Either MR or CT can be used to provide tumour volume estimations. Multiplanar MR imaging and three-dimensional reconstructions promise to provide the most accurate visualization of tumour involvement and means to estimate tumour volume.

Summary

CT and MR are the current benchmarks of laryngeal imaging. CT is faster, cheaper and more accessible. The use of an intravenous contrast agent can enhance most laryngeal tumours. It is the method of choice in the patient who cannot lie still or who swallows repeatedly. The multiplanar imaging capability of MR gives superior evaluation of tumour extent in relation to the ventricle and subglottis, and improved evaluation of the airway.

MR provides superior assessment of the tongue base and of cartilage invasion utilizing multiple pulse sequences. MR is not permitted in patients with some metal prostheses.

The indications for laryngeal CT or MR are shown in Table 22.1. MR may have the edge in evaluating the suitability for conservation surgery and in assessment of the airway providing the patient can cooperate. CT has the edge in evaluation of the neck, in the diagnosis of non-squamous tumours, and in the patient who cannot lie still.

Often the patient presents to the head and neck clinic having already had a laryngeal CT. The clinician needs to determine whether this scan answers the questions required of imaging. Directed examination is always more useful than a routine study. Above all, correct interpretation of the film with respect to critical anatomical landmarks and the correlation with the clinical examination are essential.

Technique

In performing laryngeal CT, the gantry should be angled parallel to the cords (using a lateral scout film as a guide). The standard study can be done with 5 mm thick images. Additional thinner slices may be obtained around the

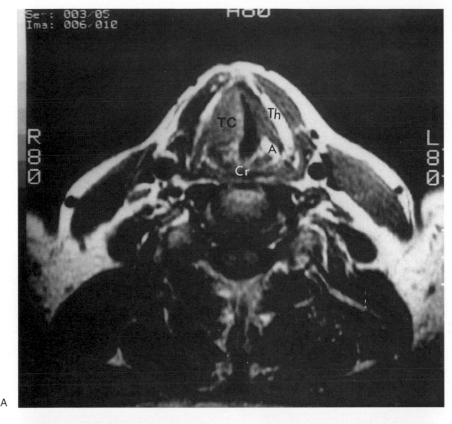

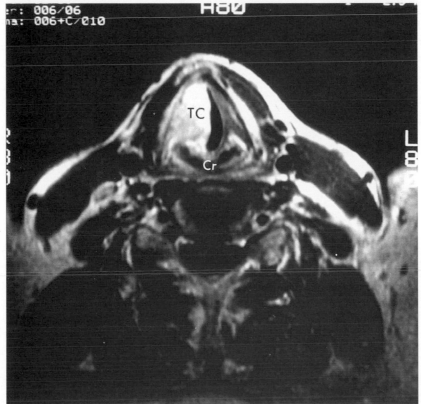

Fig. 22.10 Carcinoma of the right true cord. A. (*top*) T-1 weighted axial image at the true cord level. There is a tumour mass involving the right true cord (TC). It is difficult to assess the relationship of the mass to the cartilage as the paralaryngeal space is very thin at this level. A = arytenoid; Cr = cricoid cartilage; TC = true cord mass; Th = thyroid cartilage marrow. B. (*bottom*) Gadolinium-enhanced T-1-weighted axial image. This image is slightly caudad to that in (A). The tumour mass is again seen, but 'enhanced' by the previous administration of intravenous gadolinium. (Courtesy of A. M. Noyek, D. Fliss and H. Shulman.[18])

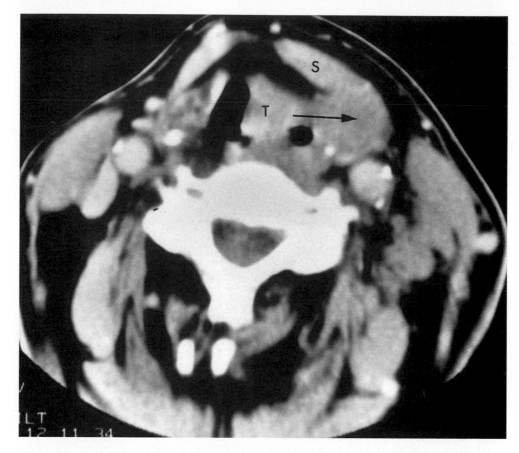

Fig. 22.11 Supraglottic carcinoma of the left false cord. The tumour is extending laterally through the thyrohyoid membrance into the neck (arrow). S = strap muscle; T = tumour. (Courtesy of A. M. Noyek, D. Fliss and H. Shulman.[18])

ventricle, and detail or bone algorithms may be used to assess the cartilage when appropriate.

Contrast enhancement can be optimized by utilizing proper timing sequences. The contrast is injected by pump at the rate of 1.5 ml/s for 20 s and then 0.5 ml/s for 2 min (a total of 90 ml). The first image is obtained 30 s after the injection has started and proceeds from the cords to the tongue base.

MR examination of the larynx requires an anterior surface coil for optimal visualization. T1-weighted spin-echo images are usually obtained in axial, sagittal and coronal planes. The sagittal images may be done first for localization and orientation. The T1 sequence is used because of the high degree of soft tissue contrast it provides. T2-weighted images may be obtained in the axial plane. While anatomical detail is inferior on the T2 sequence, it does allow tissue characterization to some degree. Tissue oedema is 'brighter' on T2 than on T1.

There is a compromise between the use of multiple excitations to increase the signal–noise ratio and the increased examination time compounding the motion artefacts due to breathing and swallowing. The T2-weighted images will be affected to a greater degree than the T1 sequence because of the longer acquisition time.

Intravenous gadolinium can be used to enhance abnormal tissue but must be used on the T1 sequence. In order to enhance the difference between fat and gadolinium on a T1 sequence, fat suppression techniques have been developed which may be of some value in the pre-epiglottic space and the paraglottic space.

BARIUM SWALLOW

The barium swallow plays a role in the evaluation of the extent of disease in piriform fossa and upper oesophagus. It is particularly of value in patients who have a tight stenosis which may limit the passage of the oesophagoscope. It can indicate the lower limit of a lesion, as well as other disease, such as strictures or possibly a second primary. It cannot detect submucosal spread, a common feature of these lesions.

Although it is non-invasive, the barium swallow can be dangerous in the patient who is aspirating due to an obstructing lesion. In these situations, the barium swallow should be modified by reducing the volume of barium given. The high-risk patient should start with 2–5 ml. The volume can be increased incrementally provided there is no aspiration. Barium has less pulmonary toxicity than does gastrograffin.

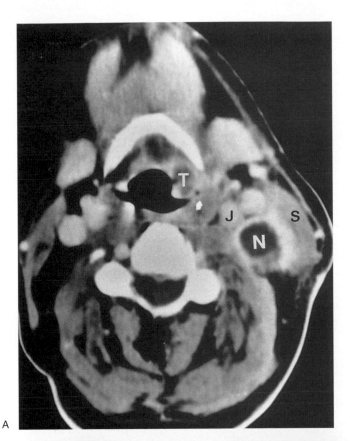

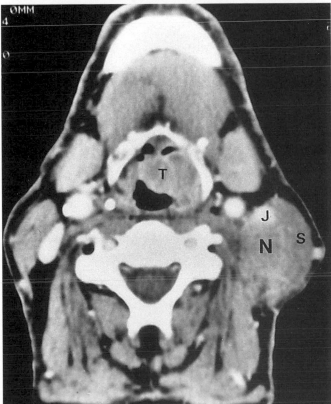

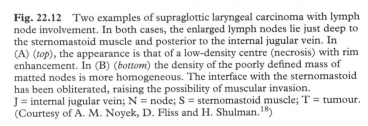

Fig. 22.12 Two examples of supraglottic laryngeal carcinoma with lymph node involvement. In both cases, the enlarged lymph nodes lie just deep to the sternomastoid muscle and posterior to the internal jugular vein. In (A) (*top*), the appearance is that of a low-density centre (necrosis) with rim enhancement. In (B) (*bottom*) the density of the poorly defined mass of matted nodes is more homogeneous. The interface with the sternomastoid has been obliterated, raising the possibility of muscular invasion.
J = internal jugular vein; N = node; S = sternomastoid muscle; T = tumour. (Courtesy of A. M. Noyek, D. Fliss and H. Shulman.[18])

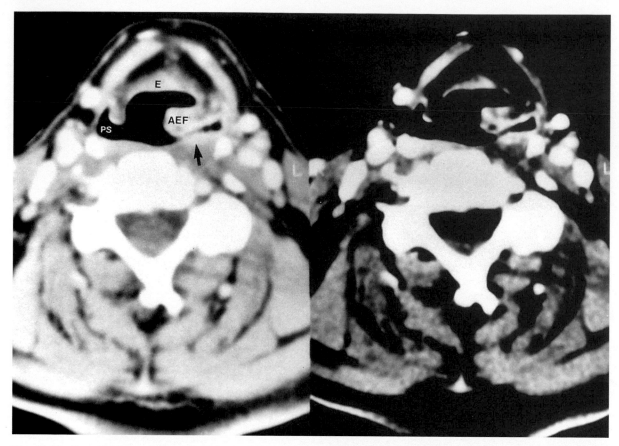

Fig. 22.13 Supraglottic carcinoma. The left aryepiglottic fold (AEF) is thickened and 'enhances' with intravenous contrast. The tumour enhancement extends around the piriform sinus to the posterior wall (arrow). The adjacent image is at the same level (narrower setting) to highlight the soft tissue differences. E = epiglottis; PS = piriform sinus. (Courtesy of A. M. Noyek, D. Fliss and H. Shulman.[18])

The examination is conducted in the lateral and frontal views. The lateral is done first, as this view permits assessment of any aspiration more readily. Spot films can demonstrate specific lesions, and the use of video-fluorsopy permits a recording of swallowing function at lower radiation risk than cinefluorscopy.

ULTRASOUND

Ultrasound is superior to clinical examination for the determination of cervical metastatic disease.[1] However, ultrasound alone cannot determine whether smaller nodes are enlarged due to tumour infiltration or by reactive changes only.

Ultrasound-guided fine-needle aspiration can provide a high degree of accuracy in staging the neck preoperatively. A recent prospective trial of ultrasound guided fine-needle biopsy in 57 necks revealed a sensitivity of 76%, a specificity of 100% and a clinical accuracy of 89%.[1] These figures exceed those of MR and CT. Nodes greater than 3 mm minimal axial diameter can be sampled, but the accuracy is less for smaller lesions.

Ultrasound can be used to assess the integrity of the thyroid cartilage in cases of suspected tumour invasion. This role has now been superseded by CT and MR, which provide a more comprehensive view of tumour invasion.

OTHER TECHNIQUES

Labelled red blood cell scan

[99m]Technetium-labelled RBC radionuclide scanning can be used to diagnose the laryngeal cavernous haemangioma.[8] Consideration of this uncommon lesion requires a high degree of clinical suspicion. The characteristic flow study can alert the surgeon to the dangers of injudicious biopsy.

Laryngography

Historically, laryngography provided the most precise imaging of the mucosal airway interface. However, it is an invasive procedure, absolutely contraindicated in cases of airway compromise. It has been superseded by newer imaging technology such as CT and MR, and by the increasing power and safety of direct laryngeal examination techniques.

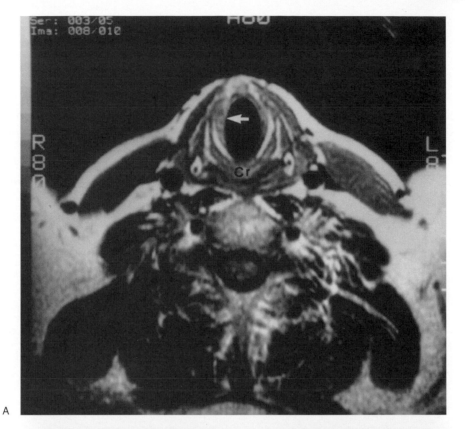

A

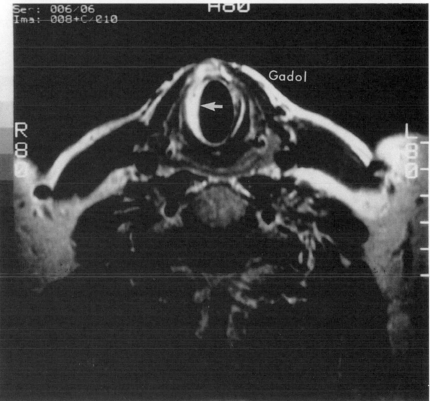

B

Fig. 22.14 T1-weighted axial images without (A) (*top*) and with (B) (*bottom*) gadolinium. The subglottic tumour extension on the right (arrow) is dramatically enhanced following gadolinium administration. Cr = cricoid cartilage (Courtesy of A. M. Noyek, D. Fliss and H. Shulman.[18])

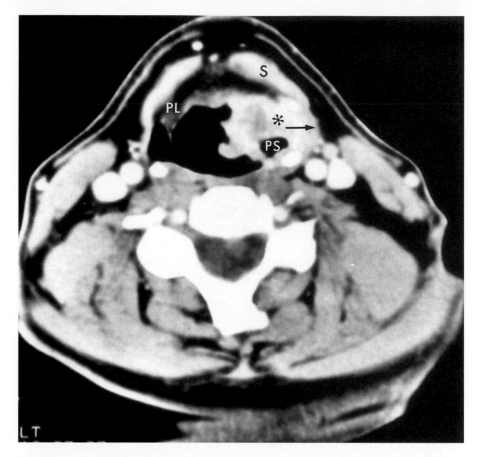

Fig. 22.15 Carcinoma of the left piriform sinus. There is a vascular tumour mass encircling the left piriform sinus with the bulk of the mass anterior to the piriform sinus. The paralaryngeal space has been replaced, and the tumour mass is impinging against the thyrohyoid membrane or may have penetrated the membrane. S = strap muscle; PL = paralaryngeal space; PS = piriform sinus; * = tumour. (Courtesy of A. M. Noyek, D. Fliss and H. Shulman.[18])

REFERENCES

1. Baatenburg de Jong R J, Rongen R J, Lameris J S, Harthoorn M, Verwoerd C D A, Knegt P 1989 Metastatic neck disease: palpation vs ultrasound examination. Arch Otolaryngol Head Neck Surg 115: 689–690
2. Birt D 1987 Observations on the size of the saccule in laryngectomy specimens. Laryngoscope 97: 190–200
3. Castelijns J A, Gerritsen G J, Kaiser M C et al 1987 Invasion of laryngeal cartilage by cancer: comparison of CT and MRI imaging. Radiology 166: 199–206
4. Celin S E, Johnson J, Curtin H, Barnes L 1991 The association of laryngocoeles with squamous cell carcinoma of the larynx. Laryngoscope 101: 529–535
5. Collins S L 1987 Controversies in management of cancer of the neck. In: Thawley S E, Panje W R, Batsakis J G, Lindberg R D (eds) Comprehensive management of head and neck tumours. Saunders, Philadelphia, pp 1386–1443
6. Curtin H 1989 Imaging of the larynx: current concepts. Radiology 173: 1–11
7. Feinmesser R, Freeman J L, Noyek A M, Birt D, Gullane P, Mullen J B 1990 MRI and neck metastases: a clinical, radiological, pathological correlative study. J Otolaryngol 19: 136–140
8. Finkelstein D M, Noyek A M, Kirsh J C 1989 Red blood cell scan in cavernous haemangioma of the larynx. Ann Otol Rhinol Laryngol 98: 707–712
9. Fletcher G H et al 1975 Reasons for irradiation failure in squamous cell carcinoma of the larynx. Laryngoscope 85: 987–1003
10. Friedman M, Mafee M, Pacella B L, Strorigl T L, Dew L L, Toriumi D M 1990 Rationale for elective neck dissection in 1990. Laryngoscope 100: 54–59
11. Gilbert R W, Birt D, Shulman H et al 1987 Correlation of tumour volume with local control in laryngeal carcinoma treated by radiotherapy. Ann Otol Rhinol Laryngol 96: 514–518
12. Kirchner J A 1989 What have whole organ sections contributed to the treatment of laryngeal cancer? Ann Otol Rhinol Laryngol 98: 661–667
13. Lawson W, Biller H F 1987 Glottic and subglottic tumours. In: Thawley S E, Panje W R, Batsakis J G, Lindberg R D (eds) Comprehensive management of head and neck tumors. Saunders, Philadelphia, pp 991–1013
14. Mancuso A A, Dillon W P 1989 The Neck. Radiol Clin North Am 27: 407–434
15. Mancuso A A, Tamakawa Y, Hanafee W N 1980 CT of the fixed vocal cord. Am J Radiol 135: 429–434
16. Rideout D F 1975 Appearances of the larynx after radiation therapy. Can J Otolaryngol 4: 98–101
17. Teresi L M, Lufkin R B, Hanafee W N 1989 Magnetic resonance imaging of the larynx. Radiol Clin North Am 27: 393–405

18. Noyek A M, Fliss D, Shulman H S 1993 Diagnostic imaging of the larynx. In: Tucker H M (ed) The larynx, 2nd edn. Thieme, New York

19. van den Brekel M W M, Castelijns J A, Stel H V et al 1991 Occult metastatic neck disease: detection with US and US-guided fine needle aspiration cytology. Radiology 180: 457–461

20. Vermund H 1970 Role of radiotherapy in cancer of the larynx as related to the TNM system of staging. Cancer 25: 485–488

21. Zinreich S J, Mattox D E, Kennedy D W et al 1988 3-D CT for cranial facial and laryngeal surgery. Laryngoscope 98: 1212–1219

ACKNOWLEDGEMENT

The authors thank Dr G. Cheung for provision of MR images.

23. TNM classification according to the UICC and AJCC

G. B. Snow, G. J. Gerritsen

HISTORY

A simple classification scheme which can be incorporated into a form for staging and universally applied is the goal of the TNM system. The two most commonly applied systems for staging are those of the Union Internationale Contre le Cancer (International Union against Cancer) (UICC) and the American Joint Committee on Cancer (AJCC).

The TNM system for the classification of malignant tumours was developed by Pierre Denoix of France in 1943. In 1953, agreement was reached between the Union Internationale Contre le Cancer (UICC) and the international congress of radiology on a general technique of classification *by anatomical extent of disease*. A special committee was set up, later known as the TNM committee. Several brochures of this committee were combined in a pocket-book. Later, in 1974 and 1978, second and third editions were published containing new site classifications and amendments. Some users, however, introduced new variations in the rules of classifications. To correct this development, the national TNM committees agreed in 1982 to formulate a single TNM system. The result is the 1987 fourth edition of the UICC TNM booklet.[51]

The AJCC was first organized in 1959 as the American Joint Committee for cancer staging and end-results reporting, for the purpose of developing a system of clinical staging of cancer by site. It decided to use the TNM system to describe the anatomical extent of the cancer at the time of diagnosis and from this information to develop a classification into stages which would be useful as a guide to treatment and prognosis and in comparing the end-results of treatment. A *Manual for Staging of Cancer* was first published in 1977. This form was revised and reprinted several times. A second edition appeared in 1983, a third in 1988 and a fourth in 1992.[2]

Until recently, these two systems displayed considerable differences, particularly regarding the staging of neck nodes. Their use of the same symbols T, N and M for, respectively, the primary tumour, neck nodes, and distant metastases, has consequently led to much confusion.

Therefore, it is gratifying to notice that the revised 1987 edition of the UICC classification and the 1988 edition of the AJCC classification systems are almost identical. Remember that both classification systems are based primarily almost exclusively on the anatomical extent of disease as determined clinically. As yet, biological tumour markers and, more importantly, characteristics of the host, are not included in these two systems.

OBJECTIVES

The TNM committee of the UICC and AJCC have been working along similar lines and with similar objectives.

The TNM system may serve a number of related objectives, namely:

1. To aid the clinician in planning treatment
2. To give some indication of prognosis
3. To assist in evaluation of results of treatment
4. To facilitate the exchange of information between treatment centres, thus providing a method of conveying clinical experience
5. To contribute to the continuing investigation of cancers.

GENERAL RULES

The TNM system for describing the anatomical extent of disease is based on the assessment of three components:

T: extent of primary tumour
N: status of regional lymph nodes
M: presence or absence of distant metastases.

The addition of numbers to these three components (e.g. T1, T2, N0, N1, etc.) indicates the extent of the malignant disease. All cases should be confirmed microscopically. All cases are identified by T, N and M categories, which must be determined and recorded *before any therapy is started*. This *clinical* classification is based on evidence acquired from physical examination, imaging, endoscopy, biopsy, surgical exploration, or other relevant examinations.

425

Events such as local spread, spread to regional lymph nodes and distant metastasis occur before they are discernible by clinical examination. Thus, examination at the time of surgical procedure, and histological examination of removed tissues may identify the significant markers of tumour growth as being different from what could be discerned clinically before therapy. So, *pathological classification carried out postsurgically* and designated as pTNM is an accurate depiction of the life history of the cancer and is therefore the most reliable parameter for prognostic purposes.

The pathological assessment of the primary tumour (pT) entails a resection of the primary tumour or biopsy adequate to evaluate the highest pT category. The pathological assessment of the regional lymph nodes (pN) entails removal of nodes adequate to validate the absence of regional lymph node metastasis (pNO) and sufficient to evaluate the highest pN category. The pathological assessment of distant metastasis (pM) entails microscopic examination.

After T, N, and M or pT, pN and pM categories have been assigned, they may be grouped into stages. The TNM classification and stage grouping, once established, must remain unchanged in the medical records. The clinical stage helps us to select and evaluate therapy, whereas the pathological stage provides useful information to estimate prognosis and calculate end-results.

If there is doubt concerning the correct T, N or M category to which a particular case should be allotted, then the lower, that is, less advanced, category should be chosen. This will also be reflected in the stage grouping. The grade of the tumour does not enter into staging of the tumour.

Therapeutic procedures alter the course and life history of cancer. Although cancers that recur after therapy may be staged with the same markers that are used in pretreatment clinical staging, the significance of these markers is not the same. Hence, the stage classification of recurrent cancer should not be considered for therapeutic guidance, prognosis and end-results reporting.

DEFINITIONS

The anatomical definitions of the various primary sites within the head and neck are now almost identical in the UICC and AJCC classifications, and the sites are listed by code numbers of the International Classification of Diseases for Oncology.[52] In Table 23.1 the division of the larynx into sites and subsites according to UICC and according to AJCC is presented. In the past there has been controversy as to the superior border of the supraglottis. This has now been settled, both UICC and AJCC including the lingual surface of the epiglottis within the supraglottis. However, UICC does not define the inferior boundary of the supraglottis, but does include

Table 23.1 Anatomical sites and subsites according to UICC and AJCC (sites are listed by ICD-O code numbers)

UICC

1. Supraglottis (161.1)
   Epilarynx (including marginal zone)
   (i) suprahyoid epiglottis (including the tip)
   (ii) aryepiglottic fold
   (iii) arytenoid
   Supraglottis excluding epilarynx
   (iv) infrahyoid epiglottis
   (v) ventricular bands (false cords)
   (vi) ventricular cavities

2. Glottis (161.0)
   (i) vocal cords
   (ii) anterior commissure
   (iii) posterior commissure

3. Subglottis (161.2)

AJCC

Site	Subsite
Supraglottis (161.1)	Ventricular bands (false cords) Arytenoids Suprahyoid epiglottis (both lingual and laryngeal aspects) Infrahyoid epiglottis Arytenoepiglottic folds (laryngeal aspect)
Glottis (161.0)	True vocal cords including anterior and posterior commissures
Subglottis (161.2)	Subglottis

the ventricular cavities in the supraglottis. In the AJCC classification the inferior boundary of the supraglottis is a horizontal plane through the apex of the ventricle. Thus, the ventricular cavities are not included in the supraglottis according to AJCC. Accordingly, the division of subsites is not completely identical for UICC and AJCC, UICC distinguishing 6 subsites as opposed to the 5 distinguished by AJCC. UICC also does not define the lower boundary of the glottis or that of the subglottis. In the AJCC classification, the lower boundary of the glottis is the horizontal plane 1 cm below the apex of the ventricle. However, many consider 5 mm below the free margin of the vocal cord, that is, approximately the line of junction between squamous and respiratory epithelium, as the border.[31] According to AJCC the subglottis is the region extending from the lower boundary of the glottis to the lower margin of the cricoid cartilage.

In Table 23.2 the current T-classification, which is now identical for UICC and AJCC, is presented. However, this does not necessarily mean that the outcome of T-staging according to UICC and AJCC will be always identical. Because of differences in definitions of laryngeal sites and subsites, as outlined in the previous paragraph, T-staging of particular tumours may be different when one or the other classification is used, and this will be further discussed under 'Comments'.

Table 23.2 Classification of primary tumour (T) for carcinoma of the larynx according to UICC and AJCC

Primary tumour (T)
TX   Primary tumour cannot be assessed
T0   No evidence of primary tumour
Tis   Carcinoma in situ

Supraglottis
T1   Tumour limited to one subsite of supraglottis, with normal vocal cord mobility
T2   Tumour invades more than one subsite of supraglottis or glottis, with normal vocal cord mobility
T3   Tumour limited to larynx with vocal cord fixation and/or invades postcricoid area, medial wall of piriform sinus or pre-epiglottic tissues
T4   Tumour invades through thyroid cartilage and/or extends to other tissues beyond the larynx, e.g. to oropharynx, soft tissues of neck

Glottis
T1   Tumour limited to vocal cord(s) (may involve anterior or posterior commissures) with normal mobility
    T1a Tumour limited to one vocal cord
    T1b Tumour involves both vocal cords
T2   Tumour extends to supraglottis and/or subglottis, and/or with impaired vocal cord mobility
T3   Tumour limited to the larynx with vocal cord fixation
T4   Tumour invades through thyroid cartilage and/or extends to other tissues beyond the larynx, e.g. to oropharynx, soft tissues of the neck

Subglottis
T1   Tumour limited to the subglottis
T2   Tumour extends to vocal cord(s) with normal or impaired mobility
T3   Tumour limited to the larynx with vocal cord fixation
T4   Tumour invades through cricoid or thyroid cartilage and/or extends to other tissues beyond the larynx, e.g. to oropharynx, soft tissues of the neck

Fortunately, the definitions of N-categories by UICC and AJCC, which have been so different in the past, are now identical, and these are presented in Table 23.3. The definitions of M-categories are listed in Table 23.4. Stage grouping, too, is now identical in the UICC and AJCC classifications and it is similar for all head and neck sites (Table 23.5).

For all head and neck sites except salivary glands and the thyroid gland, only squamous cell carcinomas are to be included in the TNM system. Although the grade of the tumour does not enter into staging of the tumour, it should be recorded. The definitions of the tumour grade (G) categories are as follows:

GX: Grade of differentiation cannot be assessed
G1:   Well differentiated
G2:   Moderately differentiated
G3:   Poorly differentiated
G4:   Undifferentiated.

STAGING PROCEDURES

A variety of procedures and special studies may be used in the process of staging a given tumour. Both UICC and AJCC are not specific and not precise in their recommendations as to the procedures for assessment of the T, N and M categories. UICC for instance states that 'the following are the procedures for assessment of T-categories: physical examination, laryngoscopy and imaging', without further indication as to the type of imaging. However, UICC recognizes an optional additional descriptor, the so-called C-factor, reflecting the validity of classification according to the diagnostic methods used. The C-factor definitions are: C1, evidence from standard diagnostic means (e.g., physical examination, standard radiography, intraluminal endoscopy); and C2, evidence obtained by special diagnostic means (e.g., CT, MRI, etc.). As all of the advanced imaging procedures are included in the same category, C2, this does not seem to make much sense. Anyhow, the C-factor does not appear to be used very often as it is usually not reported in the literature. AJCC states that 'a variety of imaging procedures are valuable in evaluating the extent of disease, particularly for advanced tumours and these include laryngeal tomograms, CT-scans and MRI-scans', but does not indicate when to use either

Table 23.3 Classification of regional lymph nodes (N) according to UICC and AJCC

NX   Regional lymph nodes cannot be assessed
N0   No regional lymph nodes metastasis
N1   Metastasis in a single ipsilateral lymph node, 3 cm or less in greatest dimension
N2   Metastasis in a single ipsilateral lymph node, more than 3 cm but not more than 6 cm in greatest dimension, or in multiple ipsilateral lymph nodes, none more than 6 cm in greatest dimension, or in bilateral or contralateral lymph nodes, none more than 6 cm in greatest dimension
    N2a Metastasis in a single ipsilateral lymph node, more than 3 cm but not more than 6 cm in greatest dimension
    N2b Metastasis in multiple ipsilateral lymph nodes, none more than 6 cm in greatest dimension
    N2c Metastasis in bilateral or contralateral lymph nodes, none more than 6 cm in greatest dimension
N3   Metastasis in a lymph node more than 6 cm in greatest dimension.

Table 23.4 Classification of distant metastases (M)

MX   Presence of distant metastasis cannot be assessed
M0   No distant metastasis
M1   Distant metastasis

Table 23.5 Stage grouping

Stage	0	Tis	N0	M0
Stage	1	T1	N0	M0
Stage	II	T2	N0	M0
Stage	III	T3	N0	M0
		T1	N1	M0
		T2	N1	M0
		T3	N1	M0
Stage	IV	T4	N0, N1	M0
		Any T	N2, N3	M0
		Any T	Any N	M1

or all of these imaging methods. The issue of staging procedures is important as it is generally recognized that *the validity of any classification is dependent on the diagnostic methods employed.* The various procedures for assessment will be briefly discussed in the following.

Assessment of the primary tumour—T

Indirect and direct laryngoscopy and conventional radiological techniques are traditionally the cornerstones in the examination of the larynx. However, these methods each have their limitations. The introduction of CT in the seventies and of MRI in the eighties have greatly enhanced our diagnostic potential for assessing the extent of laryngeal cancer in that both methods are capable of visualizing tumour extension in the horizontal or axial plane deep to the laryngeal mucosal surface.

Indirect laryngoscopy

Indirect laryngoscopy offers an excellent preliminary overall survey of the larynx. However, its limitation is the inaccessibility of certain recesses of the larynx, such as the undersurface of the ventricular bands, the lateral extent of the ventricles, the undersurface of the vocal cords, the postcricoid region and the apex and medial wall of the piriform sinuses. In addition, there are variations in patient's response to the procedure of mirror examination, and in some patients anatomical factors, such as an overhanging infantile epiglottis, interfere with mirror examination. For these patients the recent introduction of the small flexible fibreoptic laryngoscope is a break-through in our diagnostic armamentarium. After topical anaesthesia of the mucous membranes of the nose, oropharynx and larynx, this scope can be introduced readily through the nose into the larynx, permitting an adequate view of the intralaryngeal structures.

Stroboscopy

With stroboscopy a voice-synchronized light source is used to evaluate the vibratory wave pattern of the vocal cords mucosa in an ultraslow motion. Early superficial tumour infiltration will reveal disorders of vibratory mucosal wave pattern. These lesions can be treated by laser surgery without loss of functionality of the affected cord.

Radiological examinations

Radiographical studies should be done before direct laryngoscopy and biopsy because these procedures may cause anatomical changes. The following radiological techniques are most commonly used: conventional frontal tomography, CT, and MRI. In early glottic cancers, T1 and 'small' T2, conventional frontal tomography is usually still sufficient.

In larger glottic tumours, frontal tomography provides a good demonstration of tumour size. However, cartilage destruction and extralaryngeal extension cannot be visualized by this technique. Because of these limitations, frontal tomography has been superseded by CT or MRI in the evaluation of large tumours.

CT is of particular value in the visualization of the pre-epiglottic space, the thyroid cartilage, and the extra-laryngeal soft tissues and of tumour infiltration into these structures.[22] However, CT, too, has its limitations. It often fails in detecting minor cartilage invasion owing to variations in calcifications. Calcified cartilage invaded by cancer is frequently seen by CT as having an intact contour.[3,41] On the other hand, tumour approaching non-ossified cartilage may simulate cartilage invasion.[27,53]

An advantage of MRI over CT is its ability to provide multiplanar images: the laryngeal structures can be visualized in axial, sagittal, and frontal planes. Moreover, MRI appears superior to CT in detecting minor invasion of laryngeal cartilages.[14,15] MRI will therefore play an increasingly important role in the diagnostic work-up of laryngeal cancer patients. MRI images, however, are much more difficult to read than CT images, particularly for the clinician, and this will probably somewhat delay widespread acceptance of MRI as an important tool for the assessment of the extent of laryngeal cancer.

Direct laryngoscopy

Direct laryngoscopy with rigid tubes is usually performed under general anaesthesia. It is important that the anaesthetic technique provides an unobstructed view of the lesion. For small glottic cancers it may be helpful for accurate delineation of the lesion to use the operating microscope through the suspension laryngoscope, which can be fixed to the anterior chest wall. In most instances, and particularly in the more advanced tumours, a more versatile endoscope is advantageous. With the tip of the scope placed intraluminally and a hand placed externally on the thyroid cartilage, all recesses of the larynx can be inspected. By palpating the tumour mass with the tip of the suction tube, one can estimate the degree of infiltration in depth. After the extent of the tumour is assessed, the tumour is then biopsied. In supraglottic cancers spreading to the vallecula, digital palpation of the base of the tongue is important to detect submucosal tumour extension in this area; this is best done after completion of the direct laryngoscopy when the patient is still under general anaesthesia.

Assessment of regional lymph nodes—N

Although clinical palpation of the neck is still widely used for staging of the neck, it is generally accepted that this is not very accurate. More recently, computed tomography (CT), magnetic resonance imaging (MRI), ultrasound

(US) and ultrasound-guided fine-needle aspiration cytology (US-guided FNAC) have also been used in an effort to improve the results of clinical staging.

Clinical palpation

The location, consistency and size of a lymph node, as well as the type of neck and the experience of the examiner, determine whether a lymph node is clinically palpable. In experienced hands, nodes can be detected down to a size of 0.5 cm in superficial areas such as the submandibular area, and 1.0 cm in deeper areas such as the subdigastric.[39] Micrometastases can occur in nodes smaller than these, giving rise to false-negative rates of the order of 20–30%.[1] Equally, normal nodes can vary in size up to 2.0 cm and may be readily palpable.[26] Thus, clinical palpation can give rise to false-positive results in up to 20% of cases.[1] Also, palpation is unreliable in assessing the exact number and diameter of metastatic nodes.[43] Clearly, if treatment plans and prognostic information are to be based on staging of neck nodes, then an improvement in both sensitivity (so that patients who require treatment to the neck are selected to receive it) and specificity (so that patients who do not require treatment to the neck are spared the unnecessary treatment and morbidity) is desirable.

Computerized tomography

With the introduction of high-resolution CT scans came the hope and potential for detecting 'occult' (not clinically palpable) metastases. There are, however, conflicting reports in the literature as to the value of routine CT-scanning for staging of neck nodes. Feinmesser et al, from Toronto, in a retrospective study, showed similar sensitivity rates for clinical examination and CT-scanning (61.5% and 59.6% respectively).[16] The false-positive rate for clinical examination was 8.6% compared to 18.4% for CT. Feinmesser et al therefore concluded that CT offers no advantage over physical examination in staging neck nodes. Others have shown that CT-scan has a higher sensitivity than physical examination in detecting metastatic disease.[21,34,35,49,50] The criteria used for diagnosing a lymph node as malignant need to be considered. They include nodal size, central necrosis, pericapsular extensions and obliteration of perivascular fat planes.[21,34,35] Using these criteria, Friedman et al[19] reported a significantly greater sensitivity of the CT scan (87.1%) compared to clinical examination (72.3%).

Magnetic resonance imaging

MRI has better soft tissue contrast resolution than CT, and studies are now being reported on the efficacy of MRI for staging neck nodes. In a report based on 30 neck dissections in 27 patients, Feinmesser et al, from Toronto, showed that there was little advantage of MRI over clinical examination in the detection of cervical metastases.[17] Their findings are in contrast to other reports — including a recent large prospective study reported from the Free University Hospital, Amsterdam.[10] It should be noted, however, that reliable comparison of sensitivity and specificity reported in different series is difficult due to different patient populations and particularly due to the varying radiological criteria and differing imaging techniques. More accurate criteria for cervical lymph node malignancy have been reported on the basis of a pathoanatomical study.[9] Criteria for malignancy on MRI include: (i) evidence of central necrosis, (ii) minimal axial diameter greater than 11 mm in subdigastric area or greater than 10 mm in other areas, and (iii) grouping of three or more borderline nodes (minimal axial diameter 1 or 2 mm less than above) in the lymph node draining region of the tumour. With these criteria, van den Brekel et al[8] from Amsterdam, reported a sensitivity and specificity of MRI to be 81% and 88% respectively (overall error 16%) as compared with 68% and 67% respectively (overall error 32%) for clinical examination. In the clinically N0 neck, the MRI sensitivity and specificity was 60% and 89% respectively. These results indicate that contrast-enhanced MRI can be a valuable tool for cervical lymph node staging, with the overall error being half that of clinical palpation.

Ultrasound (US) and ultrasound-guided fine-needle aspiration cytology (US-guided FNAC)

There have been numerous reports on the use of US and US-guided FNAC in recent years.[4,5,7,9,11,12,24] Ultrasound does not allow differentiation between enlarged lymph nodes and enlarged metastatic nodes.[4,7] The criteria suggested for such differentiation are size (minimal axial diameter) and grouping of more than three borderline lymph nodes.[9] Sensitivity for the detection of nodes can be increased for all imaging techniques by using stricter criteria (such as a smaller minimal axial diameter), but this inevitably results in a decreased specificity for metastatic disease.[4,7] The advantage of ultrasound is that, with the addition of US-guided FNAC, the specificity too can be improved.[4,7] Thus US-guided FNAC was shown to have a sensitivity of 76% and a specificity of 100% (accuracy of 89%) in necks that were clinically negative by palpation alone.[7] These results are an improvement on those reported in the literature for CT or MRI[10,19,20,49] and are of great importance in enabling the detection of occult metastatic disease in the neck.

US-guided FNAC is a technique, requiring both expertise and experience, which is not presently available in the majority of centres. In most institutions, availability and cost considerations would preclude routine CT or

MRI scanning of the neck in all patients with head and neck malignancies. Those patients requiring CT or MRI for assessment of the primary tumour can have their necks evaluated at the same time without significant additional costs. On the balance of evidence, for laryngeal tumours, all patients with supraglottic, transglottic or large T3 and T4 lesions should have their necks evaluated by CT or MRI scans. Where the expertise is available, US-guided FNAC should be used when the results or the other modalities are doubtful.

Assessment of distant metastases—M

At the time of admission, clinically overt distant metastases are uncommon in patients with squamous cell carcinoma of the head and neck. However, distant metastases become apparent during follow-up in many more patients today than in the past as a result of more effective locoregional treatment. Therefore, interest is increasing in the early diagnosis of distant metastases,[13] particularly in patients with N2 and N3 disease, because the extent of nodal disease in the neck has been shown to be the most sensitive prognostic indicator for distant metastases.[44] The principal sites are lungs, bones (vertebrae, skull, ribs) and liver.[32]

Chest radiography allows detection of most metastases greater than 1 cm in diameter. Increased sensitivity can be obtained by CT, due to its ability to permit detection of smaller nodules and visualization of areas hidden on plain films. This increased sensitivity for small nodules is at the cost of decreased specificity.[40] A lung biopsy may be necessary to distinguish benign conditions from lung metastases.[46]

The radionuclide bone scan is the most effective whole-body screening test for bone metastases.[23] False-positive scan findings are reduced and scan specificity increased when the radionuclide bone scan and appropriate correlative radiographs are analysed and reported together. CT or MR imaging may be useful for evaluating suspicious radionuclide bone scan findings that cannot be explained radiographically and may influence the decision regarding the need for biopsy.[25]

Patients suspected of having metastatic hepatic disease must have preoperative imagings. Patients often undergo a sequence of imaging procedures including ultrasonography, nuclear medicine studies, CT and MR imaging.[36] At present, most institutions use ultrasound followed by dynamic contrast CT for the evaluation of liver lesions.

COMMENTS

The present internationally accepted TNM system for head and neck cancer in general, and cancer of the larynx in particular, provides a standardized system of categories in which it is possible to fit the tumour status of patients with these tumours. The system thus fulfils the principle purpose to be served by international agreement on the classification of cancer cases by extent of disease, that is, to provide a method of conveying clinical experience to others without ambiguity.

However, in the application of this TNM system for laryngeal cancer problems may be encountered. Firstly, tumours do not respect the anatomical borders as these have been defined: between the larynx and its neighbouring structures and between the various sites and subsites within the larynx. Also, these definitions are not always clear. For these reasons it may at times be very difficult, if not impossible, to assign a cancer in this region to the larynx or to a particular (sub)site of origin within the larynx and a specific T-category. Furthermore, because of differences in definitions of laryngeal sites and subsites between UICC and AJCC, the outcome of T-staging occasionally may be different when using one or the other classification system and this will particularly regard 'small' T1 and T2 supraglottic and glottic tumours.

Secondly, the present TNM system leaves it very much to the individual doctor to decide which procedures to use for staging, whereas it is generally recognized that the validity of any classification is dependent on the diagnostic methods employed. This holds particularly true for modern imaging methods such as CT and MRI. These methods have been a break-through in the work-up of all laryngeal cancers, except the very small ones, in that these methods are capable of visualizing the extent of submucosal disease in the axial plane. Unfortunately, the present TNM system does not accurately define — and does not even recommend — when these imaging techniques should be used for the assessment of the T- and N-categories in laryngeal cancer.

Furthermore, the present TNM system for the classification of cancer of the larynx does not always meet the other objectives of classifying malignant tumours. While, in general, good correlation with prognosis can be seen, the system is often not accurate enough to be used as a guideline for the management of a particular patient with laryngeal cancer.

In the following, T-staging and N-staging will be critically reviewed, taking into account the above-mentioned considerations.

T-staging (Table 23.2)

Glottic tumours

T1-glottic tumours. A distinction is made between tumours limited to one vocal cord, T1a, and tumours involving both vocal cords, T1b. However, this decision does not seem to have prognostic relevance, either in patients treated with radiotherapy[28,33] or in patients treated by surgery.[29] Much less experience has been gained with endoscopic CO_2 laser treatment. However, the feasibility of this treatment modality depends on the accessibility of the lesion at direct microlaryngoscopy and on the extent into — and particularly the depth of infiltration at — the anterior commissure, rather than on the extent to the contralateral vocal cord. The division between T1a and T1b therefore seems to be redundant.

T2-glottic tumours. The T2 group of glottic tumours is very heterogeneous, involving not only both small and bulky lesions, but also grouping together tumours with normal and impaired mobility.[30] It has been shown by numerous authors that the local control rate by radiotherapy — the most commonly used primary treatment modality for T2 glottic tumours — is significantly lower in patients with T2 tumours with impaired mobility as compared to patients with T2 tumours with normal mobility, and this is also reflected in a poorer survival rate. It therefore appears highly recommendable to differentiate within the T2-group between normal, T2a, and impaired, T2b, vocal cord mobility.

According to UICC, the ventricular cavities are part of the supraglottis, whereas AJCC includes the ventricular cavities in the glottis. Classification according to UICC of a given series of 'small' glottic tumours will therefore 'favour' T2 versus T1 when compared to AJCC, taking into account that T1 is limited to the glottis, whereas a tumour with extension to the supraglottis is to be designated T2.

T3-glottic tumours. This category includes tumours confined to the larynx with vocal cord fixation. The majority of these tumours are bulky, having spread to the supraglottis and/or subglottis. However, a small minority is more or less limited to the glottis. The latter group has been reported to have a significantly better prognosis as compared to the former, when treated primarily by radiotherapy.[48] *Therefore it could be considered to distinguish a T3a and a T3b group respectively.* Furthermore it is anticipated that the prognostic significance of minor or major cartilage invasion, as visualized by MRI, will be assessed in the near future. This parameter may then be included in the next edition of the TNM classification and hopefully it may be used as a guideline for the management of individual patients.

T4-glottic tumours. This group entails tumours which have extended beyond the confines of the larynx. In the 1987 UICC classification the phrasing 'tumour invades through thyroid cartilage' has been added, and this has caused confusion. It is perhaps ironic that as high-technology imaging capable of demonstrating cartilage invasion has become available, this is the only reference to cartilage invasion in the classification system.

Supraglottic tumours

Fortunately the division of the supraglottis into subsites by UICC and AJCC, which has been so different in the past, is now almost identical (Table 23.1). Both UICC and AJCC now distinguish the suprahyoid epiglottis and the infrahyoid epiglottis as separate subsites. In clinical practice the problem remains that there is no clear intralaryngeal anatomical landmark indicating the border between the suprahyoid and the infrahyoid epiglottis.

Furthermore, the marginal areas of suprahyoid epiglottis, aryepiglottic fold and arytenoids account for approximately 30% of all supraglottic tumours.[37] Tumours at these sites may, if they spread to the outer side of the larynx, become T4; if not, they remain T1. These T4 marginal tumours may be small tumours, while, for example, a T4 ventricle tumour must be large, and must be very different.

T3 supraglottic tumours. Traditionally these involve tumours confined the larynx with (vocal cord) fixation and/or other evidence of deep infiltration. In the most recent classification, the other evidence of deep infiltration has been further specified as follows: 'invasion of postcricoid area, medial wall of piriform sinus or pre-epiglottic tissues'. As the majority of supraglottic tumours originate on the laryngeal surface of the epiglottis, and as the natural fenestrae of the epiglottis below the level of the hyoepiglottic ligament predispose to anterior cancer spread, pre-epiglottic space invasion is of particular interest in this regard. Pre-epiglottic space invasion is common in 'early' epiglottic-cancer.[54] Many tumours which, on clinical grounds, would be designated T1 or T2 will be staged T3, if CT or MRI is applied. So, again, the validity of classification is dependent on the diagnostic methods used, and these should be more accurately defined than is done in the present classification system. Furthermore, it is important to assess accurately the percentage of pre-epiglottic space involvement[18] as local control rates by radiotherapy appear to decrease with increasing percentage of such involvement.

T4 supraglottic tumours. It can sometimes be very difficult, if not impossible, to define a tumour as primarily supraglottic, oropharyngeal or hypopharyngeal if the base of the tongue is infiltrated or if the hypopharynx is involved. Such advanced lesions are per se not comparable with the T4 marginal area lesion as mentioned before in terms of survival or local control rate.

N-staging (Table 23.3)

It is generally realized that the overall error in assessing the presence or absence of lymph node metastases in the neck by palpation alone is high, of the order of 25–30%,[1] and that palpation is not accurate in the assessment of size and number of metastatic lymph nodes.[43] There is a growing body of evidence that CT, and particularly MRI and US-guided aspiration cytology do much better than palpation in the detection of nodal metastases in the neck, in terms of both sensitivity and specificity.[8] Also, CT, MRI and US are far superior to palpation in size determination of involved nodes[9] and are more accurate in assessing the number of involved nodes. Furthermore, CT and MRI provide a permanent document of the status of the neck. Because of the overwhelming prognostic significance of the status of the cervical lymph nodes in head and neck cancer patients in general,[42] and in patients with cancer of the larynx in particular,[37] optimal assessment of the status of the lymph nodes in the neck is extremely important. However, even in parts of the world where CT, MRI and US are abundantly available, the neck is still widely assessed by palpation only. The use of these imaging techniques for the assessment of the cervical lymph nodes should be strongly encouraged by laryngologists and by head and neck surgeons. Furthermore, recommendations should be made to UICC and AJCC to include CT, MRI and US (guided aspiration cytology) as essential procedures for staging of the lymph nodes in the neck in their classifications.

Furthermore, it is unfortunate that the level of involvement of cervical lymph nodes is not incorporated in the UICC and AJCC staging systems, as it has been shown that the level of nodal involvement has prognostic importance.[45,47] *It is therefore highly recommended that five levels or regions of involvement be applied, as depicted in Figure 23.1.*

Region I includes the submental and submandibular triangles, regions II, III and IV include the lymph nodes adjacent to the jugular vein and the lymph nodes located medial to the sternocleidomastoid muscle. Region V includes the posterior triangle of the neck. Such a diagrammatical division may also serve a rational classification of neck dissections.[38]

PERSPECTIVES

Recently, a lot of concern has been expressed by international experts in laryngeal cancer surgery about the shortcomings of the most recent TNM classification for cancer of the larynx according to UICC and AJCC. These shortcomings are obvious and have been discussed in detail in this chapter. Some can be eliminated, but others cannot, due mainly to the limitation of any TNM classification system in that it is fundamentally a tool that has been designed to allow analysis of groups of patients.[6] Furthermore, it cannot be overemphasized that the TNM system takes into account only the anatomical extent of local invasion of the primary tumour, along with the presence of clinically detectable regional metastases or distant metastases. Other factors of the disease, such as

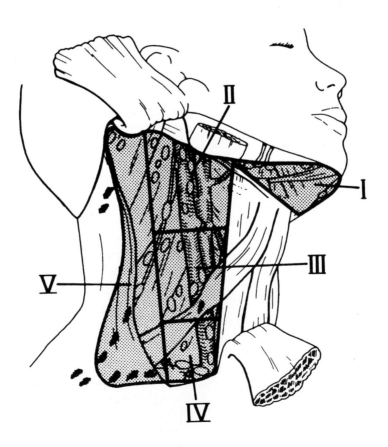

Fig. 23.1 Lymph node regions of the neck.

the growth rate of the tumour, are not reflected in the TNM system. Host factors of assumed or suggested prognostic significance, such as the patient's age and sex, and his resistance to the spread of cancer, are not taken into account. Against this background the TNM system is of great value in terms of what it can accomplish.

The biological aggressiveness of the tumour is reflected to a certain extent by its structural differentiation by the pathologist. Other prognostic histological characteristics, such as perineural spread, microvascular invasion and

extranodal spread, usually become apparent only in the surgical specimen and are therefore of no help in pretreatment staging.

It is hoped that, in the not-too-distant future, useful tumour markers will be identified in laryngeal cancer patients not only in the serum but also at the local tumour level (i. e. in biopsy material), which are predictive for the biological behaviour of the cancer. Such biological markers could then be added to those of anatomical extent in classifying head and neck cancer.

REFERENCES

1. Ali S, Tiwari R M, Snow GB 1985 False-positive and false-negative neck nodes. Head Neck Surg 8: 78–82
2. American Joint Committee on Cancer (AJCC) 1992 Manual for staging of cancer, 4th edn. Lippincott, Philadelphia
3. Archer C R, Yeager V L 1982 Computed tomography of laryngeal cancer with histopathological correlation. Laryngoscope 92: 1173–1180
4. Baatenburg de Jong R J, Rongen R J, Lameris J S 1989 Metastatic neck disease. Arch Otolaryngol Head Neck Surg 115: 689–690
5. Baatenburg de Jong R J, Rongen R J, Jong P C, Lameris J S, Knegt P 1988 Screening for lymph nodes in the neck with ultrasound. Clin Otolaryngol 13: 5–9
6. Bailey B J 1991 Beyond the 'new' TNM classification. Arch Otolaryngol Head Neck Surg 117: 369–370
7. Brekel van den M W M, Castelijns J A, Stel H V et al 1991 Occult metastatic neck disease: detection with US and US-guided fine needle aspiration cytology. Radiology 180: 457–461
8. Brekel van den M W M, Castelijns J A, Stel H V et al Computer tomography, magnetic resonance, ultrasound and ultrasound guided aspiration cytology for detecting cervical lymph node metastasis. Submitted to *Cancer*.
9. Brekel van den M W M, Stel H V, Castelijns J A et al 1990 Cervical lymph node metastases: assessment of radiologic criteria. Radiology 177: 379–384
10. Brekel van den M W M, Castelijns J A, Croll G A et al 1991 MRI versus palpation of cervical lymph node metastasis. Arch Otolaryngol Head Neck Surg 117: 666–673
11. Bruneton J N, Normand F 1987 Cervical lymph nodes. In: Bruneton J N (ed) Ultrasonography of the neck. Springer Verlag, Berlin, pp 81–91
12. Bruneton J N, Roux P, Caramella E, Demard F, Vallicioni J, Chauvel P 1984 Ear, nose and throat cancer: ultrasound diagnosis of metastasis to cervical lymph nodes. Radiology 152: 771–773
13. Castelijns J A 1991 Diagnostic radiology for head and neck oncology. Curr Opin Oncol 3: 512–518
14. Castelijns J A, Gerritsen G J, Kaiser M C et al 1987 MRI of normal or cancerous laryngeal cartilages: histopathologic correlation. Laryngoscope 97: 1085–1093
15. Castelijns J A, Gerritsen G J, Kaiser M C et al 1988 Invasion of laryngeal cartilage by cancer: comparison of CT and MR imaging. Radiology 167: 199–206
16. Feinmesser R, Freeman J L, Nojek A M, Birt B D 1987 Metastatic neck disease: a clinical/radiographic/pathologic correlative study. Arch Otolaryngol Head Neck Surg 113: 1307–1310
17. Feinmesser R, Freeman J L, Noyek A M, Birt B D, Gullane P, Mullen J B 1990 MRI and neck metastases: a clinical, radiological, pathological correlative study. J Otolaryngol 19: 136–140
18. Freeman D E, Mancuso A A, Parsons J T, Mendenhall W M, Million R R 1990 Irradiation alone for supraglottic larynx carcinoma: can CT findings predict treatment results? Int J Radiat Oncol Biol Phys 19: 485–490
19. Friedman M, Toriumi D M, Mafee M F, Strorigl T L 1990 The role of computed tomographic scanning in evaluating the clinically negative neck. In: Fee W E et al (eds) Head and neck cancer, Vol 2. Decker, Toronto; pp 138–144

20. Friedman M, Mafee M F, Pacella B L, Strorigl T L, Dew L L, Toriumi D M 1990 Rationale for elective neck dissections in 1990 Laryngoscope 100: 54–59
21. Friedman M, Shelton V K, Mafee M, Bellity P, Grybauskas V, Skolnik E M 1984 Metastatic neck disease: evaluation by computed tomography. Arch Otolaryngol 110: 443–447
22. Gerritsen G J, Valk J, van Velzen D J, Snow G B 1986 Computed tomography: a mandatory investigational procedure for the T-staging of advanced laryngeal cancer. Clin Otolaryngol 11: 307–316
23. Gold R I, Seeger L L, Bassett L W, Steckel R J 1990 An integrated approach to the evaluation of metastatic bone disease. Radiol Clin North Am 28: 471–483
24. Hajek P C, Salomonowitz E, Turk R, Tscholakoff D, Kumpan W, Czembirek H 1986 Lymph nodes of the neck: evaluation with US. Radiology 158: 739–742
25. Harbin W P 1982 Metastatic disease and the nonspecific bone scan: value of spinal computed tomography. Radiology 145: 105–109
26. Hibbert J, Marks N J, Winter P J, Shaheen O H 1983 Prognostic factors in oral squamous cell carcinoma and their relation to clinical staging. Clin Otolaryngol 8: 197–203
27. Hoover L A, Calcaterra T C, Walter G A, Larrson S G 1984 Preoperative C T-scan evaluation for laryngeal carcinoma: correlation with pathological findings. Laryngoscope 94: 310–315
28. Johansen L V, Overgaard J, Hjelm-Hansen M, Gadeberg C G 1990 Primary radiotherapy of T1 squamous cell carcinoma of the larynx: analysis of 478 patients treated from 1963 to 1985. Int J Radiat Oncol Biol Phys 6: 1307–1313
29. Kaiser T N, Sessions D G, Harvey J E 1989 Natural history of treated T1N0 squamous cell carcinoma of the glottis. Ann Otol Rhinol Laryngol 98: 217–219
30. Karim A B M F, Kralendonk J H, Yap L Y et al 1987 Heterogenity of stage II glottic carcinoma and its therapeutic implications. Int J Radiat Biol Phys 13: 313–317
31. Kirchner J A 1977 Two hundred laryngeal cancers: patterns of growth and spread as seen in serial sections. Laryngoscope 87: 474–479
32. Kotwall C, Sako K, Razack M S, Rao U, Bakamjian V, Shedd D P 1987 Metastatic patterns in squamous cell cancer of the head and neck. Am J Surg 154: 439–442
33. Krespi Y P, Meltzer C J 1989 Laser surgery for vocal cord carcinoma involving the anterior commissure. Ann Otol Rhinol Laryngol 98: 105–109
34. Mancuso A A, Harnsberger H R, Muraki A S, Stevens M H 1983 Computed tomography of cervical and retropharyngeal lymph nodes: normal anatomy, variants of normal, and applications in staging head and neck cancer. Part II: Pathology. Radiology 198: 715–723
35. Mancuso A A, Maceri D, Rice D, Hanafee W 1981 CT of cervical lymph node cancer. Am J Radiol 136: 381–385
36. Marks W M, Freeny P C 1988 Hepatic masses. In: Eisenberg R L (ed) Diagnostic imaging: an algorithmic approach. Lippincott, Philadelphia
37. Reid A P, Robin P E, Powell J, McConkey C C, Rockley T 1991 Staging carcinoma: its value in cancer of the larynx. J Laryngol Otol 105: 456–458

38. Robbins K T, Medina J E, Wolfe G T, Levine P A, Sessions R B, Pruet 1991 Standardizing neck dissection terminology — official report of the Academy's committee for head and neck surgery and oncology. Arch Otolaryngol Head Neck Surg 117: 601–605

39. Sako K, Pradier R N, Marchetta F C, Pickren J W 1964 Fallibility of palpation in the diagnosis of metastases to cervical nodes. Surg Gynecol Obstet 118: 989–990

40. Schaner E G, Chang A E, Doppman J L, Conkle D M, Flye M W, Rosenberg S A 1978 Comparison of computed and conventional whole lung tomography in detecting pulmonary nodules: a prospective radiologic–pathologic study. Am J Roentgenol 131: 51–54

41. Silverman P M, Bossen E H, Fisher S R, Cole T B, Korobkin M, Halvorsen R A 1984 Carcinoma of the larynx and hypopharynx: computed tomographic-histopathologic correlations. Radiology 151: 697–702

42. Snow G B 1989 Evaluation and staging of the patient with head and neck cancer. In: Myers E N, Suen J (eds) Cancer of the head and neck, 2nd edn. Churchill Livingstone, New York

43. Snow G B, Annyas A A, van Slooten E A, Bartelink H, Hart A A M 1982 Prognostic factors of neck node metastasis. Clin Otolaryngol 7: 185–192

44. Snow G B, Balm A J M, Arendse J W et al 1986 Prognostic factors in neck node metastases. In: Larson D L, Guillamondequi O M, Ballantyne A J (eds) Cancer in the neck. Evaluation and treatment. MacMillan, New York, pp 53–63

45. Spiro R H, Alfonso A E, Farr H W, Strong E W 1974 Cervical node metastasis from epidermoid carcinoma of the oral cavity and oropharynx. A critical assessment of current staging. Am J Surg 128: 562–567

46. Steckel R J, Kagan R A 1990 Pitfalls in the diagnosis of metastatic disease or local tumor extension with modern imaging techniques. Invest Radiol 25: 818–823

47. Stell P M, Morton R P, Singh S D 1983 Cervical-lymph node metastases. The significance of the level of the lymph node. Clin Oncol 9: 101–107

48. Stell P M, Dalby J E, Singh S D, Ramadan M F, Bainton R 1982 The management of glottic T3 carcinoma. Clin Otolaryngol 7: 175–180.

49. Stern W B R, Silver C E, Zeifer B A, Persky M S, Heller K S 1990 Computed tomography of the clinically negative neck. Head Neck 12: 109–113

50. Stevens H M, Harnsberger R, Mancuso A A, Davis R K, Johnson L P, Parkin J L 1985 Computed tomography of cervical lymph nodes staging and management of head and neck cancer. Arch Otolaryngol 111: 735–739

51. Union Internationale contre le Cancer (International Union against Cancer) 1987 TNM classification of malignant tumours, 4th edn. Springer-Verlag, Berlin

52. World Health Organization: ICD-O International Classification of Diseases for Oncology, 1st edn. 1976 WHO, Geneva

53. Yeager V L, Lawson C, Ancher C R 1982 Ossification of the laryngeal cartilages as it relates to computed tomography. Invest Radiol 17: 11–19

54. Zeitels S M, Vaughan Ch W 1991 Pre-epiglottic space invasion in 'early' epiglottic cancer. Ann Otol Rhinol Laryngol 100: 789–792

24. Perioperative medical considerations

W. E. Golden, R. C. Lavender

INTRODUCTION

Patients with head and neck cancer represent some of the most high-risk non-cardiac surgery patients in the hospital. The association of chronic alcohol and tobacco use with otolaryngological cancer, coupled with the increasing age of the general patient population, make the head and neck cancer patient likely to suffer from serious chronic conditions of the heart, lung and vascular systems. Careful preoperative assessment can identify risk-increasing medical conditions amenable to therapy, while attentive postoperative care should respond promptly to complications to avoid a prolonged and debilitating hospital stay. The following sections review important medical conditions and the principles of evaluation involved in the care of surgical patients with laryngeal cancer.

USE OF CONSULTANTS

Consultants serve different purposes for different physicians. Some surgeons request few medical evaluations and others consult several specialists on each patient.

A good perioperative consultation should be more than just a courtesy visit and should assist the surgeon and anaesthesiologist in the evaluation and treatment of an individual patient's medical conditions. Surgeons need to assess whether their clinical experience maintains, and their patterns of practice promote, the provision of efficient medical care in the postoperative period. It may be unrealistic for a busy surgeon to maintain sharp skills in the diagnosis and treatment of comorbid conditions beyond the site of abnormality. A comprehensive risk evaluation and postoperative follow-up in selected patients may help to avoid an occasional extended course. This strategy is particularly relevant in view of the increasing pressure on physicians and hospitals to reduce lengths of stay under prospective reimbursement programmes. A single holistic consultant can handle most perioperative situations. It could be useful for a surgeon to discuss with his medical consultants goals for their evaluations and thus clarify their role and responsibilities for his patients.[31] While we believe that a well-trained general internal-medicine physician can handle most perioperative problems, it is recommended that consultants be able and willing to evaluate the patient's general medical condition and avoid organ-specific consultation.[20]

EVALUATION OF MEDICAL RISKS — GENERAL PRINCIPLES

In addition to the treatment of unstable medical conditions, preoperative evaluations should assess the potential for postoperative complications. Obviously, risk needs to be weighed against the anticipated benefit of a procedure. Clinical prediction of risk, however, is not exact. Even if risk assessment were a precise exercise, the 'statistics' concerning a particular risk would not always be applicable to an individual patient. The anticipated benefit of a surgical procedure may not always be obvious. The head and neck cancer surgeon has the best understanding of the potential benefit and urgency of a particular procedure for a patient, and it is important that excellent communication exists, amongst the head and neck physician, internist, anaesthesiologist and other consultants. In addition to understanding the available literature concerning various risk factors and benefits of different surgical procedures, there is no substitute for a thorough history and physical examination. Furthermore, after an explanation of the risks and benefits of treatment, the patient's desires should always be taken into account.

PREOPERATIVE LABORATORY TESTS

In the final analysis, the most important aspect of preoperative evaluation is the history and physical examination. Several studies have demonstrated that routine preoperative screening laboratory tests, chest radiographs, and EKGs are not cost-effective in the healthy preoperative patient.[6,19,27,32,36] The best approach is to order screening tests based on the results of the history and physical examination and the nature of the proposed surgery. Obviously, a haemoglobin or haematocrit is indicated if major blood loss is anticipated during the surgery. Coagulation studies are not indicated in the absence of history or physical findings indicative of a bleeding disorder.[46] Patients with laryngeal cancer are frequently old and have chronic medical conditions reflecting chronic use of alcohol and/or tobacco products. Prior to a major operative procedure in this group of patients it would be useful to assess kidney function with a serum creatinine, liver integrity with serum amino-pepsidate and amino glutaminase, and glucose tolerance with a fasting or random glucose. A blood gas is often useful; pulmonary function tests themselves offer limited information.[25, 35] Because of the patient's malignancy, it would be wise to have a chest X-ray. Patients who have had previous neck surgery or radiation may need a TSH to rule out hypothyroidism connected with their disorder. Serum albumin is also a good indicator of the patient's preoperative nutritional status which has a major impact on the outcome of the planned procedure and post-operative management. Patients who have recently had chemotherapy may warrant more targeted haematological studies to assess the potential toxic effects of an intensive treatment regimen. EKGs in this population group are probably warranted for baseline purposes and to look for evidence of previous silent ischaemic events.

HYPERTENSION

Controlled hypertension is not itself a risk factor for surgery. Therefore, it is important that anti-hypertensive medications be continued throughout the perioperative period, including the surgery. Few medications cause concern.[12] Only guanethidine, a rarely used fourth-line antihypertensive drug, must be discontinued prior to an anaesthetic because it promotes storage of neuronal catecholamines and with anaesthetic agents can cause their massive, sudden release. Elective surgery should be postponed for one to two weeks after discontinuation of this drug. Patients who take potent diuretics should be assessed for volume depletion which can result in hypotension during the induction of anaesthesia.

Beta blockers can cause significant bradycardia, worsen heart failure, and promote bronchospasm and respiratory decompensation during the perioperative period. Physicians need to be alert for the onset of these complications. Nevertheless, the advantages of these drugs far outweigh their potential problems for most surgical patients. Patients with laryngeal cancer who also have chronic obstructive pulmonary disease are probably best served by being on an antihypertensive other than beta blockers. Angiotensive converting enzyme drugs can promote a dry cough which can be confusing in patients

with pulmonary disease or laryngeal irritation. Patients with persistent 'bronchitis' who take ace inhibitor drugs might be tried on a different agent to assess the potential for diminishing the symptoms.

Patients with longstanding, moderate hypertension should be evaluated for the presence of coexisting diseases. In particular, it is common for such individuals to have hypertrophic heart failure, atherosclerotic vascular disease, or chronic renal insufficiency. These entities are even more likely to be present if the patient smokes, has diabetes, or has a history of non-compliance with medications.

Occasional preoperative patients will present to the hospital with poorly controlled hypertension. It is important to ensure that these high readings were determined with a blood pressure cuff of appropriate size; if the occlusive bladder is less than two-thirds the circumference of the patient's arm, the recorded hypertension can be significantly erroneous. Current medical literature has failed to document increased morbidity or mortality in patients whose preoperative diastolic blood pressure is under 110.[22] Data are inconclusive for the risk to patients with more severe hypertension, but it is prudent to lower the pressure prior to the procedure. Patients with uncontrolled hypertension are relatively volume-depleted, and their blood pressure can be unpredictable under the influence of anaesthesia. Patients with ischaemic heart disease or congestive failure can have these risks reduced by control of blood pressure.

Studies attribute postoperative complications to intra-operative hypotensive and hypertensive episodes. We recommend several days of control prior to a non-emergent procedure in patients with diastolic pressures greater than 120. Rapid control is often easily attained with the use of long-acting calcium channel blockers. One must keep in mind that different types of antihypertensive agent will work differently in different ethnic groups of patients. For example, beta blockers and angiotensive converting enzyme inhibitors are somewhat less effective in black patients and should not be used if rapid control of preoperative hypertension is the goal. Asian patients, on the other hand, are very responsive to beta blockers. Clearly, patients with severe elevations of blood pressure or encephalopathic changes should not be taken directly to the operating room unless faced with dire surgical emergencies.

It is not uncommon for patients on chronic diuretic therapy to have reduced levels of serum potassium on arrival at the hospital. It is important to keep in mind that levels below 3.0–3.3 meq/ℓ may reflect loss of potassium, not just from the intravascular volume but also from intracellular stores.[51] Accordingly, a potassium level under 3 meq/ℓ reflects a significant total body depletion of potassium and could pose a risk of cardiac rhythm instability, particularly in patients with occult coronary disease. Strenuous efforts should be made to bring potassium levels above 3.0–3.3 meq/ℓ, and it may be necessary to postpone surgery for 1–3 days in order to do so.

Acute postoperative hypertension may reflect from several different conditions. In the early postoperative period, pain, fluid overload, emergence from anaesthesia, or airway obstruction can be causative factors. Patients should be evaluated for such acute reversible causations prior to the institution of parenteral antihypertensives. Most acute episodes respond to pain medications or diuresis. Should antihypertensive medicine be necessary, care should be taken to lower blood pressure in a controlled fashion, especially in the older patient. Abrupt reduction can cause stroke or cardiac ischaemia. Parenteral hydralazine in 5–10 mg doses can be effective, as is the liquid component of nifedipine capsules in 10–20 mg doses. Recent experience shows that intravenous beta blockade, with e.g. Esmolol or Labetalol, is also effective in the control of perioperative hypertension and can help reduce associated tachycardia; if used, these agents must be used with care in patients with chronic lung disease. Intravenous methyldopa does not become effective until a few hours after the initial dose and should not be used in an acute situation. Other parenteral agents are available, but they should not be used without consultation or previous experience.

Hypertensive patients who are unable to take medications by mouth during the postoperative period can pose a therapeutic and logistical challenge. The development of a weekly transdermal catapres patch can now obviate the need for parenteral therapy. This transdermal medication takes approximately 36 hours to reach effective serum levels, so it should be placed on the patient on the night prior to the surgical procedure. It is available in three strengths, and the appropriate dosage should reflect the severity of the underlying condition.

CARDIAC DISEASE

In 1977 Goldman et al published an article identifying cardiac risk factors for non-cardiac surgery.[23] Their retrospective study of 1001 non-cardiac surgery patients identified nine independent risk factors for life-threatening and fatal cardiac complications: age >70; myocardial infarction within six months; S3 gallop or jugular venous distension; significant aortic stenosis; dysrhythmias; >5 PVCs/minute; debilitated medical condition; emergency surgery; and intraperitoneal or intrathoracic surgery. Each of these risk factors received a relative point value for a total of 53 possible points. A few subsequent studies have validated or modified this index slightly to take into account severe angina or prior pulmonary oedema.[13–15] The Goldman[23] risk index appears to underestimate cardiac risk in the geriatric population.

Nevertheless, strict use of the cardiac risk index is probably not useful on a case-by-case basis. Most of the point totals reflect uncompensated congestive heart failure or recent myocardial infarction. One must assess the relative risk of each patient to the possible benefit of the surgery. Furthermore, many investigators now admit that few patients are seen in the preoperative setting with high point totals given these traditional risk indices. Indeed, the search is underway using large patient data sets to refine and identify new factors associated with postoperative morbidity and prolonged hospital stays.

Given the limitation of these risk indices, it is clear that cardiac risk assessment must focus on the data from a detailed history and physical examination. The examiner should focus on the present and past patterns of angina, exercise reserve, orthopnoea, palpitations, previous myocardial infarction, and the use of cardiac medications. Physical examination must evaluate hypertension, rhythm disturbance, signs of congestive heart failure, the presence of murmurs, an S3, and peripheral oedema.

Angina

Chronic stable angina has not been shown to represent a major risk factor for non-cardiac surgery. Nevertheless, anaesthetic technique and postoperative bedside surveillance must take the presence of coronary artery disease into account. Elective non-cardiac surgery should be postponed in patients with unstable angina until the condition is better managed.

Several studies have shown that in patients with previous CABG undergoing non-cardiac surgery, the operative mortality is close to what it is for the population as a whole.[34] Even though patients with previous CABG have a small risk of cardiac complications, this fact is not an argument for performing a CABG in patients with heart disease before non-cardiac surgery unless it is otherwise indicated. It should be remembered that there is some morbidity and mortality from CABG, especially in the elderly.

Occasionally patients are in such a frail condition that it is extremely difficult to assess exercise reserve and its ability to induce symptomatic angina pectoris. These individuals could well benefit from a dipyrimidole thallium test to assess the presence of reversible cardiac ischaemia. In addition, Doppler flow echocardiograms can identify significant valvular dysfunction as well as ejection fraction in patients whose cardiac output is unclear from history and physical examination.

In all anginal patients it is important to maintain anti-anginal therapy during the perioperative period. Beta blockers, nitrates and calcium channel blockers should be continued up to and including the morning of surgery. Topical nitroglycerine in the form of patches or paste can be particularly effective when applied on call to the OR to provide long-acting nitrate pharmacodynamics during the operative procedure. Modified-V5-lead cardiac monitoring can identify intraoperative ischaemia which often responds to IV nitroglycerine. If the patient is unable to take oral medications on the day after surgery, topical nitrates, sublingual nifedipine, and IV beta blockers can be helpful. Overnight monitoring in ICU settings is prudent in patients with fragile coronary artery disease. Serial EKG and cardiac enzymes help to identify early potential myocardial infarctions in this select subset of postoperative patients and lead to aggressive management of haemodynamic status prior to a serious cardiovascular collapse.[33]

Myocardial infarction

The risk of a postoperative myocardial infarction (MI) in adults is 0.2–2%. Studies have stratified the risk of a new postoperative MI in patients with previous infarctions by the time from the first event:

MI in previous 3 months: 30%
MI in previous 4–6 months: 15%
MI more than 6 months previously: 5%

Postponing surgery longer than six months does not result in a further decline in risk of reinfarction below 5%. The use of intraoperative invasive monitoring (A line and Swan Ganz catheter), and the use of newer drugs such as fentanyl, and cardiovascular drips, have probably lowered the risk in patients 1–6 months after a new MI.[41, 45] Nevertheless, great caution needs to be used in approaching a preoperative patient within one month of an infarction.

It is still prudent, however, to delay elective surgery until six months after an MI. If surgery is necessary in a patient with a recent MI, intraoperative haemodynamic monitoring should be utilized. In a semi-elective surgery, such as a patient with a malignancy that may not be resectable for a cure if surgery is postponed too long, each case needs to be individualized with regard to risk of postponement and assessment of other risk factors. Generally speaking, the urgent case can probably be performed as early as four weeks after a MI in the otherwise low-risk patient if appropriate precautions, planning, and monitoring are used.

A postoperative MI presents differently from that in an ambulatory patient: over 50% of cases do not manifest chest pain. Postoperative MI should be suspected in the patient with new-onset congestive heart failure, hypotension, or significant arrhythmias. Although an MI may occur intraoperatively due to stress of surgery, transient hypotension, or hypoxia, most studies report a peak incidence between the third and fifth postoperative days. Thus, patients with significant cardiac disease should be

carefully followed during the first postoperative week and assessed with electrocardiograms and cardiac isoenzymes at the first sign of impaired cardiovascular haemodynamics, even in the absence of chest pain.

Congestive heart failure

Uncompensated congestive heart failure has been found to be one of the greatest risk factors in non-cardiac surgery. Patients with uncontrolled heart failure should have all but emergent procedures postponed. Several days are usually required optimally to compensate a patient with moderate to severe congestive heart failure and to ensure that there are not side-effects of therapy such as intravascular volume depletion from over-diuresis, electrolyte abnormalities and digitalis toxicity. Factors which adversely effect cardiac performance should be searched for and corrected. Patients with perioperative congestive heart failure should be followed by a medical consultant.[5]

Valvular heart disease

Most patients with mild valvular disease present no special problems except endocarditis prophylaxis. The cardiac conditions for which endocarditis prophylaxis is recommended are listed in Table 24.1.

Significant aortic stenosis is an independent risk factor for perioperative cardiac death. Patients with critical aortic stenosis are dependent on preload to maintain cardiac output, and the loss of preload associated with the induction and maintenance of anaesthesia can produce fatal cardiac depression and unresponsive cardiac arrest.

Differentiation of important aortic stenosis from a murmur of aortic sclerosis may not always be possible from the history and physical examination. Standard M mode and two-dimensional echocardiography are insufficient to assess pressure gradients across a calcified aortic valve. Doppler echocardiography is necessary to identify critical aortic valves without cardiac catheterization.[11] Patients with haemodynamically significant aortic stenosis should have valve replacement or valvuloplasty before elective surgery. One recent study contradicted this clinical rule, but it emphasized precise haemodynamic control perioperatively.[37] Although other valvular lesions have not been proven to be independent risk factors

Table 24.1 Cardiac conditions for which endocarditis prophylaxis is recommended

Prosthetic heart valves
Congenital malformations
Surgical left-to-right shunt
Acquired valvular lesions
IHSS
History of endocarditis
Mitral prolapse with insufficiency

for fatal outcomes, many of these patients have other documented risk factors and can require careful attention to perioperative fluid management.

It is very important to identify patients with idiopathic hypertrophic subaortic stenosis. These patients are often asymptomatic, but have the characteristic harsh systolic murmur that is maximum at the lower left sternal border. The murmur is augmented when preload is reduced by having the patient stand or perform a valsalva manoeuvre —the opposite of the findings in patients with aortic stenosis or flow murmurs. Perioperative risk is low given the avoidance of conditions and drugs that decrease preload or increase myocardial contractility.[48]

The management of anticoagulation in patients with prosthetic heart valves is discussed elsewhere in this chapter.

Arrhythmias

Chronic preoperative dysrhythmias are associated with increased perioperative morbidity and mortality.[13] Most arrhythmias reflect the presence of underlying cardiac disease rather than unstable electrical systems. Underscoring this concept, the elimination of preoperative arrhythmias by pharmacological intervention has not been shown to reduce the operative risk identified by such arrhythmias. For example, a young, healthy patient with frequent PVCs but without evidence of underlying cardiomyopathy is not thought to be at increased risk for surgery. However, an older patient with arrhythmias should be carefully assessed for the presence of a significant cardiac condition. In these patients, one should be alert for undiagnosed, reversible clinical states such as electrolyte disturbances, drug toxicity, or congestive heart failure.

Intraoperative dysrhythmias are fairly common, but generally transient and benign. They rarely require antiarrhythmic treatment and usually respond to correction of the underlying cause or change in anaesthetic management. Postoperative dysrhythmias are more worrisome, but are often associated with minor postoperative complications and usually are not directly the cause of morbidity or mortality. Careful observation, fluid management and screening for infarctions are often appropriate.

Conduction abnormalities and pacemakers

A preoperative pacemaker is indicated in complete heart block, symptomatic sinus node dysfunction and Mobitz type II AV block. Left or right bundle-branch block or first degree AV block is not associated with an increased risk of perioperative complete heart block. Thus, these EKG abnormalities do not require perioperative temporary pacemakers in the absence of other arrhythmias or symptoms.

Elderly patients can present with asymptomatic sick-

sinus syndrome. Typically this condition manifests itself as a sinus bradycardia with bursts of supraventricular tachycardia. Ambulatory patients are not treated with a pacemaker unless symptomatic. Nevertheless, the literature does not document the safety of sinus node dysfunction under anaesthesia. Most patients do well with no therapy, but a transcutaneous pacemaker or central venous port should be available in case of refractory bradycardia.

Patients with permanent pacemakers are at increased risk only to the extent that they have underlying heart disease. Pacemaker type, rate, and proper function should be known before surgery. Electrocautery can potentially cause pacemaker dysfunction, and care should be taken to shield the pacemaker and place the ground plate well away from the pulse generator.

Carotid and peripheral vascular disease

Carotid bruits, if asymptomatic, do not require evaluation prior to non-cardiac surgery. There are no data documenting the safety of extensive neck resection in patients with carotid bruits. Clearly, the choice of patient for this technique must reflect the amount of tissue manipulation required and the skill of the individual surgeon. Non-invasive duplex scanning of carotid arteries has demonstrated that the presence of a bruit is not predictive of the severity of carotid disease. Indeed, the more severe lesions are often found in carotid arteries without the presence of a bruit. Nevertheless, current literature states that asymptomatic carotid bruits are not a risk factor for perioperative stroke but rather reflect the presence of diffuse atherosclerosis and the probability of significant occult coronary disease.[30, 43] Appropriate precautions should be taken to manage these patients with coronary artery impairments.

Patients who have symptomatic transient ischaemic attacks should be evaluated preoperatively with duplex scanning. These individuals could be at risk for perioperative stroke, and the severity of their lesions should be documented and appropriate therapy carried out.

In patients with asymptomatic lesions, it might be wise for a duplex scan to occur at some point in the patient's management. Evidence suggests repair of severely stenosed carotid arteries does improve patient outcome. Nevertheless, this work-up is not necessary in the preoperative setting for conditions other than the carotid artery lesion itself.

Summary — reduction of cardiac risk

Out of a possible 53 points in Goldman's risk index, 31 are potentially correctable. The risk factors worth the most points are an S-3 or a jugular venous distension— both indicative of significant congestive heart failure. Most authorities would agree that operative risk is reduced by aggressive therapy of congestive heart failure. On the other hand, suppressing preoperative arrhythmia probably does not reduce operative risk. It is important to document a recent myocardial infarction so that elective surgery can either be cancelled or urgent surgery be performed with the assistance of invasive haemodynamic monitoring. Critical aortic stenosis should be detected and corrected before elective surgery.

Attempts should be made to correct a patient's impaired non-cardiac medical conditions. As a rule, elective surgery should not be performed unless the anticipated benefit outweighs the estimated risk.

PREOPERATIVE PULMONARY EVALUATION

The evaluation of respiratory status preoperatively includes important historical aspects such as dyspnoea, wheezing, cough, sputum production, smoking habits, and prior history of pulmonary disease. On physical examination, it should be noted whether expiration is prolonged and whether wheezing, rhonchi, or crackles are present. Even with meticulous perioperative pulmonary care, some degree of atelectasis will occur with inhalational or epidural anaesthetic techniques, and breathing capacity will decrease postoperatively.[10]

Traditional perioperative literature recommends many indications for preoperative pulmonary function testing. Although the ideal study may never be done, most investigators believe that preoperative pulmonary function testing offers little in the management of non-thoracic surgery patients. Few authorities believe in a prohibitive pulmonary function test that absolutely rules out future surgery. In general, it is wise to assess the risk of postoperative morbidity in relationship to the benefits of the proposed surgery. Clearly, as FEV_1 goes below 750 ml the likelihood of postoperative morbidity from respiratory failure or postoperative pneumonia increases. In such patients, it is wise to discuss the risks amongst the surgical team, the anaesthesiologists, the medical consultant and the patients and his family prior to making a final determination about the wisdom of proposed surgery. In general, we use preoperative pulmonary function tests only to identify those high-risk pulmonary patients for whom we are giving strong consideration to the possibility that the pulmonary risks exceed the benefits of the procedure.

The patient's history of exercise tolerance, or personal observation of the patient walking down the hallway or up a flight of stairs is most useful preoperatively to assess pulmonary reserve.[38] Although a single best laboratory pulmonary function test to predict postoperative complications has not been agreed upon, measurement of FEV_1 and FVC, or of peak flow rates, is usually determined. Unfortunately, the correlation between pulmonary risk and spirometric value is not defined, and no specific values of pulmonary functions tests absolutely contra-indicate surgery. In reviewing a patient's PFTs, it is probably best to look at the percentage of predicted performance rather than absolute values of spirometry. The risk of major respiratory complications, including respiratory insufficiency, increases with an FEV_1 of less than 20% of the predicted value. Obviously, spirometry is of limited value in patients with airway obstruction secondary to a head and neck cancer.

Although arterial blood gases may help to assess risk, they can be invaluable for baseline data purposes. Knowing the patien's chronic p_aO_2 and p_aCO_2 helps in setting goals for oxygen therapy in the postoperative period. Arterial blood gases should be obtained in patients with obvious pulmonary disease, elderly patients, and patients with moderate to severely affected pulmonary function tests.

Several studies have shown that pulmonary complications after general anaesthesia are decreased with incentive spirometry, chest physiotherapy, and a variety of combined modalities. Table 24.2 lists therapeutic manoeuvres that decrease postoperative pulmonary complications. Despite poor patient compliance, the surgical candidate should be instructed to stop smoking at least two months before surgery.[53] Cessation for only one to two days preoperatively is probably less effective.

Patients with asthma should have their bronchodilators continued during the perioperative period.[28] Even if the patient does not routinely use aerosolized bronchodilators at home, inhalers should be used perioperatively. An aminophylline level can be checked preoperatively, and intravenous aminophyline can be used to obtain a therapeutic level. Patients with a history of severe asthma, severe bronchospasm, or prolonged steroid use within the last year should receive intravenous steroids. This steroid treatment should be started several hours before surgery to achieve a tissue effect. The induction of anaesthesia combined with the manipulation of the oropharynx during intubation are potent stimuli for bronchospasm. Thus, good blood levels of methylxanthines and aggressive use of aerosolized agents prior to arrival in the operating room can be useful in patients with fragile airway control. Most general anaesthetics are bronchodilators and, therefore, serve intraoperatively to reduce the propensity to bronchospasm. Nevertheless, as the effect of the anaesthetic diminishes in the postoperative

Table 24.2 Manoeuvres which decrease pulmonary risk

Preoperative cessation of cigarette smoking
Antibiotic treatment of pulmonary infection
Preoperative teaching of respiratory manoeuvres
Preoperative bronchodilators for asthmatics
Minimization of postoperative narcotic analgesia
Maximization of inspiration
Early postoperative mobilization

period, the patient may be at risk for severe bronchospasm, particularly if there are retained oropharyngeal secretions or postoperative airway irritation from tracheostomy or endobronchial tubes.

THROMBOEMBOLIC DISORDERS

Risk factors for venous thromboembolism are advanced age, previous venous thromboembolism, prolonged immobility, malignancy, obesity, oral contraceptive use, and congestive heart failure. The risk has not been well documented for most head and neck procedures but it is undoubtedly lower than that for other surgeries where postoperative ambulation does not occur as early as in the head and neck patient. However, deep-vein thrombosis prophylaxis should be considered, especially if more than one risk factor mentioned above is present.

Graduated compression stockings are inexpensive, easy to use, and can be combined with other methods of prophylaxis. However, they are probably effective only in low-risk patients. Low-dose heparin has been shown to be effective in the moderate- to high-risk general surgery patient. It is given in a dose of 5000 units subcutaneously two hours before surgery and then every 8–12 hours thereafter.[8, 9, 52] Although there is concern about bleeding, the better designed studies have shown no clinically significantly increased risk of bleeding.

Postoperative patients at times require prolonged use of an intravenous catheter placed in the subclavian vein or superior vena cava. It has been increasingly recognized that such venous access promotes thrombosis of these veins with resultant oedema of an affected upper extremity. A recent study demonstrated that the use of coumadin 1 mg p.o.q. day, while not altering levels of coagulation factors, did succeed in dramatically lowering the incidence of subclavian and superior vena cava thrombosis in patients with such intravenous catheterization.[4]

Patients with prosthetic heart valves who require surgery should be evaluated by a medical consultant. For patients with newer models of prosthetic valves, there is a low risk of embolization if coumadin is stopped a few days preoperatively and the patient goes to surgery with an INR of approximately 1.2. We recommend restarting the coumadin on the postoperative night unless there are episodes of prolonged bleeding from the surgical site. Patients who are at high risk for thromboembolism, such as patients with prosthetic mitral valves, might well benefit from discontinuation of coumadin and the use of a heparin drip pre- and postoperatively. The heparin drip has the advantage of allowing for complete anticoagulation which can be reversed within 4 hours after the discontinuation of the drip. Use of the coumadin perioperatively is recommended as it is increasingly recommended that lower doses of the drug are effective in reducing thromboembolism and careful use of the drug

can eliminate the need for a heparin drip during the perioperative period.

COAGULATION DISORDERS

Nearly all patients with a coagulation disorder can be identified from historical data. Individuals who had a previously normal prothrombin and partial thromboplastin time or who have a negative past medical history for spontaneous bleeding or postoperative haemorrhage are unlikely to have a congenital coagulopathy. Nevertheless, in patients with serious medical disorders, the examiners must also screen for coagulation impairments.

Patients taking warfarin should discontinue this medication 3–4 days before elective surgery. Coordination with a medical consultant several days prior to the chosen operative date usually improves the coordination of care and the reduction in risk of perioperative haemorrhage or thrombosis secondary to the medical condition for which the patient was taking anticoagulant medicines. Patients who are on warfarin and require emergency surgery can have their vitamin-K-dependent clotting factor returned to normal with large doses of fresh frozen plasma with or without the supplementation of subcutaneous vitamin K.

Platelet dysfunction can also result in perioperative bleeding. Aspirin causes permanent dysfunction of a platelet and requires greater than one week of elimination of the drug to restore functioning platelets to the circulation. Nevertheless, patients who are on low-dose aspirin therapy are not at significant risk for postoperative haemorrhage. Rather, studies in patients undergoing cardiac surgery have found that, on average, they require only one extra unit of packed red blood cells in transfusion for these major cases.[47] Other non-steroidal anti-inflammatory drugs cause a defect in platelet aggregation that is more readily reversible, and the effects of these medications can be reversed within 48 hours of discontinuation.

Patients with inherited clotting deficiencies (such as haemophilia) have usually sought medical attention for bleeding and are well aware of their disease.[16]

Patients with severe hepatocellular disease as a cause of a prolonged prothrombin time will not respond to vitamin K and will require fresh frozen plasma if the prothrombin time is greater than three seconds above the control. Also, disseminated intravascular coagulation (usually secondary to infection or malignancy) can cause an elevated prothrombin time. Patients with severe malabsorption or malnutrition can have vitamin K deficiency as an aetiology of a prolonged prothrombin time.

The most common iatrogenic cause of an elevated PTT is heparin therapy. Heparin has a half-life that is quite variable in different individuals, but is usually approximately 60 minutes. Therefore, if surgery can be postponed for 4–6 hours, stopping the heparin may be all that is necessary to return the partial thromboplastin time to normal. For emergency surgery, protamine sulphate can acutely reverse the effects of heparin. Patients with lupus anticoagulant have an elevated PTT, but rarely have clinically significant bleeding abnormalities.

ENDOCRINE DISORDERS

Only a few of the many varied endocrinological disease processes are encountered with frequency on the head and neck service. Accordingly, concentration should be focused on diabetic, thyroid and adrenal dysfunction as these conditions will comprise nearly the entirety of one's exposure to endocrinological problems.

Diabetes mellitus

Diabetes mellitus is now classified as either requiring or not requiring insulin in its management. In the older population groups, most diabetics will be non-insulin-dependent and pose fewer management problems. If a patient with diabetes has good control of the blood sugar by dietary and oral hypoglycaemic agents, most authorities advise discontinuing the oral agent one or two days prior to surgery depending on the half-life of the agent in use. Earlier discontinuation is particularly important for patients on chlorpropamide, as this agent has a very long half-life and can promote the syndrome of inappropriate antidiuretic hormone secretion. In fact, chlorpropamide's awkward pharmacokinetics and side-effects make it an undesirable choice for long-term management of an elderly, diabetic patient.

While uncontrolled diabetes has been shown to impair wound healing and promote postoperative infections, tight control during the surgical procedure puts the patient at risk for hypoglycaemia under anaesthesia. The potential neurological sequelae of this event dictates a preference for looser control of the blood glucose during the operative day. While the preoperative orders for a diabetic are often managed by the anaesthesiologist, several different techniques are acceptable for the non-insulin-dependent patient. Perhaps the simplest technique is to withhold the oral agent on the day of surgery, give non-glucose-containing intravenous fluids during the procedure, and check a glucose level in the recovery room. Withholding insulin and glucose is also effective for the non-brittle patient on insulin who can alternatively be managed by giving half the usual daily intermediate acting insulin, withholding short-acting preparations, and maintaining the patient on a glucose-containing intravenous drip. Most patients will not suffer impressive increases in blood glucose, and modest increases detected in the recovery room can be managed by 5–15 units of regular subcutaneous insulin. Follow-up care should monitor glucose readings every 6 hours until regular

caloric intake is resumed. Patients who fail to resume their normal intake postoperatively and who receive their chronic insulin dosage could suffer symptomatic hypoglycaemia.

Patients with longstanding insulin-dependent diabetes or brittle diabetes require extra attention. Brittle diabetics can suffer pronounced swings in their glycaemic control and can develop ketoacidosis under stress. Intraoperative monitoring of blood sugars is necessary to assure good management. Such patients should preferably have their procedures carried out early in the morning to avoid long waiting periods without oral intake. The use of portable glucose monitors in the operating suites enhances management efficiency.

Older patients with a 20- or 30-year history of diabetes have an increased likelihood of atherosclerotic disease, especially of the smaller vessels of the heart. It is probably wise to manage them as if they had diffuse coronary artery disease, even without historical symptoms of angina or congestive failure as many diabetics have clinically silent episodes of myocardial ischaemia.

Urinary measurements of glucose and ketones are not sufficiently consistent for good postoperative assessment. Patients will spill differing amounts of glucose in their urine, depending on their degree of renal insufficiency. It is far more accurate to obtain serum glucose or finger-stick determinations once a day for patients on oral agents, or at 8 am and 4 pm determinations for individuals on insulin. Sliding-scale insulin administration based on urine levels can result in inappropriate therapy and is not recommended.

In the postoperative period, physicians need to be alert for the occasional patient who develops diabetic keto-acidosis or hyperosmolarity. Warning signs of developing ketoacidosis include a decline in p_aCO_2 levels with normal pH on arterial blood gases, a harbinger of developing metabolic acidosis. Hyperosmolarity is seen in non-insulin-dependent patients; it consists of very high glucose levels and dehydration from a profound secondary osmotic diuresis. Both conditions require aggressive rehydration and judicious administration of insulin.

A large number of patients who have had surgery for laryngeal cancer will receive tube feedings during the postoperative recovery period. Management of diabetes in these individuals is especially tricky. The high carbohydrate content of most commercial tube feeding will result in significant elevations of blood glucose. Even patients who are normally controlled on oral hypoglycaemics will invariably require insulin for management. Since most tube-feeding regimens are based on a continuous feeding schedule, these patients receive a constant flow of calories throughout the day. As a result, it is frequently useful to split the entire day's insulin into two or three equal doses and deliver the material on a q.12 or q.8 hour basis. Traditional split-dose insulin techniques, in which two-thirds of the daily dose of NPH in given in the mornings, will not suffice because of this continuous caloric challenge. Blood sugar measurements every 6 hours are necessary until a stable regimen of long-acting insulin is devised.

Thyroid

Many patients with laryngeal cancer have had partial or total removal of thyroid tissue or have undergone radiation therapy to the neck. As a consequence, such patients need to be evaluated for possible hypo-thyroidism. Most clinical studies show that mild hypo-thyroidism is not a contraindication to surgery, but the more profound, chronic cases are associated with conges-tive heart failure, bradycardia, pericardial effusion, and poor wound healing. Ladenson reported that hypothyroid patients have a higher incidence of intraoperative hypo-tension and postoperative intestinal atony as well as a decreased ability to mount a febrile response.[29]

Nevertheless, rapid repletion of thyroid hormone is potentially dangerous in older individuals as large doses of thyroid hormone can aggravate angina pectoris, heart failure and occasionally overtax existing pituitary adreno-cortical reserve. Therefore, repletion in severe hypo-thyroidism should start with small doses of thyroid hormone to be increased over 2–4 weeks of therapy (surgery should be postponed if at all possible). Indivi-duals with clinically profound hypothyroidism and those who require emergency surgery are best seen in consul-tation with a medical consultant.[3]

Critically ill or debilitated patients can suffer from low serum thyroxine levels with normal thyroid-stimulating-hormone levels. This 'euthyroid sick' syndrome has several postulated aetiologies, but it does not require administration of exogenous thyroid replacement hor-mone. In fact such additional thyroid hormone could exacerbate the patient's catabolic state.

Adrenal

It is wise to assume that patients who are chronically taking corticosteroids have suppression of the adrenal–pituitary axis. Indeed, patients taking prednisone in doses as low as 7.5 mg/day for 2 weeks can have adrenal suppression for up to 6 months after the discontinuation of the drug. To avoid the possibility of acute adrenal insufficiency in the postoperative period, most clinicians have administered corticosteroids in doses equivalent to the maximum output of an intact adrenal system under stress. There is evidence in animal models that patients may require only physiological dosing and thus we may see a trend to reducing the dosage of perioperative steroids in these patients.[50] We recommend giving 100 mg intravenous hydrocortisone on call to the operating room and an additional 100 mg during the operation. Patients who are critically ill or are suffering from severe infection require the full 300 mg of hydrocortisone q.day. Most patients do not need such large replacement, neither do they need a tapering dose schedule after the operation unless complications have occurred. If a patient can take oral medications we generally restart the usual oral dose schedule on the first postoperative day unless the patient has persistent ongoing stress because of postoperative complications. For patients without oral intake, we would give between 100 and 200 mg of hydrocortisone on the first postoperative day and strive for a rapid tapering to the usual equivalent oral dose.

INFECTIOUS DISEASE

In the postoperative period, surgical drains, intravenous catheters, and urinary catheters should not be left in place any longer than is necessary. Proper catheter insertion technique and careful hand-washing by personnel involved in patient care should also be emphasized.

There are many causes of postoperative fever. Table 24.3 lists some of the more common causes.

A low-grade self-limited fever is common after major surgery. A temperature greater than 101° Fahrenheit, however, warrants bedside evaluation to search for the cause. The patient should be questioned about dysuria, productive cough, rigors, and episodes of aspiration. The management of postoperative fever depends upon the findings on history and physical examination, degree of temperature elevation, and the clinical status of the patient. With low-grade temperature elevation (less than 101°), incentive spirometry, checking intravenous catheter sites and discontinuing all non-critical medications may be all that is required. Head and neck surgery patients are prone to postoperative retention or aspiration of se-cretions in the tracheobronchial tree, and they need aggressive pulmonary toilet. Febrile patients who do not have a diagnosis for their fever should not receive anti-pyretics which could mask a continued problem. We therefore avoid the use of Tylenol during the period of diagnostic uncertainty.

Persistent temperature elevation greater than 101° in a patient who appears clinically ill warrants a CBC with differential, chest radiograph, and blood and urine cul-tures even if no obvious source is present on examination.

Table 24.3 Common aetiologies of postoperative fever

Noninfectious	Infectious
Atelectasis	Wound
Medications	Urinary tract infections
Blood transfusions	Bronchitis
Drug or ethanol withdrawal	Pneumonia
Thromboembolism	Septic IV catheter phlebitis
Catheter phlebitis	

In these patients with high fever who do not have an obvious pneumonia or urinary tract infection, consideration should be given to the following diagnosis: chemical phlebitis from an IV catheter, deep venous thrombosis, wound abscess, drug reaction, postoperative hepatitis, seroma, haematoma, and intestinal ileus.

Patients infected with the AIDS virus require cautious handling of body fluids to avoid infection of health-care personnel. Head and neck surgeons are exposed to aerosolized oral secretions and are advised to wear goggles in the care of patients infected with HIV[18, 39, 40] or of all patients if the demographics of the community bespeaks a significant incidence of silent infection with the AIDS virus.

RENAL AND ELECTROLYTE DISORDERS

Anaesthetic agents pose little threat of toxicity to the renal system. Perioperative concern, therefore, focuses on documenting the extent of perioperative physiological reserve and the awareness of the effects of potentially toxic medications during the recovery period. Glomerular filtration declines with age, and elderly patients may have normal serum creatinine levels with only one-third of normal renal function. This decline should be considered when scheduling the amount and interval of nephrotoxic medications.

Inhalational anaesthetics cause a loss of preload by a variety of mechanisms and thus profound hypotension can result in patients who are mildly dehydrated. Care should be taken to assess fluid status of operative candidates, particularly elderly individuals who have been victims of trauma. Causes of postoperative hypotension include dehydration, unreplaced blood loss, sustained effects of operative medications, allergic reactions, sepsis, and diminished myocardial function. Lack of response to a brisk fluid challenge should result in an immediate, aggressive diagnostic evaluation.

Postoperative oliguria can cause diagnostic and therapeutic dilemmas. Concern should not be overt until the urine output is consistently below 20–25 ml of urine per hour. It is helpful to obtain a spot specimen of urine for sodium and osmolarity prior to the initiation of diuretics which themselves rarely treat the underlying abnormality but merely increase urine output on a transitory basis. Loop diuretics alter urine sodium excretion even in the face of significant fluid depletion and can interfere with diagnostic decision making for almost 24 hours. Most episodes of oliguria reflects temporary decreases in intravascular volume secondary to intraoperative extracorporeal fluid losses. Therefore, additional crystalloid administration, or, if the patient has already received large quantities of saline solutions, judicious use of colloid materials such as albumin or hetastarch, can improve intravascular volume and thus renal homeostasis.

Patients whose oliguria does not respond either to fluid challenge or to 1.5 mg/kg of furosemide, or who progress to anuria, require aggressive medical management and consultation.

Hyponatraemia is also not an uncommon perioperative occurrence and usually stems from one of two causes: dilution or inappropriate secretion of antidiuretic hormone (ADH). Dilution can reflect replacement of lost intravascular volume by non-physiological concentrations of saline solutions. It is difficult to replete sodium losses by intravenous solutions that are not at least half normal in strength. Urine sodium concentration in this situation is very low and reflects efficient conservation by the kidney of sodium stores. Institution of a slow infusion of normal saline can correct the imbalance in one or two days. Inappropriate secretion of ADH results in relatively high secretion of urinary sodium and a relative excess of intravascular free water. Most patients respond to simple fluid restriction over a period of several days. Response can be frustratingly slow and may benefit from the addition of supplemental medications such as demeclocycline. Both conditions can feature serum sodium levels in the low 120s but seizures and neurological impairment usually do not occur unless the sodium decreases has been rapid or profound (<120). Aggressive partial repletion of profound hyponatraemia minimizes the risk of residual neurological injury.[2]

An occasional patient will have ongoing fluid losses from high-volume urine output or drainage sites. It is advisable to obtain fluid from the site of loss to determine the composition of electrolytes of the lost secretions in order to plan appropriate concentrations of compensatory intravenous fluids.

HAEMOPOIETIC DISORDERS

Anaemia

A patient with anaemia should have the aetiology identified before elective surgery. Few cases of anaemia of chronic disease feature a haematocrit lower than 29%. Therefore, blood counts lower than 29% in patients without a history of blood loss or renal failure should have the aetiology delineated prior to transfusion and surgery. If there is not time (i.e., surgery is not elective) or there is not an effective therapy to correct the anaemia before surgery, then the need for blood transfusion needs to be determined. Although a preoperative haematocrit of 30% is usually recommended, each case needs to be individualized. Factors important in deciding about the need for transfusion are the type of procedure and anticipated blood loss, chronicity and stability of the anaemia, and underlying cardiopulmonary status.[26]

Postoperative anaemia usually reflects blood loss during surgery and dilution from intravenous fluids. In general, the loss of one unit of blood causes the haematocrit to drop by three percentage points. The effect of dilution by intravenous fluids can be significant, but is difficult to assess. If, after taking into account the above factors, the haematocrit is lower than expected, other causes such as GI bleeding, bleeding into the wound, and haemolysis should be evaluated. Most patients tolerate the acute haemodulation of surgery well and can have good cardiovascular function with a haematocrit in the mid-twenties. The decision to transfuse should take into consideration the underlying haemodynamic status of the individual patient as well as surgical factors such as wound healing and survival of flaps used in reconstruction.

Other disorders such as erythrocytosis, leukocytosis, leukopenia, thrombocytosis, thrombocytopenia and a history consistent with a bleeding disorder should be evaluated before surgery.

Patients who undergo chemotherapy for carcinoma may frequently suffer bone marrow toxicity. Clearly, major operative procedures should be delayed until the suppressive effects of a recent course of such medication is resolved. Patients who have had longstanding chemotherapy are at risk for end organ damage depending on the agent utilized. Radiation therapy to the chest can suppress bone marrow function of the sternal marrow.

Transfusions

Use of blood products is expensive and is associated with a variety of complications. Their use should be limited and well considered.

The identification and management of the different transfusion reactions are beyond the scope of this chapter. Other potential risks of transfusions include transmission of an infectious disease. Transfusion-associated hepatitis C is rare when blood banks routinely screen for its antibody. Non-A, non-B hepatitis was a frequent complication of transfusion but the availability of antigen and antibody tests for hepatitis C should reduce this complication dramatically. Similarly, modern blood banks can screen for human immunodeficiency virus and pick up most units of blood which are tainted by this agent. More patients are opting for autologous transfusions for elective surgery.[1]

GASTROENTEROLOGY

Aside from the problems that head and neck patients encounter in maintaining oral intake, few gastroenterological problems directly affect the perioperative care of the head and neck patient. In this section, we will briefly touch upon considerations of patients with ulcer disease, adynamic ileus, and hepatic dysfunction.

It should not be surprising that many head and neck patients will have a history of active peptic ulcer disease given the frequent concomitant history of tobacco and ethanol use. Active peptic ulcers with evidence of gastrointestinal blood loss is a relative contraindication to all but emergent surgery. The perioperative stress of major surgery can promote major GI bleeding, and those patients who continue to smoke or drink to excess are particularly at risk. It is therefore prudent to maintain ulcer patients on prophylactic doses of H_2 blockers during the early stages of the postoperative recovery period. Use of sucralfate, which forms a barrier on mucosal lesions, could also be helpful, and recent evidence suggests that sucralfate, in comparison to H_2 blockers, does not alter gastric flora — thus reducing the risk of Gram-negative aspiration pneumonia in patients who are intubated.

Some patients will develop nausea and vomiting two or three days postoperatively, and auscultation of the abdomen prior to palpation may reveal the complete absence or high pitched nature of bowel sounds. In these patients, flat plate radiological examination of the abdomen will disclose dilated loops of bowel. While the patient must be examined for the possibility of a perforated ulcer or other abdominal catastrophe, the majority of such presentations represent postoperative adynamic ileus which frequently responds to conservative measures. The discontinuation of oral intake for 24 hours may be sufficient, and nasogastric suction should be reserved for those patients with persistent emesis. New research has delineated the pathophysiology of ileus and has noted that the small bowel recovers before function in the large intestine.[44] Indeed, the last intestinal segment to recover from postoperative ileus is the ascending colon. Clinical trials are evaluating medications that can expedite resolution of this intestinal problem.[49]

Postoperative diarrhoea can be a perplexing and frustrating problem. In head and neck patients, the cause can frequently stem from the osmolarity of tube feedings. A reduced concentration or slower progression of caloric increase usually resolves the problem. Nevertheless, the possibility of pseudomembranous colitis should not be overlooked in any patient who has received antibiotics. Obtaining stool smears for leukocytes is a good screening technique — as is a culture for enteric pathogens. Diarrhoea that contains blood or leukocytes and is culture-negative warrants aggressive work-up, including sigmoidoscopy.

Patients may present with abnormal liver enzymes. Transaminase elevation is associated with active destruction of hepatocytes and release of intracellular enzymes. Increased alkaline phosphatase can be seen with many systematic problems but, when applied to the liver, is indicative of biliary tract obstruction and is usually seen with concomitant increase in γ-glutamyl transpeptidase levels. Increased bilirubin can be associated with biliary tract obstruction, intrahepatic cholestasis and intravascular haemolysis. If a patient is otherwise asymptomatic, has an unremarkable clinical history, and the elevation is modest, anaesthetic risk is not seriously increased.

The existing medical literature probably overstates the risk to the patient of a surgical procedure in the face of hepatitis. Nevertheless, patients with acute hepatitis from either viral or chemical aetiologies are best handled by avoiding elective surgery until resolution of the active process. Chronic hepatitis which results in debilitation of the patient increases surgical risk, and each patient requires individual clinical decision making. It should be kept in mind that cirrhosis can present with minimal changes in liver enzymes, and impaired hepatic reserve can cause significant postoperative morbidity. Finally, inhalational — and, at times, spinal anaesthesia — can cause diminished blood flow to the liver and result in a mild, transient postoperative increase in serum transaminase levels. Observation and follow-up blood work should be sufficient in most cases.

While definitive studies are not available concerning operative risk and cirrhosis, correlation with Child's Classification of cirrhosis is adequate.[17] Patients whose liver disease results in albumin less than 3, ascites, and elevated prothrombin and partial thromboplastin times are at increased risk. Cirrhotic patients with frank evidence of hepatic failure carry a mortality rate of up to 76%, and surgery in these patients should be approached cautiously, if at all. Even if the patient survives the procedure, there is high risk of postoperative morbidity and a prolonged hospital stay.

MISCELLANEOUS TOPICS

Postoperative delirium

Impaired cognition in the postoperative patient, especially those individuals of advanced age or debilitated health, can pose challenging diagnostic problems.[7] Questions arise as to the need of aggressive diagnostic testing or the permanence of the impairment.

Clearly, the intensity of the hospital environment in an individual with serious medical conditions can result in confusion and inappropriate behaviour. This 'ICU psychosis' is possible in any location in the hospital and responds to quiet, supportive care and the presence of individuals and objects that are familiar to the patient.

Nevertheless, the presence of other serious disease states requires thorough work-up of the confused postoperative patient. Hypoxaemia is a frequent cause and stems from postoperative atelectasis, pulmonary infections or emboli, or congestive heart failure. Arterial blood gases should be obtained on every postoperative patient who develops confusion. Occult myocardial infarction can also

Table 24.4 Common causes of confusion

Congestive heart failure
Electrolyte abnormalities
Fever
Glucose abnormalities
Hepatic insufficiency
Hypotension
Hypoxaemia
Infection
Intracranial hypertension
Medications
    Sedatives
    Narcotics
    Scopolamine
    Metaclopromide
    Cimetadine
    L Dopa
Psychiatric dysfunction
Stroke

cause confusion, and an EKG is prudent as well. Elderly patients especially can have impaired mentation in the presence of infections even as trivial as mild urinary tract colonization. Silent bacteraemia can occur and will be detected only if surveillance blood cultures are obtained. Hyper- and hypoglycaemia can alter mental status as can hyponatraemia, hypercalcaemia and dehydration. Patients with Parkinson's disease are especially at risk for postoperative delirium.[21] Computed tomography of the head, and possibly lumbar puncture, should be reserved for patients with focal neurological findings or persistent confusion.

Drugs can certainly play a major role in the pathogenesis of confusion. Patient records should be reviewed to assess the extent of administration of pain and sedative medications. Effort should be made to reduce the dose or frequency of such drugs in the confused individual. Commonly used drugs that can cause perioperative confusion, particularly in elderly patients, include Metaclopromide, Cimetadine, narcotics, sedatives, antipsychotics and Methylxanthene. Table 24.4 indicates other medical causes of confusion.

An occasional patient will suffer frank delirium and will be difficult to control despite having no obvious sign of underlying metabolic abnormality. Many of these cases reflect inadequate pain relief in a confused patient. Administration of sedative drugs such as benzodiazepams or antipsychotic agents without judicious pain relief could worsen the situation. Clearly, these patients require insightful, careful and restrained management.

Seizure disorders

Most patients who suffer from chronic seizure disorders are maintained on dilantin, which is fortunately a drug with a long half-life. Preoperative patients should be assessed as to whether their seizure disorder is currently under control and dilantin can be given once a day to maintain adequate blood levels. If necessary, it can be given intravenously by slow infusion (50 mg/min) to avoid hypotension associated with rapid administration.

Patients who suffer new seizures in the postoperative period must be assessed for a variety of metabolic abnormalities. Problem with glucose regulation, calcium, sodium, and magnesium should be assessed. Ethanol withdrawal reactions are common. In addition, one must rule out the possibility of a cerebrovascular embolism or stroke. The possibility of a new central nervous system lesion, such as a tumour or infection, must also be considered. Patients can receive a gram of dilantin intravenously over 20 minutes to assure adequate loading with antiseizure medication. Status epilepticus can be treated acutely with intravenous benzodiazepines or phenobarbitol.

Ethanol and drug abuse

Since ethanol is a risk factor for significant head and neck diseases, it is not surprising that the complications of ethanol addiction are seen on a head and neck surgery unit. All alcoholic patients should receive supplemental thiamine on admission. Patients who begin to experience the hallucinosis of acute withdrawal are best treated with benzodiazepam sedation.[42] Oxazepam, which has reduced hepatic elimination, may be especially useful. In patients who can tolerate the drugs, B blockade to reduce the autonomic effects of withdrawal, such as tachycardia and diaphoresis, can be useful. Potent tranquilizers such as haloperidol may be required to achieve control of the patient's behaviour in resistant cases. Standing orders can result in oversedation and subsequent aspiration, so the drug therapy for a patient in withdrawal needs constant review and modification.

An occasional patient who admits to the intake of large quantities of ethanol daily will present for significant surgery that will require several days without oral intake in the postoperative period. Of course, it would be ideal to require the attainment of abstinence, but the achievement of this goal can be elusive and result in prolonged delay of needed surgical intervention. One method of dealing with this problem is to use continuous sedation in the perioperative period. The use of intravenous ethanol is controversial. While some individuals have condemned its use because of the potential negative implications of providing alcohol to alcoholics in a hospital setting, the toxicity of intravenous ethanol in D_5A_5 infusions is not well documented in the medical literature. It is being used successfully on several major head and neck units. One study demonstrated effectiveness when using the infusion to maintain a low level of circulating ethanol during the postoperative period.[24]

Geriatric patients

Many of the comments throughout this chapter make special mention of the susceptibility of the elderly to postoperative morbid events. Nevertheless, age alone is not a barrier to operative intervention. It is particularly important to assess patients for their organ system reserve. Indeed, there are patients in their late 80s who enjoy better physiological health than individuals 10–20 years younger. Therefore, decisions need to be made on an individual basis. It must be noted that Ziffren discovered a six-fold increased risk in radical neck dissection when a patient was in his ninth decade.[54]

Parkinson's syndrome is not uncommon in the elderly population. It is characterized by a resting tremor, rigidity, bradykynesia, and impaired postural reflexes. Autonomic dysfunction is common. Patients with significant Parkinson's syndrome are at risk for aspiration during the perioperative period during which time they are frequently sedated. Muscle rigidity may increase restrictive disease of the lungs which further limits pulmonary reserve. Patients with severe disease should be assessed to assure that they are on optimal anti-Parkinson medication, and efforts should be made to maintain the dosing schedule.

In handling patients of advanced age, it must be remembered that diminished organ reserve is a normal condition of well-functioning individuals. Recovery may be somewhat slow and drug metabolism slowed. The appearance of morbidity in one organ system could result in concomitant failure of other organs as a delicate homeostasis is disrupted. In general, we advise that patients of advanced age have a medical consultant participate in their perioperative care. Discharge planning should take into consideration the fact that home care and recovery could be impaired by the lack of suitable and physically able individuals in the household to assist with the activities of daily living. Arrangements for visiting nurses or health aides should be made prior to admission to the hospital and not in the 24 hours prior to discharge, if at all possible.

REFERENCES

1. AuBuchon J P, Popovsky M A 1991 The safety of preoperative autologous blood donation in the nonhospital setting. Transfusion 31: 523–517
2. Ayus J C, Krothapalli R K, Arieff A I 1987 Treatment of symptomatic hyponatremia and its relation to brain damage: a prospective study. NEJM 317: 1190
3. Baeza A, Aguayo J, Barria M, Paneda G 1991 Rapid preoperative preparation in hyperthyroidism. Clin Endocrinol 35: 439–442
4. Bern M M, Lokich J J, Wallach S R et al 1990 Very low doses of warfarin can prevent thrombosis in central venous catheters: a randomized prospective trial. Ann Int Med 112: 423–428
5. Charlson M E, MacKenzie C R, Gold J P, Ales K L, Topkins M, Shires G T 1991 Risk for postoperative congestive heart failure. Surg Gynecol Obstet 172: 95–104
6. Charpak Y, Blery C, Chastang C L et al 1988 Usefulness of selectively ordered preoperative tests. Medical Care 26: 95
7. Chung F, Seyone C, Dyck B et al 1990 Age-related cognitive recovery after general anesthesia. Anesth Analg 71: 217–224
8. Clagett G P, Reisch J S 1988 Prevention of venous thromboembolism in general surgery patients. Ann Surg 208: 227–240
9. Collins R, Scrimgeous A, Yusuf S, Peto R 1988 Reduction in fatal pulmonary embolism and venous thrombosis by perioperative administration of subcutaneous heparin: overview of results of randomized trials in general, orthopaedic, and urologic surgery. NEJM 318: 1162–1173
10. Craig D B 1981 Postoperative recovery of pulmonary function. Anesth Analg 60: 46–52
11. Currie P J, Seward J B, Reeder G S et al 1985 Continuous wave doppler echocardiographic assessment of severity of calcific aortic stenosis: a simultaneous doppler-catheter correlative study in 100 adult patients. Circulation 71: 1162
12. Cygan R, Waitskin H 1987 Stopping and restarting medications in the perioperative period. J Gen Intern Med 2: 270–283
13. Detsky A S et al 1986 Predicting cardiac complications in patients undergoing non-cardiac surgery. J Gen Intern Med 1: 211
14. Eagle K A, Boucher C A 1992 Cardiac risk of noncardiac surgery. NEJM 321: 1330–1332
15. Freeman W K, Gibbons R J, Shub C 1989 Preoperative assessment of cardiac patients undergoing noncardiac surgical procedures. Mayo Clin Proc 64: 1105–1117
16. Fuente B, Kasper C K, Rickles F R et al 1985 Response of patients with mild and moderate hemophilia A and von Willebrand's disease to treatment with desmopressin. Ann Int Med 103: 6
17. Garrison R N, Cryer H M, Howard D A 1984 Clarification of risk factors for abdominal operations in patients with hepatic cirrhosis. Ann Surg 199: 648
18. Gerberding J L, Schecter W P 1991 Surgery and AIDS: reducing the risk. JAMA 265: 1572–1573
19. Goldberger A L, O'Konski M 1986 Utility of the routine electrocardiogram before surgery and on general hospital admission. Ann Int Med 105: 552–557
20. Golden W E, Lavender R C 1989 Preoperative cardiac consultation. Southern Med J 82: 252–259
21. Golden W E, Lavender R C, Metzer W S 1989 Postoperative psychosis in Parkinson's disease patients. Ann Int Med 11(3) 218–222
22. Goldman L, Caldera D L 1979 Risks of general anesthesia and elective operation in the hypertensive patient. Anesthesiology 50: 285–292
23. Goldman L, Caldera D L, Nussbaum S R et al 1977 Multifactorial index of cardiac risk in noncardiac surgical procedures. NEJM 297: 845
24. Hansbrough J F, Zapata-Sirvent R L, Carrol W J 1984 Administration of intravenous alcohol for prevention of withdrawal in alcoholic burn patients. Am J Surg 148: 266
25. Jackson C V 1988 Preoperative pulmonary evaluation. Arch Int Med 148: 2120–2127
26. Jobes D R, Gallagher 1982 Acute normovolemia hemodilution. Int Anesth Clin 20(4): 77–95
27. Kaplan E B, Sheiner L B, Boeckmann A J et al 1985 The usefulness of preoperative laboratory screening. JAMA 253: 3576
28. Kingston H G G, Hirshman C A 1984 Perioperative management of the patient with asthma. Anesth Analg 63: 844–855
29. Ladenson P W, Levin A A, Ridgway E C et al 1984 Complications of surgery in hypothyroid patients. Am J Med 77: 261
30. Landercasper J, Merz B J, Cogbill T H et al 1990 Perioperative stroke risk in 173 consecutive patients with a past history of stroke. Arch Surg 125: 986–989
31. Lee T, Papius E M, Goldman L 1983 Impact of inter-physician communication on the effectiveness of medical consultations. Am J Med 74: 106–112
32. Macpherson D S, Snow R, Lofgren R P 1990 Preoperative screening: value of previous tests. Ann Int Med 113: 969–973
33. Mangano D T, Hollenberg M, Fegert G et al 1991 Perioperative myocardial ischemia in patients undergoing noncardiac surgery — 1. Incidence and severity during the 4 day perioperative period. J Am Coll Card 17: 843–850
34. Michel L A, Jamart J, Bradpiece H A, Malt R A 1990 Prediction of risk in noncardiac operations after cardiac operations. J Thorac Cardiovasc Surg 100: 595–605
35. Mohr D N, Jett J R 1988 Preoperative evaluation of pulmonary risk factors. JGIM 3: 277–287
36. Narr B J, Hansen T R, Warner M A 1991 Preoperative laboratory screening in healthy Mayo patients: cost-effective elimination of tests and unchanged outcomes. Mayo Clin Proc 99: 587–590
37. O'Keefe J H, Shub C, Rettke S R 1989 Risk of noncardiac surgical procedures in patients with aortic stenosis. Mayo Clin Proc 64: 400–405
38. Olsen G N, Bolton J W R, Weiman D S, Hornung C A 1991 Stair climbing as an exercise test to predict the postoperative complications of lung resection; two years' experience. Chest 99: 587–590
39. Popejoy S L, Fry D E 1991 Blood contact and exposure in the operating room. Surg Gynecol Obstet 172: 480–483
40. Quebbeman E J, Telford G L, Hubbard S et al 1991 Risk of blood contamination and injury to operating room personnel. Ann Surg 214: 614–620
41. Rao T L K, ElEtr A A 1981 Myocardial reinfarction following anesthesia in patients with recent infarction. Anesth Analg 60: 271
42. Romach M K, Sellers E M 1991 Management of the alcohol withdrawal syndrome. Ann Rev Med 42: 323–340
43. Roper A H, Wechsler L R, Wilson L S 1982 Carotid bruit and the risk of stroke in elective surgery. NEJM 307: 1388
44. Schippers E, Hölscher A H, Bollschweiler E, Siewert J R 1991 Return of interdigestive motor complex after abdominal surgery: end of postoperative ileus. Dig Dis Sci 36: 621–626
45. Shah K B, Kleinman B S, Sami H, Patel J, Rao T L K 1990 Reevaluation of perioperative myocardial infarction in patients with prior myocardial infarction undergoing noncardiac operations. Anesth Analg 71: 231–235
46. Suchman A L, Griner P F 1986 Diagnostic uses of the activated partial thromboplastin time and prothrombin time. Ann Int Med 104: 810
47. Taggart D P, Siddiqui A, Wheatley D J 1990 Low-dose preoperative aspirin therapy, postoperative blood loss, and transfusion requirements. Ann Thorac Surg 50: 425–428
48. Thompson R C, Liberthson R R, Lowenstein E 1985 Perioperative anesthetic risk of noncardiac surgery in hypertrophic obstructive cardiomyopathy. JAMA 254: 2419
49. Tollesson P O, Cassuto J, Rimbäck G, Fax'n A, Bergman L, Mattsson E 1991 Treatment of postoperative paralytic ileus with cisapride. Scand J Gastroenterol 26: 477–482
50. Undelsman R, Ramp J, Gallucci W T et al 1986 Adaptation during surgical stress: a reevaluation of the role of glucocorticoids. J Clin Invest 77: 1377

51. Vaughan R S 1991 Potassium in the perioperative period. Br J Anaesth 67: 194–200
52. Hyers T M, Hull R D, Weg J G 1989 Antithrombotic therapy for venous thromboembolic disease. Chest Supplement 95: 37S–51S
53. Warner M A, Divertie M B, Tinker J H 1984 Preoperative cessation of smoking and pulmonary complications in coronary artery bypass patient. Anesthesiology 60: 380
54. Zeffren S E, Hartford C E 1972 Comparative mortality for various surgical operations in older versus younger age groups. J Am Geriatric Soc 20: 485

25. Surgical therapy

C. E. Silver, I. I. Moisa, W. B. R. Stern

INTRODUCTION

Surgical management of laryngeal and hypopharyngeal malignancy involves a spectrum of procedures ranging through the entire armament of current techniques. Early-stage lesions, relatively confined in extent, may be resected with preservation of sufficient laryngeal tissue to preserve the functions of speech, respiration and deglutition. Extensive lesions require total extirpation of the larynx, often in association with adjacent portions of hypopharynx and cervical oesophagus. Such ablative procedures often require reconstruction involving transfer or reimplantation of musculocutaneous tissue, or of abdominal viscera. The procedure chosen depends on the site and extent of the tumour, the general medical condition of the patient, and the preference of the surgeon. Important considerations in management of laryngeal cancer include the place of radiation or laser therapy, management of cervical metastases, and rehabilitation of the patient. These issues have been discussed in other portions of this volume.

'CONSERVATION' PROCEDURES

Anatomical and physiological basis

The aim of conservation surgery is adequate tumour excision with preservation of the essential laryngeal functions. Anatomically and pathologically the basis of such surgery is the tendency of many laryngeal tumours to remain confined within the various fibrocartilaginous compartments of the larynx during early stages of development. The physiological basis lies in the fact that most individuals are able to adapt to loss of substantial portions of the larynx while retaining the ability to breathe, swallow and speak. Many of the conservation techniques currently employed had their origins in the late 19th and early 20th centuries, but did not become clinically useful until the advent of modern anaesthesiology, antibacterial therapy and comprehension of the natural history of laryngeal carcinoma.

Barriers to spread of cancer from one side of the larynx to the other, and from supraglottic to glottic regions have been demonstrated by numerous authors. Frazer[19] observed the separate embryological derivation of supraglottic structures from buccopharyngeal anlage and of glottic and infraglottic structures from pulmonary anlage. Hajek[25] and Pressman[49] employed dye-injection studies to demonstrate the anatomical compartmentation of this organ. Tucker and Smith[73] identified the connective tissue structures that form these compartmental barriers by studying whole-organ serial sections in the human fetus. These consist of the laryngeal cartilages and associated fibroelastic tissues, the conus elasticus with its thickened upper rim comprising the vocal ligaments, the anterior commissure (Broyle's) tendon, the ventricular connective tissue, and the quadrangular membrane with its ventricular ligaments.

In performing conservation surgery, resection is established in either the vertical or horizontal plane, according to the location of the tumour. A vertical approach is employed for glottic tumours, while supraglottic tumours are resected by horizontal section of the larynx. As exploration may reveal extension of tumour beyond preoperatively estimated limits, consent for total laryngectomy should be obtained prior to attempted conservation surgery.

Selection of patients

The lesions most suitable for conservation surgery are those that, due to local invasiveness or proximity to cartilage, are not readily curable with radiation but are small enough for adequate resection without sacrifice of the entire larynx. Conservation procedures are usually not feasible for patients with significant chronic pulmonary or neurological disorders and should be considered with caution for older patients who may find adaptation difficult.[1] The quality of life, for such patients, may be more satisfactory after successful total laryngectomy than after a functionally unsatisfactory conservation operation complicated by chronic aspiration of food and saliva. Conservation laryngectomy may be employed after irradiation failure, provided that the lesion was amenable to the same resection prior to therapy.[71] It is most important to avoid compromising a patient's chance for cure by attempting to preserve laryngeal function with a tumour too large for adequate resection by partial laryngectomy.

Tracheotomy, performed as an initial step in conservation laryngeal procedures, allows safe, unimpeded access to the larynx and a secure postoperative airway. The tracheotomy is decannulated when the surgical wound has healed, postoperative oedema has subsided, and the patient is able to swallow with minimal aspiration of food.

Vertical hemilaryngectomy

Laryngofissure

Laryngofissure, or cordectomy via thyrotomy, is suitable for small, relatively superficial carcinomas (T_1) confined to the membranous portion of the vocal cord. The operation is rarely employed for treatment of laryngeal cancer at the present time, as suitable lesions are most often treated by radiation therapy, endoscopic laser surgery, or hemilaryngectomy. Occasionally, however, laryngofissure may be useful for treatment of recurrent or persistent tumour following irradiation, particularly in severely debilitated individuals. In laryngofissure, resection is confined to mucosal and submucosal tissue. Cartilage is not removed in continuity with the tumour. The technique is demonstrated in Fig. 25.1. The defect heals by re-epithelialization with formation of a functional 'pseudocord'. The voice may be improved by sub-perichondrial resection of a portion of thyroid cartilage to permit better approximation of the pseudocord with its opposite member, or by transposition of a bipedicled flap of sternohyoid muscle into the laryngeal interior.[2] Cure rates for laryngofissure performed in the modern era have varied widely, from 60% to 98%, depending on the percentage of radiation failures in each series.[14,37,56]

Modified frontolateral laryngectomy

Lesions of any stage that approach or involve the anterior commissure should be resected with the overlying vertical midline segment of thyroid cartilage. The anterior commissure is included with the resection by making the mucosal incision through the anterior portion of the contralateral vocal cord (Fig. 25.2). If one-third or less of the contralateral cord is resected, the laryngeal mucosa of that side may be advanced to the external perichondrium without need of grafts, skin flaps or prostheses to maintain an adequate laryngeal lumen. A varying amount of ipsilateral thyroid cartilage is resected subperichondrially.

The bipedicled flap of sternohyoid muscle, described above, may be inserted beneath the preserved perichondrium in order to replace the resected portion of vocal cord.

Anterior frontal partial laryngectomy (anterior commissure technique)

Some tumours involve the anterior commissure extensively, often with significant portions of both vocal cords. Such lesions may extend sub- or supraglottically in the midline. Adequate resection necessitates removing a vertical midline segment of thyroid cartilage as well as significant portions of both vocal cords (Fig. 25.3A) The surgical defect may appear formidable, with only posterior commissure mucosa remaining in the endolarynx. Although a variety of reconstructive techniques including skin grafts, skin flaps, perichondrium and muscle flaps have been employed, the simple technique described in 1968 by Som and Silver[67] avoids the need for complex resurfacing procedures by utilizing a temporary midline partition, as developed by McNaught[38] for treatment of laryngeal webs. The partition permits both sides to re-epithelialize independently with resultant satisfactory airway and voice.

Following tracheostomy and exposure of the larynx, bilateral vertical thyrotomy incisions are made. Laryngeal soft tissues are separated from the internal aspect of each thyroid ala as far as the vocal process of arytenoid. In order to avoid compromise of the resection margin it is important to assess accurately the extent of tumour involvement prior to laryngeal entry. After initial anterior entry through the cricothyroid membrane, the mucosa is retracted superolaterally as the incision extends posteriorly on the side of lesser involvement, and then vertically at the posterior resection limit, immediately anterior to the vocal process. At the superior limit of the posterior vertical incision, the mucosal cut is carried back horizontally to the anterior midline traversing the thyrohyoid membrane. At this point the mobilized portion of the larynx can be retracted forward, affording a panoramic view of the endolarynx and the tumour (Fig. 25.3B). Resection is completed by appropriate circumcision of mucosa and muscle around the tumour. The operation may be extended to include ipsilateral arytenoid and/or the superior half of anterior cricoid cartilage, to assure a tumour-free margin.

A prosthesis is now inserted to partition the larynx (Fig. 25.3C). A semi-rigid silicone-rubber 'keel' may be employed, as shown here. This type of prosthesis is secured to the thyroid cartilage and requires a second operation, in approximately 6 weeks, for removal. A soft silicone-rubber sheet, secured with sutures through the skin, may be used in place of the rigid prosthesis. The soft partition may be removed endoscopically.

Reported results of several series of anterior frontal partial laryngectomy are summarized in Table 25.1.

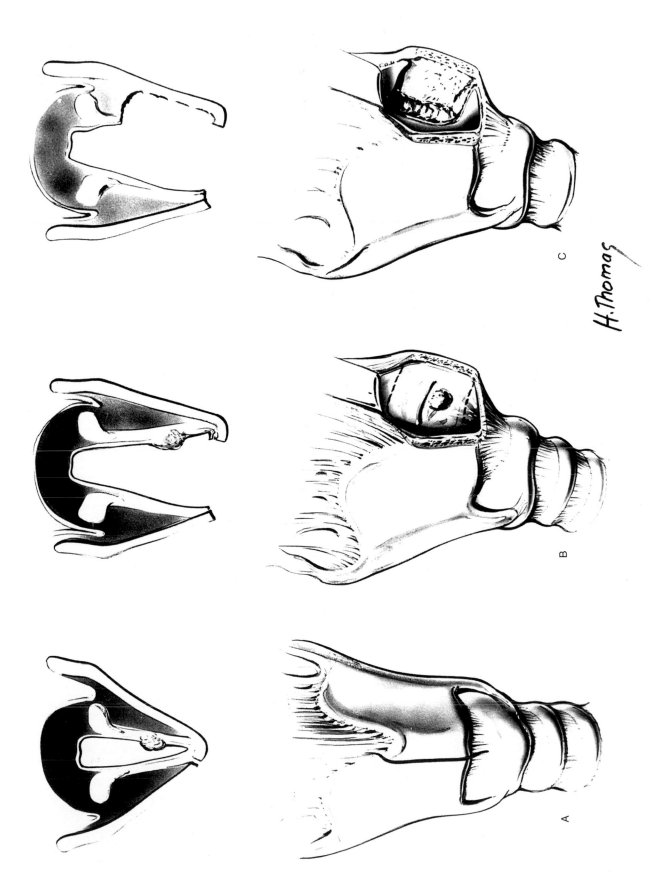

Fig. 25.1 Laryngofissure. A. (*left*) Suitable lesion. Placement of thyrotomy incision. B. (*centre*) Endolarynx exposed. Resection outlined. C. (*right*) Larynx after completion of resection. (Reprinted from Silver,[60] with permission.)

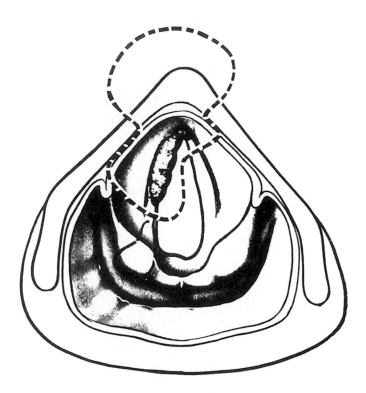

Fig. 25.2   Modified frontolateral laryngectomy — outline of resection. (Reprinted from Silver, with permission.[61])

Three-year cure in 111 of 157 (70%) cases was reported.[30,57,67]

Extended frontolateral laryngectomy (hemilaryngectomy)

The conventional 'vertical hemilaryngectomy' includes removal of a thyroid ala, arytenoid and mucosa from aryepiglottic fold to cricothyroid membrane in a sagittal plane, and from anterior commissure to posterior midline in a coronal plane (Fig. 25.4). This operation is indicated for carcinoma of the glottis with posterior extension to involve the vocal process and anterior surface of arytenoid or with involvement of the floor of the ventricle laterally with infiltration of the thyroarytenoideus muscle. The operation may be extended to include resection of various portions of the contralateral vocal cord (extended fronto-lateral laryngectomy).

The most important factors in determining suitability for conventional hemilaryngectomy are the degree and

location of subglottic extension. If subglottic extension does not exceed 8–9 mm anteriorly or 5–6 mm posteriorly, hemilaryngectomy is feasible. Limitation of vocal cord mobility, including complete fixation in some cases, does not prevent hemilaryngectomy if immobility has not been caused by subglottic extension beyond the limits mentioned, or by invasion of the cricoarytenoid joint.

Various techniques for glottic and vestibular reconstruction after hemilaryngectomy employ cartilage, muscle, skin and other tissues. Use of a pedicled thyroid cartilage flap to replace the resected arytenoid is demonstrated in Fig. 25.5. The procedure is commenced by transverse skin incision, elevation of skin flaps, and tracheostomy. The anterior two-thirds of thyroid ala is skeletonized by separating thyrohyoid and sternothyroid muscles from the oblique line, leaving inferior constrictor muscle attached posteriorly. Vertical thyrotomy incisions are made anterior to the attachment of inferior constrictor muscle and, on the contralateral side, far enough from the midline to permit adequate resection of the anterior commissure (Fig. 25.5A). After transection of superior laryngeal vessels and nerves, the posterior third of thyroid ala is separated from underlying pyriform sinus mucosa, avulsing the cricothyroid joint to permit retraction of this cartilaginous segment posteriorly.

The laryngeal interior is exposed by retraction of the thyroid alae. Horizontal incisions are made at the level of

Table 25.1   Anterior frontal (anterior commissure) partial laryngectomy

Series	Years	Stage	Tumour-free	
Som & Silver[67]	3	T_2	26/38	(68%)
Kirchner & Som[30]	4	T_2	40/58	(69%)
Sessions et al[57]	3	T_1–T_2	45/61	(74%)
Total			111/157	(70%)

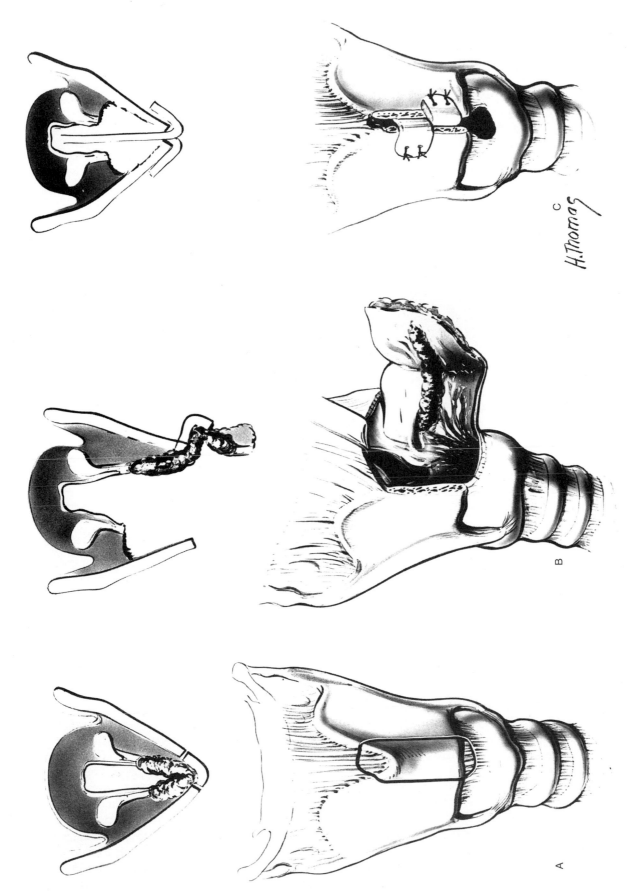

Fig. 25.3 Anterior commisure partial laryngectomy. A. (*left*) Lesion involving both vocal cords. Bilateral thyrotomy incisions. B. (*centre*) Larynx entered and lesion exposed. C. (*right*) Placement of midline partition ('keel') to prevent stricture formation. (Reprinted from Silver,[60] with permission.)

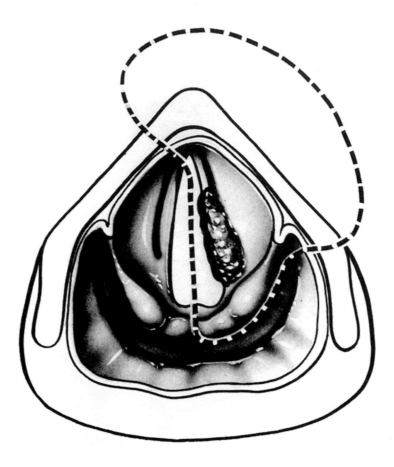

Fig. 25.4 Lesion and outline of resection for hemilaryngectomy, with resection of arytenoid. (Reprinted from Silver, with permission.[61])

cricothyroid and thyrohyoid membranes, and continued posteriorly to the midline (Fig. 25.5B). The inferior incision will traverse the cricoarytenoid joint, while the superior incision is placed in the aryepiglottic fold as it progresses posteriorly. These are joined in the posterior midline by a vertical incision that will transect the interarytenoideus muscle but not hypopharyngeal mucosa. Control of this incision is facilitated by insertion of a finger or instrument into the hypopharynx, pulling the tissue to be incised anteriorly, placing it under moderate tension. With a finger in the pyriform sinus, the cricoarytenoid joint is palpated as it is transected. This manoeuvre liberates the specimen from its last cartilaginous attachment. The pyriform sinus mucosa is preserved while remaining loose attachments are divided, completing the resection.

Reconstruction is commenced by excision of inferior and superior portions of the preserved posterior third of ipsilateral thyroid ala, leaving a central portion of cartilage, pedicled on the inferior constrictor muscle, that will be used to replace the resected arytenoid thus re-establishing, at least in part, the vestibule and posterior glottis (Fig. 25.5C). The cartilage 'flap' is fixed to the cricoid rostrum with polyglactin sutures (Fig. 25.5D), following which the endolarynx is resurfaced by advancement of hypopharyngeal mucosa, including the preserved pyriform sinus (Fig. 25.5E). The cut edge of aryepiglottic fold should be thinned prior to advancement, in order to facilitate mobility of mucosa and avoid creation of an obstructive flap of tissue within the lumen. Suture of hypopharyngeal to subglottic mucosa is carried as far anteriorly as possible, covering the cartilage flap, and resurfacing most of the hemilarynx. Anteriorly the mucosa is sutured to sternohyoid muscle, and the infrahyoid muscles reapproximated in the midline. While there is insufficient mucosa for complete resurfacing of the endolarynx, the defect heals without difficulty by secondary intention.

Following hemilaryngectomy the voice is often hoarse, breathy or weak despite various forms of glottic reconstruction. Nevertheless, vocal rehabilitation is considerably superior to what may be achieved after total laryngectomy. Reconstruction of the vestibule and posterior glottis reduces the incidence of postoperative aspiration and enables performance of this procedure in a more elderly group of patients than may otherwise be possible.

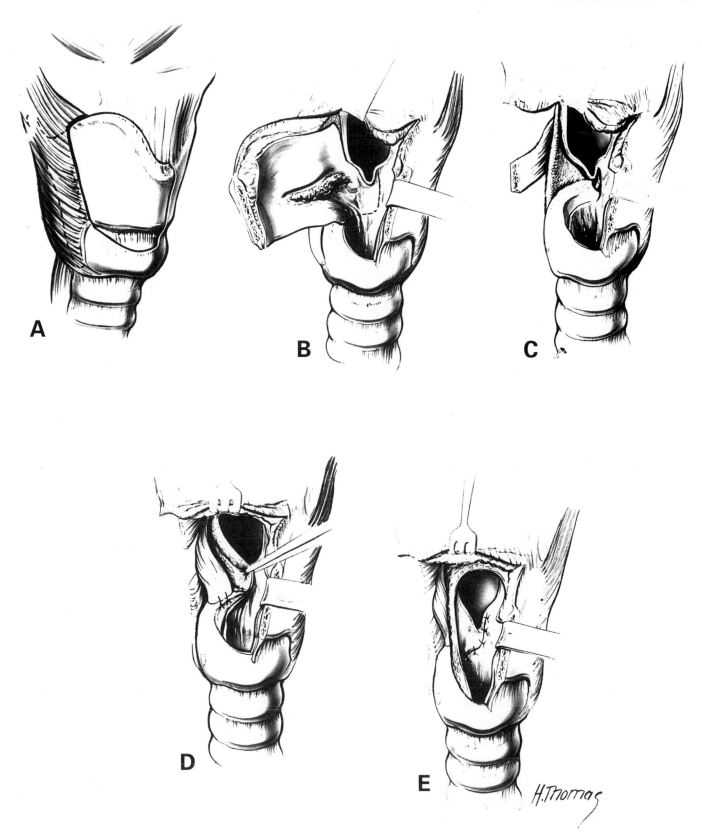

Fig. 25.5 Hemilaryngectomy technique. A. Cartilage cuts. B. Mucosal incisions. C. Specimen removed. Flap of posterior thyroid cartilage pedicled on inferior constrictor muscle. D. Cartilage flap rotated to replace arytenoid. E. Hypopharyngeal mucosa advanced to resurface hemilarynx. (Reprinted from Silver,[60] with permission.)

Biller and Lawson have reported satisfactory results with an oversized thyroid cartilage flap for replacement of cricoid cartilage in highly selected cases of glottic carcinomas with posterior subglottic extension exceeding the limitations discussed earlier.[5] Results of the effectiveness of vertical hemilaryngectomy for cure of T_2 and T_3 glottic carcinomas reported by several authors are summarized in Table 25.2.[3,6,29,35,39,43,64,66] These indicate an approximately 82% cure rate for T_2 carcinomas and 64% for T_3 carcinomas.

Subtotal laryngectomy with epiglottic reconstruction

Lesions of the glottis which involve at least half of each vocal cord result in large defects which require extensive reconstruction. When the lesion involves only the anterior halves, an anterior frontal partial laryngectomy may be performed, as described above. Reconstruction may be accomplished with a midline partition or with skin grafts or flaps. When the glottic lesion extends far enough posteriorly on one side to require sacrifice of the arytenoid cartilage, these reconstructive methods will prove insufficient to restore adequate laryngeal lumen and competence. This extensive resection of an entire hemilarynx and the mobile portion of the contralateral cord, with preservation of only a single arytenoid, has been termed (vertical) subtotal laryngectomy. The use of epiglottis for reconstruction of glottic defect was first reported in the European literature by Bouche et al.[9] Tucker et al[74] introduced his adaptation of the procedure for very large glottic defects, in the United States, in 1979.

The epiglottis provides several reconstructive advantages. Its mucosal lining is similar to that of the larynx, enhancing mucous transport and voice production. Its cartilaginous structure provides rigidity in order to maintain the anterior-posterior diameter of the larynx while still remaining flexible enough to allow for movement of the remaining arytenoid and pseudocord. It provides tissue bulk for glottic competence and reconstruction may be accomplished in one stage. Rehabilitation following subtotal laryngectomy with epiglottic reconstruction is more difficult than after more conventional vertical hemilaryngectomy. Disruption of the epiglottis interferes with the process of deglutition, as the epiglottis no longer diverts the food bolus. Its new position tethers the tongue base, and the surgical manipulation may produce some degree of superior laryngeal denervation. Thus, patient selection must be stringent; only highly motivated individuals with good pulmonary function are suitable for this procedure.

This procedure, as with other conservation operations, may be performed in selected patients after radiation failure, provided their lesions were suitable for the same resection prior to irridation, although a higher incidence of complications and greater difficulty with adaptation may be expected. An outline of the proposed resection is shown in Fig. 25.6A.

In performing the reconstruction, the epiglottis is mobilized by separating the anterior soft tissue and ligamentous attachments to the tip of the epiglottis (Fig. 25.6B). The epiglottis is then pulled inferiorly, with the aid of retraction sutures, to reach the cricoid without tension. This is abetted by removing the shoulder roll, increasing flexion of the neck. The epiglottis is then sutured with long-acting absorbable sutures laterally to the cut edges of the thyroid ala and inferiorly to the cricothyroid membrane or cricoid cartilage (Fig. 25.6C). Tucker, in his original technique, did not suture the intralaryngeal mucosal edges, feeling that this created a better pseudocord. Schechter[53] observed that suture of the mucosa created a higher pitched voice, more suitable for female patients.

Tucker et al[75] recently reported their experience with 48 patients, with a 96% 2-year survival. Five patients required total laryngectomies for recurrence; one of these five patients died of disease. All patients were decannulated, but nine required minor surgical procedures (i.e. laser surgery) prior to decannulation. All experienced some degree of aspiration. Nine patients required feeding supplementation beyond two months, and only one required assistance after six months. Approximately one-third had good voices, while two-thirds had 'functional' voices. Schechter[53] reported a 71% 3-year survival in 38 patients. All deaths occurred in previously irradiated patients. Four of the surviving patients required total laryngectomy for salvage. All patients were decannulated by the sixth postoperative week. Although all experienced some degree of aspiration for the first few postoperative weeks, only four patients required feeding tubes longer than three months, and all were free of feeding tubes by six months. Voice quality was generally 'satisfactory'.

Table 25.2 Extended frontolateral partial laryngectomy (hemilaryngectomy)

Series	Years	Stage	Tumour-free	
Ogura et al[43]	3	T_2	45/55	(82%)
Som[66]	3	T_2	79/105	(74%)
	3	T_3	15/26	(58%)
Mohr et al[39]	5	T_2	25/27	(94%)
	5	T_3	5/5	(100%)
Bauer et al[3]	5	T_3	12/18	(67%)
Leroux-Robert[35]	5	T_2	187/215	(87%)
	5	T_3	55/95	(58%)
Biller et al[6]	5	T_2	23/33	(69%)
Skolnik et al[64]	5	T_2	23/32	(72%)
	5	T_3	2/5	(40%)
Kessler et al[29]	2	T_3	23/27	(85%)
Total		T_2	382/466	(82%)
		T_3	112/176	(64%)

Conservation surgery for supraglottic tumours

Supraglottic subtotal laryngectomy (SSL)

Supraglottic carcinomas usually originate at the junction of the epiglottis and false cords. Most of these tumours are exophytic, well differentiated, and circumscribed, with 'pushing' rather than infiltrating margins. These tumours rarely involve the glottis and rarely invade thyroid cartilage. Involvement is usually confined above the anterior commissure. The pre-epiglottic space, however, is frequently infiltrated. As the entire pre-epiglottic space is removed by SSL, this operation will excise suitable lesions in a sound oncological fashion. A few supraglottic carcinomas have infiltrative margins. Such tumours are usually poorly differentiated, tend to be transglottic, and are rarely amenable to adequate resection by supraglottic laryngectomy.

Supraglottic carcinomas that do not involve the vocal cord represent the main indication for surgical management by SSL (Fig. 25.7). The procedure may be extended to include resection of various portions of the hypopharynx and tongue base. As a result of the barrier to spread of tumour from supraglottic to glottic levels, only a small margin of uninvolved mucosa is necessary inferiorly. Even when tumours appear laryngoscopically to extend close to the vocal cord, several millimetres of uninvolved ventricular mucosa are usually found in the resected specimen and constitute an adequate resection margin. Both arytenoids may be preserved in resecting lesions confined to the laryngeal surface of the epiglottis or anterior part of the false vocal cord, thus preserving vocal cord mobility. For lesions extending further posteriorly, the ipsilateral arytenoid is included in the specimen and the vocal cord surgically fixed in the midline, thus maintaining adequate glottic competence. The epiglottis may be reconstructed in situations where one-third or more of its substance can be preserved, further helping to decrease aspiration.[11] Cricopharyngeal myotomy may help improve deglutition and is often performed at the time of SSL. Glottic reconstruction after arytenoid resection may also improve deglutition.[28]

The technique of SSL is demonstrated in Fig. 25.8. After incision, elevation of skin flaps and tracheostomy, the infrahyoid muscles are transected superiorly, near their insertions on the hyoid, and reflected sufficiently to expose the upper half of the ipsilateral thyroid ala as well as the anterior half of the contralateral ala. Suprahyoid muscles are severed from their attachments to the body and ipsilateral greater cornu of the hyoid bone (Fig. 25.8A). The joint between body and contralateral greater cornu is transected with a small bone cutter. External perichondrium is separated from the ipsilateral and anterior contralateral thyroid alae, creating a flap of tissue that is reflected inferiorly as far as the estimated location of the vocal cord. Thyroid cartilage is transected horizontally at this level and the incision continued obliquely upward to the midpoint of the superior edge of the contralateral thyroid ala. If the valleculae are free of tumour, the hypopharynx is entered in this region by incising the pharyngeal wall superior to the hyoid bone, immediately anterior to the epiglottis. This incision is enlarged transversely and the epiglottis secured with a suture and retracted forward into the pharyngotomy (Fig. 25.8B). The mucosal incision is enlarged inferolaterally through the ipsilateral pyriform sinus until both aryepiglottic folds and arytenoids are exposed.

Resection of the supraglottis is now commenced by incising the aryepiglottic folds immediately in front of the arytenoids (Fig. 25.8C). These incisions are extended inferiorly into the ventricles, then anteriorly, immediately above the vocal cords, to the anterior commissure (Fig. 25.8D). The mucosal incisions are carried through full thickness of the larynx, corresponding externally with the previously placed cartilage cuts. Mucosa superior to the vocal cords should not be preserved, even if widely free of tumour, as excessive supraglottic mucosa tends to become oedematous, producing postoperative glottic obstruction. For small tumours, resection of the supraglottis may commence on either side. For more extensive resections, particularly if arytenoid is included, exposure is facilitated by mobilizing the lesser involved side initially.

After insertion of a nasogastric feeding tube, reconstruction is commenced by suturing the cut edges of pyriform sinus and supraglottic mucosa to each other (Fig. 25.8E), creating new aryepiglottic folds. The hypopharyngeal defect is closed by direct suture, commencing posteriorly and continuing as far anteriorly as possible. As the region of resected supraglottis is approached, the mucosal edges can no longer be approximated directly. The previously created perichondrial flap is reflected upward, and sutured to the cut edge of base of tongue, in order to provide tissue for closure (Fig. 25.8F). Preserved infrahyoid muscles, approximated to cut edges of suprahyoid and inferior constrictor muscles, constitute a second layer.

Results of treatment of endolaryngeal supraglottic carcinoma by supraglottic laryngectomy, reported in a number of large series, are summarized in Table 25.3.[7,8,10,36,42,44,51,65] Cure rates reported by the authors cited are comparable to those obtained by treatment of similar lesions with total laryngectomy.

Subtotal laryngectomy for supraglottic-glottic carcinoma

The applications of SSL have been extended to include supraglottic carcinomas with extension inferiorly to involve the glottis. In 1965, Ogura and Dedo[41] described an infolded flap of thyroid cartilage for glottic replacement, for T_2 supraglottic cancers involving the arytenoids, and/or glottis, with minimal subglottic extension. More recently

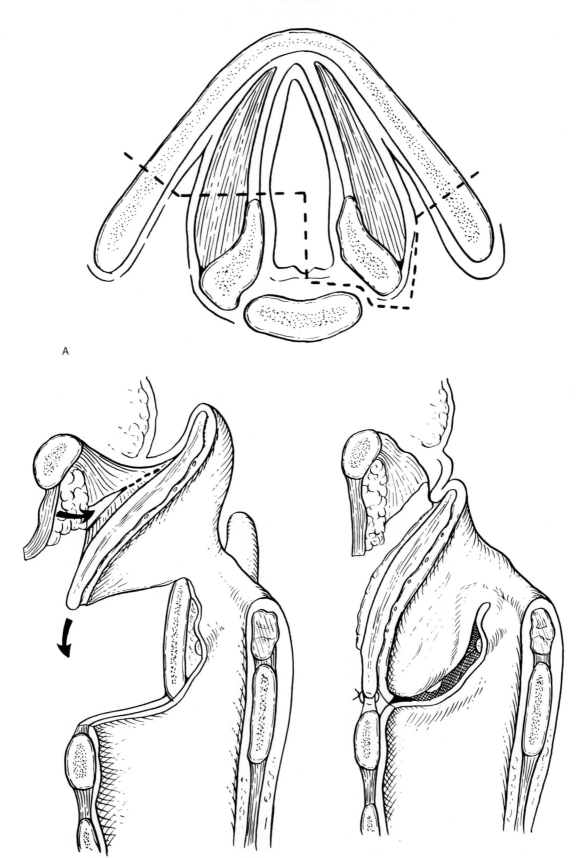

A

B

C

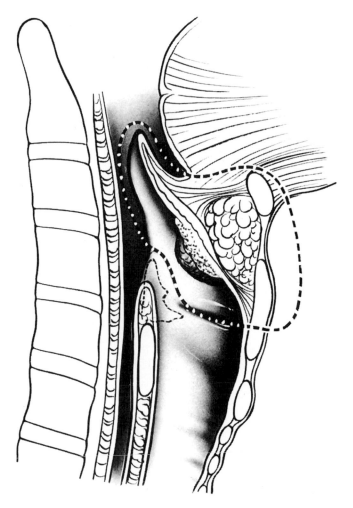

Fig. 25.7   Lesion suitable for subtotal supraglottic laryngectomy with outline of planned resection. (Reprinted from Silver, with permission.[61])

this concept has been extended to include resection of an entire vertical half of the larynx, in addition to the supraglottis: the so-called 'three-quarter' laryngectomy. Such resection has been employed for supraglottic

Table 25.3   Results of supraglottic conservation surgery

Series	Years	Patients	Tumour-free
Supraglottic subtotal laryngectomy			
Ogura et al[44]	3	177	76%
Bocca et al[7]	5	467	75%
Som[65]	5	75	68%
Burnstein & Calcaterra[10]	2	41	90%
Maceri et al[36]	2	25	80%
Robbins et al[51]	5	34	89%
Bocca et al[8]	5	74	75%
Extended supraglottic laryngectomy			
Ogura et al[42]	3	59	75%

carcinomas involving glottis as well as for transglottic carcinomas with minimal extension either subglottically or supraglottically. The prime deterrents to such procedures are major subglottic extension, cartilage invasion, extensive pyriform fossa involvement and poor pulmonary function. As with other conservation procedures, radiation failure is not a contraindication.

Reconstruction is the key to successful surgical treatment in these cases. Most techniques described have used portions of posterior thyroid cartilage to restore glottic competence and maintain the anteroposterior diameter of the larynx. Friedman et al[21] have employed a long segment of contralateral thyroid cartilage, including the superior cornu, with 'greenstick' fracture of the cartilaginous strip thus created, to reconstitute the glottis. This group reported a 3-year survival of 70% in a series of 24 patients.[20] Biller and Lawson[4] have employed a large ipsilateral thyroid

Fig. 25.6   (*opposite page*) Subtotal laryngectomy with epiglottic reconstruction. A. (*top*) Extent of planned resection shown in cross section. B. (*bottom, left*) Mobilization of epiglottis. C. (*bottom, right*) Epiglottis fixed to cricoid. The mucosa approximates well without suture. (Adapted from Tucker et al.[74])

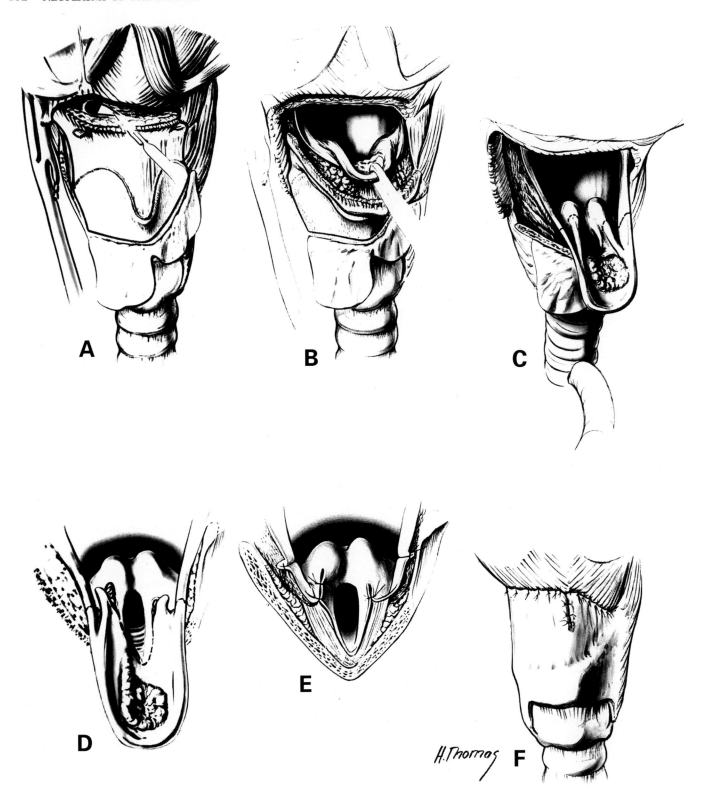

Fig. 25.8 Supraglottic subtotal laryngectomy. A. Cartilage cuts and perichondrial flap. B, C. Hypopharyngeal entry exposing supraglottic structures. D. Supraglottis resected through aryepiglottic folds and ventricles. E. True vocal cords remain. Intralaryngeal mucosa is re-approximated. F. Perichondrial flap sutured to base of tongue for anterior closure. (Reprinted from Silver,[60] with permission.)

cartilage flap, pedicled on the inferior constrictor muscle, for this purpose. Their procedure is illustrated in Fig. 25.9. Five patients operated on by these authors were free of tumour for periods greater than 1.5 years, at the time of their report.

Conservation surgery for hypopharyngeal cancer

Some localized hypopharyngeal tumours may be treated by conservation procedures. Tumours confined entirely to the pharyngeal wall may be resected without involving the larynx; other lesions are managed by extended partial laryngectomy. The entire supraglottis, except for one arytenoid, various amounts of the base of tongue, and one pyriform sinus with adjacent pharyngeal wall may be excised with preservation of laryngeal function. The procedures demonstrated here are based on the 'lateral pharyngotomy' approach employed for SSL. The term 'partial pharyngolaryngectomy' (PPL) is often used to describe such operations.

PPL for superior hypopharyngeal tumours

Suitable lesions for this approach are confined predominantly to the valleculae and lingual surface of the epiglottis, should be less than 3 cm in diameter, and should not infiltrate extensively into the base of the tongue. Lesions involving both valleculae with extension to the circumvallate papillae cannot be treated by conservation surgery.

Mobilization of the larynx, development of the perichondrial flap and bone and cartilage cuts are similar to the manoeuvres described for treatment of supraglottic carcinoma, but may include the upper halves of both thyroid alae and the entire hyoid, if necessary. The pharynx is entered through the pyriform sinus and the incision enlarged superiorly permitting exposure of the base of tongue. This incision is continued upward, creating a 2 cm margin of normal mucosa around the tumour (Fig. 25.10A). It is important to preserve at least one lingual artery. The remainder of the procedure is the same as for supraglottic carcinoma (Fig. 25.10B).

Closure of the hypopharyngeal defect is accomplished with the perichondrial flap, as described for SSL, but is more difficult because of resection of the base of tongue. Suspension of the larynx from the mental area by heavy polyglactin sutures (Fig. 25.10C) will minimize the surgical defect and relieve tension on the suture line. Elevation of the larynx in this manner helps restore the normal 'hyomandibular' apparatus, and may assist in postoperative deglutition.

PPL for pyriform sinus tumours

Pyriform sinus carcinomas are suitable for PPL if the true cord and arytenoid are freely mobile without gross tumour involvement, the apex of the pyriform sinus is uninvolved and there is no thyroid cartilage invasion.

Bone and cartilage cuts are similar to those for SSL, modified for increased exposure of the pyriform sinus. The hypopharynx is entered in the valleculae, or through the posterolateral pharyngeal wall. The pyriform sinus is retracted outward, exposing the tumour (Fig. 25.11A), and the resection procedes inferiorly beneath the tumour and through the cricoarytenoid joint, vocal process, and ventricle (Fig. 25.11B,C). The remainder of the operation is similar to SSL. Sufficient mucosa usually remains to achieve closure with local tissue. Lesions large enough to need a pedicled cutaneous or myocutaneous flap for closure require total or 'near total' laryngectomy for adequate resection and postoperative function.

Posterolateral pharyngeal wall

The lateral pharyngotomy approach may be employed for excision of tumours of the posterolateral pharyngeal wall not in continuity with the larynx. Suitable lesions may extend from above the cricopharyngeus to the level of the tip of the epiglottis or slightly higher.

The thyrotomy is made in a slightly oblique vertical direction over the posterior third of ala and extends through the junction of body and greater cornu of the hyoid bone (Fig. 25.12A). The hypopharynx is entered superiorly and mucosal incision extended laterally and inferiorly to expose posterolateral pharyngeal wall and tumour. The lesion is circumscribed with a safe margin of uninvolved mucosa (Fig. 25.12B). The method of hypopharyngeal repair varies according to the extent of resection. Primary closure may be possible by mobilization and direct approximation of pharyngeal tissue. Larger defects have been repaired with a split thickness skin graft placed on the prevertebral muscles, rotated to close the defect (Fig. 25.12C). More extensive defects may be repaired with myocutaneous flaps, or various 'free flaps' of skin or jejunum, as will be discussed below.

SURGERY FOR ADVANCED LARYNGEAL AND HYPOPHARYNGEAL CANCER

Total laryngectomy

Total extirpation of the larynx was first accomplished by Billroth[24] in 1873, and developed in the early twentieth century by Gluck and Sorenson[22] into a relatively safe and reliable procedure. Nevertheless because of difficulties with anaesthesia, infection control and lack of blood replacement, radiation therapy was employed almost exclusively during the period between the two World Wars for treatment of laryngeal cancer. The advent of modern techniques of anaesthesia, antibiotic therapy and blood transfusion in the succeeding era, coupled with the disappointing results achieved in treatment of advanced

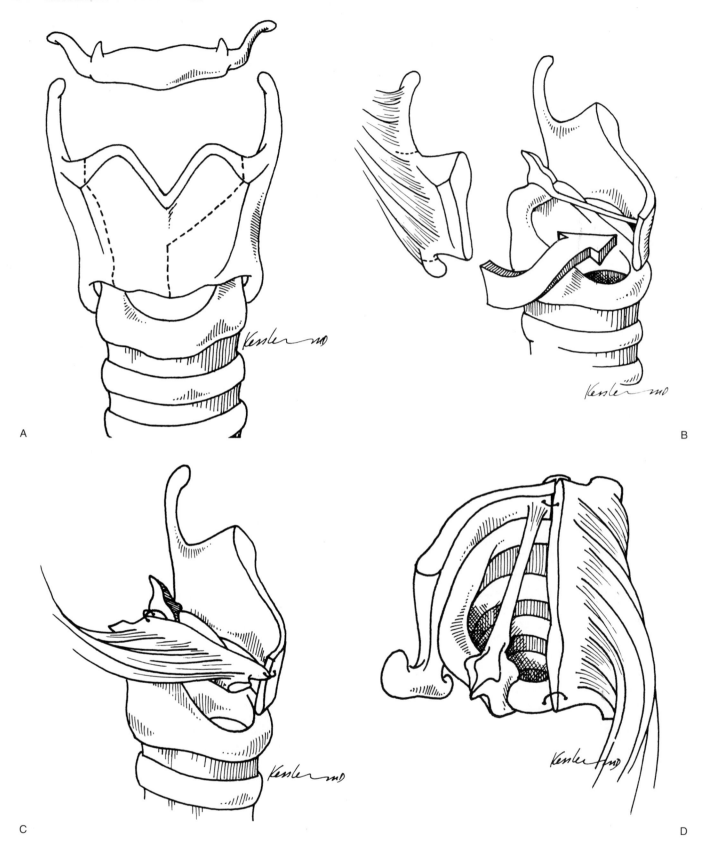

A

B

C

D

Fig. 25.9   Subtotal laryngectomy — the technique of Biller and Lawson. A. (*top, left*) Cartilage cuts for resection. B. (*top, right*) Preparation and movement of cartilage flap pedicled on inferior constrictor muscle. C, D. (*bottom left, right*) Final position of flap to replace resected portion of glottis. (Reprinted from Biller and Lawson,[4] with permission.)

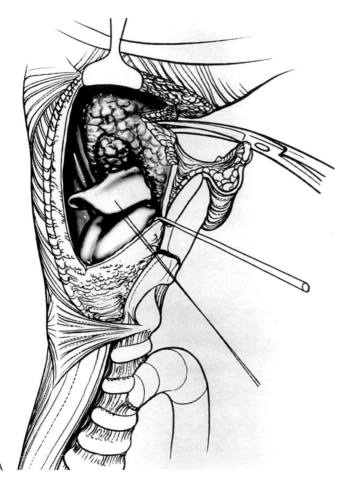

A

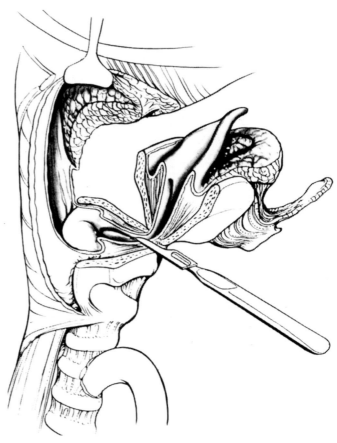

B

Fig. 25.10 Partial pharyngolaryngectomy for superior hypopharyngeal tumour. A. (*top, left*) Incision through tongue base. B. (*above*) Incision through ventricles completes the resection. C. (*bottom*) Laryngeal suspension sutures minimize the defect, relieve tension on closure and assist postoperative deglutition. (Reprinted from Silver, with permission.[61])

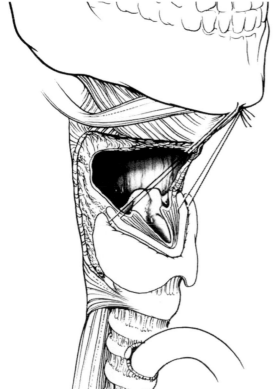

C

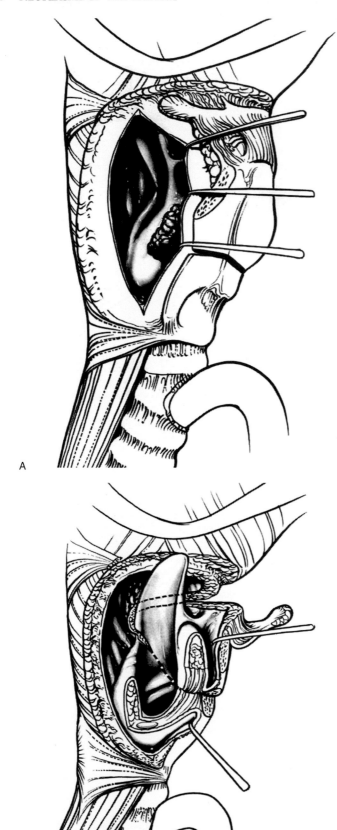

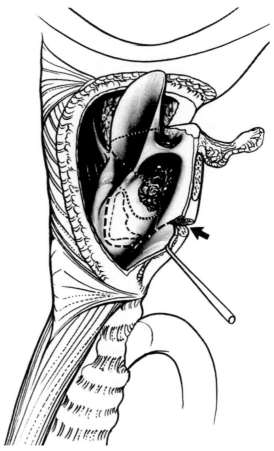

Fig. 25.11 Partial pharyngolaryngectomy for pyriform sinus tumour. A. (*top, left*) Exposure of tumour through incision of posterolateral pharyngeal mucosa. B. (*above*) Outline of mucosal resection. C. (*bottom*) Supraglottis is resected with medial and lateral walls of pyriform sinus. Resection does not include the apex of pyriform sinus. (Reprinted from Silver, with permission.[61])

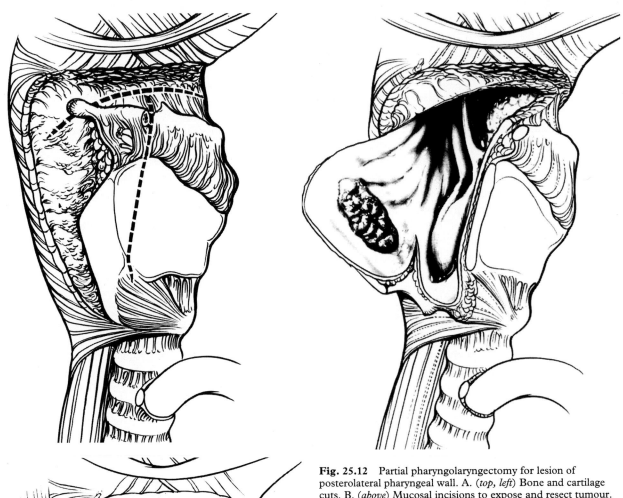

A

B

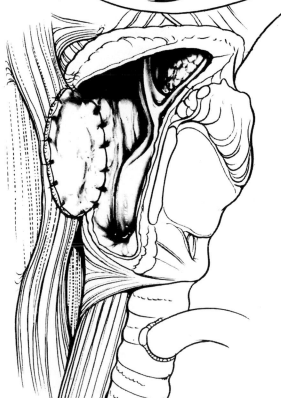

C

Fig. 25.12 Partial pharyngolaryngectomy for lesion of posterolateral pharyngeal wall. A. (*top, left*) Bone and cartilage cuts. B. (*above*) Mucosal incisions to expose and resect tumour. C. (*bottom*) Closure with skin graft based on prevertebral muscles. (Reprinted from Silver, with permission.[61])

laryngeal cancer by radiation therapy alone, served to institute successful and widespread employment of total laryngectomy as the mainstay of treatment for advanced laryngeal and hypopharyngeal cancer.

Total laryngectomy for treatment of laryngeal cancer remains the standard against which other operations and modalities must be judged with regard to cure rates. As techniques of radiation therapy and conservation surgery have developed, however, the indications for total laryngectomy have become controversial. Advocates of the more extended conservation operations, as well as proponents of 'near total' laryngectomy have demonstrated results with selected lesions that are comparable to those that would be obtained by total laryngectomy. The indications for total laryngectomy thus differ among surgeons. Total laryngectomy is currently the treatment of choice for the more extensive laryngeal cancers, including most subglottic, the majority of T_3 and most T_4 glottic, and most T_3 or T_4 supraglottic carcinomas involving the glottis. Extensions of total laryngectomy to include resection of contiguous portions of the pharynx are employed for most hypopharyngeal carcinomas. Although conservation surgery may be employed selectively after radiation failure, total laryngectomy remains the safest procedure for salvage in the majority of instances. A summary of indications for total laryngectomy is shown in Table 25.4.

Technique of total laryngectomy for endolaryngeal tumour

The conventional wide-field total laryngectomy includes resection of the entire larynx from the hyoid bone to the second tracheal ring including the prelaryngeal (strap)

Table 25.4 Indications for total laryngectomy

Glottic
  T_3 carinoma with cord fixation and subglottic extension beyond limits suitable for hemilaryngectomy
  T_4 carcinoma

Supraglottic
  T_3 tumours with pre-epiglottic space invasion and vocal cord involvement
  T_3 tumours with vocal cord fixation (exceptions noted in text)
  T_4 carcinoma

Subglottic
  All primary subglottic tumours
  Glottic tumours with fixaton and extensive subglottic extension

Transglottic
  Carcinoma with paraglottic space invasion, particularly with vocal cord fixation

Pyriform sinus
  Carcinoma with involvement of apex of pyriform sinus, vocal cord fixation or paraglottic space invasion

All laryngeal carcinomas
  Following tracheotomy performed as an independent procedure prior to definitive resection

muscles, varying amounts of pyriform sinus and hypopharyngeal mucosa, and the ipsilateral thyroid lobe.

The incisions for total laryngectomy vary, depending on whether a neck dissection is done in continuity (Fig. 25.13A), if a previously placed tracheotomy is present (Fig. 25.13B), or if there is to be no neck dissection—in which case the superior and lateral extensions of the skin flaps are not necessary. The ipsilateral side is mobilized by separating the carotid sheath vessels from the laryngotracheal structures and transecting the infrahyoid muscles low in the neck, revealing thyroid gland, trachea and oesophagus. The thyroid lobe is resected in continuity with the larynx and is mobilized by dividing inferior thyroid artery as well as the paratracheal structures inferior to the thyroid lobe, including the recurrent laryngeal nerve. If a previous tracheotomy is in place, it is necessary to include the entire tracheotomy site within the resected block. The trachea is exposed, cleared, and will eventually be transected below that level (Fig. 25.13C).

The superior thyroid artery is divided and suprahyoid muscles severed along the superior border of the body and greater cornu of the hyoid bone. Care must be taken not to injure the hypoglossal nerve or lingual artery which are on superficial and deep aspects of hyoglossus muscle, in close proximity to the cornu. Muscles that originate from the body of the hyoid bone are thick and must be transected completely before the external aspect of hypopharyngeal mucosa is uncovered. If tumour is suspected within the valleculae, the suprahyoid muscles are left attached to the body of the hyoid bone (Fig. 25.13D).

The contralateral side is mobilized in a similar manner, although with greater conservation of tissue. After division of the thyroid isthmus, the thyroid lobe on this side will be separated from the trachea, preserving its blood supply (Fig. 25.13E).

If the contralateral pyriform sinus is free of tumour, mucosa on this side may be saved. The inferior constrictor muscle fibres are incised along the posterior edge of the thyroid ala, exposing pyriform sinus which is dissected from the inner aspect of the thyroid cartilage to liberate as much tissue as possible. (Fig. 25.13F).

With the larynx now mobilized, the trachea is transected at least 2 cm below the inferior limit of the tumour (or tracheotomy site). If possible, the tracheal incision should be bevelled upwards posteriorly, to increase the diameter of the tracheostoma. The posterior tracheal wall and cricoid are separated from the oesophagus. A cuffed endotracheal tube (not shown) is inserted in the the distal trachea for control of airway. The hypopharynx is usually entered through the contralateral pyriform sinus. It may be entered through the valleculae or through the postcricoid mucosa if necessary. The site of entry should be planned as far from the tumor margin as possible (Fig. 25.13G).

After entry into the hypopharynx, the mucosal incision is extended superiorly through the valleculae. As it is enlarged, the entire hypopharynx can be visualized and the remaining resection line planned (Fig. 25.13H). The mucosal incision is completed through the postcricoid region and remaining attachments of the larynx severed (Fig. 25.13I).

The large triangular hypopharyngeal defect is closed with interrupted sutures of 00 or 000 polyglactin, with knots tied on the inside. In order to correct the discrepancy in length between superior and inferior flaps, sutures are placed in closer proximity through the superior than the inferior flap (Fig. 25.13J). In this manner, it is usually possible to achieve a transverse linear closure after resection of endolaryngeal tumours (Fig. 25.13K). This is preferable to a trifurcated closure line, as it is less susceptible to postoperative fistulization. The tracheostoma is constructed by suture to the skin edges with interrupted sutures of polyglactin or nylon. The tracheostoma is placed either in the main incision (with a downward vertical extension if feasible), or through a separate small incision in the inferior flap, as shown (Fig. 25.13). The latter is preferable, as there is less likelihood of postoperative stenosis, but it is usually not possible if a previous tracheostomy site has been excised.

Total laryngectomy produces cure rates of 60–70% for T_3N_0 laryngeal carcinomas and 45–50% for T_4N_0 tumours.[61] Lower cure rates are usually obtained in patients after radiation failure or in those with cervical lymph node metastases. Approximately 30–50% of patients regain oesophageal speech following total laryngectomy, and a large percentage of the remaining patients can be rehabilitated either with a variety of surgical prostheses or by use of a hand-held electrolarynx. Thus, although disability is incurred, most patients are able to adapt reasonably well to total laryngectomy, and the operation offers many patients with advanced laryngeal tumours the best available chance for cure.

'Near-total' laryngectomy

A new concept of conservation surgery developed by Pearson[46] involves performing a 'true' hemilaryngectomy including cricoid cartilage and perilaryngeal tissues for extensive but unilateral transglottic, fixed glottic and advanced supraglottic carcinomas. The procedure may also be useful for tumours that require extensive hypopharyngeal resection but involve the larynx minimally. A prerequisite for this procedure is that the posterior commissure, one arytenoid and the ipsilateral ventricle must be free of tumour. Although the laryngeal tissue preserved is insufficient to maintain an intact airway, salvage of contralateral laryngeal mucosa with an arytenoid cartilage, intrinsic musculature, and the recurrent laryngeal nerve, allows the creation of a dynamic phonatory shunt. This procedure prevents aspiration, permits restoration of a

lung powered voice, and may have wider applicability in elderly patients as well as for more extensive tumours than operations that attempt to preserve respiratory as well as phonatory and deglutitory function of the larynx. The oncological feasibility of this procedure has recently been reinforced by whole-organ studies.[50] The technique has been utilized for resection of hypopharyngeal and base-of-tongue carcinomas without extensive laryngeal involvement, including lesions that require flap reconstruction.[15,16]

The ipsilateral (right) larynx is mobilized in the same manner as for total laryngectomy, with the thyroid lobe, prelaryngeal muscles and adjacent lymphoareolar structures included in the resected specimen. On the contralateral (left) side, the larynx is skeletonized as for vertical hemilaryngectomy. The central portion of thyroid cartilage is outlined, and will be removed (Fig. 25.14A). This exposes the ventricular mucosal defect through which the larynx will be entered, at about the midportion of the contralateral vocal cord (Fig. 25.14B). In resection of hypopharyngeal tumours that do not involve the endolarynx, the laryngotomy may be performed in the midline to preserve the entire contralateral mucosa. The mucosal incision is extended superiorly (Fig. 25.14C) and inferiorly (Fig. 25.14D) until the endolarynx is exposed and an adequate resection margin outlined (Fig. 25.14E). The deep structures in the posterior midline, the interarytenoideus muscle and cricoid lamina are incised, with care not to injure the anterior hypopharyngeal mucosa (Fig. 25.14F). Fracture of the cricoid lamina is facilitated by scoring the anterior perichondrium, and placing a finger in the hypopharynx, as shown. The specimen, consisting of the entire right hemilarynx, with the tumour and adequate mucosal margins is now excised (Fig. 25.14G). As the entire paraglottic space has been included, adequate extirpation of transglottic carcinoma is achieved.

The reconstructive phase of the procedure commences with submucosal dissection and piecemeal removal of a sufficient amount of residual (left) cricoid cartilage to permit tubing of the subglottic mucosa (Fig. 25.14H). The defect in right pyriform sinus is sutured as far as the reflection of postcricoid mucosa (Fig. 25.14I). In most cases of endolaryngeal tumour there will be insufficient laryngeal mucosa remaining to form a shunt of adequate diameter (the mucosal tube should accommodate a 14F —5 mm diameter—catheter). The mucosa available for tubing may be augmented with a flap of pyriform sinus mucosa sutured to the remaining laryngeal mucosa (Fig. 25.14J). This new mucosal structure, with its overlying muscle, is now tubed, using the 14F catheter as a temporary template (Fig. 25.14K). After closure of the remaining pharyngeal defect, a second layer is provided by suture of the preserved left infrahyoid to suprahyoid musculature. An anterior wall tracheotomy, placed through the third tracheal ring, is 'matured' to the skin.

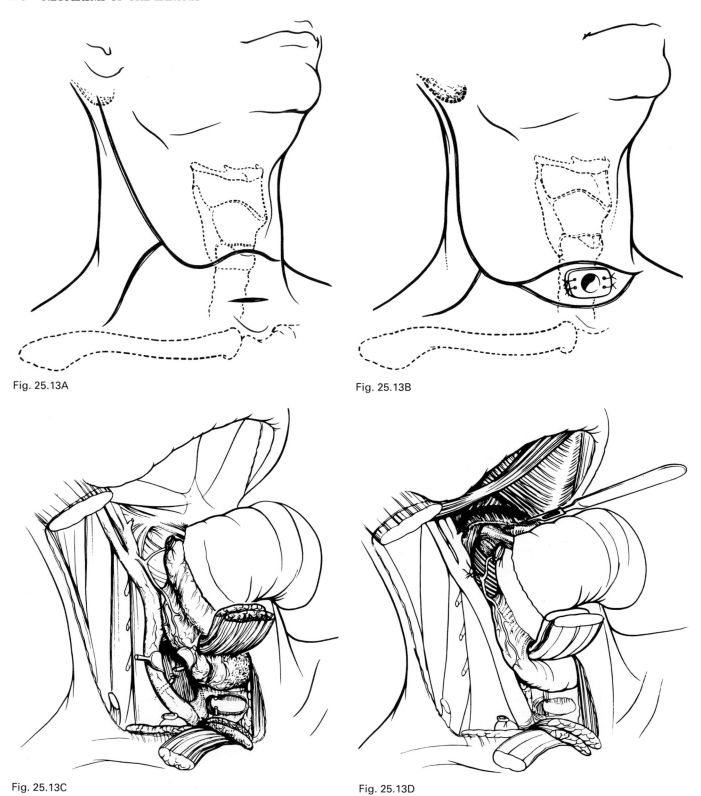

Fig. 25.13A

Fig. 25.13B

Fig. 25.13C

Fig. 25.13D

Fig. 25.13 A–L. Total laryngectomy. See text for explanation. (Reprinted from Silver, with permission.[61])

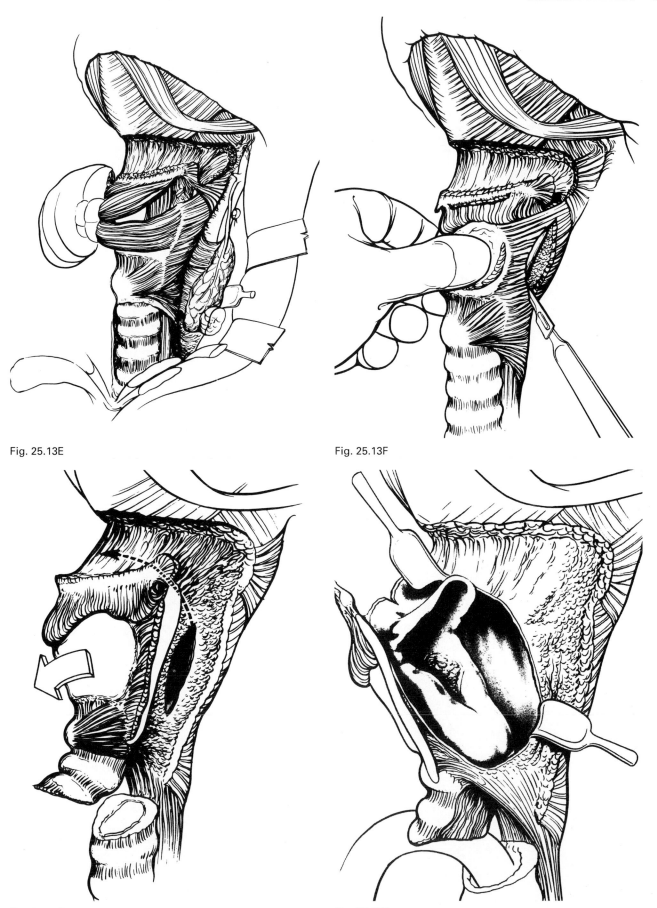

Fig. 25.13E

Fig. 25.13F

Fig. 25.13G

Fig. 25.13H

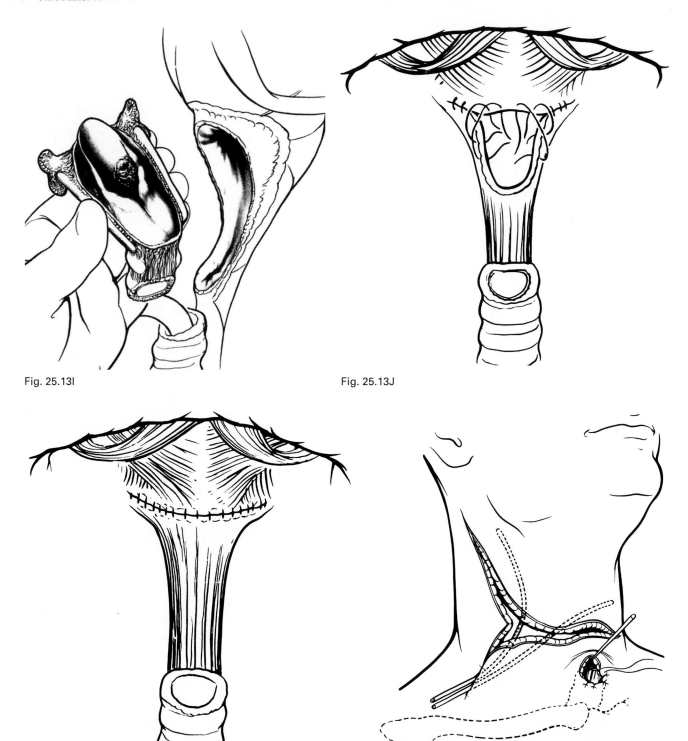

Fig. 25.13I

Fig. 25.13J

Fig. 25.13K

Fig. 25.13L

The resulting configuration is shown in sagittal section (Fig. 25.14L).

A recent literature review indicated short-term (1–3-year) cure in 76 of 120 (63%) patients, with local recurrence in only 6 (5%). Satisfactory voice was achieved in 81% of patients. Fewer than 10% of patients developed complications of aspiration or shunt stenosis.[62]

Extended total laryngectomy for hypopharyngeal tumours

Tumours of the hypopharynx, or laryngopharynx, were formerly termed 'extrinsic' laryngeal carcinomas. Nineteenth- and early twentieth-century surgeons recognized that these tumours were associated with a more rapid clinical course, frequent local and regional recurrence and considerably poorer prognosis than 'intrinsic' (endolaryngeal) laryngeal tumours. The hypopharynx consists of the superior hypopharynx (valleculae and lingual surface of epiglottis), posterior pharyngeal wall, pyriform sinuses and postcricoid region. Surgical treatment of most of these tumours requires laryngectomy (total or partial as described above) with contiguous resection of the involved hypopharyngeal mucosa. The tendency for submucosal spread of hypopharyngeal tumours creates a need for wide resection of mucosa beyond grossly evident margins. In many cases, insufficient local tissue will remain for primary closure after adequate resection, and tissue must be transferred from remote regions for reconstruction. Most postcricoid carcinomas, particularly those involving the cervical oesophagus, require circumferential resection of the entire larynx, pharynx and cervical oesophagus (pharyngolaryngectomy–oesophagectomy). Methods of reconstructing this segmental defect will be discussed in a later section.

Technique of extended total laryngectomy for pyriform sinus carcinoma

Initial mobilization of the larynx is similar to the procedure described above for endolaryngeal tumours. The hypopharynx is entered as far from the tumour as is feasible, usually through the contralateral pyriform sinus, and the mucosal incision extended to encompass the lesion with a wide margin of uninvolved mucosa (Fig. 25.15A). The specimen is removed as resection is completed. Margins should not be limited by concern for tissue available for closure of the hypopharynx (Fig. 25.15B). Reconstruction of the hypopharynx is usually possible by direct suture if no more than 50% of its mucosal circumference has been resected. The defect often extends posteriorly, where closure is commenced by suturing inferior to superior margins of the defect with interrupted suture of 00 or 000 polyglactin (Fig. 25.15C). Closure continues anteriorly, correcting the discrepancy between flaps by appropriate

suture placement (Fig. 25.15D). In many cases, a simple transverse closure cannot be achieved and an inferior vertical extension is required (Fig. 25.15E).

If too much mucosa has been excised to permit primary closure without tension, a mucosal defect remains anteriorly (Fig 25.15F). In the past, this problem was often managed by exteriorization of the defect, creating a temporary pharyngostome that would be closed at a second stage. Recently available methods of reliable tissue transfer have rendered this two-stage approach unnecessary in most instances. Use of a pectoralis major myocutaneous flap will be shown here. Other methods, employing free transfer of jejunum or radial forearm flap will be discussed in conjunction with reconstruction after total pharyngolaryngectomy–oesophagectomy.

An appropriate skin 'paddle' is outlined on the chest and the pectoralis major muscle exposed by elevation of overlying skin (Fig. 25.15G). The muscle is rotated on its vascular pedicle, transferring the skin island to the hypopharyngeal defect which is now repaired (Fig 25.15H). The donor site defect on the chest wall can usually be repaired by direct suture. Occasionally a skin graft may be necessary (Fig 25.15I).

RECONSTRUCTION FOLLOWING TOTAL LARYNGOPHARYNGO-OESOPHAGECTOMY

Complete resection of the larynx, hypopharynx and part or all of the cervical oesophagus is indicated for annular postcricoid carcinomas, extensive pyriform sinus carcinomas with involvement of more than two-thirds of the hypopharyngeal circumference, extensive lesions of the posterior pharyngeal wall that involve the larynx, and carcinomas of the cervical oesophagus. Such tumours produce severe dysphagia with aspiration of food and saliva. Starvation and aspiration pneumonia are the inevitable result of this highly symptomatic obstruction.

Adequate resection produces a circumferential defect in the upper alimentary tract, sometimes including the entire oesophagus. Single-stage restoration of alimentary continuity with minimal postoperative morbidity and mortality is required in order to achieve rapid and satisfactory palliation. Numerous reconstructive methods employed in the past have included multistaged operations employing skin and mucosal flaps as well as transposition of abdominal viscera. All too often these resulted in prolonged hospitalization, persistent salivary fistulae, and tumour recurrence before reconstruction was completed.[58] Newer reconstructive methods have been far more successful in achieving single-stage reconstruction with minimal morbidity and palliation in a significant percentage of patients.

The methods most often employed for immediate pharyngo-oesophageal reconstruction after pharyngolaryngo-oesophagectomy, or for other major hypopharyngeal

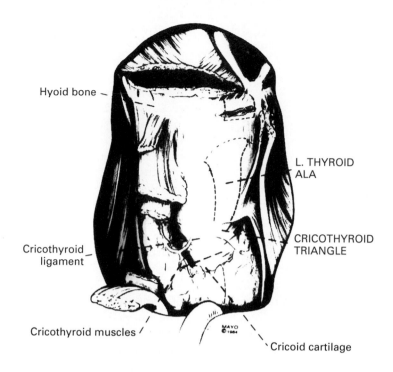

Hyoid bone

L. THYROID
ALA

CRICOTHYROID
TRIANGLE

Cricothyroid
ligament

Cricothyroid muscles

Cricoid cartilage

Fig. 25.14A

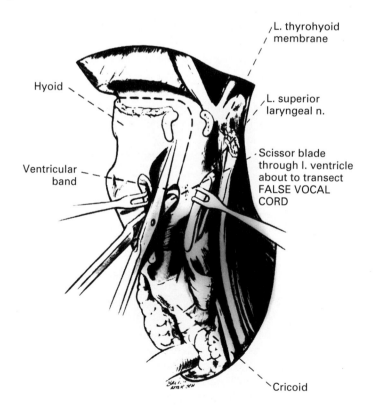

L. thyrohyoid
membrane

Hyoid

L. superior
laryngeal n.

Scissor blade
through l. ventricle
about to transect
FALSE VOCAL
CORD

Ventricular
band

Cricoid

Fig. 25.14B

Fig. 25.14   A–L. Near total laryngectomy. See text for explanation.
(Reprinted from Pearson,[47] with permission.)

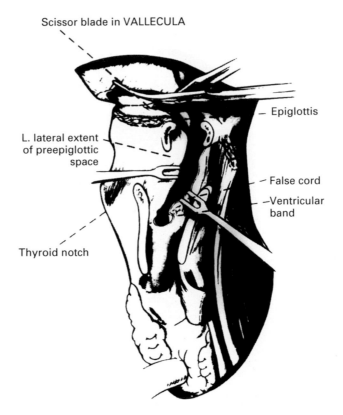

Scissor blade in VALLECULA

Epiglottis

L. lateral extent
of preepiglottic
space

False cord

Ventricular
band

Thyroid notch

Fig. 25.14C

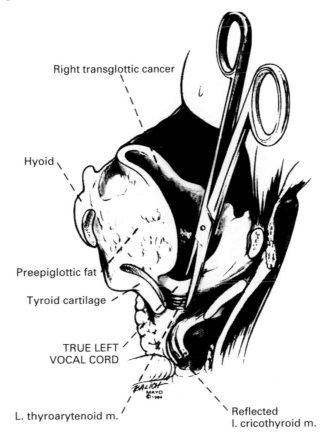

Right transglottic cancer

Hyoid

Preepiglottic fat

Tyroid cartilage

TRUE LEFT
VOCAL CORD

L. thyroarytenoid m.

Reflected
l. cricothyroid m.

Fig. 25.14D

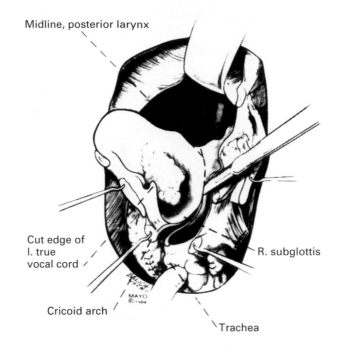

Midline, posterior larynx

Cut edge of
l. true
vocal cord

Cricoid arch

R. subglottis

Trachea

Fig. 25.14E

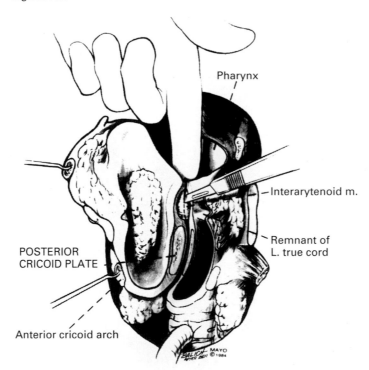

Pharynx

Interarytenoid m.

Remnant of
L. true cord

POSTERIOR
CRICOID PLATE

Anterior cricoid arch

Fig. 25.14F

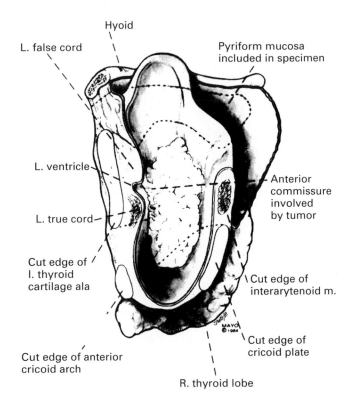

Hyoid

L. false cord

Pyriform mucosa
included in specimen

L. ventricle

Anterior
commissure
involved
by tumor

L. true cord

Cut edge of
l. thyroid
cartilage ala

Cut edge of
interarytenoid m.

Cut edge of
cricoid plate

Cut edge of anterior
cricoid arch

R. thyroid lobe

Fig. 25.14G

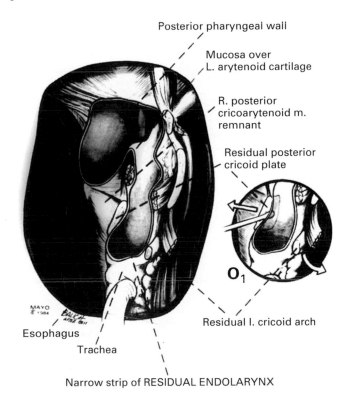

Posterior pharyngeal wall

Mucosa over
L. arytenoid cartilage

R. posterior
cricoarytenoid m.
remnant

Residual posterior
cricoid plate

O₁

Residual l. cricoid arch

Esophagus

Trachea

Narrow strip of RESIDUAL ENDOLARYNX

Fig. 25.14H

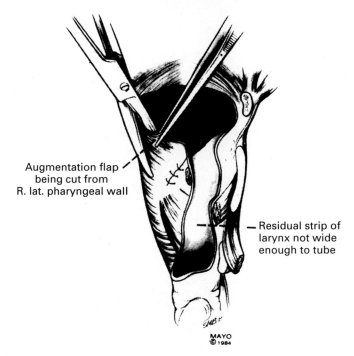

Augmentation flap
being cut from
R. lat. pharyngeal wall

Residual strip of
larynx not wide
enough to tube

Fig. 25.14I

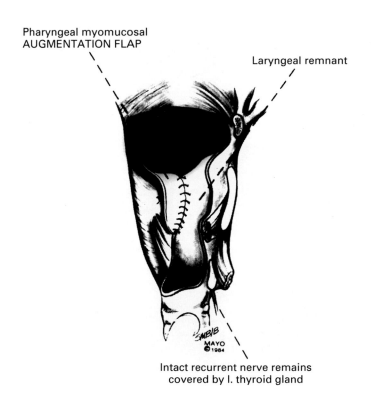

Pharyngeal myomucosal
AUGMENTATION FLAP

Laryngeal remnant

Intact recurrent nerve remains
covered by l. thyroid gland

Fig. 25.14J

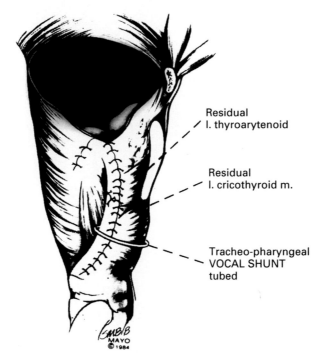

Residual
l. thyroarytenoid

Residual
l. cricothyroid m.

Tracheo-pharyngeal
VOCAL SHUNT
tubed

Fig. 25.14K

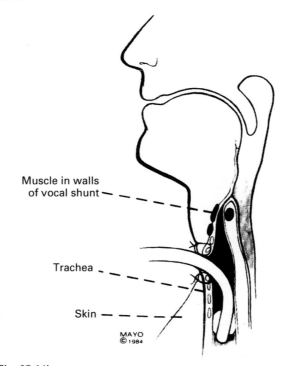

Muscle in walls
of vocal shunt

Trachea

Skin

Fig. 25.14L

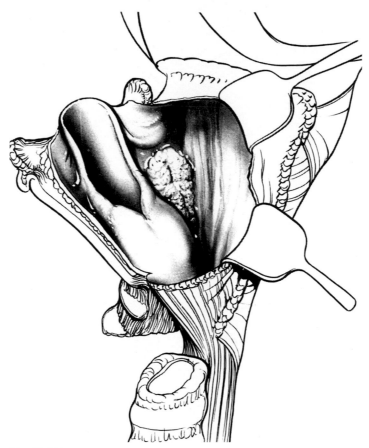

Fig. 25.15A

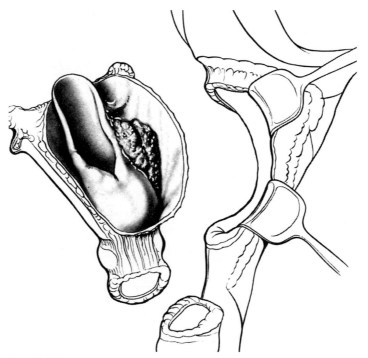

Fig. 25.15B

Fig. 25.15   A–I. Extended total laryngectomy for pyriform sinus carcinoma. See text for explanation. (Reprinted from Silver, with permission.[61])

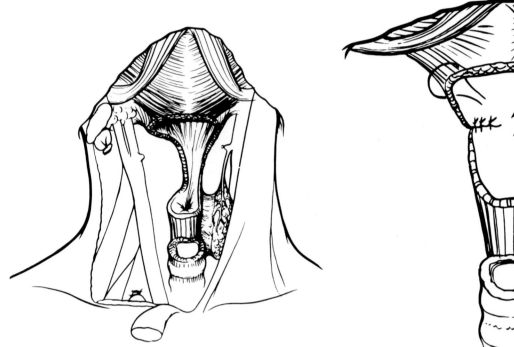

Fig. 25.15C

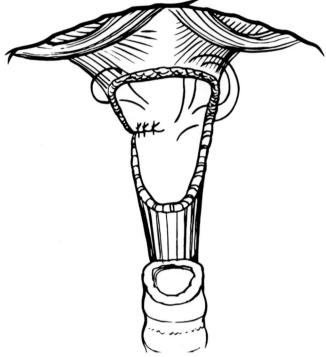

Fig. 25.15D

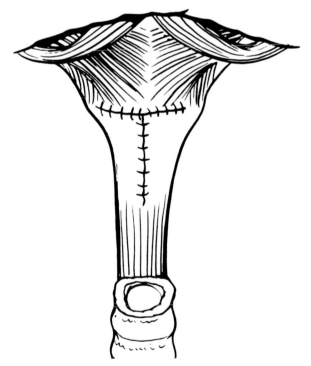

Fig. 25.15E

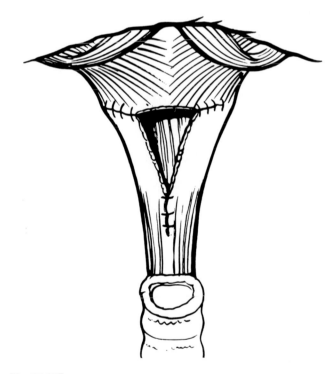

Fig. 25.15F

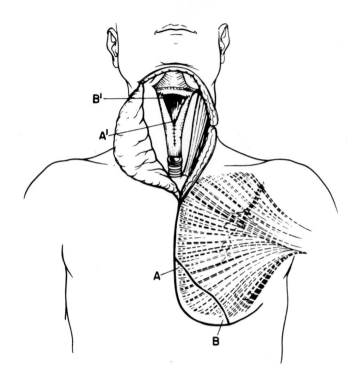

Fig. 25.15G

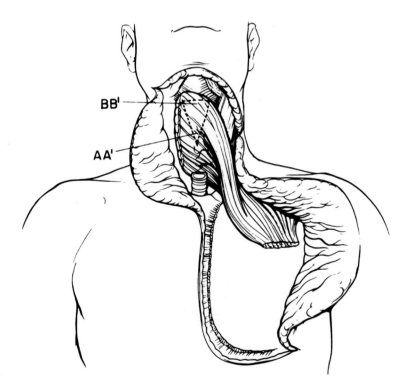

Fig. 25.15H

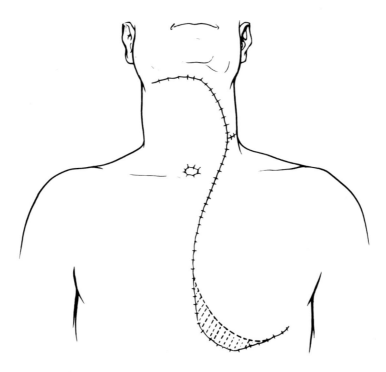

Fig. 25.15I

defects, are gastric transposition, the tubed pectoralis major myocutaneous flap and free transplantation of jejunum. Recently, free transfer of forearm skin based on the radial artery, has been employed with success.

Gastric transposition

Single-stage pharyngolaryngectomy with 'blunt,' closed chest total oesophagectomy and replacement by transposition of the mobilized stomach through the posterior mediastinum was developed and reported in 1960 by Ong and Lee.[45] The procedure was modified and experience widened by Lequesne and Ranger,[34] Stell,[69] Silver,[59] and Harrison.[26] The transposed stomach has an excellent blood supply, and can easily reach the level of the superior hypopharynx where only a single anastomosis is required. The procedure is most useful for oesophageal replacement after resection of carcinomas of the cervical oesophagus and post cricoid carcinomas (Fig. 25.16A). Resection of the entire oesophagus entailed by this operation will assure an adequate distal resection margin without concern as to the amount of oesophagus available for distal anastomosis. Transposed stomach may also be employed for oesophageal replacement or bypass after resection of thoracic oesophageal carcinomas, oesophageal strictures and tracheal stomal recurrence of laryngeal carcinoma with pharyngo-oesophageal involvement. It is less useful for replacement after resection of hypopharyngeal carcinomas that extend superiorly, as the intact stomach will not reach beyond the level of the hyoid bone without

modifications that increase greatly the possibility of postoperative fistula and other complications.

A two-team approach is employed. After resectability of the lesion has been established, the larynx, trachea and cervical oesophagus are mobilized. The abdomen is entered through an upper midline incision and the stomach freed along greater and lesser curvatures, preserving right gastroepiploic and right gastric vessels with their arcades. Left gastric and left gastroepiploic vessels are transected near their origins (Fig. 25.16B). The gastro-oesophageal junction is dissected free and the vagus nerves divided. The hiatus is enlarged by dilatation and transection of muscle until the surgeon's hand can be passed well into the mediastinum. The lower third of the oesophagus can now be liberated by blunt digital dissection, without difficulty.

After mobilization of the stomach, the cervical trachea and superior hypopharynx are transected. With upward traction on larynx and hypopharynx, downward dissection of oesophagus from the cervical field is commenced. Lateral attachments of oesophagus are divided under direct vision, with haemostatic clipping, for a distance of several centimetres into the posterior mediastinum. Anteriorly, the oesophagus is dissected sharply from the posterior tracheal wall, with care taken to deflate the endotracheal balloon prior to separation of trachea and oesophagus. Posteriorly the oesophagus is easily freed by blunt dissection.

At this point, the central third of the oesophagus is mobilized by blunt digital dissection contributed by both abdominal and cervical surgeons (Fig. 25.16C), until the entire oesophagus is free and can be extracted by gentle upward traction into the cervical field, while the stomach is guided and pushed into the posterior mediastinum. The gastric fundus is pulled upward at this point, until it reaches the stump of oropharynx (Fig. 25.16D). The cardio-oesophageal junction is transected and closed with a stapling device, and the specimen removed from the field. An incision is made in the gastric fundus and a pharyngogastrostomy created in one or two layers (Fig. 25.16E).

Harrison[27] recently reported results of gastric transposition in a series of 140 patients. There were 13 (9.3%) operative deaths in the series, and only two instances of pharyngogastric fistula among the surviving patients. The most common serious problem encountered was a rather high (15%) incidence of postoperative pulmonary problems. Most patients were able to swallow liquids by the fifth postoperative day and had excellent deglutition by the tenth. The average period of hospitalization was two weeks. Similar results have been noted in other recent reports; a review of 134 cases by five authors[31,40,48,54,63] revealed 10% postoperative deaths, 16% pharyngogastric fistulae, and satisfactory postoperative deglutition in at least 75% of patients. Delayed gastric emptying and regurgitation was an occasionally reported problem, that invariably resolved spontaneously. The need for only a single anastomosis, the wide resection of oesophagus made possible by this approach, the virtual absence of stenosis and the good cosmetic results obtained are all factors that favour the employment of this procedure, particularly for resection of lesions that extend inferior to the cricopharyngeus.

Pectoralis major myocutaneous flap

The utility of the pectoralis major myocutaneous flap for replacement and repair of hypopharyngeal defects has been demonstrated above. We have found this flap to be most useful for repair of circumferential defects in the hypopharynx and cervical oesophagus, when the defects are confined to the cervical region. In order to assure blood supply of the neo-oesophagus a trapezoidal skin island, with no 'random' portion, is created directly over the pectoralis major muscle (Fig. 25.17A). The flap is designed so as to conform to the length of the defect as well as to the circumferences of oropharyngeal and distal oesophageal stumps. As the flap will be inverted when it is rotated into the cervical wound, the larger (oropharyngeal) parallel side of the trapezoid is placed inferiorly.

After mobilization of the pectoralis major muscle on its vascular pedicle, the flap is tunnelled beneath a 'bridge' of superior pectoral skin into the neck where it is fitted into the oesophageal defect (Fig. 25.17B). The flap may be 'tubed' prior to anastomosis to oropharynx and oesophagus, or it may be partly sutured into the alimentary defect and tubed as anastomosis progresses (Fig. 25.17C). We have not taken measures to enlarge the distal anastomosis by bevelling or interdigitating the mucosa, as we feel that such measures, by decreasing the vertical length of the flap, serve to increase the degree of anastomotic tension —the primary cause of disruption with resultant fistula, scar formation and stenosis. The bulky pectoralis major muscle serves to cover the carotid artery and the oesophageal skin tube. If cervical skin cannot be readily closed over the flap, a meshed skin graft is placed on the pectoralis muscle to resurface the neck (Fig. 25.17D). The donor site, despite its size and odd shape, can usually be closed primarily by advancement of surrounding skin, even in male patients.

We have reported the technique and results of our experience with tubed pectoralis major myocutaneous flap for pharyngo-oesophageal reconstruction in ten severely debilitated patients.[13] Six had primary reconstruction following total pharyngolaryngo-oesophagectomy for carcinoma; the other four had long segments of pharyngo-oesophageal stenosis requiring resection and total replacement after previous laryngectomy. Six patients were over 80 years of age, and six had received previous high-dose radiation therapy.

No technical difficulties were encountered in tubing the flaps, which all retained viability, and none were too bulky for placement into the cervical wound. Distal anastomotic fistulae developed in four patients, all previously irradiated. Two of these fistulae healed with conservative management; the other two occurred in patients who died of unrelated medical complications before their wounds healed completely. One instance of mild stenosis responded to a single dilatation.

Satisfactory and lasting deglutatory function was achieved with the eight surviving patients. While four non-irradiated patients in this group commenced oral feeding within 1–3 weeks following surgery, three of four previously irradiated patients required 4 weeks or longer before normal deglutition was possible. Two of five patients, operated on for cancer more than two years ago, remained free of tumour for at least two years. All secondarily reconstructed patients have remained free of disease since surgery.

Our results are similar to others reported in the literature.[33,70,72] A review of 67 reported cases revealed adequate restoration of deglutition in 68.7%, mortality of 8.9%, fistula in 35.8% and stenosis in 25.4%. The tubed pectoralis major myocutaneous flap has proven to be a relatively safe, simple and reliable technique for pharyngo-oesophageal reconstruction that is particularly useful for elderly and debilitated patients.

Free jejunal transplantation

The feasibility of replacement of cervical oesophagus by freely transplanted jejunum was first demonstrated at our institution in 1959.[55] Reliable application of this technique

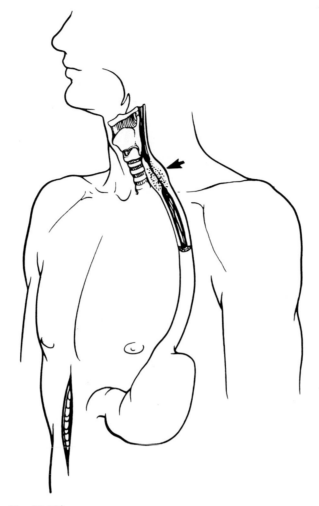

Fig. 25.16A

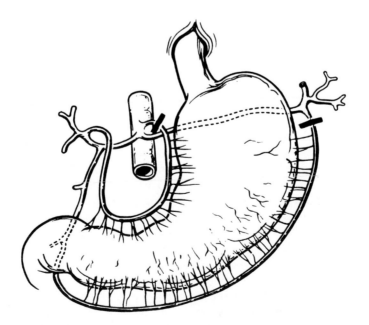

Fig. 25.16B

Fig. 25.16   A–E. Oesophageal replacement by gastric transposition. See text for explanation. (Reprinted from Silver, with permission.[61])

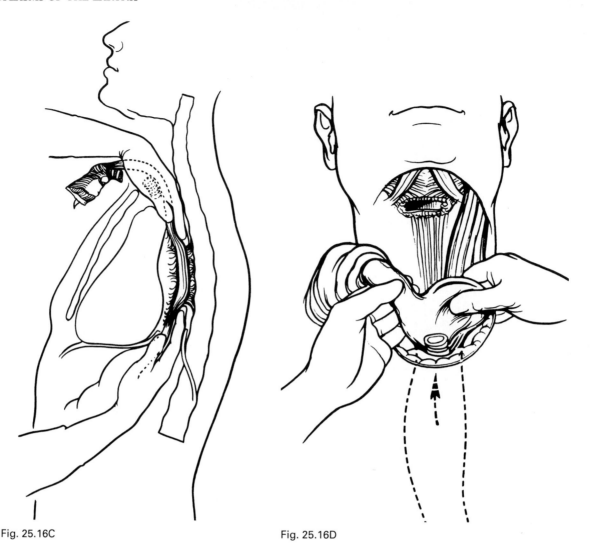

Fig. 25.16C   Fig. 25.16D

had to await developments in microvascular anastomosis and free tissue transfer, which emerged during the 1970s. By the 1980s, free jejunal transfer was employed by many surgeons who reported results and complications comparable to or better than previously employed reconstructive methods.[12,17,18] Use of transplanted jejunum has several advantages over other reconstructive methods. The tissue obtained has excellent blood supply, is pliant and adaptable to defects of varying size and shape, and is similar in nature to the tissue that has been removed. Less dissection is required to transfer the tissue to the neck, as contrasted with pedicled abdominal viscera which require development of a pathway to the neck. On the other hand, the complication rate is fairly high,[12,17,18] numerous vascular and intestinal anastomoses are required, and operating time is longer than with the methods described above. Freely transplanted jejunum cannot be used to replace the entire oesophagus; for pharyngo-oesophageal replacement its use is limited to resections confined above the thoracic inlet.

The technique is demonstrated in Fig. 25.18. A loop of jejunum is chosen that can be isolated on a single artery and vein, and will conform to the cervical defect when oriented in an isoperistaltic direction (Fig. 25.18A). After transfer to the neck, the mesenteric artery is anastomosed to a cervical vessel, most often external carotid artery; although common carotid, superior thyroid, facial, lingual and transverse cervical vessels have been employed (Fig. 25.18C). The mesenteric vein is anastomosed to an appropriate available vessel. If necessary, anastomosis may be made to vessels from the contralateral side of the neck. Segmental vein grafts may be employed for either arterial or venous anastomoses if available pedicle length does not permit vascular union free of tension. After anastomosis, it is important to shorten the bowel segment appropriately to avoid redundancy.

Colemen et al[12] reported results of 96 free jejunal transfers performed in 88 patients. Initial operation was successful in 78 (89%) of the patients. Five more eventually underwent successful second jejunal transfers, producing

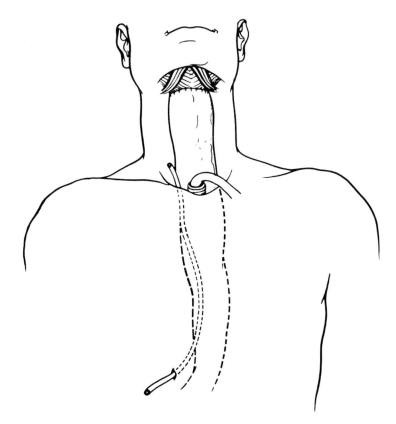

Fig. 25.16E

ultimate repair of the defect by jejunal autograft in 83 (94%) of the 88 patients. Anastomotic fistulae occurred in 28 patients, 12 of whom required further surgery for closure. Other swallowing difficulties were caused by stenosis (six cases) or redundant jejunum. Evaluation of ultimate swallowing function was possible in 68 patients, and considered 'good' in 52 (76%). Review of 64 additional cases reported in the literature[17,18,54] revealed five (8%) flap failures, four (6%) deaths, and other complications including fistula, intestinal obstruction, and gastrointestinal and carotid artery haemorrhage.

'Patches' of revascularized free jejunum, split along the antimesenteric border, have been employed for reconstruction after partial excision of oro- and hypopharynx, with or without total laryngectomy.[32,52] These flaps have the advantage of being pliant, fitting more easily into the defect than bulkier pedicled flaps, and providing a natural mucosal surface.

Free radial forearm flap

Skin flaps based on the radial artery have been employed for partial patched and segmental tubed replacement of oral, pharyngeal and cervical oesophageal defects. The radial artery is a large-calibre vessel that may provide a long pedicle, allowing considerable variation in flap design. Inclusion of the medial or lateral antebrachial cutaneous nerves, or the superficial branch of the radial nerve may provide sensation to the flap by anastomosis to the superior laryngeal, cervical plexus or greater auricular nerves. Bone may be included in the flap if necessary.

The flap is designed on the volar forearm in order to maximize the hairless skin obtainable (Fig. 25.19). The paratenon covering the flexor carpi radialis and palmaris longus tendons should be preserved in order to facilitate skin grafting of the donor site. Preoperatively, an Allen test or angiography must be performed to assure adequate collateral circulation.

Souter et al[68] reported successful use of the radial forearm flap in all ten of their patients. Urken et al[76] presented evidence, in a preliminary report, that postoperative swallowing in a patient, reconstructed with a re-innervated flap after partial pharyngectomy and partial supraglottic laryngectomy, was superior to that obtained in patients reconstructed by methods employing insensate tissue. Other advantages of this reconstruction are that the replacement tissue is thin, pliant, and may be obtained without an abdominal procedure. The donor site is pain-free, and hand and wrist function are not affected. Significant cosmetic deformity, however, is usually produced at the donor site.

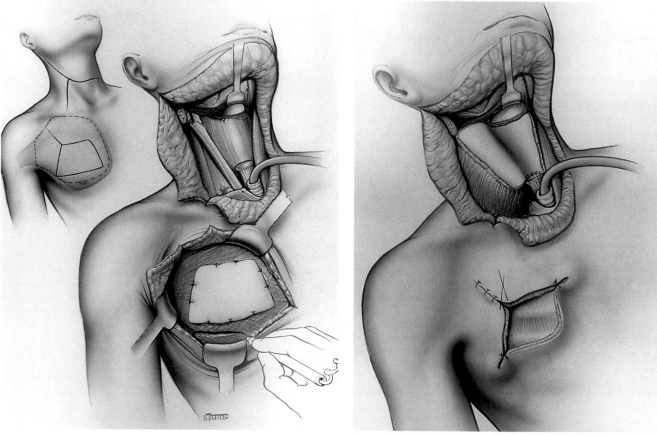

Fig. 25.17A   Fig. 25.17B

Fig. 25.17   A–D. Oesophageal replacement with tubed pectoralis major myocutaneous flap. See text for explanation. (Reprinted from Cusumano et al,[13] with permission.)

Authors' preferences

On our service, we have preferred to employ gastric transposition for most tumours involving cervical oesophagus, and the pectoralis myocutaneous flap for relatively confined lesions involving only the hypopharynx. Free jejunal transplantation has been reserved for specific problems where, because of previous surgery, unusual defects or the need to preserve the larynx, this method proved particularly advantageous. Free radial forearm flaps have not been employed, although this method appears to have merit, particularly for replacement of partial hypopharyngeal defects in cases where the larynx has been preserved.

CONCLUSIONS

Current management of laryngeal cancer provides the surgeon with a variety of options for treatment of early and advanced lesions. Conventional and extended conservation surgery permits surgical cure of early and selected moderately advanced laryngeal and hypopharyngeal cancers while preserving the essential functions of the larynx. Total laryngectomy is an effective operation for control of advanced laryngeal carcinomas as well as many instances of radiation failure. The operation may be extended to include resection and replacement of varying amounts of adjacent tissue for treatment of hypopharyngeal cancers. The near-total laryngectomy, suitable for selected advanced lesions, offers a physiological method of preserving vocal function in patients whose lesions require resection of more laryngeal tissue than will permit preservation of an intact airway. Several reliable alternatives are available for replacement of the pharyngo-oesophageal segment after resection of tumours that require partial or complete circumferential segmental removal of larynx, pharynx and oesophagus.

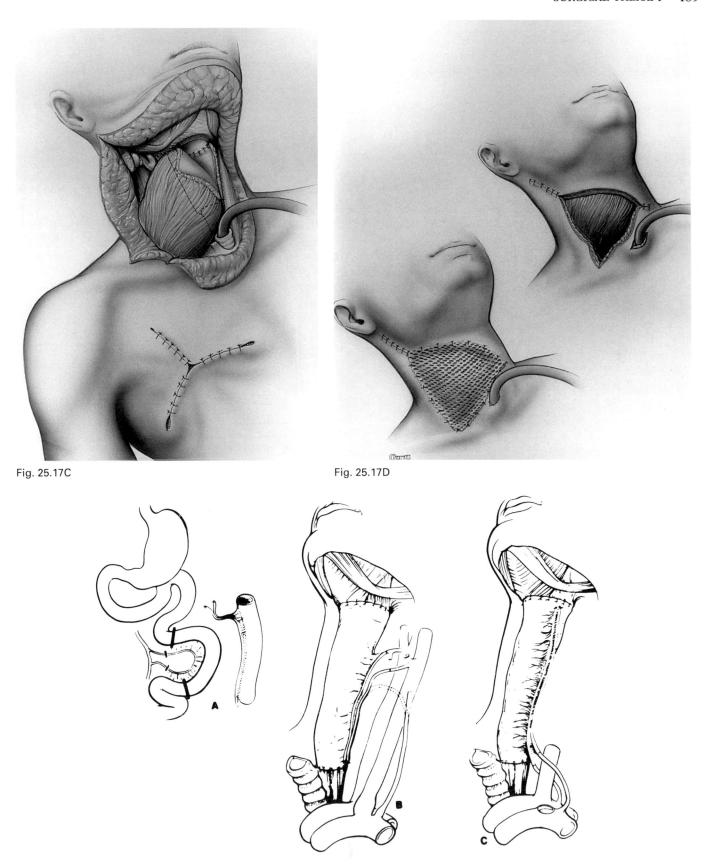

Fig. 25.17C

Fig. 25.17D

Fig. 25.18   Oesophageal replacement with free revascularized jejunum. A. Loop of jejunum with vascular arcade. B. Anastomosis to superior thyroid artery. C. Anastomosis to branch of thyrocervical axis. (Reprinted from Silver, with permission.[61])

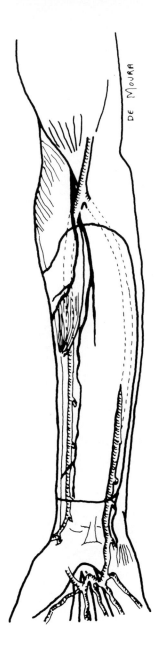

Fig. 25.19   Design and blood supply of free radial forearm flap. (Reprinted from Greenstein et al,[23] with permission.)

REFERENCES

1. Alajmo E, Fini-Storchi O, Agostini V, Polli G 1985 Conservation surgery for cancer of the larynx in the elderly. Laryngoscope 95: 203–205
2. Bailey B J 1975 Glottic reconstruction after hemilaryngectomy: bipedicle muscle flap laryngoplasty. Laryngoscope 85: 960–977
3. Bauer W C, Lesinski S G, Ogura J H 1975 The significance of positive margins in hemilaryngectomy specimens. Laryngoscope 85: 1–13
4. Biller H F, Lawson W 1984 Partial laryngectomy for transglottic cancers. Ann Otol Rhinol Laryngol 93: 297–300
5. Biller H F, Lawson W 1986 Partial laryngectomy for vocal cord cancer with marked limitation or fixation of the vocal cord. Laryngoscope 96: 61–64
6. Biller H F, Ogura J H, Pratt L L 1971 Hemilaryngectomy for T_2 glottic cancers. Arch Otolaryngol 93: 238–243
7. Bocca E, Pignataro O, Oldini C 1983 Supraglottic laryngectomy: 30 years of experience. Ann Otol Rhinol Laryngol 92: 14–18
8. Bocca E, Pignataro O, Oldini C, Sambataro G, Cappa C 1987 Extended supraglottic laryngectomy. Review of 84 cases. Ann Otol Rhinol Laryngol 96: 384–386
9. Bouche J, Freche Ch, Husson Y 1965 L' hémi-laryngectomie avec épiglottoplastie. Nouvelle application de l' épiglottoplastie. Ann Otolaryngol Chir Cervicofac 82: 421–428
10. Burnstein F D, Calcaterra T C 1985 Supraglottic laryngectomy: series report and analysis of results. Laryngoscope 95: 833–836
11. Calcaterra T C 1985 Epiglottic reconstruction after supraglottic laryngectomy. Laryngoscope 95: 786–789
12. Coleman J J III, Searles J M Jr, Hester T R, Nahai F, Zubowicz V, McConnel F M S, Jurciewicz M J 1987 Ten years experience with the free jejunal autograft. Am J Surg 154: 394–398
13. Cusumano, R J, Silver C E, Brauer R J, Strauch B 1989 Pectoralis myocutaneous flap for replacement of cervical esophagus. Head Neck 11: 450–456
14. Daly J F, Kwok F N 1975 Laryngofissure and cordectomy. Laryngoscope 85: 1290–1297
15. DeSanto L W, Pearson B W, Olsen K D 1989 Utility of near-total laryngectomy for supraglottic, pharyngeal, base-of-tongue, and other cancers. Ann Otol Rhinol Laryngol 98: 2–7
16. Dumich P S, Pearson B W, Weiland L H 1984 Suitability of near-total laryngopharyngectomy in piriform carcinoma. Arch Otolaryngol 110: 664–669
17. Ferguson J L, DeSanto L W 1988 Total pharyngolaryngectomy and cervical esophagectomy with jejunal auto transplant reconstruction: complications and results. Laryngoscope 98: 911–914
18. Flynn M B, Banis J, Acland R 1989 Reconstruction with free bowel autografts after pharyngoesophageal or laryngopharyngo-esophageal resection. Am J Surg 158: 333–336
19. Frazer F J 1910 The development of the larynx. J Anat Physiol 44: 156–191
20. Friedman W H, Katsantonis G P 1991 Subtotal laryngectomy with contralateral laryngoplasty. In: Silver C E (ed) Laryngeal cancer. Thieme, New York, pp 183–191
21. Friedman W H, Katsantonis G P, Siddoway J R, Cooper M H 1981 Contralateral laryngoplasty after supraglottic laryngectomy with vertical extension. Arch Otolaryngol 107: 742–745
22. Gluck T, Sorenson J 1931 Die Resektion und Extirpation des Larynx, Pharynx und Esophagus. In: Katz L, Presing H, Bumenfeld F (eds) Handbuch der Spez. Chir. Ohres und der Obereu. Lefwege, Vol IV, C. Kabizch, Wurzburg
23. Greenstein B, de Moura W G, Strauch B 1986 Free flaps. In: Silver C E (ed) Atlas of head and neck surgery. Churchill Livingstone, New York, pp 60–70
24. Gussenbauer C 1874 Über die erste durch Th. Billroth am Menschen ausgeführte Kehlkopf. Extirpation und die Anwendung eines künstlichen Kehlkopfes. Arch Klin Chir 17: 343–356
25. Hajek M 1891 Anatomische Untersuchungen über das Larynxödem. Arch Klin Chir 42: 46–93
26. Harrison D F N 1979 Surgical management of hypopharyngeal cancer. Particular reference to the gastric 'pull-up' operation. Arch Otolaryngol 105: 149–152
27. Harrison D F N 1991 Replacement of cervical esophagus by gastric transposition. In: Silver C E (ed) Laryngeal cancer. Thieme, New York, pp 260–267
28. Hirano M, Kurita S, Tateishi M, Matsuoka H 1987 Deglutition following supraglottic horizontal laryngectomy. Ann Otol Rhinol Laryngol 96: 7–11
29. Kessler D J, Trapp T K, Calcaterra T C 1987 The treatment of T_3 glottic carcinoma with vertical partial laryngectomy. Arch Otolaryngol Head Neck Surg 113: 1196–1199
30. Kirchner J A, Som M L 1975 The anterior commissure technique of partial laryngectomy: clinical and laboratory observations. Laryngoscope 85: 1308–1317
31. Krespi Y P, Wurster C F, Sisson G A 1985 Immediate reconstruction after total laryngopharyngoesophagectomy and mediastinal dissection. Laryngoscope 95: 156–161
32. Lam K H, Ho C M, Lau W F, Wei W I, Wong J 1989 Immediate reconstruction of pharyngoesophageal defects: preference or reference. Arch Otolaryngol Head Neck Surg 115: 608–612
33. Lau W F, Lam K H, Wei W I 1987 Reconstruction of hypopharyngeal defects in cancer surgery: Do we have a choice? Am J Surg 154: 374–380
34. LeQuesne L P, Ranger D 1966 Pharyngolaryngectomy with immediate pharyngogastric anastomosis. Br J Surg 53: 105–109
35. Leroux–Robert J 1975 A statistical study of 620 laryngeal carcinomas of the glottic region personally operated upon more than five years ago. Laryngoscope 85: 1440–1452
36. Maceri D R, Lampe H B, Makielski K H, Passamani P P, Krause C J 1985 Conservation laryngeal surgery — a critical analysis. Arch Otolaryngol 111: 361–365
37. McGavran M H, Spjut H, Ogura J 1959 Laryngofissure in the treatment of laryngeal carcinoma. A critical analysis of success and failure. Laryngoscope 69: 44–53
38. McNaught R C 1950 Surgical correction of anterior web of the larynx. Laryngoscope 60: 264–272
39. Mohr R M, Quenelle D J, Shumrick D A 1983 Vertico-frontolateral laryngectomy (Hemilaryngectomy). Indications, technique, and results. Arch Otolaryngol 109: 384–395
40. Moores D W O, Ilves R, Cooper J D, Todd T R J, Pearson F G 1983 One-stage reconstruction for pharyngolaryngectomy: esophagectomy and pharyngogastrostomy without thoracotomy. J Thorac Cardiovasc Surg 85: 330–336
41. Ogura J H, Dedo H H 1965 Glottic reconstruction following subtotal glottic-supraglottic laryngectomy. Laryngoscope 75: 865–878
42. Ogura J H, Sessions D G, Ciralsky R H 1975 Supraglottic carcinoma with extension to the arytenoid. Laryngoscope 85: 1327–1331
43. Ogura J H, Sessions D G, Spector G J 1975 Analysis of surgical therapy for epidermoid carcinoma of the laryngeal glottis. Laryngoscope 85: 1522–1530
44. Ogura J H, Session D G, Spector G J 1975 Conservation surgery for epidermoid carcinoma of the supraglottic larynx. Laryngoscope 85: 1808–1815
45. Ong G B, Lee T C 1960 Pharyngogastric anastomosis after oesophagopharyngectomy for carcinoma of the hypopharynx and cervical oesophagus. Br J Surg 48: 193–200
46. Pearson B W 1981 Subtotal laryngectomy. Laryngoscope 91: 1904–1912
47. Pearson B W 1986 Near total laryngectomy. In: Silver C E (ed) Atlas of head and neck surgery. Churchill Livingstone, New York, pp 235–245
48. Pradhan S A, Rajpal R M 1984 Gastric pull-up for cancers of the hypopharynx and cervical esophagus: our experience. J Surg Oncol 26: 149–152
49. Pressman J 1956 Submucosal compartmentation of the larynx. Ann Otol Rhinol Laryngol 65: 766–771

50. Robbins K T, Michaels L 1985 Feasibility of subtotal laryngectomy based on whole-organ examination. Arch Otolaryngol 111: 356–360

51. Robbins K T, Davidson W, Peters L J, Geopfert H 1988 Conservation surgery for T2 and T3 carcinomas of the supraglottic larynx. Arch Otolaryngol Head Neck Surg 114: 421–426

52. Sasaki T, Baker H, McConnel D, Vetto, R M 1982 Free jejunal mucosal patch graft reconstruction of the oropharynx. Arch Surg 117: 459–462

53. Schechter G L 1991 Subtotal laryngectomy with epiglottic reconstruction. In: Silver C E (ed) Laryngeal cancer. Thieme, New York, pp 193–196

54. Schechter G L, Baker J W, Gilbert D A 1987 Functional evaluation of pharyngoesophageal reconstructive techniques. Arch Otolaryngol Head Neck Surg 113: 40–44

55. Seidenberg B, Rosenak S S, Hurwitt E S, Som M L 1959 Immediate reconstruction of the cervical esophagus by a revascularized isolated jejunal segment. Ann Surg 149: 162–71

56. Sessions D G, Maness G M, McSwain B 1965 Laryngofissure in the treatment of carcinoma of the vocal cord: a report of forty cases and a review of the literature. Laryngoscope 75: 490–502

57. Sessions D G, Ogura J H, Fried M P 1975 The anterior commissure in glottic carcinoma. Laryngoscope 85: 1624–1632

58. Silver C E 1976 Reconstruction after pharyngolaryngectomy-esophagectomy. Am J Surg 132: 428

59. Silver C E 1976 Gastric pull-up operation for replacement of the cervical portion of the esophagus. Surg Gynecol Obstet 142: 243–245

60. Silver C E 1977 Surgical management of neoplasms of the larynx, hypopharynx and cervical esophagus. Curr Prob Surg 14: 2–69

61. Silver C E 1981 Surgery for cancer of the larynx. Churchill Livingstone, New York

62. Silver C E, Moisa II 1991 Near-total laryngectomy. In: Silver C E (ed) Laryngeal cancer. Thieme, New York, pp 232–239

63. Silver C E, Cusumano R J, Fell S C, Strauch B 1989 Replacement of upper esophagus: results with myocutaneous flap and with gastric transposition. Laryngoscope 99: 819–821

64. Skolnik E M, Yee K F, Wheatley M A, Martin L O 1975 Carcinoma of the laryngeal glottis: therapy and end results. Laryngoscope 85: 1453–1466

65. Som M L 1970 Conservation surgery for carcinoma of the supraglottis. J Laryngol Otol 84: 655–678

66. Som M L 1975 Cordal cancer with extension to vocal process. Laryngoscope 85: 1298–1307

67. Som M L, Silver C E 1968 The anterior commissure technique of partial laryngectomy. Arch Otolaryngol 87: 138–145

68. Souter Ds, Scheker L R, Tanner N S, McGregor I A 1983 The radial forearm flap: a versatile method for intra-oral reconstruction. Br J Plast Surg 36: 1–8

69. Stell P M 1970 Esophageal replacement by transposed stomach. Following pharyngolaryngo-esophagectomy for carcinoma of the cervical esophagus. Arch Otolaryngol 91: 166–170

70. Stell P M 1984 Replacement of pharynx after pharyngolaryngectomy. Ann Royal Coll Surg Engl 66: 388–390

71. Strauss M 1988 Hemilaryngectomy rescue surgery for radiation failure in early glottic carcinoma. Laryngoscope 98: 317–320

72. Surkin M I, Lawson W, Biller H F 1984 Analysis of the methods of pharyngoesophageal reconstruction. Head Neck Surg 6: 953–970

73. Tucker G, Smith H 1962 A histological demonstration of the development of laryngeal connective tissue compartments. Trans Am Acad Ophthalmol Otolaryngol 66: 308–318

74. Tucker H M, Wood B G, Levine H, Katz R 1979 Glottic reconstruction after near total laryngectomy. Laryngoscope 89: 609–619

75. Tucker H M, Benninger M S, Roberts J K, Wood B G, Levine H L 1989 Near-total laryngectomy with epiglottic reconstruction: long-term results. Arch Otolaryngol Head Neck Surg 115: 1341–1344

76. Urken M L, Weinberg H, Vickery C, Biller H F 1990 The neurofasciocutaneous radial forearm flap in head and neck reconstruction: a preliminary report. Laryngoscope 100: 161–1739

26. Rationale for evaluation and treatment of the neck

M. Friedman, A. D. Mayer

INTRODUCTION

Formulating rational decisions for treatment of the neck in patients with primary laryngeal squamous cell carcinoma is complex. When palpable lymph nodes are present, the question of the validity of neck treatment is moot. Deciding on the type of neck dissection, modified or radical, becomes the issue at hand. The presentation of a patient with primary laryngeal cancer without clinically evident nodes poses a greater dilemma to the head and neck surgeon. Treatment options include (i) no treatment, (ii) elective neck irradiation, (iii) elective neck dissection, and (iv) a combination of irradiation and surgery. With the availability of multiple treatment modalities together with their unique costs and benefits, a surgeon must be capable of making sound scientific management choices tailored to each patient's needs.

The purpose of this chapter is to present the principles essential for the decision-making process in treating the clinically negative neck and the techniques available for treatment. It includes discussion of the application and value of current radiological techniques to the evaluation of the clinically negative neck, as well as descriptions of modified neck dissections. This chapter is limited to the rationale for evaluation and treatment of squamous cell carcinoma of the larynx only, and its contents do not apply to other primary laryngeal tumours.

PROPHYLACTIC NECK TREATMENT AND OCCULT DISEASE

Prophylactic or elective neck dissection is an operation performed in the absence of clinically evident cervical lymph nodes. The premise for performing elective neck dissection is based on the concept of occult disease, which is defined as regional micrometastatic nodal tumour that is undetectable by clinical evaluation (false-negative nodal disease). The importance of occult disease is its potential to become clinically apparent cervical metastatic disease, possibly leading to unresectable tumour or other, distant metastases. MacKenzie,[40] one of the initial proponents of elective neck dissection, stated that 'early extirpation of the entire [larynx] with its tributary lymphatics and glands, whether the latter are apparently diseased or not, is the only possible safeguard against local recurrence or metastasis'. Crile[18] also promoted dissection, 'whether the glands are or are not palpable'. Elective neck dissection is ultimately performed with the goal of improving survival.

Unfortunately, no definitive evidence supports prophylactic neck treatment as a superior management strategy over 'watchful waiting'. Opponents of elective neck dissection point out the high percentage of unnecessary surgical procedures and the comparable survival rates when therapeutic dissection is performed for neck disease detected clinically at a later time.

Rationale for treating occult disease is based on empiric evidence and logic alone. As long as morbidity and mortality rates for elective neck treatment can be maintained at a reasonably low level, it is sensible to overtreat rather than undertreat the neck. Treatment of neck disease is never 100% successful, but recurrence rates are lower when a clinically negative neck is treated versus recurrence after treatment of a positive neck.[22,62] Also, smaller lymph nodes are easier to resect. Risks of watchful waiting include decreasing prognosis due to extracapsular nodal invasion and inadequate follow-up in an unreliable patient.

When making any treatment decision, the clinician cannot overlook the pragmatic considerations. Although the necessity for prophylactic neck dissection in every instance is unclear, the widespread application of this procedure has permitted the accumulation of a statistical record of the occurrence of occult disease for a variety of head and neck cancers. The incidence of occult metastases ranges from 3 to 60%, with the majority of recorded values between 20 and 40% (see Table 26.1). Analysis of the occult rate for a specific lesion can help a physician determine a cut-off point between electively treating the clinically negative neck (N0) and abstaining from treatment. A 25 to 30% incidence of occult disease is generally an acceptable cut-off point for rationalizations of elective neck dissection (see Table 26.2), and no author has recommended elective neck dissection for an occult rate less than 15%. By using occult disease rate specific to tumour location and stage, together with clinical examination of the head and neck, as well as surgical knowledge and past experience, patients have historically been divided into high- and low-risk groups. High-risk N0 laryngeal cancer patient groups include patients with T3–T4 glottic lesions, patients with T2–T4 supraglottic lesions, and patients with any subglottic lesions (Table 26.3). Patients who satisfy the criteria for the high-risk groups have traditionally been candidates for elective treatment, while those in low-risk groups have not.

PROGNOSTIC CONSIDERATIONS IN SQUAMOUS CELL CARCINOMA OF THE LARYNX

The treatment and prognosis of squamous cell carcinoma of the larynx depend on several factors and cannot be based solely on the site and extent of the lesion.[27] Other factors for consideration include the presence of cervical node metastases, the histological grading and growth rate of the neoplasm, the health and immunocompetence of the host, the presence of synchronous or metachronous

Table 26.1 Incidence of occult disease for head and neck carcinoma: clinical N0 necks upstaged by histological evaluation

Source, Year	Number of cases (%)
O'Keefe[51] 1959	16/68 (23.5)
Southwick et al[66] 1960	29/68 (42.6)
Beahrs & Barber[4] 1962	48/234 (20.5)
McGavran et al[45] 1961	11/68 (16.2)
Sako et al[58] 1964	34/123 (27.6)
Ogura et al[50] 1971	23/181 (12.7)
Spiro et al[68] 1974	107/305 (35.1)
Martis et al[44] 1979	42/112 (37.5)
Brandenburg & Lee[9] 1981	36/99 (36.4)
Ali et al[1] 1985	15/71 (21.1)
Farrar et al[23] 1988	338 RNDs (32.3)*

*RND indicates radical neck dissection.

Table 26.2 Recommended cut-off point for justification of elective neck treatment

Source, Year	Occult (%)
O'Keefe[51] 1959	>25
McGavran et al[45] 1961	>16
Reed & Rabuzzi[56] 1969	>30
Ogura et al[50] 1971	>28
Lee & Krause[36] 1975	>15
Bocca & Pignataro[7] 1984	>30
Ali et al[1] 1985	>20
Mendenhall & Million[46] 1986	>20 (with irradiation)
Friedman et al[31] 1990	>25

Table 26.3 The rate of false-negative lymph nodes on physical examination by T stage of laryngeal cancer*

T Stage	Source	Occult (%)	Number of cases
Glottic			
T1–T2	Byers et al[13]	21.4	14
T2	Mendenhall et al[47]	3	75
T2–T4	O'Keefe[51]	11.1	18
T3–T4	Byers et al[13]	14	80
Supraglottic			
T1	Mendenhall & Million[46]	20–30	–
T1–T2	Byers et al[13]	30.8	13
T1–T2	Levendag et al[37]	35	79
T2–T4	Mendenhall & Million[46]	>30	
T2–T4	O'Keefe[51]	32	28
T3–T4	Byers et al[13]	25	80
Subglottic			
T2–T4	O'Keefe[51]	23	22
Tx	McGavran et al[45]	22	16

*When interpreting this table, one must take into consideration the changing AJCC[2] definitions of the T staging of laryngeal carcinoma over the years. Also note that we are not discussing subglottic carcinoma in this chapter because of its low incidence rate.

primary cancers of the head and neck, and the age of the patient.

The presence of cervical lymph node metastases is relatively common in laryngeal carcinoma and occurs more frequently in neoplasms with a poorly differentiated cell type than in those with well-differentiated or moderately differentiated cell types. Prognosis is affected by the presence of extracapsular spread, the number of nodes involved, and the level of cervical nodal involvement. Extracapsular spread increases the potential for distant metastases and justifies the use of combined surgical and radiation therapy. Metastatic involvement of the anterior inferior and the posterior inferior cervical triangles is associated with a poor prognosis.[27]

Metastases via the bloodstream are a late finding in the course of laryngeal squamous cell carcinoma, and most commonly involve the lungs, liver, bones, brain, skin and mediastinal lymph nodes.

ELECTIVE NECK RADIATION

Several authors have advocated the use of radiation for treatment of the N0 neck as an alternative to surgical neck treatment.[3,15,43,46,55] It is generally felt that 4500–5000-rad doses of external radiation to the clinically negative neck sterilize occult tumour cells with success equal to that achieved by dissection. Radiation is administered to the neck either together with radiation therapy for the primary tumour or following excision of the primary. The rate of lymph node recurrence in the irradiated neck is often the measure of success, reportedly ranging from 1 to 6.4% in several studies,[3,15,43,46,55] when the primary tumour is controlled. The argument for elective neck dissection versus elective neck irradiation[67] is beyond the scope of this chapter. The chapter will deal with the criteria for determining the need for treatment and the type of surgical treatment. One important factor in determining which treatment is chosen is the type of treatment administered for the primary; surgical treatment of the primary may then make surgical treatment of the neck a logical choice once treatment of the neck is deemed necessary. Radiation therapy of the primary can be combined with radiation treatment of the neck.

THE NECK AT RISK

When discussing risk factors for N0 neck disease, the laterality of the primary tumour must be taken into account. Ipsilateral 'high-risk' lesions always place the ipsilateral neck at risk, while 'high-risk' tumours that cross the midline endanger the ipsilateral and the contralateral neck. If bilateral neck dissection is warranted, a two-stage operation is advisable. Removal of the primary tumour together with dissection of the dominant neck, followed by subsequent dissection of the contralateral neck after a 4- to 6-week interval, gives the body time to accommodate to the ensuing cerebral, corneal, and facial haemodynamic insult. The vertebral venous system should be adequate to handle the increased blood flow if removal of both internal jugular veins is necessary. If both necks can be treated with modified neck dissection, simultaneous neck dissection with preservation of the internal jugular vein is an option.

A midline tumour with one clinically positive neck and one clinically negative neck is a common occurrence. The clinically negative second neck is truly a 'high-risk negative' neck and should be treated no differently than a high-risk ipsilateral neck for a unilateral tumour. In all cases in which bilateral neck dissection is planned, modified neck dissection with preservation of the internal jugular vein should be planned on both sides if there is no evidence of extracapsular invasion. It is much more difficult to preserve the internal jugular vein on the second side if a classical radical neck dissection was performed earlier on the first side. The increased collateral flow to the second side makes inadvertent injury to the internal jugular vein more common. A planned modified procedure on the second neck must often be converted to a classical radical neck dissection.

ADVANCED RADIOLOGICAL TECHNIQUES IN HEAD AND NECK CANCER

In the 1990s advanced radiological studies of the head and neck have served as a powerful non-invasive diagnostic aid for the surgeon.[30-32,42,51,54,69,70] With these new tools, the high-risk N0 neck has been redefined with improved accuracy of diagnosis. There is great variability in reported occurrences of lymph node dissection upon

clinical examination, reflecting both diversity in patients' neck anatomy and the difference in the techniques of individual examiners. The neck can be particularly difficult to palpate in patients with short fat necks, in whom the anatomy is obscured by excessive fatty tissues, and in necks that have sustained previous radiation treatment or surgery, distorting the natural contours of the soft tissues. Examination of the neck by palpation is also limited to nodes within reach, excluding deeper structures. Several studies have demonstrated the accuracy of palpation of the neck to range between 65 to 76.9% (see Table 26.4), leaving a significant margin for diagnostic error and its consequences.

Both CT scanning and MR imaging can detect and localize regional lymph node metastasis with relatively greater accuracy, ranging from 86.5 to 95%. When used for a defined high-risk patient population, CT and MRI neck evaluation combined with physical examination diminished the incidence of occult metastases to 6–12%.[31,42,70] Diagnostic scans used for preoperative evaluation of the clinically positive neck serve as a valuable baseline for later detection of tumour recurrence or for following the nodal response to radiation or chemotherapy. Further, information about the nodal status of the contralateral neck, the extent of tumour invasion, and the presence of jugular vein thrombosis or involvement of the carotid artery may influence the extent of operative resection and prognosis.

Recently, one study has demonstrated the value of high-resolution B-mode ultrasound as a reliable method for detection of occult neck disease and staging of head and neck cancer.[54] The potential advantages of using ultrasound over CT or MRI include (i) decreased financial expense to the patient, (ii) widespread availability of the equipment, and (iii) the re-allocation of CT or MRI resources for other purposes. One disadvantage is that ultrasound cannot be used to evaluate the primary tumour. Certainly the utility of ultrasound in head and

Table 26.4 Comparison between sensitivity and specificity of palpation versus CT/MRI

Source, Year	Sensitivity (%)		Specificity (%)
	Palpation	CT/MRI	CT/MRI
McGavran et al[45] 1961	71*	–	–
Sako et al[58] 1964	72.4*	–	–
DeSanto et al[22] 1982	65	–	–
Mancuso et al[41] 1983	–	91.3	–
Stevens et al[70] 1985	70	93–95	82
Feinmesser et al[24] 1987	61.5	59.6	85
Close et al[16] 1989	76.9	86.5	71
van den Brekel et al[10] 1990	68**	87	–
Feinmesser et al[25] 1990	67	76	78
Lee & Krause[36]	64**	–	–
Friedman et al[31] 1990	71.7	91.1	77

*Accuracy rate implies sensitivity.
**Sensitivity has been estimated by subtracting the error rate from 100.

neck cancer warrants further investigation and extensive comparison with other radiological modalities.

CT OR MRI

Both CT and MRI have similar sensitivity rates in identifying cervical lymph node metastasis[31] and similar error rates.[10,24,69,70] Both MR and CT have proven valuable in upstaging disease.[10,16,24,31,41,71]

There are several differences between CT and MRI worthy of further discussion. MRI has advantages over CT in its ability to show contrast between soft tissues and to generate multiplanar imaging. No ionizing radiation or iodinated contrast infusion is usually needed, making MRI less invasive than CT. On the other hand, CT scanning has better sensitivity to calcifications and bony detail and has the advantage of less distortion and motion artefact relative to MRI. Both CT and MRI often predict lymph node size to be smaller than pathologically determined lymph node size. Friedman et al[31] found node size with CT to be 24% smaller, and van den Brekel et al[11] found node size with MRI to be 25% smaller to 12% larger than actual physical dimensions. Node size may be inappropriately estimated by CT and MRI because of transection of nodal tissue in an oblique or off-centre plane.

Evaluation of the neck by CT or MRI is not a substitute for clinical examination, but rather an adjunct limited to high-risk cases or low-risk patients who happen to receive CT or MRI evaluation of their primary lesion. The addition of CT/MRI results to findings on physical examination maximizes the accuracy of diagnosis.[31]

The CT and MR studies of the neck are not warranted for all patients. A determination to use CT or MRI should include consideration of the anatomy of the patient, the characteristics of the primary laryngeal tumour, and the likelihood of the neck harbouring occult disease. The decision ultimately depends on the surgeon's discretion and may be affected by the opinion of the surgeon that a particular tumour may be acting in a more aggressive fashion than usual and cannot be approached in a 'cookbook' manner. In general, indications for CT or MRI evaluation of the neck include the following situations: (i) high-risk necks (as previously defined); (ii) all patients scanned for a primary tumour (the neck should be included and usually can be at no additional expense to the patient); (iii) unusual or aggressive tumour presentation; (iv) physical examination of the neck is limited by anatomical features that make palpation unreliable. By maximizing sensitivity, or the capacity to diagnose metastatic neck disease more precisely, both accuracy of patient assessment and cost-effectiveness are improved.[30] CT and MRI can also apply to the official American Joint Committee on Cancer[2] staging of laryngeal cancer, improving subsequent accuracy of prognosis. The surgeon

is provided with a more scientific basis for determining proper patient management.

The application of varying criteria for malignancy, multiple models and types of scanners, and differences in the training and technique of evaluating radiologists have all contributed to the confusion over the efficacy of the use of CT or MRI in the investigation of neck disease.[24,25] Some investigators consider nodes larger than 1.5 cm on CT to be positive for malignancy,[24,70] while others cite 1 cm as their cut-off point.[31,32] Some consider nodes just under the assigned size limit to constitute malignancy if they are found as a group, while others do not consider this criterion at all. Most radiologists agree that central necrosis within a lymph node may be the most specific criterion for malignancy.[10,32,69] Other morphological characteristics of abnormal nodes include pericapsular extension and obliteration of perivascular and fat planes.[41,42] It is suggested that a standard subset of criteria for malignancy be developed; however, the particular attributes and deficiencies of each centre must be factored into the equation. When using CT to evaluate a high-risk neck the criteria that maximize sensitivity should be applied. These include any neck with a node larger than 1.0 cm, central necrosis, a node with perivascular invasion, and groups of nodes.

ELECTIVE NECK TREATMENT

Sensitivity can be maximized at the expense of reduced specificity when scanning the neck of a patient who is considered to be 'committed' to elective treatment. The balance between sensitivity (the ability to predict correctly the presence of positive lymph nodes) and specificity (the ability of predict correctly the absence of lymph node metastases) can be manipulated by adjusting radiological criteria for malignancy. Establishing strict criteria (i.e., considering any node larger than 1.0 cm as positive) improves sensitivity thereby minimizing the number of false-negative results. Concurrently, specificity is diminished, causing some increment in the number of false-positive scans. Since it is in our interest to err on the side of treatment of any radiologically suspicious nodes, the fewest false-negatives, together with some additional false-positives, is optimal for finding patients with disease who require treatment while identifying those patients who do not warrant treatment of the neck.

Using high-sensitivity criteria for CT and MRI scans, many so-called clinically negative necks will be transformed to CT/MR-positive necks, and essentially no lesions have an occult rate greater than 14%. In the high-risk patient, any positive CT or MRI is considered a true positive finding and, of course, warrants treatment. The decision to operate on a CT/MR-negative neck is based on several factors: (i) the belief that even an occult rate of 14% necessitates treatment; (ii) pragmatic considerations based on the site of the primary tumour, the reliability of the patient, the aggressive nature of the tumour, and the options between the surgeon and the patient.

TREATMENT OF THE POSITIVE NECK

Once the neck has been evaluated appropriately, the question of how to treat the patient remains. Basic management goals include (i) control regional disease; (ii) increase survival rate; (iii) minimize morbidity and cosmetic deformity; and (iv) maintain a reasonable financial cost for the patient.

Options for surgery and irradiation must be considered, keeping in mind the different surgical procedures and the various doses and schedules for irradiation. It is generally accepted that necks deemed clinically positive require therapeutic dissection, possibly with preoperative or postoperative radiation. Determining whether such neck dissection should be radical or modified is an issue replete with differing surgical and oncological philosophies. The costs and benefits of combined therapy have also been studied extensively with few clear conclusions.

NECK DISSECTION

The concept of radical neck dissection for the treatment of cancer of the head and neck was first described by Crile.[18] En bloc dissection was intended to control metastatic disease by completely resecting involved lymphatic tissues between the superficial and deep cervical fascia, together with all neck structures in close proximity (sparing the phrenic, vagus, hypoglossal, and lingual nerves) from the base of the skull to the level of the clavicle.

Since Crile's time, several surgeons have developed modifications of his technique designed to avoid side-effects of the original procedure by sparing certain neck structures.[5,6,20,53,64] The modifications range from the most minimal modification, sparing only the spinal accessory nerve, to a maximal modification, such as the functional neck dissection, where all muscles, nerves, and major vessels are preserved. All of the various modified dissections, of which there are many,[12,13] fall between these two extremes. Since the details of radical neck dissection can be found elsewhere the focus here will be on descriptions of the maximal and minimal modified neck dissections.

The Subcommittee for Neck Dissection Nomenclature of the Committee for Head and Neck Surgery and Oncology of the American Academy of Otolaryngology–Head and Neck Surgery has classified neck dissection into four categories: (i) radical, considered to be the standard procedure for cervical lymphadenopathy; (ii) modified radical, or any alteration of the radical procedure that involves preservation of one or more non-lymphatic structures of the neck; (iii) selective, including supraomohyoid, posterolateral, lateral and anterior, each representing a specific procedure that preserves one or more lymph node groups routinely removed in radical dissection; and (iv) extended, or any alteration involving removal of additional lymph node groups or non-lymphatic structures relative to the radical procedure.[57]

The Sloan–Kettering Memorial Group has defined six anatomic levels of cervical lymph nodes.[63] This classification is designed to standardize the terminology used to describe lymph node groups at risk for tumour metastases and to define clearly the boundaries of lymph node groups.

Level I. Submental group: lymph nodes within the triangular boundary of the anterior belly of the digastric muscles and hyoid bone. Submandibular group: lymph nodes within the boundaries of the anterior and posterior bellies of the digastric muscle and the body of the mandible. The submandibular gland is included in the specimen when the lymph nodes within this triangle are removed.

Level II. Upper jugular group: lymph nodes located around the upper third of the internal jugular vein and adjacent spinal accessory nerve extending from the carotid bifurcation (surgical landmark) and hyoid bone (clinical landmark) to the skull base. The posterior boundary is the posterior border of the sternocleidomastoid muscle and the anterior boundary is the lateral border of the sternohyoid muscle.

Level III. Middle jugular group: lymph nodes located around the middle third of the internal jugular vein extending from the carotid bifurcation superiorly to the omohyoid muscle (surgical landmark) or cricothyroid notch (clinical landmark) inferiorly. The posterior boundary is the posterior border of the sternocleidomastoid muscle, and the anterior boundary is the lateral border of the sternohyoid muscle.

Level IV. Lower jugular group: lymph nodes located around the lower third of the internal jugular vein extending from the omohyoid muscle superiorly to the clavicle inferiorly. The posterior boundary is the posterior border of the sternocleidomastoid muscle and the anterior boundary is the lateral border or the sternohyoid muscle.

Level V. Posterior triangle group; this group comprises predominantly the lymph nodes located along the lower half of the spinal accessory nerve and the transverse cervical artery. The supraclavicular nodes are also included in this group. The posterior boundary is the anterior border of the trapezius muscle, the anterior boundary is the posterior border of the sternocleidomastoid muscle, and the inferior boundary is the clavicle.

Level VI. Anterior compartment group; this group comprises lymph nodes surrounding the midline visceral structures of the neck extending from the level of the hyoid bone superiorly to the suprasternal notch inferiorly.

On each side, the lateral boundary is the medial border of the carotid sheath. Located within this compartment are the perithyroidal lymph nodes, paratracheal lymph nodes, lymph nodes along the recurrent laryngeal nerves, and precricoid lymph nodes.

Of the types of selective neck dissection listed above, there is evidence to support the use of selective neck dissection with preservation of the level I lymph nodes[26] and for selective neck dissection with preservation of the level V lymph nodes,[65] as oncologically sound and successful procedures for treatment of laryngeal carcinoma. As a routine, standard or modified neck dissection should be used, with selective procedures reserved for certain cases, based on the individual patient and the philosophy of the surgeon.

Absolute indications for classical radical neck dissection include suspicion of extracapsular nodal disease based on physical examination and CT or MRI, fixed lymph nodes that seem to be invading neck structures, particularly large nodes, and those with irregular borders. Relative indications can include any patient presenting with a suspicion of neck metastases. The ability to preserve anatomy and function while effectively removing cancer generally requires the experience and skilled hands of a physician who specializes in head and neck surgical oncology.

Suarez must be credited as the first to define the anatomic basis and surgical criteria for functional neck dissection[32a] which has been the standard for comparison since the 1960s (see illustrations). This procedure is often mentioned as 'Bocca neck dissection' because it was Bocca and his coworkers who popularized the method in the English language.[6-8] Suarez[72] explicitly described the aponeurotic system of the neck as being compartments filled with areolar tissue and lymphatics, distinct from the muscular, vascular, and neural structures of the neck. Removal of the entire fibrofatty lymphatic system by dissecting the anterior and lateral neck compartments in continuity and stripping the sheaths from the overlying and underlying structures along the whole extension of the neck is carried out with preservation of the sternocleidomastoid, the internal jugular vein, the submandibular gland, and the spinal accessory nerve. Suarez called the procedure 'functional neck dissection'[32a] and stated that the extent of a radical approach should be conceived against cancer and not against the neck.

Although there are no absolute indications for performing a functional neck dissection, relative indications are numerous. For example, functional neck dissection can be used when nodal disease is less than 2 cm in size by palpation and CT shows no evidence of extracapsular invasion, in young patients who are concerned about cosmesis and shoulder function, and in patients who are potentially at risk for bilateral neck disease. Bocca considers the only contraindications to include fixed nodes, fixed nodes that become mobile after radiation treatment, or recurrence of metastatic disease in the lymph nodes following radiation or previous surgery.[7]

The spinal accessory nerve-sparing dissection has no absolute indications, but may be the preferred treatment for clinically positive lymph nodes without CT evidence of extracapsular nodal invasion or direct involvement of the nerve with disease, and when no node is greater than 3 cm in size in the jugulodigastric area or spinal accessory chain.[12,14] This dissection is quicker and easier than a functional neck dissection and can be used when criteria for the functional neck dissection are lacking. Preservation of the spinal accessory nerve is comparable to preservation of the vagus nerve and the carotid artery in the classic dissection, where proximity to the jugulodigastric nodes for all three structures is identical. Other arguments for the preservation of the spinal accessory nerve are based on the low incidence of metastases in the posterior triangle,[45,64,65] and on studies demonstrating the direction of lymphatic flow away from the spinal accessory nodal group, toward the jugular or transverse cervical nodes, without retrograde flow.[26,28,73] Opponents[59] feel that preservation of the spinal accessory nerve cannot be justified based on a 90% rate of involvement of the spinal accessory nodes at the superior jugular portion of the nerve, outside of the posterior triangle. When the modified neck dissection is properly performed, the spinal accessory nerve is dissected up to the jugular foramen, leaving no nodal disease behind, thereby obviating this concern.

The basic principles of oncologically sound surgery remain the same for modified and radical dissection: all adjacent lymph nodes must be removed. Criticism of modified techniques comes from fear of leaving behind potentially resectable disease in the neck[17] and from anatomical considerations. Beahrs and Barber[4] questioned the value of non-radical dissections, stating that 'the first surgical attack on an anatomic region is the golden opportunity for doing the safest and most thorough operation. To operate secondarily in the neck is a surgeon's nightmare'.

Several surgeons have critically compared radical to modified neck dissection based on disease recurrence in the neck[9,12,14,35,38] and found no difference in the rate of recurrent neck disease between patients receiving radical or conservative dissections. The overall rate of tumour recurrence in the N1 and N0 neck treated with radical neck dissection ranged from 12–19% versus 6–7% recurrence rate following modified dissection. These numbers may reflect the fact that modified neck dissections are performed in lower-risk patients. Lingeman et al[38] evaluated 445 neck dissections and concluded that conservative neck dissection should be used for subclinical and N1 disease, reserving the classic en bloc procedure for N2 and N3 situations.

Surgical technique

Standard radical neck dissection is a procedure well known to every head and neck surgeon and is well illustrated in many surgical atlases. Selective neck dissection is based on the same principles as radical neck dissection with preservation of selected areas of the neck. Functional neck dissection as described removes all the lymphatics normally removed with radical neck dissection with preservation of certain nonlymphatic structures. The functional neck dissection preserves the sternocleidomastoid muscle, the internal jugular vein, the submandibular gland, the spinal accessory and greater auricular nerves. The most commonly preserved structure is the spinal accessory nerve.

Figure 26.1 illustrates commonly used incisions for neck dissections associated with laryngectomy. Skin incisions for modified dissection are identical to those used for radical neck dissection.

Figures 26.1 through 26.6B illustrate the technique for preservation of the spinal accessory nerve.

Figures 26.1 through 26.3, and 26.7 through 26.14, illustrate the technique of the functional neck dissection. In all dissections, a Shaw haemostatic scalpel is used.

Sequelae and complications of surgery

Classic radical neck dissection results in patient discomfort, morbidity, and mortality.[45,48,49,53] Even if only one side is involved, the patient may be a candidate for secondary neck dissection at a later time and therefore may suffer the sequelae of bilateral neck dissection. Common consequences of dissection include the 'shoulder syndrome' or trapezius palsy with limited arm abduction secondary to loss of enervation of the trapezius muscle by the spinal accessory nerve, inability to move the head well without the sternocleidomastoid muscle, disfigurement of the neck, chronic discoloration of the lower face from compensatory vasodilation of the subcutaneous venous network, chronic swelling of the lower face, anaesthesia, pain or paresthesia of the cervical region, and the risk of adverse circulatory effects on the brain and cornea due to change in the venous drainage, especially with bilateral radical neck dissection.[56] These side-effects can limit the patient's ability to work, engage in sports, and may interfere with psychosocial well-being. Schuller et al[62] compared the impact of radical neck dissection versus modified neck dissection on total patient disability and found that more radical neck dissection patients experienced difficulty lifting their arms after surgery and were more disturbed by the appearance of their necks. These factors had a negative influence on patients' social activity. Most of these sequelae are diminished or eliminated with modified neck dissection.

All neck dissections entail risks and possible complications. As with any operation there is a risk of infection and haemorrhage. Bleeding within 4–5 days after surgery may require reopening of the wound with evacuation of clots or securing of bleeding points. Infection, wound dehiscence, and sloughing of skin flaps due to poor vascularization of healing tissues can occur, with the risk of flap necrosis with subsequent carotid blow-out and shock with hemiplegia. Once again, the risk is diminished by preservation of the sternocleidomastoid muscle if a modified neck dissection is done. Fistula formation can occur, including chylous fistula from perforation of the thoracic duct. Also, neck dissection does not ensure definitive cure. DeSanto et al[22] found 2-year recurrence rates of 7.5, 20.2 and 37.4% in N0, N1 and N2 necks, respectively, after dissection alone.

COMBINATION TREATMENT

Combination treatment of the neck in patients with laryngeal cancer is another hotly debated issue.[60] In the positive neck, the rationale for combination therapy is based on high recurrence rates in the dissected neck and such treatment has become standard in some institutions.[33] It is hoped that added therapeutic radiation will destroy any microscopic disease inadvertently left behind by the surgeon, and thereby decrease neck recurrence. Radiation therapy, however, is associated with well-known adverse effects, such as the 'spitting cotton syndrome'[23] from the destruction of salivary glands and neck fibrosis and contracture. The advantage of prophylactic radiation to the N0 neck following dissection has not been widely investigated.

Several surgeons have suggested that the overall cure rate is not improved by combination treatment, which may relate to an increase in the rate of distant metastases when neck disease is controlled.[29,34,61,71] There is also some increased morbidity associated with radiation therapy. Few authors recommend the use of preoperative radiation treatment[3,52] because the complications, although equal in frequency to those found with postoperative radiation treatment, are more severe.[19] Patients receiving preoperative radiation may experience delayed primary healing or skin sloughs. Patients are at a higher risk for carotid blow-out and pharyngeal fistulization complications. Lutz et al[39] found that the overall neck failure rate was higher for patients with supraglottic carcinoma receiving combination therapy versus surgery alone (15 versus 12%) secondary to a lessened salvage rate in patients who received radiation. DeSanto et al,[21] in a large study at the Mayo Clinic, found that combination therapy was not superior to operation alone in decreasing rates of recurrence in all stages of neck disease.

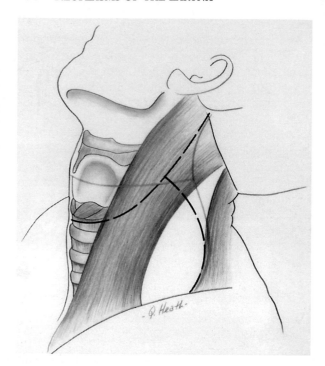

Fig. 26.1 Option 1 (dashed line) is used for neck dissection associated with total laryngectomy. This combines an apron incision with a posterior limb as shown. Option 2 (solid line) is used for supraglottic laryngectomy combined with neck dissection. The horizontal limb is at the level of the midportion of the thyroid cartilage. The vertical limb is S-shaped and it is important to avoid any acute angles at the trifurcation.

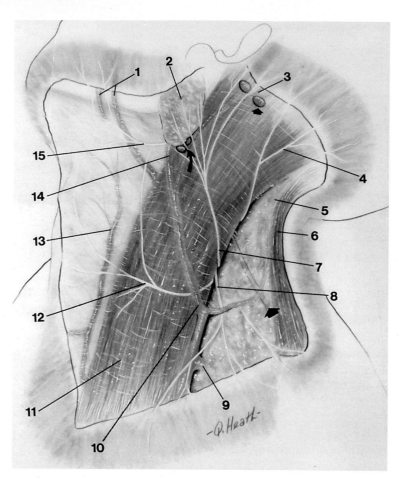

Fig. 26.2 The flaps are elevated in a subplatysmal plane to expose the neck as illustrated. Note the proximity of the spinal accessory nerve (large arrowhead) to the skin flaps. This is especially important since there is no platysma over the posterior triangle in this area. Inadvertent dissection in this area can injure the nerve before it is identified. Similarly, the marginal mandibular branch of the facial nerve (number 15) can be injured with flap elevation. It should be identified with a nerve stimulator and carefully dissected. Note that the marginal mandibular branch of the facial nerve crosses the facial vein at a variable distance from the mandible. Ligation of the facial vein does not guarantee protection of the nerve unless the vein is ligated below the level of the nerve. Number 1 indicates the facial artery and vein; 2, parotid gland; 3, posterior auricular vein; 4, lesser occipital nerve; 5, posterior external jugular vein; 6, trapezius muscle; 7, great auricular nerve; 8, supraclavicular nerve; 9, transverse cervical vein; 10, external jugular vein; 11, sternocleidomastoid muscle; 12, transverse cervical nerve; 13, anterior jugular vein; 14, retromandibular vein; and 15, facial nerve. The small arrowhead shows the retroauricular lymph nodes, and the arrow the superficial parotid lymph nodes.

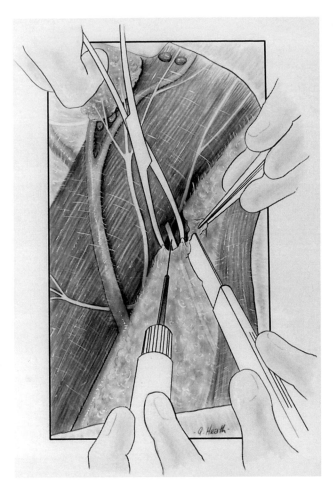

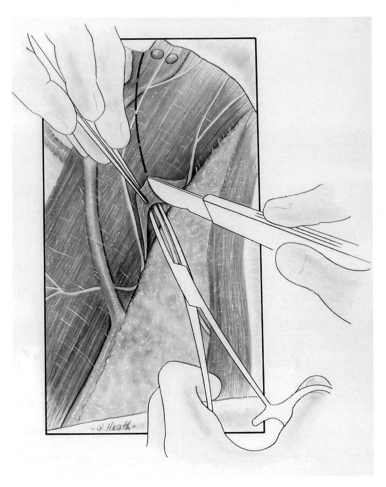

Fig. 26.3   The spinal accessory nerve is identified at the posterior border of the sternocleidomastoid. Although it is preferable not to have the patient paralysed, there is usually some response to direct stimulation even in the paralysed patient. The nerve is then traced distally by placing a haemostat over the nerve and then cutting the posterior fat. Vessels that are seen are coagulated with a bipolar cautery. Unipolar cauterization is never used near nerves. The nerve is traced until it enters the trapezius muscles. The undersurface of the nerve is dissected with scissors.

Fig. 26.4   The nerve is traced proximally as it enters the sternocleidomastoid muscle. The muscle is cut with a knife over the haemostat protecting the nerve. The nerve is traced up to the base of the skull.

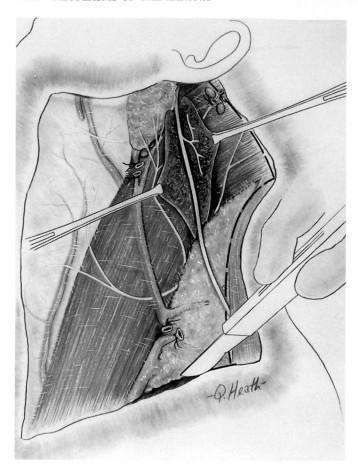

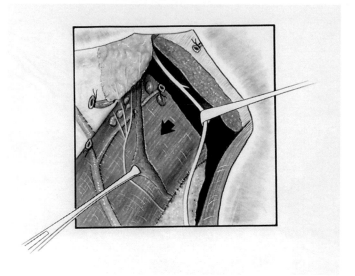

A

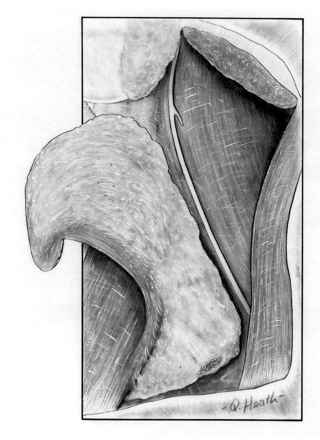

B

Fig. 26.5   Once the nerve is traced to the jugular foramen, the undersurface of the proximal portion is freed and the branch to the sternocleidomastoid muscle is cut. The dashed line indicates the line of incision where the sternocleidomastoid is cut at the mastoid tip and down along the trapezius muscle.

Fig. 26.6   A. The upper lateral aspect of the sternocleidomastoid is dissected along with the surrounding fat and this portion is moved under the spinal accessory nerve so that it can be removed with the rest of the specimen. B. The entire sternocleidomastoid muscle is now anterior to the spinal accessory nerve.

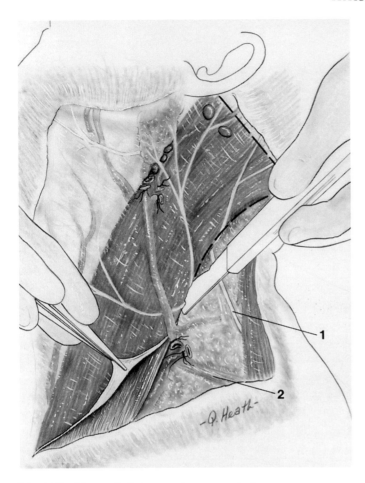

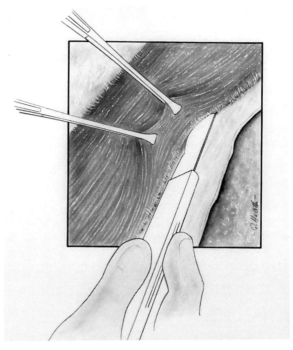

Fig. 26.8   The muscle is retracted and the fascia peeled away from the deep surface.

Fig. 26.7   The cervical plexus and greater auricular nerve are sacrificed. The external jugular vein is first ligated just above the clavicle. The posterior facial vein is then identified as it exits the parotid gland and is ligated. This can be easily done by tracing the marginal mandibular branch of the facial nerve through the parotid. Although not shown in the illustrations, the parotid tissue caudal to the nerve is transected and the vein is identified at the level of the parotid lymph nodes and is removed with the specimen. The superficial cervical fascia is then cut along the posterior border of the sternocleidomastoid muscle with a knife as shown. The fascia is then peeled off the surface of the muscle. Number 1 indicates the spinal accessory nerve; 2 indicates the omohyoid muscle (inferior belly).

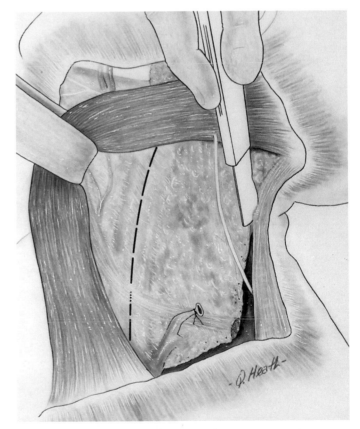

Fig. 26.9   The posterior triangle fat is freed from the trapezius superior and inferior to the spinal accessory nerve. The fat is also freed above the clavicle. The omohyoid muscle is avulsed at its distal attachment. After the posterior and inferior borders are mobilized, the sternocleidomastoid muscle is retracted and the carotid sheath is identified. The dashed line indicates the incision to open the carotid sheath.

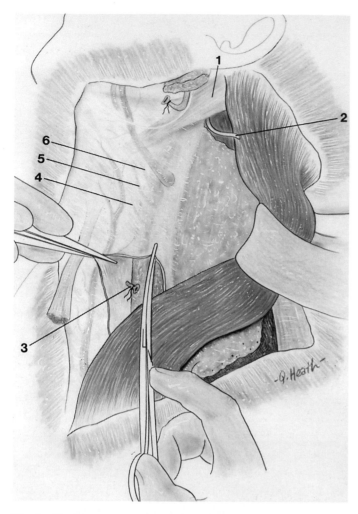

Fig. 26.10   The carotid sheath is opened with scissors. Number 1 indicates the stylohyoid muscle; 2, spinal accessory nerve; 3, inferior thyroid vein; 4, superior thyroid vein; 5, ascending pharyngeal vein; and 6, lingual vein.

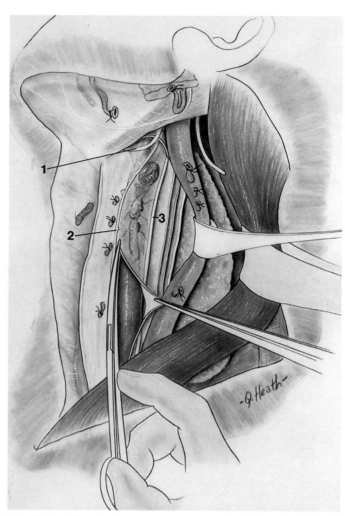

Fig. 26.12   The vein is retracted and all the fascia and surrounding nodes are left to be removed with the specimen. The fascia overlying the carotid with nodes is dissected away from the artery and the vagus. Number 1 indicates the hypoglossal nerve; 2, ansa cervicalis; and 3, vagus nerve.

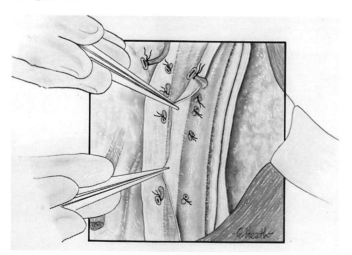

Fig. 26.11   The fascia over the internal jugular vein is dissected and the vein is unwrapped. The branches of the vein are ligated as shown. The fascia is dissected completely away from the vein so that the vein can be retracted in a similar fashion as the sternocleidomastoid muscle.

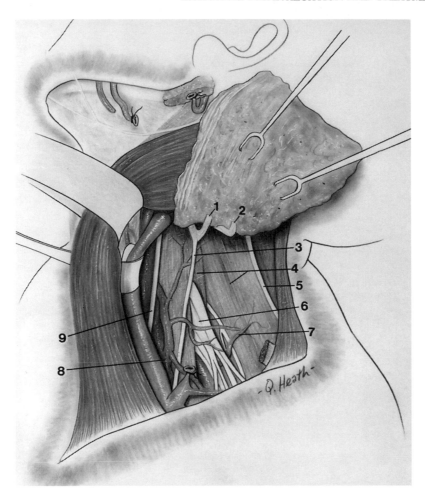

Fig. 26.13 The lateral fat is elevated away from the splenus and levator scapulae. The cervical plexus is cut after the phrenic nerve is identified and preserved. The dissection is carried up to the jugular foramen. Number 1 indicates the fourth cervical nerve (cut); 2, third cervical nerve (cut); 3, phrenic nerve (saved); 4, scalene muscles; 5, spinal accessory nerve; 6, brachial plexus; 7, transverse cervical artery; 8, subclavian artery; and 9, vagus nerve.

CONCLUSIONS

1. The primary modality for evaluation of the neck in laryngeal cancer is clinical examination.

2. A positive clinical finding is considered to be metastatic neck disease and warrants treatment.

3. Positive necks should be treated surgically with lymphadenectomy. Procedures can range from selective neck dissection in some cases and modified or classical radical neck dissection depending on multiple factors. Suspicion of extracapsular nodal disease, fixed lymph nodes that seem to be invading neck structures, lymph nodes greater than 2 cm, or those with irregular borders warrant treatment with classical radical neck dissection. Modified neck dissection, with either preservation of the spinal accessory or a functional neck dissection is relatively indicated when nodal disease is less than 2 cm, there is no evidence of extracapsular invasion, when cosmesis is an issue, and especially in patients who are potential candidates for bilateral dissection, e.g., a patient who presents with a primary tumour that crosses the midline or a patient who presents with bilateral metastases.

4. Negative necks are divided into low-risk and high-risk groups. High-risk N0 laryngeal cancer patient groups include those with T3–T4 glottic lesions, T2–T4 supraglottic lesions, or any subglottic lesion. Low-risk patients require no further radiological evaluation and are followed closely with clinical examination. High-risk patients require further neck evaluation with CT, MRI, and/or ultrasound. Radiologically positive necks are treated like positive necks, as described above. Treatment of the radiologically negative neck is left to the discretion of the physician. Options include (i) no treatment; (ii) elective neck irradiation; (iii) elective neck dissection; and (iv) a combination of irradiation and dissection.

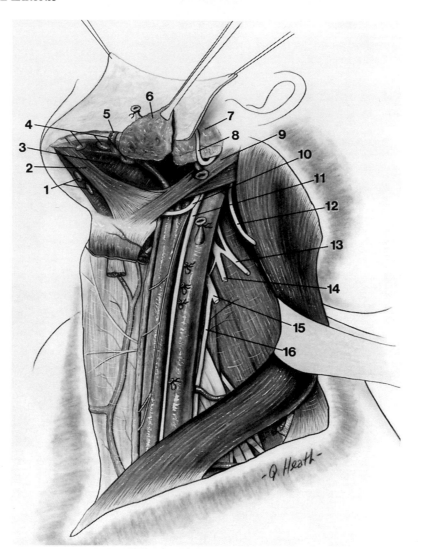

Fig. 26.14 The fascia over the submandibular gland is incised and stripped with surrounding nodes. The submandibular and submental nodes are removed with the rest of the specimen. This figure illustrates these nodes still in place prior to removal. The rest of the neck is illustrated after completion of the dissection. Drainage and closure of the modified neck vary only slightly from standard radical neck dissection. Suction drains should be used in all cases, and one drain should be deep to the sternocleidomastoid muscle and one superficial to the muscle. Haematoma formation is more difficult to detect with the preservation of the sternocleidomastoid, since the neck always has a much fuller appearance postoperatively compared with the appearance after classical radical neck dissection where the skin flaps are flat against the carotid and deep muscles. Number 1 indicates the submental nodes; 2, digastric muscle; 3, mylohyoid muscle; 4, submandibular nodes; 5, facial artery; 6, submandibular gland; 7, parotid gland; 8, facial nerve; 9, stylohyoid muscle; 10, hypoglossal nerve; 11, vagus nerve; 12, spinal accessory nerve; 13, second cervical nerve (cut); 14, third cervical nerve (cut); 15, fourth cervical nerve (cut); and 16, phrenic nerve.

REFERENCES

1. Ali S, Tiwari R M, Snow G B 1985 False positive and false negative nodes. Head Neck Surg 8: 78–82

2. American Joint Committee on Cancer (AJCC) 1992 Manual for staging of cancer, 4th edn, Lippincott, Philadelphia, 39–44

3. Barkley H T, Fletcher G H, Jesse R H, Lindberg R D 1972 Management of cervical lymph node metastases in squamous cell carcinoma of the tonsillar fossa, base of tongue, supraglottic larynx, and hypopharynx. Am J Surg 124: 463–466

4. Beahrs O H, Barber K W 1962 The value of radical neck dissection of structures of the neck in the management of carcinoma of the lip, mouth and larynx. Arch Surg 85: 49–56

5. Bocca E 1953 Functional problems connected with bilateral neck dissection. J Laryngol Otol 67: 567–577

6. Bocca E, Pignataro O 1967 A conservative technique in radical neck dissection. Ann Otol Rhinol Laryngol 76: 975–980

7. Bocca E, Pignataro O 1984 Functional neck dissection: an evaluation and review of 843 cases. Laryngoscope 94: 942–945

8. Bocca E, Pignataro O, Sasaki C 1980 Functional neck dissection: a description of operative technique. Arch Otolaryngol 106: 524–527

9. Brandenburg J H, Lee C Y S 1981 The eleventh nerve in radical neck surgery. Laryngoscope 91: 1851–1859

10. Brekel van den M W M, Castelijns J A, Stel H V et al 1991 Detection and characterization of metastatic cervical adenopathy by MR imaging: comparison of different MR techniques. J Comput Assist Tomogr 14: 581–589

11. Brekel van den M W M, Stel H V, Castelijns J A et al 1990 Cervical lymph node metastasis: assessment of radiologic criteria. Radiology 177: 379–384

12. Byers R M 1985 Modified neck dissection: a study of 967 cases from 1970 to 1980. Am J Surg 150: 414–421

13. Byers R M, Wolf P F, Ballantyne A J 1988 Rationale for elective modified neck dissection. Head Neck Surg 10: 160–167

14. Carenfelt C, Eliasson K 1980 Cervical metastases following radical neck dissection that preserved the spinal accessory nerve. Head Neck Surg 2: 181–184

15. Chow J M, Levin B C, Krivit J S, Applebaum E L 1989 Radiotherapy or surgery for subclinical cervical node metastases. Arch Otolaryngol Head Neck Surg 115: 981–984

16. Close L G, Merkel M, Vuitch M F, Reisch J, Schaefer S D 1989 Computed tomographic evaluation of regional lymph node involvement in cancer of the oral cavity and oropharynx. Head Neck 11: 309–317

17. Conley J J 1975 Radical neck dissection. Laryngoscope 85: 1344–1352

18. Crile G W 1906 Excision of cancer of the head and neck. JAMA 47: 1780–1786

19. Cummings C W, Johnson J, Chung C K, Sagerman R 1977 Complications of laryngectomy and neck dissection following planned preoperative radiotherapy. Ann Otol Rhinol Laryngol 86: 745–750

20. Dargent M, Papillon J 1945 Resultats eloignes de l'evidement gang du cou avec conservation du filet mentonier et du spinal. Lyon Chir 41: 715

21. DeSanto L W, Beahrs O H, Holt J J, O'Fallon W M 1985 Neck dissection and combined therapy: study of effectiveness. Arch Otolaryngol 111: 366–370

22. DeSanto L W, Holt J J, Beahrs O H, O'Fallon W M 1982 Neck dissection: is it worthwhile? Laryngoscope 92: 502–509

23. Farrar W B, Finkelmeier W R, McCabe D P, Young D C, O'Dwyer P J, James A G 1988 Radical neck dissection: is it enough? Am J Surg 156: 173–176

24. Feinmesser R, Freeman J L, Noyek A M, Brit B D 1987 Metastatic neck disease: a clinical, radiographic, pathologic correlative study. Arch Otolaryngol Head Neck Surg 113: 1307–1310

25. Feinmesser R, Freeman J L, Noyek A M, Brit B D, Gullane P, Mullen J B 1990 MRI and neck metastases: a clinical, radiological, pathological correlative study. J Otolaryngol 19: 136–140

26. Feldman D E, Applebaum E L 1977 The submandibular triangle in radical neck dissection. Arch Otolaryngol 103: 705–706

27. Ferlito A 1987 Malignant laryngeal epithelial tumors and lymph node involvement: therapeutic and diagnostic considerations . Ann Otol Rhinol Laryngol 96: 542–548

28. Fisch U P, Siegel M E 1964 Cervical lymphatic system as visualized by lymphography. Ann Otol Rhinol Laryngol 73: 869–882

29. Fletcher G H 1979 Basic principles of the combination of irradiation and surgery. Int J Radiat Oncol Biol Phys 5: 2091–2096

30. Friedman M, Roberts N 1990 Computed tomography in the diagnosis of head and neck tumors. In: Schuller D, Cummings C (eds) Cost-effective head and neck surgery. Decker, Toronto

31. Friedman M, Mafee M F, Pacella B L, Strorigl T L, Dew L L, Toriumi D M 1990 Rationale for elective neck dissection in 1990. Laryngoscope 100: 54–59

32. Friedman M, Shelton V K, Mafee M, Bellity P, Grybauskas V T, Skolnik E M 1984 Metastatic neck disease: evaluation by computed tomography. Arch Otolaryngol 110: 443–447

32a. Gávilan J, Gávilan C, Herranz J 1992 Functional neck dissection: three decades of controversy. Ann Otol Rhinol Laryngol 101: 339–341

33. Jesse R H, Fletcher G H 1977 Treatment of the neck in patients with squamous cell carcinoma of the head and neck. Cancer 39: 868–872

34. Jesse R H, Lindberg R D 1975 The efficacy of combining radiation therapy with a surgical procedure in patients with cervical metastases from squamous carcinoma of the oropharynx and hypopharynx. Cancer 35: 1163–1166

35. Jesse R H, Ballantyne A J, Larson D 1978 Radical or modified neck dissection: a therapeutic dilemma. Am J Surg 136: 516–519

36. Lee J G, Krause C J 1975 Radical neck dissection: elective, therapeutic, and secondary. Ann Otol Rhinol Laryngol 101: 656–659

37. Levendag P, Sessions R, Bikram B, Strong E W, Shah J P, Spiro R, Gerold R 1989 The problem of neck relapse in early stage supraglottic larynx cancer. Cancer 63: 345–348

38. Lingeman R E, Helmus C, Stephens R, Ulm J 1977 Neck dissection: radical or conservative. Ann Otol Rhinol Laryngol 86: 737–744

39. Lutz C K, Johnson J T, Wagner R L, Myers E N 1990 Supraglottic carcinoma: patterns of recurrence. Ann Otol Rhinol Laryngol 99: 12–17

40. MacKenzie J N 1900 A plea for early naked-eye diagnosis and removal of the entire organ, with the neighboring area of possible lymphatic infection, in cancer of the larynx. Trans Am Laryngol Assoc: 56

41. Mancuso A A, Harnsberger H R, Muraki A S, Stevens M H 1983 Computed tomography of cervical and retropharyngeal lymph nodes: normal anatomy, variants of normal and applications in staging head and neck cancer. Radiology 148: 715–723

42. Mancuso A A, Maceri D, Rice D, Hanafee W 1981 C T of cervical lymph node cancer. A J R 136: 381–385

43. Mantravadi R, Katz A, Haas R, Liebner E J, Sabato D, Skolnik E M, Applebaum E L 1982 Radiation therapy for subclinical lymph nodes. Arch Otolaryngol 108: 108–111

44. Martis C, Karabouta I, Lazaridis N 1979 Incidence of lymph node metastasis in elective (prophylactic) neck dissection for oral carcinoma. J Maxillofac Surg 7: 182–191

45. McGavran M H, Bauer W C, Ogura J H 1961 The incidence of cervical lymph node metastasis from epidermoid carcinoma of the larynx and their relationship to certain characteristics of the primary tumor: a study based on the clinical and pathological findings in 96 patients treated by primary en bloc laryngectomy and radical neck dissection. Cancer 14: 55–66

46. Mendenhall W M, Million R R 1986 Elective neck irradiation for squamous cell carcinoma of the head and neck: analysis of time–dose factor and causes of failure. Int J Rad Oncol Biol Phys 12: 741–746

47. Mendenhall W M, Parsons J T, Brant T A, Stringer S P, Cassisi N J, Million R R 1989 Is elective neck treatment indicated for T2N0 squamous cell carcinoma of the glottic larynx? Radiother Oncol 14: 199–202

48. Nichols R T, Greenfield L J 1968 Experience with radical neck dissection in the management of 426 patients with malignant tumors of the head and neck. Ann Surg 167: 23

49. Ogura J H 1960 Cancer of the larynx, pharynx and upper cervical esophagus. Arch Otolaryngol 72: 66

50. Ogura J H, Biller H F, Wette R 1971 Elective neck dissection for pharyngeal and laryngeal cancers. Ann Otol Rhinol Laryngol 80: 646–651

51. O'Keefe J J 1959 Evaluation of laryngectomy with radical neck dissection. Laryngoscope 69: 914–920

52. Parsons J T, Mendenhall W M, Cassisi N J, Stringer S P, Million R R 1989 Neck dissection after twice-a-day radiotherapy: morbidity and recurrence rates. Head Neck 11: 400–404

53. Pietrantoni L, Fior R 1958 Clinical and surgical problems of cancer of the larynx and hypopharynx: review of 570 consecutive cases operated on in ear, nose and throat clinic of Milan between 1948 and 1954 with special regard to problems of metastases. Acta Otolaryngol suppl 142

54. Quetz J U, Rohr S, Hoffman P, Wustrow J, Mertens J 1991 Die B-Bildsonographie biemt Lymphtenostaging im Kopf-Hals-Bereich: ein Vergleich mit der Palpatron, Computer- und Magnetresonanztomographie. HNO 39: 61–63

55. Rabuzzi D D, Chung C T, Sagerman R H 1980 Prophylactic neck irradiation. Arch Otolaryngol 106: 454–455

56. Reed G F, Rabuzzi D D 1969 Neck dissection. Otolaryngol Clin North Am 4: 547–563

57. Robbins R T, Medina J E, Wolfe G T, Sessions R B, Pruet C W 1991 Standardizing neck dissection terminology: official report of the Academy's Committee for Head and Neck Surgery and Oncology. Arch Otolaryngol Head Neck Surg 117: 601–605

58. Sako K, Pradier R N, Marchetta F C, Pickren J W 1964 Fallibility of palpation in the diagnosis of metastases to cervical nodes. Surg Gynecol Obstet 118: 989–990

59. Schuller D E, Platz C E, Krause C J 1978 Spinal accessory lymph nodes: a prospective study of metastatic involvement. Laryngoscope 88: 439–450

60. Schuller D E, Laramore G, Al-Sarraf M, Jacobs J, Pajek T F 1989 Combined therapy for resectable head and neck cancer. A phase 3 intergroup study. Arch Otolaryngol Head Neck Surg 115: 364–368

61. Schuller D E, McGuire W F, Krause C J, McCabe B F, Pflug B K 1979 Adjuvant cancer therapy of head and neck tumors: increased survival with surgery alone versus combined therapy. Laryngoscope 89: 582–594

62. Schuller D E, Reiches N A, Hamaker R C et al 1983 Analysis of disability resulting from treatment including radical neck dissection or modified neck dissection. Head Neck Surg 6: 551–558

63. Shah J P, Stiang E, Spiro R J, Vikiam B 1981 Neck dissection: current and future possibilities. Clin Bull 11: 25–33

64. Skolnik E M, Tenta L T, Wineinger D M 1967 Preservation of XI cranial nerve in neck dissection. Laryngoscope 77: 1304–1314

65. Skolnik E M, Yee K F, Friedman M, Golden T A 1976 The posterior triangle in radical neck surgery. Arch Otolaryngol 102: 1–4

66. Southwick H W, Slaughter D P, Trevino E T 1960 Elective neck dissection for intraoral cancer. Arch Surg 80: 905–909

67. Spiro R H, Strong E W 1973 Epidermoid carcinoma of the oral cavity and oropharynx: elective vs therapeutic radical neck dissection as treatment. Arch Surg 107: 382–384

68. Spiro R H, Alfonso A E, Farr H W 1974 Cervical node metastases from epidermoid cancer of the oral cavity and oropharynx. Am J Surg 128: 562–567

69. Stern W B R, Silver C E, Zeifer B A, Persky M S, Heller K S 1991 Computed tomography of the clinically negative neck. Head Neck 13: 73–75

70. Stevens M H, Harnsberger R, Mancuso A A, Davis R K, Johnson L P, Parkin J L 1985 Computed tomography of cervical lymph nodes: staging and management of head and neck cancer. Arch Otolaryngol 111: 735–739

71. Strong E W 1969 Preoperative radiation and radical neck dissection. Surg Clin North AM 49: 271–276

72. Suarez O 1963 El problema de las metastasis linfaticas y alejdas del cancer de larynge e hipolaringe. Rev Otorrinolaringol 28: 83–99

73. Welsh L W, Welsh J P 1966 Cervical lymphatics: pathologic conditions. Ann Otol Rhinol Laryngol 75: 176–191

27. Treatment with the CO$_2$ laser

S. M. Shapshay, E. E. Rebeiz

INTRODUCTION

Carcinoma of the larynx most commonly involves the glottis and, in general, can be diagnosed early. Many therapeutic options are available, including radiotherapy, endoscopic excision, or partial laryngectomy.

Conservative treatment of patients with these lesions is based on the fact that the tumour is usually confined to the laryngeal structure. Radical surgery, which can usually be avoided, is reserved for patients with advanced lesions. The role of the carbon dioxide (CO$_2$) laser in the endoscopic treatment of patients with laryngeal disease emerged in the 1970s when Strong and Jako[6] reported their first experience. They used the CO$_2$ laser in the canine larynx and then in humans for excision of benign and malignant tumours. Although the technique was controversial at first, the CO$_2$ laser has been used successfully for the management of patients with benign and malignant laryngeal lesions. It is a precise surgical tool, particularly when coupled to an operating microscope with a variable-spot-size micromanipulator. The role of the CO$_2$ laser in the treatment of patients with carcinoma of the larynx includes excisional biopsy of T1 lesions, incisional biopsy and biological staging of T2 to T3 lesions, removal of as much obstructing tumour as possible to secure an airway and to avoid tracheotomy, palliation of disease in poor surgical candidates or in patients with terminal disease, and destruction of as much of the tumour as possible before radiotherapy.

When good operative technique is used, damage to the surrounding tissue at the margins of laser excision is only 50–100 μm, which provides a good specimen for the pathologist. A narrow zone of laser-induced char at the margins of the specimen may be beneficial because it marks the edges of excision and outlines the surgical margin for the pathologist.

Excellent function of the vocal cords can be preserved with voice quality comparable to that after radiotherapy alone, although controlled studies are needed to compare results after laser excision with results after radiotherapy on a prospective basis.

Many surgeons and patients view the laser as a magical tool, leading to overextension of its applications to include excision of advanced lesions or to the inappropriate use of excessive energy. The laser has occasionally been used inappropriately for excision of T2 laryngeal carcinoma, for lesions of the anterior commissure, and for vaporization of laryngeal lesions. Understanding the biological behaviour of laryngeal carcinoma and the physical properties of the laser is an important consideration in the endoscopic treatment of patients with this condition.

EXCISIONAL BIOPSY WITH THE CO$_2$ LASER

One of the main applications of the CO$_2$ laser in laryngeal carcinoma is the excision of early tumours of the true vocal cords. The lesions most suitable for transoral laser excisional biopsy are hyperkeratosis, dysplasia, carcinoma in situ, and early invasive squamous cell carcinoma (T1 tumours). Studies[1,2] have shown excellent rates of cure for patients with T1 squamous cell carcinoma using this approach; such rates are comparable to results achieved with radiotherapy.

Strict criteria for endoscopic excision need to be emphasized when managing early invasive carcinoma with the laser. The lesion should be minimally invasive, localized to the midportion of the true vocal cord, and should not extend to the anterior commissure, vocal process of the arytenoid cartilage, or the supraglottic or subglottic larynx. Extension of the tumour does not permit complete controlled excision, although some degree of involvement, up to 1–2 mm along the floor of the ventricle, may be managed endoscopically. Mobility of the vocal cords should be normal—indicating minimal invasiveness of the carcinoma. A tumour of the anterior commissure should not be excised because the distance between the tumour and the thyroid perichondrium is small, making it difficult to obtain good surgical margins.

When the tumour extends into the region of the anterior commissure, recurrence is likely with any endoscopic technique[3] (Fig. 27.1).

Endoscopic management of laryngeal neoplasia presupposes adequate laryngoscopic exposure with a wide-bore laryngoscope. In about 10–20% of our patients, the larynx has been difficult to expose because of a narrow dental arch, large tongue, and previous surgery of the neck or radiotherapy-induced tissue contracture. An example of difficult laryngoscopy is the examination of an obese patient with a short thick neck, underdeveloped mandible, and full dentition. Difficulty with flexion of the neck can also be encountered during laryngoscopy on patients with cervical arthritis, a condition prevalent in patients with rheumatoid arthritis, and in elderly patients.

Usually, we prefer to use the Dedo–Jako laryngoscope with an anterior commissure design (Pilling Company, 420 Delaware Drive, Fort Washington, PA 19034) or the Kleinsasser laryngoscope of similar design (Karl Storz Endoscopy-America, Inc., 10111 West Jefferson Blvd, Culver City, CA). Although we first attempt to place the largest possible laryngoscope for the best exposure, only about 60% of patients can tolerate this type of instrument. We also prefer the Boston University suspension system (Pilling Company) that requires a specially adapted laryngoscope. When the suspension is in place, the entire table can be moved in various positions without changing the exposure. The Boston University system also prevents torque-like movement on the suspension, such as that encountered with the Lewy system.

The CO_2 laser is not a magical tool for this type of surgical treatment because excision can be performed using 'cold' microsurgical techniques with microscissors and microforceps. The advantage of using the laser is non-contact microprecision in a bloodless field. The potential disadvantage is the risk of thermal damage, a problem that, for superficial lesions, such as keratosis and dysplasia, puts an extra burden on the clinician with regard to the need for meticulous technique. Undoubtedly, wound healing following excision of tissue by thermal effects (laser or electrocautery) is slower than it is after non-thermal surgical treatment.

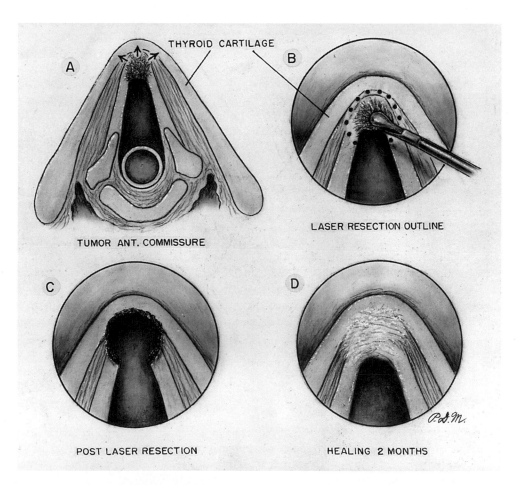

Fig. 27.1 Surgical excision of an anterior commissure lesion. The mucosa is close to the thyroid cartilage, and good margins cannot be obtained.

The CO_2 laser can be used in laryngology for the diagnosis and treatment of selected lesions. True lesions of the vocal cords that can be treated successfully by excision with the CO_2 laser are keratosis, carcinoma in situ, and T1 invasive carcinoma. The technique and extent of excision depend on the nature, size and location of the lesion.

Staining with toluidine dye is used to determine areas of dysplasia and is especially helpful in the presence of multicentricity.[7] Staining is helpful to outline the areas selected for biopsy, and it decreases the percentage of false-negative biopsies. Care should be taken to avoid abrasion of the surfaces of the vocal cords because they would then stain positively. A positive stain with toluidine blue is deep purple rather than the lighter blue seen with respiratory epithelium (false cords and subglottis). A cottonoid pledget saturated with toluidine blue is applied liberally to the surfaces of the vocal cords. After 5 seconds, a suction–irrigation microlaryngeal instrument is used vigorously to remove excess toluidine blue from the vocal cords, using about 20 ml of saline solution.

Laryngeal hyperkeratosis is a premalignant lesion. The lesion is usually superficial, and excision should be conservative. The false vocal cords are retracted to expose the ventricular surfaces. Keratotic areas should be excised completely down through the mucosa without exposing the vocal ligament or muscle. Using the 25× magnification of the operating microscope, the larynx is examined carefully with the aid of fine microlaryngeal probes and mirrors to inspect the undersurface of the vocal cord and subglottic region of the anterior commissure. The operating microscope is switched to an optimum 16× magnification, and the CO_2 laser microspot is used to outline the lesion using a 0.1-second pulsed mode. About 2 W of energy at 0.1-second exposures is used with the 300 μm spot size. When the depth of excision is reached with the outlining technique, the keratotic area separates from the surrounding tissue. A 1-mm laryngeal forceps is used to grasp the lesion, and a straight 1-mm laryngeal scissors is used to free the specimen from its base. This technique of excision is preferred to laser excision because it diminishes the effect of heat near the vocalis muscle for better function of the vocal cords. Because the specimen is thin, minimal heat coagulation is desired, particularly at the base and margins of the specimen.

When areas of carcinoma in situ are identified, a deeper excision exposing the vocalis muscle is required, and a 2–3-mm margin around the tumour is obtained. This margin is important for proper assessment of the depth of invasion and for complete excision. When the lesion violates the vocal ligament, the diagnosis is changed to invasive carcinoma.

Excision should be carried out in an even plane, respecting the vocal ligament, and stripping of the mucosa should be avoided. Care with this technique prevents scarring and adhesions and therefore poor voice quality (Fig. 27.2). The lesion should be oriented carefully for the pathologist for the determination of frozen-section margins. A full-thickness specimen should be obtained because the pathologist needs to determine whether the basal epithelial membrane has been invaded. Invasion cannot be determined from a shallow specimen. When this microprecise technique is used, both vocal cords can be treated simultaneously, taking care not to strip the epithelium in the region of the anterior commissure.

The use of the CO_2 laser for endoscopic excision can be extended to T1 invasive squamous cell carcinoma. Although these lesions can be treated successfully with radiotherapy, laser excision offers many benefits. A small exophytic lesion that is limited to the midcord, not reaching the anterior commissure or the vocal process of the arytenoid, can be excised totally transorally.

Endoscopic excision with the CO_2 laser offers a 90% rate of cure[1] that is comparable to radiotherapy. In addition, it offers treatment in one session compared with the many treatment sessions required with radiotherapy. Treatment with the CO_2 laser is associated with less morbidity, can be repeated, and can be used as a biopsy procedure for examination of the margins of the tumour. Radiotherapy should be employed for failures of treatment and for recurrent or for second primary tumours frequently present in patients with carcinoma of the head and neck. When the lesion extends to the anterior commissure or to the arytenoid cartilage, excision with the CO_2 laser is contraindicated.

Surgical excision of an early carcinoma of the vocal cord demands meticulous technique. Good exposure and constant tension on the specimen are the key points for successful excision. The lesion should be outlined with a margin of at least 2–3 mm of healthy surrounding mucosa. A pulsed mode is used to diminish the effects of heat on the margins of the tumour as well as postoperative heat-induced swelling and subsequent scarring; 6 W of energy is used in a pulsed 0.1-second exposure. The specimen is hand-carried to the pathologist, and the margins are properly oriented. The specimen is pinned to a strip of moist non-adherent dressing to avoid contraction. Longitudinal serial sections are taken for adequate orientation and sampling of the margins. When the margins are insecure or too close, laser excision is repeated, using the base of the new specimen as the deep margin rather than taking random deep biopsies. The next layer excised is considered the new margin and, therefore, should be properly oriented again. A negative random deep biopsy may give the clinician a false sense of security. Histological specimens and margins are reviewed by the clinician and the pathologist for treatment to be successful.

The quality of the voice is satisfactory in general, depending on the depth of laser resection, and is usually

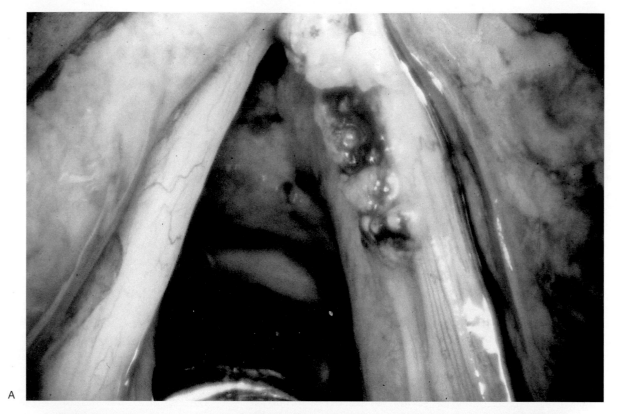

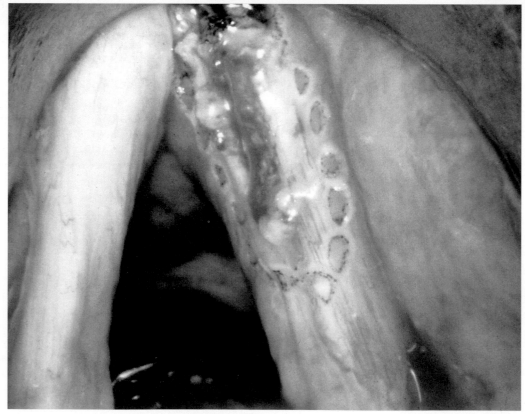

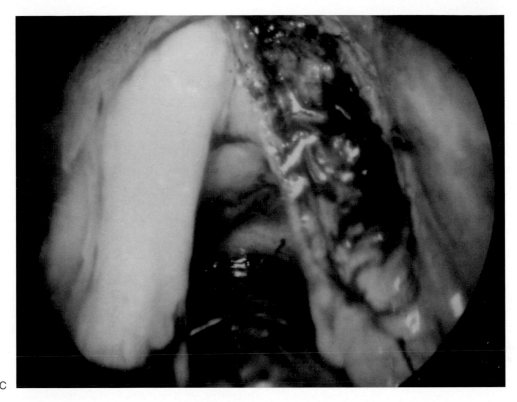

C

Fig. 27.2   A. Stage T1 carcinoma of the midvocal cord excised with the CO_2 laser. B. The lesion is delineated with a 1–2 mm margin using the microspot CO_2 laser. C. The defect shown after complete excision of the tumour. (Reprinted with permission from Shapshay et al.[5])

comparable to that obtained after radiotherapy. Unfortunately, the literature lacks a prospective randomized study to compare the quality of voice after endoscopic excision and after radiotherapy. A recent study by McGuirt et al[4] on patients treated for T1 laryngeal carcinoma by endoscopic laser excision only showed that the quality of the voice was acceptable and was rated by the patients as normal to nearly normal.

Aspiration is not usually a problem when the arytenoid cartilage is not resected.

Diagnosis and staging

Although not suitable for excision of advanced lesions, the CO_2 laser offers some benefits when used for diagnosis and staging of these lesions. When performing excisional biopsy, the clinician sometimes finds that the tumour has invaded to an unexpected depth. With the aid of an operating microscope at 16× — or sometimes 25× —magnification, the clinician can determine definite invasion of the vocal ligament and muscle even when invasion is not expected clinically because the mobility of the vocal cords may be unimpaired.

The unique features of the CO_2 laser in a relatively bloodless operative field have generated the concept of biological staging. From a biological standpoint, this would appear to upgrade the tumour from T1 carcinoma of the vocal cord to a somewhat more aggressive biological T3 lesion of the vocal cord, thus greatly affecting the treatment plan, prognosis, and quality of the voice. In this situation, the surgeon is often tempted to localize the tumour and excise it completely; however, this action is not recommended. When deep muscle invasion is noted, the clinician should be satisfied with incisional biopsy because the function of the vocal cords may be less impaired if radiotherapy is chosen as the definitive modality of treatment. Deep excision often leads to scarring and retraction and adhesions between the remaining vocalis muscle and the mucosa.

Some situations may arise in which the tumour is found to be invading the thyroid cartilage at the anterior commissure (Fig. 27.1). The lesion can then be staged correctly as T4 squamous cell carcinoma when, clinically, a T1 lesion had been suspected. Because computed tomography does not accurately determine invasion of the thyroid cartilage, particularly at the anterior commissure, endoscopic diagnosis is valuable. The CO_2 laser is used as an excisional or biopsy tool for more accurate determination of the depth of invasion by the tumour. Open surgical techniques can then be planned for the patient with a lesion of the anterior commissure that involves the thyroid cartilage, and radiotherapy can be chosen for the patient with a lesion deeply invasive into the vocalis muscle.

Use of the CO_2 laser for reduction of tumour size

The use of the CO_2 laser to reduce the size of the tumour has been helpful in many situations. This technique has been used for reduction of the tumour in an attempt to facilitate radiotherapy, to avoid tracheotomy before definitive treatment begins, for palliation in unresectable disease, or in patients in whom general anaesthesia is not possible.

Microlaryngeal reduction of the tumour by use of the laser before definitive radiotherapy is an attractive although not proved concept. This technique is desirable in the management of patients with bulky tumours, particularly when the depth of invasion is not easy to determine clinically. In these situations, the laser is used for staging, for assessing invasion, and for reducing the size of the tumour. As a treatment modality, reducing the size of the tumour has not proved of benefit over radiotherapy alone. A prospective randomized study comparing this technique of tumour reduction with radiotherapy alone would be of interest. Whether reduction of carcinomatous cells before radiotherapy has any deleterious effects on the voice or whether it slows the deliverance of radiotherapy is unknown. Reduction of the tumour is performed routinely in our practice. Patients are usually happy with some improvement in their voice. Even when some delay in initiating radiotherapy occurs, a satisfactory airway is maintained and the quality of the voice is adequate.

Endoscopic laser excision is a useful technique for advanced exophytic lesions of the vocal cord that cause obstruction of the airway. Although obstruction is not common, such tumours are usually extensive. They are often associated with supraglottic or subglottic extension and fixation of the vocal cords and can present an airway emergency. The patient should be intubated awake with a small (5–5.5 mm) laser-resistant endotracheal tube, and the laser can be used to reduce the size of the obstructing tumour, thereby avoiding tracheotomy as a preliminary stage before laryngectomy. This procedure theoretically reduces the possibility of a recurrent lesion at the stoma, although not definitively proved as a causative factor, and avoids a contaminated field, thereby reducing the possibility of an infection associated with tracheotomy before laryngectomy. When most of the tumour in the anterior portion of the larynx has been removed with the laser, a Venturi jet ventilation system is placed on the laryngoscope. Laryngeal examination without the endotracheal tube is helpful for exposure of the subglottic and posterior larynx. With large vascular tumours, intermittent spot electrocautery of large blood vessels may be needed when haemostasis is a problem.

Although not a common situation, elderly patients, often in their 80s, can present with recurrent laryngeal carcinoma after radiotherapy. Endoscopic laser palliation is an attractive treatment modality to maintain an airway and some voice and to delay the use of tracheotomy for as long as possible. Laser treatment for palliation is also useful for patients who are high medical risks for open partial or total laryngectomy after failure of radiotherapy. In five of our patients, all in their 80s, this endoscopic approach has proved to be useful.[5]

Salvage treatment with the laser for recurrence after radiotherapy

Endoscopic laser excision for salvage treatment of recurrent tumour after radiotherapy is difficult and somewhat risky. Recurrent tumours after radiotherapy may be multicentric and submucosal. Nests of tumour cells may be hidden between areas of radiation-induced fibrosis, leading to the presence of skip areas that can be missed and misinterpreted as free margins. When the recurrent tumour is superficial and is detected at an early stage, it is worthwhile to attempt a salvage technique with the laser. Subtotal cordectomy for control of the tumour is preferred, and, again, careful orientation and preparation of the specimen are extremely important for the proper determination of margins. Unfortunately, in these situations, it is extremely difficult to judge the margin of endoscopic excision. In a series reported by Blakeslee et al,[1] the rate of control of recurrent tumour after radiotherapy was only 50%. When control of the margins of the tumour is believed to be good after laser excision, a deep nest of tumour cells, not detected at the time of excision, may be the cause of fixation of the vocal cord later. When a hidden tumour is not detected as a relatively early recurrent lesion, the fixed cord places the patient in great jeopardy, necessitating salvage by total laryngectomy.

SUPRAGLOTTIC CARCINOMA

The role of CO_2 laser excision for supraglottic carcinoma is limited. In rare situations, a small T1 epiglottic carcinoma involving the suprahyoid portion of the epiglottis or the rim of the arytenoepiglottic fold, or both, can be treated by endoscopic laser excisional techniques. The supraglottic larynx is abundantly supplied by lymphatic vessels that require consideration when planning treatment. Supraglottic T1 and T2 carcinomas are usually considered to be in the same category because early T1 tumours are discovered only rarely. Radiotherapy is the treatment of choice for patients with these tumours because both the primary carcinoma and high-risk lymph nodes are treated simultaneously. Selected patients with T2 supraglottic carcinomas are best managed by open supraglottic partial laryngectomy techniques and modified neck dissections, depending on the extent of metastasis of lymph nodes to the neck.

Indications for laser excision in advanced lesions, such as a large T1 carcinoma or a T2 lesion, are limited to T2 lesions or to situations in which standard treatment modalities are not possible, such as when the patient has refused radical treatment or is a high-risk surgical candidate for palliation of symptoms. In these instances, the laser can be used for staging and to secure an airway.

Laser excision can also be performed in a patient who has a limited recurrent tumour in the supraglottis after radiotherapy. Two such patients, who use their voice professionally, have been treated by endoscopic laser supraglottic partial laryngectomy or by extended epiglottidectomy, preserving sensory innervation to the larynx. This concept can be extended to patients who are poor medical risks with accessible supraglottic tumours that have recurred after radiotherapy.

Endoscopic supraglottic partial laryngectomy is associated with little risk of aspiration compared with open partial techniques, especially when performed after radiotherapy, and can be attempted in selected patients. The gold standard for control of carcinoma is total laryngectomy, and this operation should always be considered.

REFERENCES

1. Blakeslee D, Vaughan C W, Shapshay S M, Simpson G T, Strong M S 1984 Excisional biopsy in the selective management of T1 glottic cancer: a three-year follow-up study. Laryngoscope 94: 488–494
2. Koufman J A 1986 The endoscopic management of early squamous carcinoma of the vocal cord with the carbon dioxide surgical laser: clinical experience and a proposed subclassification. Otolaryngol Head Neck Surg 95: 531–537
3. Krespi Y P, Meltzer C J 1989 Laser surgery for vocal cord carcinoma involving the anterior commissure. Ann Otol Rhinol Laryngol 98: 105–109
4. McGuirt W F, Blalock D, Koufman J A, Feehs R S 1992 Voice analysis of patients with endoscopically treated early laryngeal carcinoma. Ann Otol Rhinol Laryngol 101: 142–146.
5. Shapshay S M, Hybels R L, Bohigian R K 1990 Laser excision of early vocal cord carcinoma: indications, limitations, and precautions. Ann Otol Rhinol Laryngol 99: 46–50
6. Strong M S, Jako G J 1972 Laser surgery in the larynx: early clinical experience with continuous CO_2 laser. Ann Otol Rhinol Laryngol 81: 791–798.
7. Strong M S, Vaughan C W, Incze J 1970 Toluidine blue in diagnosis of cancer of the larynx. Arch Otolaryngol 91: 515–519

28. Radiation therapy

W. M. Mendenhall, J. T. Parsons, S. P. Stringer, N. J. Cassisi, R. R. Million

INTRODUCTION

The following is a discussion of the role of radiation therapy, either alone or in combination with surgery, in the management of squamous cell carcinoma of the larynx. The primary surgical management of laryngeal cancer is presented elsewhere in the text.

At the University of Florida, the treatment of laryngeal cancer has been relatively consistent over the past 27 years. Patients with head and neck cancer are presented at a weekly disposition conference attended by otolaryngologists, radiation oncologists, plastic surgeons, pathologists, diagnostic radiologists, and dentists who specialize in the management of head and neck cancer. A joint treatment recommendation is rendered, and the patient is usually treated accordingly. Unless otherwise specified, the data presented in this review are from the University of Florida. Tumours were staged according to the 1983 AJCC staging system.[2]

If a lesion is suitable for irradiation or total laryngectomy, with a similar chance of cure, the former treatment is preferred. Many patients, when faced with a total laryngectomy for a moderately advanced lesion, choose irradiation in an attempt to preserve the voice, even if the chance of cure is slightly lower. Although significant advances have been made in voice rehabilitation, only about 70% regain a useful voice following total laryngectomy.

When evaluating treatment complications, it is worthwhile to recall that total laryngectomy is not considered a complication if it is the initial form of treatment, whereas radiation sequelae that necessitate a total laryngectomy are regarded as severe complications.

SUPRAGLOTTIC LARYNX

Selection of treatment modality

For purposes of treatment planning, patients may be considered to be in either an early or favourable group, which is suitable for radiation therapy or supraglottic laryngectomy, or an unfavourable group, often requiring total laryngectomy. For the unfavourable group, treatment with radiation therapy results in a relatively low cure rate, and the larynx may not function well afterward. Neck nodes are commonly involved and influence the overall treatment plan.

Early and moderately advanced supraglottic carcinoma

These lesions include T1, T2, and favourable T3 cancers. A favourable T3 lesion is one that is relatively exophytic, and is staged T3 on the basis of pre-epiglottic-space invasion or minimal extension to the medial wall of the pyriform sinus; the patient should have mobile vocal cords and an adequate airway. Treatment of the primary lesion for the early group is either by external-beam irradiation or supraglottic laryngectomy.[32,48] Total laryngectomy is reserved for treatment failure.

Irradiation and supraglottic laryngectomy are both highly successful modes of therapy for early lesions. Supraglottic laryngectomy became an option at our institution in 1973. Before that time, all patients with early or moderately advanced carcinoma of the supraglottic larynx were treated with irradiation. Approximately 50% of supraglottic laryngectomies performed at the University of Florida are followed by postoperative radiation therapy because of positive or close margins or because of indications secondary to neck disease.

Our guidelines for selection of supraglottic laryngectomy or radiation therapy are described. However, the patient and family are sometimes instrumental in making the decision based on previous experience with surgery or radiation therapy. Approximately half of the patients with T1, T2, or favourable T3 supraglottic larynx cancer seen at the University of Florida were not suitable for supraglottic laryngectomy because of anatomical tumour extensions (e.g., to the vocal cords, ventricle, etc.).

Approximately half the patients seen in our clinic whose lesions are technically suitable for a supraglottic laryngectomy are not eligible for the operation because of medical reasons (for example, inadequate pulmonary status or other major medical problems), and these patients are treated by radiation therapy. Poorly motivated or elderly patients are often not good candidates for supraglottic laryngectomy. Among the remaining patients who are technically and medically suitable for supraglottic laryngectomy, irradiation is preferred in many because of the ease of managing subclinical neck disease in patients at high risk for bilateral lymph node involvement (e.g., those with poorly differentiated midline primary lesions).

Analysis of local control by anatomical subsite within the supraglottic larynx shows no significant differences in local control rates with radiation therapy when comparing similar-stage lesions. Lesions extending to the true vocal cords are not suitable for supraglottic laryngectomy, but they may be managed by radiation therapy in favourable cases. Invasion of the pre-epiglottic space is not a contraindication to supraglottic laryngectomy or radiation therapy. A large, bulky infiltrative lesion filling more than 50% of the pre-epiglottic space is a common reason to select supraglottic laryngectomy. However, irradiation alone is often successful in controlling lesions that involve more than half of the pre-epiglottic space, and should be used if a total laryngectomy is the only other treatment option.

The status of the neck often determines the selection of treatment of the primary lesion. Patients with clinically negative neck nodes and a high risk for occult bilateral neck disease may be treated by radiation therapy because of the ease of bilateral elective neck irradiation (for example, a patient with poorly differentiated carcinoma of the suprahyoid epiglottis with midline base-of-tongue involvement). Alternatively, supraglottic laryngectomy and bilateral conservation neck dissections may be done.

For patients with early-stage primary lesions but advanced neck disease (N2B or N3), combined treatment is frequently necessary to produce a high rate of control of the neck disease. In these cases, the primary lesion is usually treated for cure by irradiation, with surgery added to the involved hemineck(s). If such a patient were treated by supraglottic laryngectomy, neck dissection, and postoperative irradiation, the radiation therapy portals would unnecessarily irradiate the primary site as well as the neck. If the patient has early, resectable neck disease (N1 or N2A) and surgery is elected for the primary site, postoperative irradiation is added only in the case of unexpected findings (such as positive margins, multiple positive nodes, or extracapsular extension). We generally prefer to avoid routine high-dose preoperative or postoperative irradiation in conjunction with a supraglottic laryngectomy, because the lymphoedema of the remaining larynx may be considerable, although it will eventually subside. However, good results have been reported from the M. D. Anderson Cancer Center with combined supraglottic laryngectomy and postoperative irradiation for patients with moderately advanced lesions.[15,39]

Advanced supraglottic carcinoma

These lesions include unfavourable T3 and T4 cancers. An unfavourable T3 lesion is a bulky endophytic cancer, often with vocal cord fixation and/or airway compromise. The treatment of choice is total laryngectomy combined with adjuvant irradiation in selected cases. Preoperative irradiation is administered if the lesion is not thought to be completely resectable, usually based on fixation of clinically positive neck nodes.[47] Postoperative irradiation is added after surgery for the following reasons: positive or close margins, subglottic extension, thyroid or cricoid cartilage invasion, extension of the primary tumour to the soft tissues of the neck, perineural invasion, two or more positive nodes, and extracapsular extension.[1]

Irradiation technique

Irradiation alone

A detailed presentation of the irradiation technique used for the treatment of laryngeal cancer may be found elsewhere.[19] Briefly, the primary lesion and both sides of the neck are treated with approximately 4500 cGy; the portals are then reduced in size to avoid the spinal cord and to treat the primary site as well as any clinically positive neck nodes, depending on whether a neck dissection is planned to follow the course of radiotherapy. The neck is irradiated electively even if no suspicious nodes are palpable because of the relatively high risk of occult nodal disease.[16,18,24] The final dose to the primary tumour varies with the T stage, disease volume within that stage, and growth pattern (exophytic versus endophytic). For example, the following doses would be prescribed for a once-a-day fractionation schedule using 200 cGy per fraction: T1, 6000 to 6400 cGy; T2, 6400 to 6800 cGy; T3 and T4, 6400 to 7000 cGy. Since 1978, twice-a-day irradiation has been used to treat T2–T4 supraglottic carcinomas at our institution.[37]

Patients with one or two mobile nodes that are less than 3 cm in diameter and located in the primary portals are usually treated with irradiation alone to the neck.[17] Patients with more advanced neck disease are considered for a neck dissection 4–6 weeks following irradiation;[20] if regression is complete by the first follow-up visit, the possibility of withholding neck dissection and proceeding with close follow-up is considered if the initial lymph nodes were 3–4 cm in maximum diameter. However, if the patient has a neck node recurrence after irradiation alone for positive neck nodes, the probability of salvage is less than 5%.[17] If it is necessary to perform bilateral neck dissections, they may be staged 3–4 weeks apart. The need to stage bilateral neck dissections may be less critical if functional dissections, which spare the jugular vein, are planned.

Following treatment, patients are seen monthly for 1 year, every 2 months for the second year, every 3 months for the third year, every 4–6 months for the fourth and fifth years, and annually after 5 years. Chest roentgenograms are obtained every 6–12 months following treatment. If there is a question of a local recurrence on follow-up examination, a computed tomography (CT) scan is obtained and direct laryngoscopy may be performed. It is unwise to perform biopsies of the larynx following irradiation unless a definite abnormality consistent with recurrent tumour is noted, because such biopsies may precipitate a necrosis or severe oedema that could result in laryngectomy. It is not unusual to observe persistent anatomic distortion with a smooth mucosa or even a mass effect that may persist for many months or even years after successful treatment, especially for the larger lesions. Oedema, usually symmetrical, may persist for a year or more after successful irradiation. In patients who have undergone a postirradiation neck dissection, pronounced ipsilateral oedema is very common. If the patient is pain-free, the findings are not progressive, and the CT suggests no focal abnormality, close follow-up without direct laryngoscopy is our usual approach. In some cases, it is impossible to distinguish post-treatment changes from recurrent cancer, and if a patient has major oedema and pain, it may be necessary to recommend a laryngectomy, realizing that the specimen may be negative for tumour on pathological examination. This is particularly true after irradiation for a locally advanced lesion. In most cases, the follow-up care after radiation therapy for moderately advanced lesions is the most difficult part of the treatment, and considerable judgement and experience are essential.

Adjuvant irradiation

Patients treated with preoperative irradiation receive 4600–5000 cGy at 180–200 cGy per fraction to the primary lesion and neck; the dose to fixed nodes is boosted to 6000–7000 cGy based on the initial size of the node, the degree of fixation, and the response to irradiation.[47]

Postoperatively, the dose is 6000–7000 cGy at 180–200 cGy per fraction, depending on the status of the margins and the presence and extent of known residual disease.[1] Postoperative irradiation is the generally preferred sequence in our institution for patients who require combined treatment.

Results

Irradiation alone

The rates of disease control at the primary site with irradiation alone at the University of Florida are shown in Table 28.1[30] Twenty-three patients with local recurrence underwent salvage surgery, which was successful in 15 (65%). Three patients underwent supraglottic laryngectomy for salvage, and the operation was successful in all three.

Overall, 33% of patients were initially suitable (technically and medically) for a supraglottic laryngectomy, 22% had anatomically suitable lesions but would have been unable to tolerate the procedure, and 45% had lesions anatomically situated in such a way that a total laryngectomy would have been necessary. In 50 of 73 patients (68%) who would have required a total laryngectomy if the initial treatment had been surgery, the disease was locally controlled with irradiation alone (Table 28.2).

Most of the patients with T2 and T3 lesions treated with irradiation alone had normal vocal cord mobility at diagnosis. The local control rate in the small subset of patients presenting with impaired vocal cord mobility was

Table 28.1 Supraglottic larynx carcinoma: local control* (129 patients with 131 lesions)

Stage	Local control after radiotherapy	No. salvaged/ no. attempted[†]	Ultimate local control
T1	13/13 (100%)	ND	13/13 (100%)
T2	34/42 (81%)	3/7	37/42 (88%)
T3	25/41 (61%)	9/13	34/41 (83%)
T4	3/9 (33%)	3/3	6/9 (67%)

ND = no data.
*Continuous-course irradiation, once-a-day or twice-a-day fractionation. Excludes 26 patients who died less than 2 years after treatment with primary site continuously disease-free.
[†]Surgical salvage implies continuous local control for at least 12 months following salvage procedure.
  Modified from Mendenhall et al 1990 Carcinoma of the supraglottic larynx: a basis for comparing the results of radiotherapy and surgery. Head Neck 12: 204–209, Table 1, p 205.

Table 28.2 Supraglottic larynx carcinoma: local control with radiotherapy as related to suitability for operation: 103 patients with 105 evaluable lesions (no. controlled/no. treated)*

| Stage | Anatomically suitable for supraglottic laryngectomy | | | Anatomically unsuitable for supraglottic laryngectomy |
	Medically suitable	Medically unsuitable	Total	
T1	7/7	5/5	12/12	1/1
T2	14/17 (82%)	8/9	22/26 (85%)	12/16 (75%)
T3	3/5	3/7	6/12 (50%)	19/29 (66%)
T4	1/3	0/1	1/4	2/5

*Excludes 26 patients who died within 2 years of radiotherapy with primary site continuously disease-free.
  From Mendenhall et al 1990 Carcinoma of the supraglottic larynx: a basis for comparing the results of radiotherapy and surgery. Head Neck 12: 204–209, Table 3, p 206.

lower compared to those with normally mobile vocal cords (Table 28.3).

Local control is also related to the extent of pre-epiglottic space invasion and to primary tumour volume, as demonstrated by computed tomography.[6] However, in almost half the patients treated with irradiation alone for high-volume (≥6cc) primary tumours, the disease is locally controlled with radiotherapy (Table 28.4).

Control above the clavicles refers to disease control at the primary site and in the neck. The rate of disease control above the clavicles as a function of AJCC stage is given in Table 28.5[30] Stage IV is subdivided into a favourable subset, IVA (T1–T3, N2A–N3A), and an unfavourable subset, IVB (T4 and/or N3B).[26] The control rate for stage IVA lesions was similar to that for stage III disease.

The rates of absolute survival and cause-specific survival (that is, survival excluding deaths due to intercurrent disease) at 5 years are presented in Table 28.6[30]

Adjuvant irradiation

The results at the M. D. Anderson Cancer Center for surgery alone (total laryngectomy in almost all cases) and for total laryngectomy plus postoperative irradiation for resectable stage IV squamous cell carcinoma of the supraglottic larynx are outlined in Tables 28.7 and 28.8.[5,8]

Table 28.3 Supraglottic larynx carcinoma: local control with radiotherapy; 83 patients with 83 evaluable lesions (no. controlled/no. treated)

Stage	Cord mobility			
	Mobile	Decreased	Fixed	Not stated
T2	29/33 (88%)	2/5	ND	3/4
T3	18/28 (64%)	3/6	3/6	1/1

ND = no data.

From Mendenhall et al 1990 Carcinoma of the supraglottic larynx: a basis for comparing the results of radiotherapy and surgery. Head Neck 12: 204–209, Table 4, p 207.

Table 28.4 Supraglottic larynx carcinoma: local control as a function of T stage for low-volume and high-volume lesions (31 patients)

Stage	Local control by tumour volume	
	<6 cc	≥6 cc
T1	3/3	—
T2	3/4	0/1
T3	9/11 (82%)	6/11 (55%)
T4	—	0/1
Total*	15/18 (83%)	6/13 (46%)

*P = 0.038

From Freeman et al 1990 Irradiation alone for supraglottic larynx carcinoma: can CT findings predict treatment results? Int J Radiat Oncol Biol Phys 19: 485–490, Table 3, p 488.

Table 28.5 Supraglottic larynx carcinoma: control above the clavicles (129 patients)*

Modified AJCC stage	Control with initial treatment	No. salvaged/ no. attempted	Ultimate control
I	8/8 (100%)	ND	8/8 (100%)
II	18/23 (78%)	4/5	22/23 (96%)
III	20/34 (59%)	8/10	28/34 (82%)
IVA	8/14 (57%)	2/4	10/14 (71%)
IVB	13/30 (43%)	4/8	17/30 (57%)

ND = no data.

*Continuous-course irradiation, once-a-day or twice-a-day fractionation. Two patients with synchronous primary lesions were staged according to the more advanced lesion. Excludes 20 patients who died less than 2 years after treatment and who had been continuously disease-free above the clavicles.

Modified from Mendenhall et al 1990 Carcinoma of the supraglottic larynx: a basis for comparing the results of radiotherapy and surgery. Head Neck 12: 204–209, Table 7, p 208.

Table 28.6 Supraglottic larynx carcinoma: survival at 5 years in 84 patients*

Modified AJCC stage	Absolute survival	Cause-specific survival
I	2/6 (33%)	2/2 (100%)
II	10/20 (50%)	10/12 (83%)
III	9/20 (45%)	9/13 (69%)
IVA	4/9 (44%)	4/6 (67%)
IVB	7/29 (24%)	7/22 (32%)

*Continuous-course irradiation, once-a-day or twice-a-day fractionation. One patient with synchronous primary lesions was staged according to the more advanced lesion.

From Mendenhall et al 1990 Carcinoma of the supraglottic larynx treated with radiotherapy: a basis for comparing the results of radiotherapy and surgery. Head Neck 12: 204–209, Table 8, p 208.

Table 28.7 Supraglottic larynx carcinoma: recurrence above the clavicles after initial surgery (total laryngectomy) in resectable stage IV lesions* (M. D. Anderson Cancer Center)

Result	Surgery only	Surgery + postoperative radiation therapy
Definite failure above the clavicles (2-year minimum follow-up after rescue surgery, if needed)	28/116 (24%)	7/53 (13%)

*Stage IV = T4 N0–N1, T1–T4 N2–N3.

Adapted from Goepfert et al 1975 Optimal treatment for the technically resectable squamous cell carcinoma of the supraglottic larynx. Laryngoscope 85: 14–32, Table 9, p 28.

Complications

Irradiation alone

During the course of irradiation, the patient experiences sore throat, loss of taste, and a variable degree of xerostomia, depending on how much of the parotid gland is irradiated. Approximately 10% of patients require a nasogastric feeding tube for nutritional support during treatment; it is very unusual to require an unplanned

Table 28.8 Stage IV* supraglottic carcinoma: event-free survival rates† (M. D. Anderson Cancer Center)

	Surgery only††	Surgery + radiation therapy
Two years	34/87§ (39%)	37/54§ (69%)
Five years	19/78 ‡ (24%)	16/38 ‡ (42%)

*Stage IV = T4 N0–N1, T1–T4 N2–N3.
†Living, free of cancer.
††All patients had a total laryngectomy.
§P = <0.005.
‡ P = <0.08.
  From Fletcher G H, Goepfert H 1980 Larynx and pyriform sinus. In: Fletcher G H (ed) Textbook of radiotherapy, 3rd edn, pp 330–363, Table 3–31, p 357, Lea & Febiger, Philadelphia

treatment interruption. If ^{60}Co is used, most patients develop dry desquamation of the skin within the treatment portals. Moist desquamation of the skin rarely occurs if care is taken to avoid tangential irradiation of the skin of the anterior neck. With advanced lesions, there is a small risk of laryngeal oedema leading to airway compromise that would necessitate a temporary tracheostomy.

Late side-effects of irradiation include xerostomia and an increased risk of dental caries. Caries can usually be prevented with the use of prophylactic fluoride carriers and periodic dental evaluation. Usually, xerostomia is minimal to moderate because only the tail of the parotid and part of the submaxillary gland are irradiated, but this may still be enough to lead to caries. Osteoradionecrosis of the mandible is rare, because usually only the angle of the mandible is included in the treatment field. Late complications may include severe laryngeal oedema, osteochondronecrosis, and a remote risk of radiation myelitis. The risk of inducing a second malignancy is negligible.[14,36,40] Severe late complications developed in eight (6%) of 129 patients treated at the University of Florida: 4 of 115 with T1, T2, and T3 lesions (3%) and 4 of 14 with T4 cancers (29%).[30]

Adjuvant irradiation

The complications of preoperative irradiation are essentially those observed following surgery, except that they occur at an increased incidence. The major complication of postoperative irradiation following supraglottic laryngectomy is worsening of laryngeal oedema, with resultant aspiration and airway compromise. It may not be possible to decannulate the patient or to remove the feeding tube if significant laryngeal oedema or difficulty in swallowing persists after treatment. An occasional patient may experience aspiration pneumonia, which may be fatal. A recent update from Lee and coworkers included 60 patients who underwent supraglottic laryngectomy, which was followed by postoperative irradiation in 50 patients (83%).[15] An additional three patients who underwent supraglottic laryngectomy for salvage after a local recurrence following irradiation (two patients) or following neoadjuvant chemotherapy (one patient) were included in the analysis of postoperative complications and sequelae. The authors noted that 80% of patients had normal deglutition by 4 months postsurgery; patients who underwent postoperative irradiation required more time to discontinue nasogastric feeding than those treated with surgery alone. Seven patients required a gastrostomy tube; all seven received postoperative radiotherapy. The gastrostomy tube remained in place for an average of 5 months, except in one patient who had the gastrostomy tube until death at 7 years. Approximately 80% of patients were decannulated within 5 months of the operation. The overall incidence of significant complications was 14%. Two patients died in the immediate postoperative period, and three patients required a total laryngectomy for intractable aspiration. An additional patient (one of seven who required a gastrostomy) died of aspiration pneumonia at 7 years.

Postoperative irradiation after local laryngectomy is associated with a remote risk of pharyngeal stricture and stomal stenosis.[1]

GLOTTIC LARYNX

Selection of treatment modality

The goal of treatment is cure with the best functional result and the least risk of a serious complication. For purposes of treatment planning, patients may be considered to be in one of the following groups: (i) an early group, where there is a high rate of cure with voice preservation, (ii) a moderately advanced group, where the cure rate is still good but larynx preservation is possible in only 60–70% of cases, or (iii) an advanced group, where there is a moderate chance of cure and a remote possibility of voice preservation. At our institution, the early group is treated initially by irradiation or, in a few selected cases, by partial laryngectomy. We have no experience with laser excision. The moderately advanced group is treated with irradiation, with laryngectomy reserved for failure, or with total laryngectomy, with or without radiation therapy. The advanced group is treated with total laryngectomy alone or combined with adjuvant irradiation; irradiation is occasionally used for patients who refuse laryngectomy or who are medically inoperable.

Carcinoma in situ

A lesion diagnosed as carcinoma in situ may sometimes be controlled by stripping the cord. However, it is difficult to exclude the possibility of microinvasion on these specimens. Recurrence is frequent, and the cord may become thickened and the voice hoarse with repeated stripping.

We have come to recommend irradiation much earlier for carcinoma in situ because most such patients would eventually need this treatment, and earlier use of irradiation means a better chance of preserving a good voice.

Many patients treated for carcinoma in situ have obvious lesions that probably contain invasive carcinoma. We have occasionally proceeded with radiation therapy rather than put the patient through a second biopsy.

Early vocal cord carcinoma

Early vocal cord cancer is defined as the subset of lesions that can be cured with larynx preservation in a substantial number of cases. In most centres, irradiation is the initial treatment prescribed for early (T1 and T2) lesions, with surgery reserved for salvage of irradiation failures. While hemilaryngectomy or cordectomy produces a comparable cure rate for selected T1 and T2 vocal cord lesions, irradiation is generally the preferred initial therapy. Cordectomy can be accomplished by laryngofissure or endoscopically with the laser. There is limited short-term information available pertaining to the efficacy of laser excision.[10] The procedure is suitable only for carefully chosen patients; unacceptably high failure rates following laser resection have been reported by some, particularly if the anterior commissure is involved. Voice quality is worse than after irradiation, but generally better than after hemilaryngectomy.

The major advantages of irradiation over hemilaryngectomy or laryngofissure and cordectomy are that the quality of the voice is better, and that an operation is avoided.[23,45] The voice after hemilaryngectomy remains hoarse; we tell the patient that the voice will be 'as hoarse as it is now or even worse'. The voice after successful irradiation is usually better than before the therapy, but in occasional patients there is no improvement or, uncommonly, a worsening. Another advantage is that irradiation is less expensive than a surgical procedure.[33,41] Hemilaryngectomy finds its major use as a salvage operation in suitable cases after irradiation failure. Even if the patient has a local recurrence after a salvage hemilaryngectomy, there is a third chance in the form of total laryngectomy, which may still be successful.

Neel and coworkers, from the Mayo Clinic, reported a series of 182 patients with early vocal cord cancer who underwent laryngofissure and cordectomy.[34] Two patients were operated on for recurrence following irradiation; the remainder underwent surgery as the initial treatment for cancer. The authors noted a 26% incidence of complications; none was fatal. Twenty patients required direct laryngoscopy for removal of granulation tissue and to evaluate the possibility of recurrence, delayed wound healing and cartilage sequestration occurred in two patients, laryngeal stenosis was noted in two patients, and one patient developed an obstructing web. Gall and associates, from Washington University, reported a 16% incidence of complications in 237 patients undergoing hemilaryngectomy for vocal cord cancer.[7] Complications included the following: infection (0.4%), wound slough (0.8%), haemorrhage (0.8%), and carotid artery exposure and/or blowout (3.8%). Two patients (0.8%) experienced fatal complications.

Moderately advanced and advanced vocal cord carcinoma

Fixed-cord lesions (T3) may be subdivided into relatively favourable lesions and unfavourable lesions, the latter usually consisting of extensive bilateral disease with a compromised airway. Lesions considered favourable are confined mostly to one side of the larynx and are found in patients who have a good airway, are relatively easy to examine, and are reliable for follow-up.[21,38] Women have a better chance of cure overall and should always be seriously considered for conservative treatment.

The patient with a favourable lesion is advised of the alternatives of either radiation therapy with surgical salvage or immediate total laryngectomy. Once radiation therapy has begun, it might seem logical to make a decision to continue radiotherapy or stop and perform a laryngectomy based on the return of vocal cord mobility at 5000 cGy. However, in our experience this parameter has not been predictive of local control with irradiation.[28,38] The patient must be willing to return for follow-up every month for the first year and every 6–8 weeks for the second year. He or she must understand that total laryngectomy may be recommended purely on clinical grounds without biopsy-proven recurrence, that the risk of laryngeal osteochondronecrosis is about 5%, and that surgical salvage is associated with a slightly higher morbidity compared with initial total laryngectomy. Very few patients will choose total laryngectomy over irradiation when presented with these alternatives. The percentages of patients presenting with T3 vocal cord cancer who were subsequently treated with irradiation alone at our institution since 1965 have been: 1965–1969, 4/20 (20%); 1970–1979, 13/44 (30%); and 1980–1988, 36/54 (67%).[28]

The patient with an unfavourable lesion is advised to undergo total laryngectomy; preoperative or postoperative irradiation may be added for the indications previously outlined.[1] Occasionally patients with limited thyroid cartilage invasion or limited exolaryngeal extension (through the thyrohyoid membrane) have been offered primary irradiation; the local control rate in these patients is approximately 40%.

The major difficulty in the use of irradiation for the more advanced lesions is in distinguishing between radiation oedema and local recurrence during follow-up examinations. Progressive laryngeal oedema, persistent throat pain, otalgia, and/or fixation of a previously mobile vocal cord frequently predict recurrent disease in the larynx, although an occasional patient with these findings will remain disease-free with long-term follow-up.

Extended hemilaryngectomy has been used by a few surgeons in the treatment of well-lateralized fixed-cord lesions.[3,4,13,44] This alternative is suitable for approximately 5–10% of patients presenting with T3 vocal cord cancers.[4] A permanent tracheostomy may be required for some cases if a portion of the cricoid cartilage is resected, but a useful voice may be retained.

Irradiation technique

Irradiation alone

Patients with T1 and T2 vocal cord cancers are treated with limited ^{60}Co fields covering the primary lesion; the lymph nodes are not electively irradiated.[22] At our institution, the physician draws the portal lines on the patient each day, using anatomical landmarks to determine the field borders.[27,31] Patients are treated with 225 cGy per fraction, one fraction per day, 5 days a week, using continuous-course irradiation. The final tumour dose is as follows: Tis or very early T1 cancer, 5625 cGy in 25 fractions; T1 and early T2 cancer, 6300 cGy in 28 fractions; late T2 cancer, 6525 cGy in 29 fractions. For the last 4 years, twice-daily irradiation has been used at our institution for T2 vocal cord cancer (120 cGy per fraction to 7440 cGy total dose with a 6-hour interfraction interval).

Patients with T3 and, occasionally carefully chosen T4 lesions are treated with parallel opposed fields covering the primary lesion and upper neck, a technique similar to that employed for carcinomas of the supraglottic larynx.[21] The field size is reduced once or twice during the course of treatment. At the University of Florida, patients are treated with twice-a-day irradiation, 120 cGy per fraction, to a total dose of 7440–7680 cGy.

Adjuvant irradiation

The recommendations for adjuvant irradiation and the follow-up policy for patients with true vocal cord cancer are the same as those previously outlined for patients with supraglottic larynx cancer.

Results

Tis

In a study of 13 patients with carcinoma in situ of the glottic larynx treated with definitive irradiation at the University of Florida, one patient died of intercurrent

disease within 2 years of treatment and thus was not evaluable for local control. Of the remaining 12 patients, local control with irradiation was obtained in 11 (92%), with follow-up ranging from 2 to 16 years.[25] The patient who had a local recurrence was salvaged with a total laryngectomy and is alive and well 11.5 years following irradiation (7.5 years since salvage surgery).

T1, T2

Radiation therapy was used to treat 304 patients with invasive, previously untreated T1 and T2 squamous cell carcinomas of the glottic larynx between 1964 and 1984 at the University of Florida.[29] All patients had been observed for at least 2 years, and 82% had a minimum follow-up of 5 years. T1 lesions were stratified into two groups based on whether the tumour involved one (T1a) or both (T1b) vocal cords. T2 lesions were stratified based on vocal cord mobility: normal (T2a) and impaired (T2b).

The rates of local control after irradiation and ultimate local control, including patients successfully salvaged after a local recurrence, are given in Table 28.9.[29] Involvement of the anterior commissure did not adversely affect the likelihood of local control. Local control with irradiation was obtained in 15 of 16 T1 lesions (94%) and 45 of 63 T2 lesions (71%) that would have required a total laryngectomy had the initial treatment been surgery. Thirty-eight patients underwent a salvage operation, which was successful in 27 (71%): 6 of 10 (60%) who had a hemilaryngectomy and 21 of 28 (75%) who had a total laryngectomy. Four patients who had not been suitable for a hemilaryngectomy before radiotherapy later had a hemilaryngectomy for a local recurrence, and the surgical procedure was successful in two of four cases.

Twice-daily irradiation has been used to treat T2 true vocal cord cancer at our institution over the last 5 years. The local control rate with twice-daily irradiation is 26 of 28 (93%) compared to 80 of 107 (75%) with once-daily irradiation.

When the primary lesion was controlled, the rate of recurrent disease in the neck was 0% for T1 lesions and

Table 28.9 T1–T2 carcinoma of the glottic larynx: local control — 279 patients (no. controlled/no treated)

Stage	Excluded*	Local control	No. salvaged/ no. attempts	Ultimate local control
T1a	11	130/140 (93%)	7/10	137/140 (98%)
T1b	2	29/31 (94%)	0/2	29/31 (94%)
T2a	7	50/65 (77%)	13/15	63/65 (97%)
T2b	5	31/43 (72%)	7/11	38/43 (88%)

*Died less than 2 years after treatment with the primary site continuously disease-free.
Modified from Mendenhall et al 1988 T1–T2 vocal cord carcinoma: a basis for comparing the results of radiotherapy and surgery. Head Neck Surg 10: 373–377, Table 2, p 375.

3% for T2 lesions.[22] However, when tumour recurred at the primary site, the rate of neck recurrence increased to 20% for T1 tumours and 22% for T2 lesions. An elective neck dissection is advised for patients who have operations for recurrent T1 and T2 vocal cord carcinoma. Four of eight patients who developed recurrent disease in the neck were successfully salvaged by further treatment.

The absolute and cause-specific survival rates are shown in Table 28.10.[29] Eleven of the 213 patients (5%) at risk for ≥5 years died as a result of vocal cord cancer.

T3

Between 1965 and 1988, 118 patients with T3 squamous cell carcinoma of the glottic larynx were treated with curative intent at the University of Florida by irradiation alone (53 patients) or by surgery with or without irradiation (65 patients).[28] Table 28.11 shows the pretreatment characteristics of the two groups; the laryngectomy group had a higher proportion of advanced disease cases, as judged by the percentage of patients who

Table 28.10 T1–T2 carcinoma of the glottic larynx: 5-year survival*

Stage	Absolute survival	Cause-specific survival
T1a N0	107/122 (88%)	107/110 (97%)
T1b N0	23/29 (79%)	23/24 (96%)
T2a N0	43/57 (75%)	43/46 (93%)
T2b N0	29/38 (76%)	29/33 (88%)

*Excludes three patients with synchronous primary head and neck cancers and one patient with clinically positive neck nodes at presentation.
From Mendenhall et al 1988 T1–T2 vocal cord carcinoma: a basis for comparing the results of radiotherapy and surgery. Head Neck Surg 10: 373–377, Table 4, p 376.

Table 28.11 T3 squamous cell carcinoma of the glottic larynx: patient population

Parameter	Irradiation alone (53 patients)	Surgery ± irradiation (65 patients)
AJCC Stage		
T3N0	40 (75%)	49 (75%)
T3N1	10 (19%)	9 (14%)
T3N2–3	3 (6%)	7 (11%)
Supraglottic extension		
Present	46 (87%)	51 (78%)
Absent	7 (13%)	10 (15%)
No data	0	4 (6%)
Subglottic extension		
Present	37 (70%)	48 (74%)
Absent	15 (28%)	14 (22%)
No data	1 (2%)	3 (4%)
Pretreatment tracheostomy		
Present	4 (8%)	16 (25%)

From Mendenhall et al 1992 Stage T3 squamous cell carcinoma of the glottic larynx: a comparison of laryngectomy and irradiation. Int J Radiat Oncol Biol Phys 23: 725–732, Table 1, p 726.

required a pretreatment tracheostomy. Of those patients treated surgically, 63 underwent a total laryngectomy and two patients underwent a hemilaryngectomy. Thirty-three surgically treated patients received adjuvant radiation therapy, preoperatively in seven patients and postoperatively in 26 patients. All patients were observed for at least 2 years, and 83% had a minimum follow-up of 5 years. The rates of local–regional control, local–regional control with voice preservation, survival, and severe complications for the two treatment groups are listed in Table 28.12. Local–regional control is evaluated rather than local control because it is sometimes difficult to distinguish a local failure from a nodal recurrence following a total laryngectomy.[1] A severe complication is defined as one that requires surgical intervention or prolonged hospitalization that results in death. The rates of severe complications include those secondary to the initial treatment as well as those following salvage treatment. No patient treated with irradiation alone experienced a fatal complication compared to one of 65 patients managed surgically. Initial local–regional control was higher in the group treated with surgery alone or with adjuvant irradiation. There were no differences in the rates of ultimate local–regional control, survival, cause-specific survival, or severe complications between the two treatment groups. The incidence of local–regional control with voice preservation was significantly higher in patients treated with irradiation alone.

The probabilities of local control versus treatment technique for patients treated with irradiation alone are outlined in Table 28.13. The rate of local control is somewhat better after twice-daily irradiation compared to once-daily irradiation (Fig. 28.1). The relationship between vocal cord mobility assessed at various points in the treatment course and subsequent local control with irradiation alone is depicted in Table 28.14. Persistent vocal cord fixation during or following irradiation does not appear to be associated with a higher likelihood of local recurrence.

Table 28.12 T3 squamous cell carcinoma of the glottic larynx: 5-year results*†

Parameter	Irradiation alone (53 patients)	Surgery ± irradiation (65 patients)	Significance level
Local–regional control	62%	75%	0.10
Ultimate local–regional control	84%	82%	0.95
Local–regional control with voice preservation	63%	6%	<0.01
Absolute survival	55%	45%	0.12
Cause-specific survival	75%	71%	0.26
Severe complications	16%	15%	0.56

*Calculated by the Kaplan–Meier product limit method.
†Of recurrences, 98% were noted within 5 years of treatment.
Data from Mendenhall et al 1992.[28]

Table 28.13 T3 squamous cell carcinoma of the glottic larynx: local control with irradiation alone according to treatment technique (no. controlled/no. treated)

Treatment technique		Local control
Once-daily fractionation		9/17 (53%)*
Continuous-course	8/15 (53%)	
Split-course	1/2	
Twice-daily fractionation		20/28 (71%)*
Total		29/45 (64%)

*P = 0.17.

Excludes six patients who died within 2 years of irradiation with the primary site continuously disease-free, one patient who underwent total laryngectomy at 5 months for suspected local recurrence (laryngectomy specimen negative for tumour), and one patient who underwent a total laryngectomy at 8 months for a chondronecrosis.

From Mendenhall 1992 Stage T3 squamous cell carcinoma of the glottic larynx: a comparison of laryngectomy and irradiation. Int J Radiat Oncol Biol Phys 23: 725–732, Table 3, p 728.

Table 28.14 T3 squamous cell carcinoma of the glottic larynx: local control with irradiation versus vocal cord mobility (no. controlled/no. treated)

Vocal cord mobility assessed	Vocal cord mobility	Local control
At 5000 cGy	Mobile	7/9
	Impaired	5/12 (42%)
	Fixed	15/21 (71%)
	No data	2/3
End of irradiation	Mobile	12/18 (67%)
	Impaired	3/7
	Fixed	13/18 (72%)
	No data	1/2
1 month following radiation therapy	Mobile	14/20 (70%)
	Impaired	4/7
	Fixed	11/18 (61%)

Excludes six patients who died within 2 years of treatment with the primary site continuously disease-free, one patient who underwent a total laryngectomy at 5 months for suspected local recurrence (laryngectomy specimen negative for tumour), and one patient undergoing a total laryngectomy at 8 months for a chondronecrosis.

From Mendenhall et al 1992 Stage T3 squamous cell carcinoma of the glottic larynx: a comparison of laryngectomy and irradiation. Int J Radiat Oncol Biol Phys 23: 725–732, Table 4, p 728.

T4

The results of treatment of T4 vocal cord cancer from four surgical series and two irradiation series are presented in Table 28.15.[11]

Complications

Irradiation alone

During the course of irradiation, patients with T1 or T2 glottic cancers will experience transient worsening of their voices, dry desquamation of the skin within the treatment fields, a mild-to-moderate sore throat, and a sensation of a 'lump' in the throat.

The likelihood of long-term complications for patients with T1 or T2 lesions is low. Five of 305 patients (less than 2%) developed moderate-to-severe treatment complications. The incidence was lower for T1 lesions (one of 184 patients, or less than 1%) than for T2 cancers (four of 120 patients, or 3%). The incidence of complications is also related to total dose of irradiation and the dose per fraction.[29] Two patients developed complications that responded to conservative management: an osteochondronecrosis in one patient and a fat necrosis in the other. Three patients developed severe laryngeal oedema that necessitated a tracheostomy. One of these patients was thought to have a local recurrence and underwent a total laryngectomy, with no tumour found in the specimen. In the other two patients, the tracheostomy was temporary in one patient and permanent in the other.

Patients with T3 or T4 carcinomas of the glottic larynx treated with irradiation alone experience acute effects secondary to treatment that are similar to those observed in patients irradiated for carcinoma of the supraglottic larynx. Late complications include laryngeal oedema that may necessitate a tracheostomy and osteochondronecrosis that may result in a laryngectomy. There is a very remote risk of radiation myelitis.

Three patients treated with irradiation alone for T3 glottic cancer at the University of Florida developed severe complications due to radiotherapy: laryngeal oedema requiring a temporary tracheostomy, laryngeal oedema necessitating a permanent tracheostomy, and laryngeal chondronecrosis requiring total laryngectomy. This last patient required a pretreatment tracheostomy and, following irradiation, underwent multiple deep blind biopsies for a suspected local recurrence prior to developing the chondronecrosis; both the biopsy specimens and the laryngectomy specimen were negative for tumour. Five patients who underwent a salvage procedure for a recurrence after irradiation alone developed a severe complication (one wound dehiscence necessitating a split-thickness skin graft and four pharyngocutaneous fistulae requiring flap reconstruction).

In contrast to patients treated with irradiation alone, patients who developed a severe complication after surgery alone or combined with irradiation at our institution did so after the initial treatment and not after salvage procedures.

Adjuvant irradiation

The complications of adjuvant irradiation are the same as those described for patients with supraglottic larynx cancer.

SUBGLOTTIC LARYNX

Selection of treatment modality

Primary cancer of the subglottic larynx is rare; most patients have dyspnoea and stridor due to locally advanced

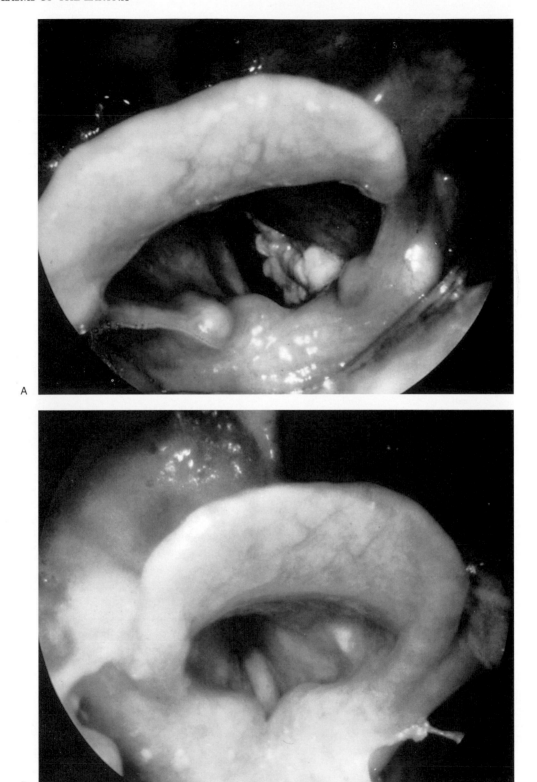

Fig. 28.1 A. A 66-year-old male presented with a 1-year history of hoarseness. Physical examination revealed a bulky lesion involving the entire right true vocal cord with complete fixation of the cord. Direct laryngoscopy revealed involvement of the ventricle; computed tomography demonstrated 8 mm of subglottic extension. Airway was adequate. He was diagnosed as having a T3ON0 squamous cell carcinoma of the right true vocal cord and received 7440 cGy in 62 fractions with twice-daily, continuous-course irradiation. B. The patient has remained disease-free for 4 years 4 months and has not experienced any treatment complications.

Table 28.15 Stage T4 glottic carcinoma: literature review

Author and date of publication	Stage	Number of patients	Method of treatment	Results (no evidence of disease)
Jesse, 1975[12]	T4 N0–N+	48	Laryngectomy	54% at 4 years
Ogura et al, 1975[35]	T4 N0	11	Laryngectomy	45% at 3 years
Skolnick et al 1975[42]	T4 N0	7	Laryngectomy	30% at 5 years
Vermund, 1970[46]	T4 N0	31	Laryngectomy	35% at 5 years
Stewart & Jackson, 1975[43]	T4 N0	13	Irradiation with surgery for salvage	38% at 5 years
Harwood et al 1981[11]	T4 N0	56	Irradiation with surgery for salvage	49% at 5 years*

*Life-table method; uncorrected for deaths due to intercurrent disease.

Modified from Harwood et al 1981 T4N0M0 glottic cancer: an analysis of dose-time volume factors. Int J Radiat Oncol Biol Phys 7: 1507–1512, Table 4, p 1511.

disease. Patients with T1 and T2 lesions have a high probability of cure with irradiation alone and are treated with this modality. Patients with T3 and T4 cancers are usually treated with a total laryngectomy followed by postoperative irradiation. Selected patients with locally advanced lesions are treated with irradiation alone if the cancer is relatively low volume, the patient is medically inoperable, or if the patient refuses surgery. If the patient is a borderline candidate for irradiation alone, irradiation is given and the patient is re-evaluated at 5000 cGy. If there is marked tumour regression, the treatment is continued to high-dose. If not, irradiation is discontinued and a laryngectomy is performed. Because most patients with T3 and T4 cancers require combined modality treatment, little is lost with this approach.

Irradiation technique

The irradiation treatment techniques are as described for carcinoma of the true vocal cord. If it is not possible to cover adequately the inferior extent of the primary tumour with parallel opposed lateral fields, the lateral fields may be angled 5 to 10 degrees inferiorly or, alternatively, a four-field box technique may be employed.[21]

Results

There are limited published data pertaining to the use of irradiation alone for carcinoma of the subglottic larynx. Between 1964 and 1985, six patients were treated with irradiation alone with curative intent at the University of Florida.[9] Local control was obtained with irradiation in four of six patients: TisN0, one of one; T2N0, one of two; and T4N0, two of three. One patient is alive and disease-free 4 years following treatment. Three patients died disease-free due to intercurrent illness at 3.5 years, 4 years, and 5 years following irradiation.

Two patients who developed a local recurrence after radiotherapy underwent a salvage total laryngectomy. One died of lung cancer 3 years after salvage surgery and the other died due to a stomal recurrence 15 months after salvage laryngectomy.

Complications

The complications associated with treatment of carcinoma of the subglottic larynx are the same as those described for the glottic larynx. Of the six patients treated at the University of Florida, one patient required a temporary tracheostomy during irradiation due to laryngeal oedema and airway compromise.[9] No other significant complications were observed.

REFERENCES

1. Amdur R J, Parsons J T, Mendenhall W M, Million R R, Stringer S P, Cassisi N J 1989 Postoperative irradiation for squamous cell carcinoma of the head and neck: an analysis of treatment results and complications. Int J Radiat Oncol Biol Phys 16: 25–36
2. American Joint Committee on Cancer 1983 Manual for staging of cancer, 2nd edn. Lippincott, Philadelphia
3. Biller H F, Lawson W 1986 Partial laryngectomy for vocal cord cancer with marked limitation or fixation of the vocal cord. Laryngoscope 96: 61–64
4. DeSanto L W 1984 T3 glottic cancer: options and consequences of the options. Laryngoscope 94: 1311–1315
5. Fletcher G H, Goepfert H 1980 Larynx and pyriform sinus. In: Fletcher G H (ed) Textbook of radiotherapy, 3rd edn. Lea & Febiger, Philadelphia, pp 330–363
6. Freeman D E, Mancuso A A, Parsons J T, Mendenhall W M, Million R R 1990 Irradiation alone for supraglottic larynx

carcinoma: can CT findings predict treatment results? Int J Radiat Oncol Biol Phys 19: 485–490
7. Gall A M, Sessions D G, Ogura J H 1977 Complications following surgery for cancer of the larynx and hypopharynx. Cancer 39: 624–631
8. Goepfert H, Jesse R H, Fletcher G H, Hamberger A 1975 Optimal treatment for the technically resectable squamous cell carcinoma of the supraglottic larynx. Laryngoscope 85: 14–32
9. Guedea F, Parsons J T, Mendenhall W M, Million R R, Stringer S P, Cassisi N J 1992 Primary subglottic cancer: results of radical radiation therapy. Int J Radiat Oncol Biol Phys 21: 1607–1611
10. Haraf D J, Weichselbaum R R 1988 Treatment selection in T1 and T2 vocal cord carcinoma. Oncology 2: 41–47
11. Harwood A R, Beale F A, Cummings B J, Keane T J, Payne D, Rider W D 1981 T4N0M0 glottic cancer: An analysis of dose–time volume factors. Int J Radiat Oncol Biol Phys 7: 1507–1512

12. Jesse R H 1975 The evaluation of treatment of patients with extensive squamous cancer of the vocal cords. Laryngoscope 85: 1424–1429
13. Kessler D J, Trapp T K, Calcaterra T C 1987 The treatment of T3 glottic carcinoma with vertical partial laryngectomy. Arch Otolaryngol Head Neck Surg 113: 1196–1199
14. Kogelnick H D, Fletcher G H, Jesse R H 1975 Clinical course of patients with squamous cell carcinoma of the upper respiratory and digestive tracts with no evidence of disease 5 years after initial treatment. Radiology 115: 423–427
15. Lee N K, Goepfert H, Wendt C D 1990 Supraglottic laryngectomy for intermediate stage cancer: UTMD Anderson Cancer Center experience with combined therapy. Laryngoscope 100: 831–836
16. Mendenhall W M, Million R R 1986 Elective neck irradiation for squamous cell carcinoma of the head and neck: analysis of time–dose factors and causes of failure. Int J Radiat Oncol Biol Phys 12: 741–746
17. Mendenhall W M, Million R R, Bova F J 1984 Analysis of time–dose factors in clinically positive neck nodes treated with irradiation alone in squamous cell carcinoma of the head and neck. Int J Radiat Oncol Biol Phys 19: 639–643
18. Mendenhall W M, Million R R, Cassisi N J 1980 Elective neck irradiation in squamous cell carcinoma of the head and neck. Head Neck Surg 3: 15–20
19. Mendenhall W M, Million R R, Cassisi N J 1984 Squamous cell carcinoma of the supraglottic larynx treated with radical irradiation: analysis of treatment parameters and results. Int J Radiat Oncol Biol Phys 10: 2223–2230
20. Mendenhall W M, Million R R, Cassisi N J 1986 Squamous cell carcinoma of the head and neck treated with radiation therapy: the role of neck dissection for clinically positive neck nodes. Int J Radiat Oncol Biol Phys 12: 733–740
21. Mendenhall W M, Million R R, Sharkey D E, Cassisi N J 1984 Stage T3 squamous cell carcinoma of the glottic larynx treated with surgery and/or radiation therapy. Int J Radiat Oncol Biol Phys 10: 357–363
22. Mendenhall W M, Parsons, J T, Brant T A, Stringer S P, Cassisi N J, Million R R 1989 Is elective neck treatment indicated for T2N0 squamous cell carcinoma of the glottic larynx? Radiother Oncol 14: 199–202
23. Mendenhall W M, Parsons J T, Cassisi N J, Stringer S P 1990 The role of hemilaryngectomy in the management of T1 vocal cord cancer. Arch Otolaryngol Head Neck Surg 116: 107–108
24. Mendenhall W M, Parsons J T, Million R R 1988 Elective lower neck irradiation: 5000 cGy in 25 fractions versus 4050 cGy in 15 fractions. Int J Radiat Oncol Biol Phys 15: 439–440
25. Mendenhall W M, Parsons J T, Million R R, Cassisi N J 1988 The article reviewed (commentary). Oncology 2: 59–61
26. Mendenhall W M, Parsons J T, Million R R, Cassisi N J, Devine J W, Greene B D 1984 A favorable subset of AJCC stage IV squamous cell carcinoma of the head and neck. Int J Radiat Oncol Biol Phys 10: 1841–1843
27. Mendenhall W M, Parsons J T, Million R R, Fletcher G H 1988 T1-T2 squamous cell carcinoma of the glottic larynx treated with radiation therapy: relationship of dose-fractionation factors to local control and complications. Int J Radiat Oncol Biol Phys 15: 1267–1273
28. Mendenhall W M, Parsons J T, Stringer S P, Cassisi N J, Million R R 1992 Stage T3 squamous cell carcinoma of the glottic larynx: a comparison of laryngectomy and irradiation. Int J Radiat Oncol Biol Phys 23: 725–732
29. Mendenhall W M, Parsons J T, Stringer S P, Cassisi N J, Million R R 1988 T1–T2 vocal cord carcinoma: a basis for comparing the results of radiotherapy and surgery. Head Neck Surg 10: 373–377
30. Mendenhall W M, Parsons J T, Stringer S P, Cassisi N J, Million R R 1990 Carcinoma of the supraglottic larynx: a basis for comparing the results of radiotherapy and surgery. Head Neck 12: 204–209
31. Million R R, Cassisi N J. Larynx 1984 In: Million R R, Cassisi N J (eds) Management of head and neck cancer: a multidisciplinary approach. Lippincott, Philadelphia, pp 315–364
32. Million R R, Cassisi N J, Parsons J T, Mendenhall W M 1988 Radiation therapy in the management of carcinoma of the larynx. In: Fried M P (ed) The larynx: a multidisciplinary approach. Brown, Boston, pp 557–589
33. Mittal B, Rao D V, Marks J E, Ogura J H 1983 Comparative cost analysis of hemilaryngectomy and irradiation for early glottic carcinoma. Int J Radiat Oncol Biol Phys 9: 407–408
34. Neel H B III, Devine K D, DeSanto L W 1980 Laryngofissure and cordectomy for early cordal carcinoma: outcome in 182 patients. Otolaryngol Head Neck Surg 88: 79–84
35. Ogura J H, Sessions D G, Spector G J 1975 Analysis of surgical therapy for epidermoid carcinoma of the laryngeal glottis. Laryngoscope 85: 1522–1530
36. Parker R G, Enstrom J E 1988 Second primary cancers of the head and neck following treatment of initial primary head and neck cancers. Int J Radiat Oncol Biol Phys 14: 561–564
37. Parsons J T, Mendenhall W M, Cassisi N J, Isaacs J H Jr, Million R R 1988 Hyperfractionation for head and neck cancer. Int J Radiat Oncol Biol Phys 14: 649–658
38. Parsons J T, Mendenhall W M, Mancuso A A, Cassisi N J, Stringer S P, Million R R 1989 Twice-a-day radiotherapy for T3 squamous cell carcinoma of the glottic larynx. Head Neck 11: 123–128
39. Robbins K T, Davidson W, Peters L J, Goepfert H 1988 Conservation surgery for T2 and T3 carcinomas of the supraglottic larynx. Arch Otolaryngol Head Neck Surg 114: 421–426
40. Seydel H G 1975 The risk of tumor induction in man following medical irradiation for malignant neoplasm. Cancer 35: 1641–1645
41. Sigal M C, Million R R 1984 Cost of management in head and neck cancer. In: Million R R, Cassisi N J (eds) Management of head and neck cancer: a multidisciplinary approach. Lippincott, Philadelphia, pp 647–649
42. Skolnick E M, Yee K F, Wheatley M A, Martin L O 1975 Carcinoma of the laryngeal glottis: therapy and end results. Laryngoscope 85: 1453–1466
43 Stewart J H, Jackson A W 1975 The steepness of the dose response curve both for tumor curve and normal tissue injury. Laryngoscope 85: 1107–1111
44 Tucker H M, Benninger M S, Roberts J K, Wood B G, Levine H L 1989 Near-total laryngectomy with epiglottic reconstruction. Arch Otolaryngol Head Neck Surg 115: 1341–1344
45 Urken M L, Biller H F 1988 Management of early vocal cord carcinoma. Oncology 2: 48–59
46 Vermund H 1970 Role of radiotherapy in cancer of the larynx as related to the TNM system of staging: a review. Cancer 25: 485–504
47 Wang Z H, Million R R, Mendenhall W M, Parsons J T, Cassisi N J 1989 Treatment with preoperative irradiation and surgery of squamous cell carcinoma of the head and neck. Cancer 64: 32–38
48. Weems D H, Mendenhall W M, Parsons J T, Cassisi N J, Million R R 1987 Squamous cell carcinoma of the supraglottic larynx treated with surgery and/or radiation therapy. Int J Radiat Oncol Biol Phys 13: 1483–1487

29. Chemotherapy

P. M. Stell

INTRODUCTION

Chemotherapy may be used for the treatment of laryngeal cancer in one of several ways:

1. Adjuvant chemotherapy: The chemotherapy may be used in one or more ways:
   a. Induction chemotherapy is used to reduce the bulk of the tumour before administration of radiotherapy or surgery. If the patient has not previously received chemotherapy (so called 'chemotherapy naive') the treatment is called neoadjuvant.
   b. Concomitant (syn concurrent, synchronous) chemotherapy is given during a course of radiotherapy.
   c. Maintenance chemotherapy is given at intervals after radiotherapy or surgery.
2. Palliative chemotherapy for end-stage disease, that is, where the disease is so advanced as to be not suitable for radiotherapy or surgery, or where recurrence after prior radiotherapy or surgery is no longer suitable for these methods.
3. For organ preservation. It is thought that a tumour that responds to chemotherapy is likely to respond to radiotherapy, so that a patient with an advanced laryngeal cancer may be spared a total laryngectomy.

Before proceeding further it is necessary to define various terms. A *partial response* is a reduction by more than 50% in the product of two diameters at right-angles to each other. A *complete response* indicates complete disappearance of visible tumour.

Trials for the assessment of chemotherapy are of three types:

Phase I. Patients, usually with end-stage disease, are treated with increasing doses to assess toxicity, and to fix a suitable dose.
Phase II. A group of patients, usually about 20–30 in number, is treated to assess how many respond. There is usually no control arm in such a series.
Phase III. Many patients—usually several hundred—are divided randomly between two or more arms to allow comparison with established drugs, or no treatment at all. The end point is survival.

ADJUVANT CHEMOTHERAPY: SQUAMOUS CARCINOMA

No trial of adjuvant chemotherapy has concentrated solely on laryngeal squamous carcinoma. Therefore we must rely on trials of head and neck cancer in general and attempt to draw conclusions from these about laryngeal cancer.

The present review is based on all the trials of adjuvant chemotherapy in squamous carcinoma of the head and neck published in the English language to 1991. Several trials were excluded from the analysis for the following reasons: firstly, several well-designed studies did not report the survival rate;[3,17,31,48] secondly, one study was not randomized, as the control arm consisted of those rejected for radical treatment;[30] thirdly, one trial did not include an arm receiving conventional treatment only.[52] This left 21 randomized controlled trials that contained patients with laryngeal cancer and that quoted survival data.[4,14,15,21–24,27,28,34,36,41,47,51,53,54,56–58,60,63]

The data for dosage, timing of chemotherapy, site, stage and local treatment of the tumour are given in Tables 29.1–29.3 Seven regimens were based on cisplatinum alone or in combination, four on methotrexate and ten on miscellaneous regimens. These trials are analysed from the point of view of design of the trial, response rates, and survival.

Design of the trial

Power of the trial

The minimal difference in survival which each trial would be likely to detect was calculated from the formula given by George.[19] It is based on the number of patients in each trial, on the survival rate of the control arm, and on an assumption of a type I error of 5%, and a type II error of

Table 29.1 Patients' details: cisplatinum-based regimens

Reference	Tumour site	Tumour stage	Type of chemotherapy	Local treatment	Dose
4	M,O,H,L	III–IV	Induction	DXRT/Surg	Cisplatinum 20 mg/m^2 d 2–4 Bleomycin 12.5 mg/m^2 d 1–4 Vindesine d 1 MTX 10 g/m^2 i.v. d 2
14	M,A,N,O,L H,U, ear	III–IV	Induction/main	Surg/DXRT	Cisplatinum 20 g/m^2 d 1–5 Bleomycin 10 u/m^2 d 3–7 i.v. Methotrexate 200 mg/m^2 d 15, 22, 29, 36
23	M,O,H,L	III–IV	Induction/main	Surg + DXRT	Cisplatinum 100 g/m^2 d1 Bleomycin 15 g/m^2 d 3–7
36	M,O,H,L	I–IV	Induction	Surg/DXRT	Cisplatinum 100 mg/m^3 5-FU 1 g/m^2 120 h
41	M,O,N,H,L	III–IV	Synchronous/main	DXRT	Cisplatinum 20 mg/m^2 i.v. d. 1,2,3 Bleomycin 10 g/m^2 d1,3,5,7
51	M,O,H,L	III–IV	Induction	Surg + DXRT	Cisplatinum 50 mg/m^2 i.v. d 1 MTX 40 mg/m^2 i.v./d 1 Bleomycin 15 u/m^2 i.v. d 1,8 Vincristine 2 mg i.v. d 1
58	M,O,N,A,G,H	III–IV	Induction	DXRT/Surg	Cisplatinum 100 g/m^2 5-FU 500 g/m^2 1–5 d

Key: M = oral cavity; A = nose and sinuses; N = nasopharynx; O = oropharynx; H = hypopharynx; L = larynx; U = unknown parity; DXRT = deep X-ray therapy; MTX = methotrexate; SURG = surgery; MAIN = maintenance.

Table 29.2 Patients' details: methotrexate-based regimens

Reference	Tumour site*	Tumour stage	Type of chemotherapy	Local treatment	Dose
15	M,A,N,O,H,L,	III–IV	Induction	DXRT	25 mg i.v. d 3,6,9,12,15
22	M,O,H,N,A	III–IV	Synchronous	DXRT	100 mg/m^2 i.v. d 0 & 14
34	A,M,N,O,H,L,U	III–IV	Induction	DXRT	Escalated to 240 mg/m^2 d 1–5
47	M,O,H,L	III–IV	Induction/main	Surgery/main	40 g/m2 DXRT escalated to 80 mg/m^2 weekly × 16

*See key to Table 29.1.

20%, these being commonly regarded as the minimal acceptable values for these parameters.

The minimal difference in survival which could be detected by each trial ranged from 11 to 51% with a median of 25%. It can be assumed that any new form of treatment that produced an improvement in survival as great as 25% would be adopted rapidly, without the necessity for a trial. No trial was large enough to detect the likely increase in survival of 5–10%.

Randomization

All the trials reviewed were randomized, but many did not describe the randomization process: it may be that some used systems, such as randomizing by the date of birth, which allow the clinician to know beforehand the treatment arm to which a patient would be allocated.

Exclusion of eligible patients

Only four trials adhered to the policy of 'intention to treat',[22,54,56,60] that is, all eligible patients were randomized and included in the analysis, whether treated or not.

Only five authors[14,18,24,49,58] gave details of how many eligible patients had been excluded. These latter five trials contained a total of 648 patients; 134 (20.7%) of eligible patients were excluded before randomization.

Eight reports excluded some treated patients from the final analysis.[15,18,23,27,36,53,55,63] One hundred and thirty-eight patients were excluded from the analysis out of a total of 1849 patients in these eight trials (7.5%).

Thus, 20% of eligible patients were excluded before randomization, only about a quarter of these trials adhered to the policy of 'intention to treat', and furthermore, 7.5% of treated patients were excluded from analysis. These exclusions are an enormous source of bias because it is highly likely that excluded patients do badly. A further source of bias of any review of published trials is the fact that small trials and negative trials are unlikely to be reported (publication bias). It has been shown that positive trials are 2.5 times as likely to be reported as negative trials.[11]

Response rates

These apply only to induction trials. The response rates are summarized where they have been reported, and the survival in these trials analysed.

Table 29.3 Patient's details: miscellaneous regimens

Reference	Reference tumour site*	Tumour stage	Type of chemotherapy	Local treatment	Agent and dose
18	M,N,O,H,L	III–IV	Synchronous/main	DXRT DXRT	Bleomycin 5 u i.v. 2/wk during Bleomycin 15 u i.v. weekly × 16 main MTX 25 mg/m² i.v. weekly × 16 main
21	M,O,N,H,L,U	II–IV	Synchronous	DXRT	5-FU i.v. 10 mg/kg/daily days 1–3, then 5 mg/kg 3 times weekly
24	M,A,L,H,N,O	III–IV	Induction/main	DXRT/surg	Bleomycin 10 units/t.d.s. d 1–4 Cytotoxan 200 mg/m² d 1–5 Methotrexate 30 g/m² d 1 and 5 5-FU 400 mg/m² d 1–5
27	M,O,L,N,A,U	I–IV	Synchronous	DXRT	Hydroxyurea 60 mg/kg/3 times weekly
53	M,O,L,N,A,H		Synchronous	DXRT	Hydroxyurea 80 mg/kg orally twice weekly
54	M,L,O,N,H	III–IV	Induction/main	DXRT	Vincristine 1.5 mg/m² i.v. 0 h Methotrexate 75 g/m² 12 h Methotrexate 75 g/m² i.v. 15 h }I Bleomycin 60 mg i.v. 15 h Methotrexate 75 g/m² i.v. 18 h 5-FU 350 mg/m² i.v. 18 h Hydroxyurea 3 g/m² 0 h }II 6MP 150 g/m² orally 6 h Cyclophos 500 mg/m² i.v. 12 h
56	L,H,O,M,N, ear	III–IV	Induction/main	DXRT	Vinblastine 6 mg/m² 0 h Bleomycin 15 mg i.m. 8 h Methotrexate 40 mg/m² 24 h Cyclophos 400 mg/m² 24 h 5-FU 5 mg/kg 24 h
57	M,L,O,N,H	III–IV	Induction/main	DXRT + surg	Induction: Methotrexate 60 mg/m² 6-hourly d 1,5,9 Maintenance: Cisplatinum 40 mg/m² } 3 weeks × 4 Adriamycin 40 mg/m²
60	M,O,N,H,L,A	II–IV	Synchronous	DXRT	Bleomycin total dose 100 mg. i.v.
63	M,L,O,H,N	II–IV	Synchronous	DXRT	Mitomycin C 15 mg/m² i.v. d 5

*See key to Table 29.1.

Response rates using WHO criteria were quoted in only four of the induction studies. The results (Table 29.4) show a response rate of 47%, but the death rate was 4% *higher* in the treated patients, although this change was not significant.

Meta-analysis of survival

The appropriate data for survival were extracted from the papers quoted and were subject to meta-analysis.[45] The mathematical basis of this technique is described elsewhere.[55]

The basic principle of meta-analysis is that, for each series, the number of deaths is noted in each arm at a fixed point—usually 2 years. The number of expected deaths (E) is then calculated and is subtracted from the number of deaths observed (O). The resulting figure (O–E) will be negative if the number of deaths is reduced in the treated arm, and vice versa. If the sign for most or all of the (O–E)s is the same, this usually indicates a definite trend in favour of one arm, whereas if some are negative and some are positive it is likely that treatment is ineffective. The individual (O–E)s are summed and divided by the square root of their variances, and the result referred to tables of the normal distribution.

The death rate was 815/1443 (56.5%) in the control arms, and 893/1588 (56.2%) in the treated arms, a decrease in survival of 0.3% in the chemotherapy arms. In nine trials the death rate was higher in the treated arm, and in 12 it was lower. Meta-analysis showed that the sum of (O–E) over all trials was + 16.96 and that its variance was 175.35. This difference is not significant ($z = 1.28$).

A sub-group analysis was carried out for the different agents, irrespective of whether they were used for induction, maintenance etc. (Tables 29.5–29.8). The death rate was higher in the treated arm in four of seven

Table 29.4 Response rates and survival

Reference	Response rate	Deaths	
		Control arm	Treated arm
4	24/48	31/52	32/48
23	104/282	67/152	62/140
36	25/37	18/36	14/37
51	56/75	34/76	49/82
Total	209/442 (47%)	150/316 (47%)	157/307 (51%)

Table 29.5   Meta-analysis: cisplatinum regimens

Reference	Deaths Control arm	Chemotherapy arm	O–E	Variance	Z	P
4	31/52	32/48	+1.76	5.82	0.73	NS
14	8/20	3/26	−3.22	2.10	−1.89	NS
23	67/152	Induction 62/140	+0.15	18.03	0.04	NS
		Induction/main 59/151	−3.79	18.46	−0.88	NS
36	18/36	14/37	+2.85	3.90	1.44	NS
41	13/13	15/23	−2.89	1.48	−2.38	<0.025
51	35/76	51/82	+6.37	9.85	2.03	<0.05
59	13/33	17/30	+2.71	3.98	1.37	NS
Total	185/382 (48%)	249/537 (46%)	+3.94	63.62	0.49	NS

Table 29.6   Meta-analysis: methotrexate regimens

Reference	Deaths Control arm	Chemotherapy arm	O–E	Variance	Z	P
15	213/326	209/312	+2.63	35.76	0.44	NS
22	87/156	75/157	−6.26	19.60	−1.42	NS
34	44/48	45/48	+0.50	1.64	0.39	NS
47	9/27	8/28	−0.65	2.99	−0.38	NS
Total	353/557 (63%)	337/545 (62%)	−3.78	59.99	0.49	NS

Table 29.7   Meta-analysis: VBM (vincristine–bleomycin–methotrexate) regimens

Reference	Deaths Control arm	Treated arm	O–E	Variance	Z	P
54	22/48	30/37	+ 7.36	5.02	3.28	<0.005
56	2/35	10/33	+ 4.18	2.51	2.66	<0.01
Total	24/83 (29%)	40/70 (57%)	+11.54	7.53	4.21	<0.001
Bleomycin regimens						
18	34/52	26/52	−4.0	6.41	−1.58	N.S.
60	40/111	48/111	+4.0	13.34	1.10	N.S.
Total	74/163 (45%)	74/163 (45%)	0.0	19.75	0.00	N.S.
5-FU Regimen						
21	19/25 (76%)	21/34 (62%)	−1.41	1.87	−1.03	N.S.

Table 29.8 Meta-analysis: miscellaneous regimens

Reference	Deaths Control arm	Chemotherapy arm	O–E	Variance	Z	P
24	27/40	31/43	+0.95	4.41	0.46	NS
27	12/16	17/24	−0.4	1.96	0.28	NS
53	63/75	70/75	+4.00	3.99	2.01	NS
57	25/41	26/41	+0.50	4.88	0.23	NS
63	33/61	28/56	−1.20	7.35	0.44	NS
Total	160/233 (69%)	172/239 (72%)	+3.85	22.59	0.81	NS

cisplatinum studies, in two of four methotrexate studies, in one of two bleomycin studies, and in three of six studies with miscellaneous agents. However, this *decreased* survival was not significant. Finally, the death rate in the treated arm in two studies based on VBM was significantly *elevated* (Tables 29.5–29.8).

There were seven induction studies; the death rate in the treated arm was higher than that in the control arm in *each* of the studies, and meta-analysis showed that this difference was almost significant ((O–E) = 16.97, variance = 78.98, P = 0.056). The death rate in the treated arm was higher than that in the control arm in three of six synchronous trials ((O–E) = +1.55, variance = 48.11) and in four of seven induction plus maintenance studies ((O–E) = –1.56, variance = 48.26) but these differences were not significant.

In two synchronous/maintenance studies the treated patients fared better, and this result was significant ((O–E) = –6.89, variance = 7.89, P <0.001).

As regards site, a separate analysis for laryngeal tumours was possible in three trials only.[15,22,29] The death rate in the control arm was 56/115 (49%) and in the treated arm was 63/166 (38%). However, a meta-analysis showed no significant benefit.

Finally, subgroup analysis of the number of agents (irrespective of agent and timing of use) showed that the death rate was worse in six of nine studies in the treated arm of single agents ((O–E) = +4.03, variance = 88.50), and in eight of 12 trials using multiple agents ((O–E) = +12.93, variance = 86.85). Neither of these outcomes was significant.

Site of failure

The concept is gaining ground that adjuvant chemotherapy might be useful in reducing the proportion of patients who require salvage surgery for failed radiotherapy. Also, some believe that it might increase the rate of distant metastases,[60] and some believe that it might reduce it.[51] Therefore, data for site of failure were extracted when they were available.

Data about the site of failure were given in ten papers. The failure rate from locoregional recurrence was reduced in five of the ten studies, being 4% less in the treated groups, but this difference was not significant. The failure rate for distant metastases was lower in seven of eight studies, being 1% lower overall, but this, too, was not significant (Tables 29.9 and 29.10).

Table 29.9   Locoregional failure

Reference	Control arm	Treated arm	(O–E)	Variance	Z	P
4	24/52	24/48	+0.96	6.23	0.38	NS
15	75/173	69/164	–1.08	20.66	–0.24	NS
22	72/156	53/156	–9.50	18.79	–2.19	<0.05
23	36/144	35/135)				
		31/132)	–0.26	17.50	–0.06	NS
24	16/39	24/38	+4.26		4.87	1.93
				NS		
27	10/16	15/24	0.00	2.31	0.00	NS
34	33/48	37/48	+2.00	4.79	0.91	NS
36	12/36	10/37	–1.15	3.9	0.58	NS
58	10/33	12/27	+2.10	3.51	1.12	NS
60	70/111	61/111	–4.5	13.48	–1.22	NS
Total	358/808(44%)	371/920(40%)	–7.17	96.04	0.73	NS

Table 29.10   Distant metastases

Reference	Control arm	Treated arm	(O–E)	Variance	Z	P
4	10/52	6/48	–1.68	3.39	0.91	NS
15	27/173	16/164	–4.93	9.40	–1.61	NS
23	27/144	26/135)	–4.23	12.49	–1.20	NS
		12/132)				
24	5/39	1/38	–1.96	1.40	–1.66	NS
34	11/48	6/48	–2.50	3.53	–1.33	NS
36	4/36	2/37	–1.04	1.4	0.88	NS
58	2/33	1/27	–0.35	0.72	–0.41	NS
60	13/111	26/111	+6.50	8.07	2.29	<0.025
Total	99/636(16%)	96/620(15%)	–10.19	40.4	1.60	NS

Toxicity

Toxicity was reported fully and graded in only four papers.[14,18,23,51] Only one paper[51] used the scheme recommended by the WHO.[39]

Deaths from toxicity were mentioned in 11 series.[14,15,18,24,34,36,41,51,54,56,63] One of these did not record the number of deaths due to toxicity, but stated that serious complications, including death, occurred in 'less than 10% of all patients'.[34] In ten reports, the total mortality from chemotherapy was 37/701, that is 5%. The death rate in these ten trials totalled 400/695 (58%) in the control arm, and 422/701 (60%) in the treated arm. Thus, in these ten trials the death rate was 2% *higher* in the treated arms, to which must be added a further 5% increase in deaths due to toxicity, making a total *reduction* in survival of 7%. Seven of these ten trials were of induction chemotherapy, and three were of synchronous chemotherapy.

Most of the trials relied on analysis of cancer deaths rather than total mortality. Although chemotherapy does not affect the rate of intercurrent deaths, or the survival of patients lost to follow-up, calculation should nonetheless be based on total mortality because deaths from toxicity may be counted as intercurrent deaths, thus giving a false sense of the overall picture.

ADJUVANT CHEMOTHERAPY: NON-SQUAMOUS CARCINOMA

Three papers have recently claimed increased survival from the combination of chemotherapy with radiotherapy for small cell carcinoma of the larynx. Giddings et al reported four cases of their own and 49 from the literature.[20] Three of six patients treated by combined therapy in Ferlito's series were alive more than 6 years later.[16] Aguilar et al achieved a 2-year survival of 52%.[1]

PALLIATIVE CHEMOTHERAPY

Many phase II studies of chemotherapy for end-stage head and neck cancer have been published. Patients with end-stage disease may have disease that is too extensive at first presentation for radiotherapy or surgery, or they may have recurrent or grossly persistent disease, due to failure of surgery and/or radiotherapy with curative intent. The end-point in most of these studies has been response of the tumour, and few studies had a control arm. In contrast, few controlled (phase III) trials have been published in which survival of the patient is the end-point.

Phase II trials

No single published trial has been devoted entirely to chemotherapy for patients with end-stage laryngeal cancer. However, there have been several excellent reviews, and much of the following is based on that of Al-Sarraf.[2]

Overall disease status

In assessing the results of chemotherapy—response type, rate, duration, and survival—of patients with end-stage head and neck cancer, it is important to consider the extent of the disease as this may influence outcome (Table 29.13).

Patients with minimal disease respond better to chemotherapy, their chance of complete response (CR) is higher, and long-term palliation is possible. In randomized trials, differences between therapeutic regimens may not be observed if all patients are lumped together regardless of tumour burden.

Other aspects of disease status that may influence the effectiveness of chemotherapy include systemic disease, response to previous chemotherapy and the site of disease. Direct bone erosion due to cancer is very difficult to eradicate with local radiation therapy or with systemic chemotherapy. Patients with systemic bone metastases with hypercalcaemia, or with lymphangitic spread, especially in the skin, respond poorly to chemotherapy.

Other diseases

Patients with head and neck cancer may have additional problems (Table 29.11). Many have a long history of abuse of tobacco and alcohol. These factors can influence the quality of life and survival, they may require active supportive care, and need to be taken into account in evaluating the results of chemotherapy.

Prognostic factors

The most important prognostic factor that affects both response to chemotherapy, and the survival of these patients is the performance status. Patients with only loco-regional recurrence have a better response to chemo-

Table 29.11 Recurrent and/or systemic disease: associated disorders (from Al-Sarraf)[2]

Second primary cancer
Medical disorders
Nutritional problems
Hypercalcaemia
Meningeal invasion
Infections
    local
        aspiration pneumonia
        systemic
Local pain
Bleeding
    arterial
    venous
    capillary

therapy than those with systemic and visceral metastases. Patients with bulky disease, bone invasion (with or without hypercalcaemia), extensive skin invasion by lymphangitic spread or persistent disease after radiotherapy, respond poorly to chemotherapy, and survival is short. Patients who fail first-line chemotherapy for recurrent and/or disseminated head and neck cancer seldom respond to a second agent or combination. This is a practical problem in evaluating the effectiveness of new agent(s) which are usually tested in previously treated patients.

These prognostic factors must be allowed for, either by stratification or by using multivariate analysis of survival.

Chemotherapeutic agents

Many single agents and combination regimens have been identified as active in patients with recurrent and metastatic squamous cell carcinoma of the head and neck. The questions which need to be addressed in relation to the use of these agents include the comparative activity of the agent(s), their optimal dose, the frequency of administration, and the duration of therapy once the maximal response has been reached. The most important type of response is complete response, especially when confirmed by biopsy. Once histologically confirmed complete remission is achieved, the next question is the optimal duration of therapy to achieve cure or the longest palliation possible.

Only complete response (CR) is of any value, especially if it is confirmed histologically.

The achievement of partial response (PR) helps to identify effective drug(s), but PR does not influence the survival of patients with recurrent head and neck cancer. Unfortunately at present most patients treated with chemotherapy do not achieve complete response. Median survival is not expected to improve unless we have substantial improvement in the CR rate.

Randomized trials between agents with similar response rates and low complete response rates, are unlikely to identify meaningful advantages in survival.

Results of chemotherapeutic trials

Many single agents have been investigated, the four most active being cisplatin, methotrexate, 5-fluorouracil (FU) and bleomycin. Varying doses and schedules of administration, and many prognostic factors, can influence the outcome and make it difficult to compare the results from different reports in the literature.

The overall response rate to each of these four agents ranged from 15 to 30%, especially when used as first-line therapy for recurrent head and neck cancer (Table 29.19). Most of these responses are partial, with a median duration of 3 to 5 months; the chance of improving the

survival of these patients is very small. When these agents are used as second-line chemotherapy, the overall response rate is less than 10% and of short duration.

A wide range of combination chemotherapy regimens has been used, and the response rates seem to be higher than those for single-agent chemotherapy (Table 29.13) The complete response rate to combination chemotherapy is about 10% higher than for single agents, but sadly the duration of response and survival are not improved. The drug-induced toxicities seem to be higher than those of single-agent therapy.

Several prospective randomized phase II trials have been conducted. These trials compared single agents, especially methotrexate, with each other, or with combination chemotherapy, or compared two different combinations. All except two randomized trials have been negative. The CR rate seems to be higher with combinations than for single agents, but this difference was not statistically significant.

One trial, which compared methotrexate with the combination of methotrexate, bleomycin and cisplatin, showed a significant difference in the response rates from 35 to 48%. More importantly, the frequency of CR to the combination was higher (13 of 80) than to methotrexate alone (7 of 83). However, no significant differences were found in the duration of response or in the survival between the two groups.[62]

The use of cisplatin and a 96-hour infusion of 5-fluorouracil (5-FU) every 3 weeks achieves an overall response rate of 70% (21 of 30) and, more importantly, a CR rate of 27% (8 of 30).[33] This led to a randomized trial comparing the cisplatin and 5-FU infusion with the same dose of cisplatin and 5-FU as an intravenous (IV) bolus on days one and eight every three weeks. Patients were stratified to the following prognostic factors: performance status, previous chemotherapy (as adjuvant or

Table 29.12 Overall response rate to most commonly used single agents in recurrent cancer (from Al-Sarraf)[2]

Agents	Number of evaluable patients	Overall response (%)
Methotrexate	988	31
Bleomycin	347	21
Cisplatin	288	28
Fluorouracil	118	15

Table 29.13 Chemotherapy for recurrent head and neck cancer (from Al-Sarraf)[2]

Combination	Number of evaluable patients	Overall response (%)
Cisplatin[*]	577	43
Cytoxan	313	44
Nitrosourea	223	36
Mitomycin C	81	57
Other	282	48

[*]Other than 5-FU and cisplatin.

treatment for recurrent disease), prior radiation, previous surgery and the site of recurrent disease (systemic versus locoregional).

There were statistically significant differences in the response rate in favour of the infusion group (72%) versus the bolus group (20%). The CR rate was higher for the infusion (22%) than for the bolus arm (10%). All patients with complete response were alive at 2 years.

Although it is widely accepted that cisplatinum plus 5-FU is superior to cisplatinum alone, this view is based largely on trials where response was the end-point. When *survival* was the end-point, no difference was found in two trials.[6,9]

When 5-FU and cisplatin are used as second-line therapy the results are much worse: a 6% response rate in one series for example.[38]

The search for new agents for patients with head and neck squamous cell cancer has been very active since the mid 1970s, but unfortunately, the response rate to most of these agents is poor. The one promising new agent that needs further evaluation in combination with other agent(s) is the platinum analogue CBDCA (carboplatin). It is less nephrotoxic than cisplatin, but the results are similar. A recent report[42] of 59 patients with end-stage disease showed 4 (8%) complete responders and 12 (24%) partial responders. The median survival for all patients was 4.8 months—not vastly different from 3 months with no treatment, and less than 8.5 months achieved with cisplatinum.

Phase III trials

All the above rests on conclusions from phase II trials. Phase III trials concentrating on survival, and with an untreated arm, have been sparse. The current author has carried out two phase III trials of patients with end-stage disease, but is not aware that others have carried out such trials in this disease. One of the many important differences between a phase II study and a properly conducted phase III trial is that the latter emphasizes the number of patients unsuitable for treatment. In a phase II trial unsuitable patients are not included or reported, whereas a phase III trial conforming to 'intention to treat' shows that large numbers of these patients are unsuitable.

Our first phase III trial was a 2×2 factorial design of cisplatinum and bleomycin in 116 patients with recurrent or advanced squamous cell carcinoma of the head and neck. Patients were randomized to no chemotherapy, cisplatinum alone, bleomycin alone, or cisplatinum plus bleomycin.

Some 30% of patients proved to be unfit for chemotherapy, and, of those treated, progression of tumour was the commonest 'response'. However, 25% of patients achieved a partial or complete response, with no significant difference in response rates between the treated arms. Bleomycin reduced survival, but not significantly so, whereas cisplatinum prolonged median survival significantly by 10 weeks.[40]

In our next phase III trial of chemotherapy for patients with end-stage squamous cell carcinoma of the head and neck the four treatment arms were methotrexate alone, cisplatinum alone, cisplatinum + methotrexate, and cisplatinum + 5-fluorouracil. The response rates were: methotrexate alone 19%, cisplatinum alone 40%, cisplatinum + methotrexate 31%, and cisplatinum + 5-fluorouracil 33%. The median survival time for the cisplatinum-alone group, 260 days, was significantly longer than the 80 days for the methotrexate-alone group. The median survival times for cisplatinum + methotrexate (160 days) and for cisplatinum + 5-fluorouracil (200 days) did not differ significantly from that for cisplatinum alone.[6]

No trials have been restricted to patients with laryngeal cancer. However, there have been a few studies which have used multivariate methods to dissect out the effect of site. Site had no significant effect on survival of 152 patients treated with cisplatinum, bleomycin, vincristine and methotrexate (CABO).[8] In the above two phase III trials of chemotherapy in end-stage disease, 129 patients were treated with cisplatinum, either alone or in two-drug combination with bleomycin, methotrexate or 5-fluorouracil. The overall response was 33%, whereas it was 40% for laryngeal tumours, but this trend did not reach significant levels.[7]

PALLIATIVE CHEMOTHERAPY: NOVEL APPROACHES

In addition to the use of standard cytotoxic agents there have been a few attempts at entirely novel treatments. Panje experimented with indomethacin, an inhibitor of prostaglandin synthetase. This was based on work on experimental animals that showed that many experimental tumours produced increased amounts of prostaglandin. He treated seven patients with very advanced disease and obtained two complete and three partial responses. This method does not appear to have been taken up by others.[44]

Others have attempted to capitalize on the fact that the larynx is clearly responsive to sex hormones. Schuller et al measured the oestrogen and progesterone receptors of 65 patients with head and neck cancer, including 16 with laryngeal cancer. Only 2.7% of the patients had oestrogen receptors and none had progesterone receptors.[50] Mattox et al measured androgen receptor levels in 32 laryngeal and three oropharyngeal cancers. The median level of receptor was 0.7 femtomoles/mg. (They do not tell us the normal levels). Ten patients were treated with flutamide, an antiandrogen: three patients had a brief partial response, but there was no correlation between response and androgen receptor levels.[37]

ORGAN PRESERVATION

It has been appreciated for a long time that the combination of chemotherapy and radiotherapy may render an inoperable tumour operable, or even avoid the need for surgery. In one of the earliest reports cisplatinum plus bleomycin rendered 14 patients operable (including several with laryngeal carcinoma).[25,49] However, we are *not* concerned here with this use of chemotherapy, but rather with the use of chemotherapy plus radiotherapy as an alternative to surgery for advanced but operable disease to achieve organ preservation. The concept is based on the idea that response to chemotherapy predicts response to radiotherapy, and that chemotherapy reduces the bulk of the disease, so that response to radiotherapy is then more likely.

There has been only one controlled trial of this concept,[26] but there have been several uncontrolled studies.[10,12,28,32,43,46,61] There are several questions that must be answered.

1. Are patients who respond to chemoradiotherapy likely to retain their larynx? This does indeed seem to be the case; 71% of 265 patients reported in five series retained their larynx.[10,26,32,46,61]

2. What is the subsequent response to radiotherapy of responders to chemotherapy? Of partial responders to chemotherapy, 43% went on to achieve a complete response to radiotherapy in two trials.[12,46] It is difficult to understand how response to radiotherapy could be assessed in complete responders to chemotherapy, as was reported in some trials.[43]

   If the tumour has disappeared completely in response to chemotherapy, the only method of assessment is subsequent survival, which brings us to the next question.

3. Is the survival of responders better than that of non-responders? There was no difference in two series,[10,12] the survival of responders compared with that of non-responders was prolonged from 14 to 34 months in another,[32] and the survival at 2 years for responders was 87% compared with only 23% in another.[46]

4. Is the subsequent fate of non-responders the same as it would have been if they had undergone immediate laryngectomy? The evidence suggests that the outcome is disastrous in non-responders — a 10% failure-free rate

at 2 years in one series.[46] This is the only trial to tell us of the fate of non-responders. This is very worrying, given that 40% of patients have not responded by the end of chemotherapy and radiotherapy.[46] Presumably this poor outcome is due to delay in the institution of proper treatment, the emergence of resistant strains in response to chemotherapy,[59] and reduced general condition as a result of the chemotherapy.

5. Was radiotherapy alone a viable alternative for any of these patients? One series[10] contained a high proportion of patients with T_1 and T_2 tumours that would surely have done well with conventional radiotherapy —in fact in this series only 30% of the patients had disease that was so far advanced that it would be generally regarded as suitable only for surgery. The 2-year survival in three series[10,26,46] was 61%—probably much the same as would be achieved by modern radiotherapy for a similar group of patients.

   Furthermore, it has been shown that patients will accept a trade-off of reduced survival for an increased chance of retaining their larynx. Of healthy volunteers, 20% said that they would accept radiotherapy, rather than undergo surgery, even though the chance of survival was less.[35] However, they were told that the best result for surgery was a survival rate of 60% at 3 years, compared with 48% for radiotherapy. Had they been given the true figures of 58% for radiotherapy[5] even more might have opted for radiotherapy.

6. Is the toxicity acceptable? Three reports do not mention toxicity; the death rate was 4% in the remainder.[10,32,46,61]

7. Have the questions of informed consent been adequately addressed? The only controlled trial[26] consisted of two arms: chemoradiotherapy versus total laryngectomy. It is difficult to believe that all eligible patients accepted laryngectomy if that was the treatment to which they were randomized and they knew of the alternative. As we are not told about compliance we cannot assess the value of this trial.

8. Could other methods based on cell kinetics or ploidy, for example, be used to predict response to radiotherapy? Ensley and his colleagues have already shown that only non-diploid tumours respond to chemotherapy, so that presumably this approach should not be used for diploid tumours.[13]

REFERENCES

1. Aguilar E A, Robbins K I, Stephens J, Dimery I W, Batsakis J G 1987 Primary oat cell carcinoma of the larynx. Amer J Clin Oncol 10: 26–32
2. Al Sarraf M 1988 Head and neck cancer: chemotherapy concepts. Sem Oncol 15: 70–85
3. Bakowski M. T, Macdonald E, Mould R F, Cawte P, Sloggem J, Barrett A, Dalley V, Newton K A, Westbury G, James S E, Hellmann K 1978 Double blind controlled clinical trial of radiation plus razoxane (ICRF 159) versus radiation plus placebo in the

treatment of head and neck cancer. J Radiat Oncol Biol Phys 4: 115–119
4. Brunin F, Rodriguez J, Jaulerry C, Jouve M, Pontvert D, Point D, Mosseri V, Pouillart P, Asselain B, Brugere J, Bataini J P 1989 Induction chemotherapy in advanced head and neck cancer. Acta Oncol 28: 61–65
5. Bryce D P 1972 The role of surgery in the management of carcinoma of the larynx. J Laryngol Otol 86: 669–683
6. Campbell J B, Dorman E B, McCormick M, Miles J, Morton R P,

Rugman F, Stell P M, Stoney P J, Vaughan E D, Wilson J A 1987 A randomized phase III trial of cisplatinum, methotrexate, cisplatinum + methotrexate, and cisplatinum + 5-fluoro-uracil in end-stage head and neck cancer. Acta Otolaryngol 103: 519–528

7. Campbell J B, Dorman E B, Helliwell T R, McCormick M, Miles J, Morton R P, Rugman F, Stell P M, Stoney P J, Vaughan E D, Wilson J A 1987 Factors predicting response of end stage squamous cell carcinoma of the head and neck to cisplatinum. Clin Otolaryngol 12: 167–176

8. Cognetti F, Pinnaro P, Ruggeri E M, Carlini P, Perrino A, Impiombato F A, Calabresi F, Chilelli M G, Giannarelli D 1989 Prognostic factors for chemotherapy response and survival using combination chemotherapy as initial treatment of advanced head and neck squamous cell cancer. J Clin Oncol 7: 829–837

9. Coninx P, Nasca S, Lebrun D, Panis X, Lucas P, Garbe E, Legros M 1988 Sequential trial of initial chemotherapy for advanced cancer of the head and neck. DDP versus DDP + 5-fluorouracil. Cancer 62: 1888–1892

10. Demard F, Chauvel P, Santini J, Vallicioni J, Thyss A, Schneider M 1990 Response to chemotherapy as justification for modification of the therapeutic strategy for pharyngolaryngeal carcinomas. Head Neck 12: 225–231

11. Easterbrook P J, Berlin J A, Gopalan R, Matthews S R 1991 Publication bias in clinical research. Lancet 337: 867–872

12. Ensley J F, Jacobs J R, Weaver A, Kinzie J, Crissman J, Kish J A, Cummings G, Al-Sarraf M 1984 Correlation between response to cisplatinum-combination chemotherapy and subsequent radiotherapy in previously untreated patients with advanced squamous cell cancers of the head and neck. Cancer 54: 811–814

13. Ensley J, Maciorowski Z, Pietraszkiewicz H, Kish J, Tapazoglou E, Jacobs J, Mathog R, Sakr W, Al-Sarraf M, Metch B, Schuller D, Coltman C 1990 Prospective correlation of cytotoxic response and DNA content parameters in advanced squamous cell cancer of the head and neck (SCCHN). Proceedings of ASCO 9(No. 173) abstract 671

14. Ervin T J, Clark J R, Weichselbaum R R, Fallon B G, Miller D, Fabian R L, Posner M R, Norris C M Jr, Tuttle S A, Schoenfeld D A, Price K N, Frei E III 1987 An analysis of induction and adjuvant chemotherapy in the multidisciplinary treatment of squamous cell carcinoma of the head and neck. J Clin Oncol 5: 10–20

15. Fazekas J T, Sommer C, Kramer S 1980 Adjuvant intravenous Methotrexate or definitive radiotherapy alone for advanced squamous cancers of the oral cavity, oropharynx, supraglottic larynx or hypopharynx. Int J Rad Oncol Biol Phys 6: 533–541

16. Ferlito A, Pesavento G, Recher G, Caruso G, Dal Fior S, Montaguti A, Carraro R, Narne S, Pennelli N 1986 Long term survival in response to combined chemotherapy and radiotherapy in laryngeal small cell carcinoma. Auris-Nasus-Larynx 13: 113–123

17. Fletcher G H, Suit H D, Howe C D, Samuels M, Jesse R H, Villareal R U 1963 Clinical method of testing radiation-sensitizing agents in squamous cell carcinoma. Cancer 16: 355–363

18. Fu K K, Phillips T L, Silverberg I J, Jacobs C, Goffinet D R, Chun C, Friedman M A, Kohler M, McWhirter K, Carter S K 1987 Combined radiotherapy and chemotherapy with Bleomycin and Methotrexate for advanced inoperable head and neck cancer: update of a Northern California Oncology Group Randomized Trial. J Clin Oncol 5: 1410–1418

19. George S L 1984 The required size and length of a phase III clinical trial. In: Buyse M E, Staquet M J, Sylvester R J (eds) Cancer clinical trials — methods and practice. Oxford University Press, Oxford, p 289.

20. Giddings N A, Kennedy I L, Vrabec D P 1987 Primary small cell carcinoma of the larynx: analysis of treatment. J Otolaryngol 16: 157–166

21. Gollin F F, Ansfield F J, Brandenburg J H, Ramirez G, Vermund H 1972 Combined therapy in advanced head and neck cancer: a randomized study. Am J Roentgenol 114: 83–88

22. Gupta N K, Pointon R C S, Wilkinson P M 1987 A randomised clinical trial to contrast radiotherapy with radiotherapy and Methotrexate given synchronously in head and neck cancer Clin Radiol 38: 575–581

23. Head and neck contracts program 1987. Adjuvant chemotherapy for advanced head and neck squamous carcinoma. Cancer 60: 301–311

24. Holoye P Y, Grossman T W, Toohill R J, Kun L E, Byhardt R W, Duncavage A, Teplin R W, Ritch P S, Hoffman R G, Malin T C 1985 Randomized study of adjuvant chemotherapy for head and neck cancer. Otolaryngol Head Neck Surg 93: 712

25. Hong W K, Shapshay S M, Bhutani R, Craft M L, Ucmakli A, Yamaguchi K, Vaughan C W, Strong M S 1979 Induction chemotherapy in advanced squamous head and neck carcinoma with high dose cisplatinum and bleomycin infusion. Cancer 44: 19–25

26. Hong W K, Wolf G T, Fisher S, Spaulding M, Endicott J, Laramore G, Hillman R, McClatchey K, Fye C 1989 Laryngeal preservation with induction chemotherapy (CT) and radiotherapy (XRT) in the treatment for advanced laryngeal cancer: interim survival data. Proceedings of ASCO 9 (No. 167) abstract 650

27. Hussey D H, Abrams J P 1975 Combined therapy in advanced head and neck cancer: hydroxyurea and radiotherapy. Prog Clin Cancer 6: 79–86

28. Jacobs C, Goffinet D R, Goffinet L, Kohler M, Fee W E 1987 Chemotherapy as a substitute for surgery in the treatment of advanced resectable head and neck cancer. A report from the Northern California Oncology Group. Cancer 60: 1178–1183

29. Jacobs C, Makuch R 1990 Efficacy of adjuvant chemotherapy for patients with resectable head and neck cancer: a subset analysis of the head and neck contracts program. J Clin Oncol 8: 838–847

30. Johnson J T, Myers E N, Strodes C H, Mayernik D G, Sigler B A, Schramm V L, Nolan T A, Wagner R L 1985 Maintenance chemotherapy for high-risk patients. Arch Otolaryngol 111: 727–729

31. Kapstad B, Bang G, Rennaes S, Dahler A 1978 Combined preoperative treatment with cobalt and bleomycin in patients with head and neck carcinoma — a controlled clinical study. J Radiat Oncol Biol Phys 4: 85–89

32. Karp D, Carter R, Vaughan C, Willett B, Heeren T, Calarese P, Zeitels S, Hong W 1988 Voice preservation using induction chemotherapy (CT) plus radiation therapy (XRT) as an alternative to laryngectomy in advanced head and neck cancer: long term follow-up. Proceedings of ASCO 7 (No. 152) abstract 587

33. Kish J A, Weaver A, Jacobs J et al 1984 Cisplatin and 5-fluorouracil infusion in patients with recurrent and disseminated epidermoid cancer. Cancer 53: 1819–1824

34. Knowlton A H, Percarpio B, Bobrow S, Fischer J J 1975 'Methotrexate and radiation therapy in the treatment of advanced head and neck tumors'. Ther Radiol 116: 709–712

35. McNeill B J, Weichselbaum R, Pauker S G 1981 Speech and survival — tradeoffs between quality and quantity of life in laryngeal cancer. New Eng J Med 305: 982–987

36. Martin M D, Hazan A, Vergnes L, Peytral C, Mazeron J J, Senechaut J P, Lelievre G, Peynegre R 1990 Randomized study of 5-Fluorouracil and Cisplatin as neoadjuvant therapy in head and neck cancer — a preliminary report. Int J Radiat Oncol Biol Phys 19: 973–975

37. Mattox D E, Hoff D D von, McGuire W L 1984 Androgen receptors and antiandrogen therapy for laryngeal carcinoma. Arch Otolaryngol 110: 721–724

38. Merlano M, Conte P F, Tatorek R 1984 Ineffectiveness of 5-fluorouracil and cisplatin as a second line chemotherapy in head and neck cancer. Tumori 70: 267

39. Miller A B, Hoogstraten B, Staquet M, Winkler A 1981 Reporting results of cancer treatment. Cancer 47: 207–214

40. Morton R P, Rugman F, Dorman E B, Stoney P J, Wilson J A, Veevers A, Stell P M 1985 Cisplatinum and Bleomycin for advanced or recurrent squamous cell carcinoma of the head and neck: a randomised factorial phase III controlled trial. Cancer Chemother Pharmacol 15: 283–289

41. Nissenbaum M, Browde A, Bezwoda W R, De Moor N G, Derman D P 1984 Treatment of advanced head and neck cancer: multiple daily dose fractionated radiation therapy and sequential multimodal treatment approach. Med Pediatr Oncol 12: 204–208

42. Olver I N, Dalley D, Woods R, Aroney R, Hughes P, Bishop J F, Cruikshank D 1989 Carboplatin and continuous infusion 5-Fluorouracil for advanced head and neck cancer. Eur J Cancer Clin Oncol 25: 173–176

43. Panis X, Coninx P, Nguyen T D, Legros M 1990 Relation between responses to induction chemotherapy and subsequent radiotherapy in advanced or multicentric squamous cell carcinomas of the head and neck. Int J Rad Oncol Biol Phys 18: 1315–1318

44. Panje W R 1981 Regression of head and neck carcinoma with a prostaglandin-synthesis inhibitor. Arch Otolaryngol 107: 658–663

45. Peto R 1987 Why do we need systematic overviews of randomized trials? Stat Med 6: 233–240

46. Pfister D G, Strong E, Harrison L, Haines I E, Pfister D A, Sessions R, Spiro R, Shah J, Gerold F, McLure T, Vikram B, Fass D, Armstrong J, Bosl G J 1991 Larynx preservation with combined chemotherapy and radiation therapy in advanced and resectable head and neck cancer. J Clin Oncol 9: 850–859

47. Rentschler R E, Wilbur D W, Petti G H, Chonkich G D, Hilliard D A, Camacho E S, Thorpe R C 1987 Adjuvant Methotrexate escalated to toxicity for resectable stage III and IV squamous head and neck carcinomas — a prospective randomized study. J Clin Oncol 5: 278–285

48. Richards G J, Chambers R G 1969 Hydroxyurea: a radiosensitizer in the treatment of neoplasms of the head and neck. Am J Roentgenol 105: 555–565

49. Schuller D E, Wilson H E, Smith R E, Batley F, James A 1983 Preoperative reductive chemotherapy for locally advanced carcinoma of the oral cavity, oropharynx and hypopharynx. Cancer 51: 15–19

50. Schuller D A, Abou-Issa H, Parrish R 1984 Estrogen and progesterone receptors in head and neck cancer. Arch Otolaryngol 110: 725–727

51. Schuller D E, Metch B, Stein D W, Mattox D, McCracken J D 1988 Preoperative chemotherapy in advanced resectable head and neck cancer: final report of the Southwest Oncology Group. Laryngoscope 98: 1205–1211

52. SECOG, Cancer Research Campaign Clinical Trial Centre. 1986 A randomized trial of combined multidrug chemotherapy and radiotherapy in advanced squamous cell carcinoma of the head and neck. Europ J Surg Oncol 12: 289–295

53. Stefani A, Chung T S 1980 Hydroxyurea and radiotherapy in head and neck cancer — long term results of a double blind randomized prospective study. Radiat Oncol Biol Phys 6: 1398

54. Stell P M, Dalby J E, Strickland R, Fraser J G, Bradley P J, Flood L M 1983 Sequential chemotherapy and radiotherapy in advanced head and neck cancer. Clin Radiol 34: 463–467

55. Stell P M, Rawson N S B 1990 Adjuvant chemotherapy in head and neck cancer. Br J Cancer 61: 779–787

56. Stolwijk C, Wagener D J, Van Den Broek P, Levendag P C, Kazem I, Bruaset I 1983 Randomized adjuvant chemotherapy trial for advanced head and neck cancer. Neth J Med 28: 347

57. Taylor S G, Applebaum E, Showel J L, Norusis M., Holinger L D, Hutchinson J C Jr, Murthy A K, Caldareli D D 1985 A randomized trial of adjuvant chemotherapy in head and neck cancer. J Clin Oncol 3: 672–679

58. Toohill R J, Anderson T, Byhardt R W, Cox J D, Duncavage J A, Grossman T W, Haas C D, Haas J S, Hartz A J, Libnoch J A, Malin T C, Ritch P S, Wilson J F 1987 Cisplatin and Fluorouracil as neoadjuvant therapy in head and neck cancer. A preliminary report. Arch Otolaryngol Head Neck Surg 113: 758–761

59. Toohill R J, Duncavage J A, Grossman T W, Malin T C, Teplin R W, Wilson J F, Byhardt R W, Haas J S, Cox J D, Anderson T, Holoye P Y, Ritch P S, Haas C D, Libnoch J, Hoffman R G 1987 The effects of delay in standard treatment due to induction chemotherapy in two randomised prospective studies. Laryngoscope 97: 407–412

60. Vermund H, Kaalhus O, Winther F, Trausio J, Thorud E, Harang R 1985 Bleomycin and radiation therapy in squamous cell carcinoma of the upper aero-digestive tract: a phase III clinical trial. Int J Radiat Oncol Biol Phys 11: 1877–1886

61. Vikram B, Bosl G J, Pfisterd, Strong E W, Spiro R H, Sessions R B, Gerold F P, Shah J P 1988 New strategies for avoiding total laryngectomy in patients with head and neck cancer. NCI Monogr 6: 361–364

62. Vogl S E, Schoenfeld D A, Kaplan B H, Lerner H J, Engstrom P F, Horton J 1985 A randomised prospective comparison of methotrexate with a combination of methotrexate, bleomycin and cisplatin in head and neck cancer. Cancer 56: 432–442

63. Weissberg J B, Son Y H, Papac R J, Sasaki C, Fischer D B, Lawrence R, Rockwell S, Sartorelli A C, Fischer J J 1989 Randomised clinical trial of mitomycin C as an adjunct to radiotherapy in head and neck cancer. Int J Radiat Oncol Biol Phys 17: 3–9

30. Voice rehabilitation after total laryngectomy

M. I. Singer

INTRODUCTION

Historically, patients suffering from laryngeal cancer face survival without the intrinsic human characteristic of voice and verbal communication. Laryngeal cancer gradually erodes the sound-generating glottis, and surgical treatment frequently sacrifices this structure. The prospect of voicelessness is terrifying, and it often complicates the effective treatment of this disease by causing delay and risking cure in order to preserve voice.

The first reported total laryngectomy for laryngeal carcinoma was that carried out by Billroth in 1873.[3] This was accomplished by the placement of a pharyngostoma to divert secretions from the tracheostoma with planned delayed closure of the pharynx. It was known that expired air, when directed to the pharynx through a special tracheal cannula, would produce voice. The initial Billroth report included a description of one of these devices.

American and European surgeons later refined the laryngectomy procedure by eliminating the pharyngostoma and requiring another rehabilitation method for speech referred to as 'oesophageal voice'. Patients are taught to insufflate the oesophagus and stomach with injected or inhaled air. Gradual release of the air vibrates regions of the upper oesophageal sphincter to produce sound or vicarious voice. It is generally held that 60% of alaryngeal speakers will develop oesophageal speech that is intelligible, although recent prospective studies suggest an oesophageal speech acquisition rate of 30% or less.[2]

Modern surgical innovations for voice conservation include partial laryngectomy procedures. These techniques reduce the laryngeal framework by sacrifice of portions of the glottis and are referred to as vertical laryngectomies, or they remove the epiglottis and related supraglottic structures and are considered horizontal laryngectomies.[4] The conservation laryngectomy procedures permit intelligible voice and avoid a permanent tracheostoma. They may be complicated by problems with deglutition and chronic tracheal aspiration.

The determination of the type of laryngectomy is based on the extent of disease as described by the TNM classification. Total laryngectomies are often required after radiotherapy failure, or for T[3] lesions. This obligates the patient to a permanent tracheostoma, and sacrifices the laryngeal voicing mechanism. A number of shunt techniques have been devised to direct tracheal air into the pharyngo-oesophagus analogous to the approach described by Billroth. These procedures have been called 'reconstructive laryngectomies', 'laryngoplasties', 'neoglottic methods', and, recently, 'tracheo-oesophageal punctures'.[5]

The puncture procedures use a small channel measuring 3.3 mm in diameter between the trachea and oesophagus for air passage through the upper oesophageal sphincter. A silicone valve is placed in the puncture to stent it permanently and to allow tracheo-oesophageal airflow without oesophageal reflux into the trachea. This valve is unidirectional and is referred to as a 'voice prosthesis'. The valves are disposable, inexpensive, and changeable by the patients.

RATIONALE FOR PUNCTURE

The tracheo-oesophageal puncture is a simple midline 'stab' perforating the membranous trachea and the anterior oesophageal wall. The fibrous connective tissue of the common wall and the two layers of oesophageal muscle and single layer of trachealis muscle support the prosthesis. The puncture tract eventually epithelializes and ranges between 1.5 cm and 2.5 cm in overall length (Fig. 30.1).

Occlusion of the tracheostoma with the prosthesis in place permits intratracheal pressures of 20 mmHg to 100 mmHg which will drive air through the valve and inflate the oesophagus. In successful speakers, the air will exit the oesophagus across the upper oesophageal sphincter. This exiting airflow vibrates the mucus membrane and produces a low pitched sound. The vocal tract is intact after laryngectomy with preservation of the articulatory structures of the tongue, teeth, palate and lips. The

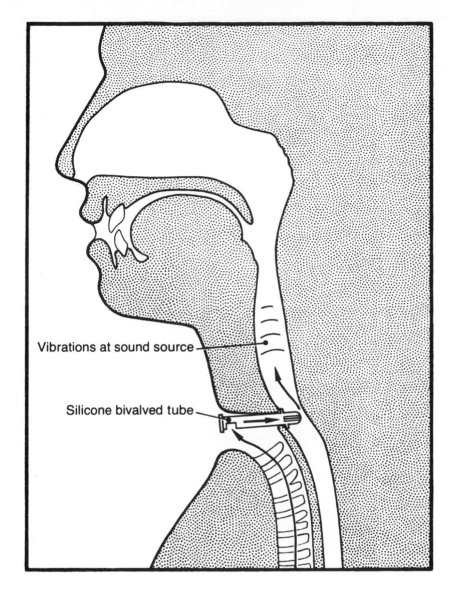

Fig. 30.1 Voice prosthesis in the tracheo-oesophageal puncture with sound-producing vibration in the laryngectomized pharynx.

pharyngo-oesophageal sound is articulated in the vocal tract as understandable speech.

During deglutition the valve is closed against the oesophageal contents, and nothing is regurgitated into the trachea. The puncture and prosthesis permit a phonatory fistula with little risk of tracheal soiling. Earlier shunt and neoglottic procedures were complicated by stenosis of the passage requiring excessive air pressures for speech generation, or by the problem of aspiration into the unprotected airway.

The puncture method introduces air flow at the upper oesophagus producing mucosal vibration for the sound production. Significant numbers of patients are not capable of fluent voice production by this method without modification of the upper oesophageal sphincter.[6] It is estimated that 40% of oesophageal speech failures will also fail by the puncture method as well.

Oesophageal distention of the intact patient will produce a reflexive rise in the resting tension of the upper oesophageal sphincter zone.[1] This is mediated by the vagus nerve through the pharyngeal plexus, and may receive contributions from the IXth nerve and sympathetics. Pressure rises over 40 mmHg usually result in dysfluent speech in the laryngectomized patient. Laryngectomized patients have varying residual innervation of this region which is presumably determined by the extent of resection and the operative technique. The better speakers are not capable of generating high pharyngo-oesophageal pressures during oesophageal distention.

Alteration of the pharyngeal closure is required to eliminate this detriment to speech acquisition. Typically, the pharynx is closed in a variety of configurations after laryngectomy which include vertical 'I', 'T', or transverse suture lines. The suture line is supported with one or two more layers, the last including the pharyngeal constrictor muscles. The supporting layer of muscle is generally considered a good technique to avoid suture line leaks or fistulae; however, the residual musculature will form a sphincter. If the innervation is intact, and a moderate muscle bulk remains, the sphincter will be capable of air-trapping and prevent fluent speech production.

For the development of effective tracheo-oesophageal phonation, the pharyngeal constrictors require management different from simple closure to ensure a high rate of speech acquisition. Initially we suggested the addition of a constrictor myotomy at the time of the pharyngeal closure. This myotomy extended from the base of the tongue to include the middle pharyngeal constrictor muscle, the inferior pharyngeal constrictor, and the cricopharyngeus which represents 3–6 cm in vertical dimension.

A further refinement of this muscle relaxation technique is a pharyngeal plexus neurectomy which decreases the risk of uncontrolled fistulization, reflux, and pharyngeal wall devascularization, while it preserves the intrinsic elasticity of the pharyngeal constrictor muscles. This may eventuate in a wider fundamental frequency range of the resultant voice which will more closely approximate normal laryngeal voice.

OPERATIVE TECHNIQUE FOR PRIMARY VOICE RESTORATION

The following discussion describes the modifications of the conventional total laryngectomy that are used for the development of tracheo-oesophageal phonation. These techniques include the method for tracheostoma construction, the tracheo-oesophageal puncture procedure and the pharyngeal constrictor muscle relaxation procedures, consisting of the middle and inferior pharyngeal constrictor myotomy or the pharyngeal plexus neurectomy.

The preferred laryngectomy incisions are either an apron or low collar, and at the inferior limb an 'X' is outlined. The skin triangles superiorly and inferiorly are excised, preserving the lateral triangles. After the laryngectomy specimen has been removed, the transected trachea is fixed to the inferior skin, with a monofilament suture placed circumferentially around the cartilaginous ring of the trachea, and to the skin as a vertical mattress suture. This resurfaces the de-epithelialized cartilage. The posterior trachea is incised bilaterally at the junction of the membranous wall and the cartilage for a distance of 1

cm, which permits advancement of the trachea anteriorly. The resulting defect in the tracheal wall is closed by interposition of the lateral triangular skin flaps described with the incision. The rest of the trachea is sutured to the inferior skin flap as previously described with the monofilament suture.

After the tracheostoma has been established the puncture is placed. A right-angled clamp is introduced into the open pharyngotomy to the level of the tracheostoma in the cervical oesophagus. The clamp tips are pressed anteriorly against the posterior membranous trachea at 8 to 10 mm from the superior margin of the stoma. A knife is placed over the impression of the clamp tips on the tracheal side of the membranous wall and a 3 mm incision is made allowing the clamp tips to exteriorize in the tracheostoma. A silicone Foley catheter, Fr. 14, is grasped with the clamp and brought retrograde into the pharyngo-oesophageal lumen. The balloon is inflated with 1.5 ml of water, and is directed into the distal oesophagus for later use as a cervical oesophageal feeding tube. The catheter stents the tracheo-oesophageal puncture for 2–3 weeks, when it is replaced with the appropriately sized voice prosthesis.

The pharyngeal constrictor myotomy is carried out before the pharyngotomy has been closed. The lateral edge of the pharyngeal mucosa is grasped with a Babcock clamp at the level of the tongue base and inferiorly at the level of the oesophagus. The pharynx is rotated away from the operator with traction on the clamps while the retropharyngeal plane is developed with scissors dissection to the midline. A tunnel is fashioned with fine scissors between the fibres of the middle pharyngeal constrictor in the midline posterior pharynx. The tunnel is dissected in the midline inferiorly to the level of the cervical oesophagus. One blade is withdrawn from the muscular tunnel and the tunnel is incised its entire length, dividing the muscle fibres to the submucosa. Bleeding is controlled effectively by bipolar cautery. Following the myotomy, the pharynx is then closed in layers as previously discussed.

The alternative technique to myotomy is the pharyngeal plexus neurectomy. The exposure is the same as that for the myotomy. Pharyngeal rotation with the grasping clamps permits dissection of the retropharynx. The great vessels are retracted laterally, and the middle pharyngeal constrictor muscle is identified in the field. The fibres of the plexus run on the surface of this muscle and its inferior edge immediately subjacent to the investing fascia. Identification of the plexus is confirmed by electrical stimulation.

The plexus fibres branch from two descending trunks and radiate obliquely in the direction of the concentric fibres of the pharyngeal constrictors. The nerve fibres are dissected from the muscle fibres, electrocoagulated, and sharply divided. This reduces the reflexive pharyngeal wall tension during oesophageal distention, with minimal trauma to the underlying pharyngeal wall and preserves the elasticity of the circumferential constrictor muscles.

DISCUSSION

The method of alaryngeal voice restoration, referred to here as tracheo-oesophageal puncture and voice prosthesis, was originally developed as a secondary method for oesophageal voice failures. The success rate is variable, but 90% of the patients can acquire voice by this method, with failures resulting from difficulties managing the voice prosthesis, extrusions, and excessive voicing efforts from unrecognized pharyngeal constrictor reflex hypertension. Some patients experience puncture dilatation or granuloma formation, representing 1–2% of our 600-case experience. They will require minor revision procedures to continue long-term prosthetic use.

The procedure is applicable to radiated patients, unless the dose exceeds 65 Gy to the midline and stoma. It has been successfully applied to patients years after laryngectomy, and requires an adequate tracheostoma, minimal reflexive hypertension, and proper instruction for the use of the voice prosthesis. The presence of radical neck dissection or a reconstructive flap does not impede the successful use of the voice prosthesis. Although the experience is limited to date with pharyngeal replacement procedures, i.e., gastric interposition or free jejunal grafts, intelligible speech has been reported for this patient population.

As experience was acquired with the secondary application of this rehabilitative method, we initiated its use with the laryngectomy for several reasons. The operative exposure for the puncture and the myotomy or neurectomy is clearly better than the secondary setting. The tracheostoma can be better designed for prosthesis use, and the patients are psychologically prepared for voice restoration as soon as they recover from the laryngectomy. The only complicating factors of significance are the possibility of stoma inflammation from the stent with secondary breakdown or stenosis, or patient difficulty managing the new tracheostoma and tracheo-oesophageal puncture early in the postoperative recovery period.

Selective application of these techniques provides an easily reproducible method for alaryngeal speech rehabilitation. The modifications described here are simple, safe, and present no alteration of accepted surgical oncology approaches to laryngeal cancer. The resultant speech is highly intelligible, preferable to oesophageal speech and artificial larynx speech, and is acquired rapidly without prolonged therapy or excessive expense. The voice prosthesis as described costs no more than the batteries used in the conventional electrolarynx.

Tracheo-oesophageal phonation as a primary or secondary method for rehabilitation of the voice after laryngectomy has been used for over 13 years, and has become widely accepted as a method of choice for rehabilitation of the laryngectomee. The concepts are simple, little additional cost is encountered, and the success rates are high. This adjunctive modality for the treatment of laryngeal cancer presents new rehabilitative and research directions for laryngectomized patients.

REFERENCES

1. Creamer B, Schlagel J F 1957 Motor responses of the esophagus to distention. J Applied Physiol 10: 498–504
2. Gates G A, Ryan W J, Cooper J C 1982 Current status of laryngectomee rehabilitation: results of therapy. Am J Otolaryngol 3: 1–14
3. Gussenbauer C 1874 Ueber die erste durch Th. Billroth am Menschen ausgeführte Kehlkopf Exstirpation und die Anwendung eines künstlichen Kehlkopfes. Arch Klin Chir 17: 343–356
4. Lawson W, Biller H F 1981 Cancer of the larynx. In: Suen J Y, Myers E N (eds) Cancer of the head and neck. Churchill Livingstone, New York, p 200
5. Singer M I, Blom E D 1980 An endoscopic technique for restoration of voice after laryngectomy. Ann Otol Rhinol Laryngol 89: 529–533
6. Singer M I, Blom E D, Hamaker R C 1981 Further experience with voice restoration after total laryngectomy. Ann Otol Rhinol Laryngol 90: 498–502

31. Stomal recurrence after total laryngectomy

Y. Murakami

INTRODUCTION

Stomal recurrence is a troublesome malignancy of the tracheal stoma which is occasionally seen after total laryngectomy and which always offers one of the most difficult problems for surgeons.

Primary tumour of almost all stomal recurrences is squamous cell carcinoma of the larynx, and only a few cases originate from carcinomas of the hypopharynx.

INCIDENCE

In 1979 Myers and Ogura[15] analysed previous reports on stomal recurrence in laryngectomized patients and reported that the average incidence seen in five different institutes was 8.3%; the highest was 14.7% (Keim et al)[8] and the lowest was 4.1% (Stell and Broek)[28]. In 1981 Mantravadi et al[13] reported a 5% incidence among 507 total laryngectomies, and in 1990 Rubin et al[17] reported the much lower incidence of 3.4% among 444 patients. The author's own experience showed a 6.4% incidence among 525 total laryngectomies between 1971 and 1985, but only 3.6% among 142 total laryngectomies between 1986 and 1990.

These data may indicate that the incidence of stomal recurrence after total laryngectomy is decreasing at around 4–5% per year, which is probably due to increasing information on the characteristics of stomal recurrence and subsequent improvements in treatment modalities for prevention — such as surgical procedures, including thorough extirpation of regional lymph nodes for patients with transglottic carcinoma and/or subglottic involvement.

RISK FACTORS

It is generally accepted that the incidence of stomal recurrence after total laryngectomy has been significantly higher in patients who had previously had transglottic carcinoma with extensive subglottic invasion and metastasis in the regional lymph nodes.

The other risk factors responsible for stomal recurrence may include tumour size, oncological aggressiveness, preoperative/emergency tracheotomy, previous conservation laryngeal surgery, cell implantation to the trachea, cell dissemination to the surgical field, and so on.

In the treatment of obstructive laryngeal carcinomas, an association has often been noted between emergency tracheotomy for air-way relief and subsequent post-laryngectomy stomal recurrence,[1,17,18] though it remains unclear whether this is due to tumour implantation in the tracheotomy truck or the involvement of regional lymph nodes.

Mantravadi et al[13] stated that an initial subglottic extension of the tumour and metastatic paratracheal nodes are the most significant risk factors, but the primary tumour size, prior emergency tracheotomy and conservation laryngeal surgeries have no effect on the incidence of stomal recurrence. Rubin et al[17] reported that 80% of patients with stomal recurrence had tumours in the subglottic region, and this is significant in comparison to those cases in which different sites were involved; these authors came to the same conclusion as Mantravadi et al, emphasizing that tumour involvement of the subglottic region is statistically the single most important risk factor.

In 1991 Rockley et al,[16] on the other hand, investigated 26 T3N0 glottic carcinomas treated with emergency tracheotomy followed by total laryngectomy; these were compared with 65 stage-matched cases treated with laryngectomy alone. The 'emergency tracheotomy' group was reported to have a very poor prognosis with a much higher incidence of recurrence at the tracheal stoma and also in the regional lymph nodes. These authors concluded that paratracheal lymph node metastasis is an important mechanism in the development of stomal recurrence.

However, it is noteworthy that, in 1990, Barr et al[3] analysed 14 stomal recurrences and compared them with 15 other types of aggressive recurrences in the neck for factors implicated in stomal recurrence; these authors stated that stomal recurrence has a greater association with subglottic extension, but that this difference is not statistically significant and that stomal recurrence can be considered a part of the group of aggressive neck recurrences associated simply with more advanced disease prior to laryngectomy. It may be the case that, when laryngeal carcinomas have an oncologically aggressive character, they can invade far down the subglottis to make the air-way stenosed for subsequent tracheotomy, and that they can metastasize to regional lymph nodes at higher incidence.

The author has experienced a small recurrence localized in tracheal mucosa slightly apart from the mucocutaneous junction of the tracheal stoma. This case may indicate that tumour cell implantation at the time of total laryngectomy can lead to a type of stomal recurrence. In the other patient with an extensive lingual carcinoma, stomal recurrence with invasion in the neighbouring skin was observed 7 months after total glossectomy and laryngectomy with bilateral neck dissection. This case may indicate that tumour cell dissemination into surgical wounds can also originate the other type of stomal recurrence, since the extirpated larynx and regional lymph nodes had been completely free from carcinoma.

According to these data, it seems most likely that the most common cause of stomal recurrence may be the involvement of the regional lymph nodes enhanced by the aggressiveness of the tumour showing remarkable subglottic extension, and that tumour cell implantation into the trachea, or dissemination into surgical wounds, may offer a rare but possible chance of stomal recurrence. These various causes are summarized in Table 31.1.

CLASSIFICATION

Type

Stomal recurrence can be grouped into several types by clinically characteristic presentations probably based on the variety of causes.

Type A

This type of stomal recurrence is the one most frequently experienced. It usually begins as an invisible, diffuse, peristomal, subcutaneous induration with or without swelling

Table 31.1 Various causes of stomal recurrence*

1. Residual metastatic carcinoma in regional lymph node(s)
2. Residual carcinoma in the trachea in the case of extensive subglottic invasion
3. Implantation of carcinoma cells into the trachea by surgical procedures
4. Dissemination of carcinoma cells into the surgical wound (by tracheotomy, laryngectomy or neck dissection)

*All may be related to oncological aggressiveness of the carcinoma.

of the tracheal wall, and may often be misdiagnosed as postoperative fibrosis containing hyaline degeneration. It often remains undetected and spreads insidiously, resulting in a gradual discoloration and ulceration of the skin neighbouring the tracheal stoma, and is finally diagnosed by a 'too late' biopsy. This type of clinical presentation is designated type A; it probably originates from cause 1 or 4 (Table 31.1) (Fig. 31.1).

Type B

This type of stomal recurrence is also common. It usually begins as a mild ulceration in a quadrant of the stoma, progressing to a friable mass that may clinically be misdiagnosed as granulation tissue — though it is visible from the earliest stage, in contrast to the A type. If it remains undetected, it also spreads subcutaneously, resulting in a gradual constriction of the tracheal stoma and subsequent asphyxiation. This type of clinical presentation is designated type B; it is probably due to cause 2 (Table 31.1).

Type C

This is a rare type of stomal recurrence which begins as a small, visible tumour in the tracheal wall slightly apart from the mucocutaneous junction of the tracheal stoma; it is usually detected and properly diagnosed in the initial stage. If it remains untreated, however, it may spread submucosally far down into the thoracic trachea, or extraluminally into the surrounding mediastinal tissues. This clinical presentation is designated type C; it may be attributable to cause 3 (Table 31.1), or it may be evaluated as a second primary (Fig. 31.2).

Stage

TNM classification has not yet been used for staging stomal recurrence. In 1989 Sisson[22] proposed a staging system and grouped stomal recurrences into four stages for the purpose of sorting out lesions which were too far advanced and non-resectable. This staging system was based on his experience with a great number of patients; if up-to-date imaging systems are used, the staging system can be applied in assessing the resectability of the stomal recurrence by mediastinal dissection. Sisson's four proposed stages were as follows. Stage 1 lesions are those superior to the tracheal stoma in clock-area nine to three (Fig. 31.3). On scan, the trachea, but not the oesophagus, may show possible disease. Patients have no difficulty in swallowing, have normal oesophagoscopic findings, and can be treated by mediastinal dissection, showing the best results. Stage 2 lesions may be above or below the stoma in clock-area nine to three (Fig. 31.4). When below, they may or may not involve the oesophagus, but when above,

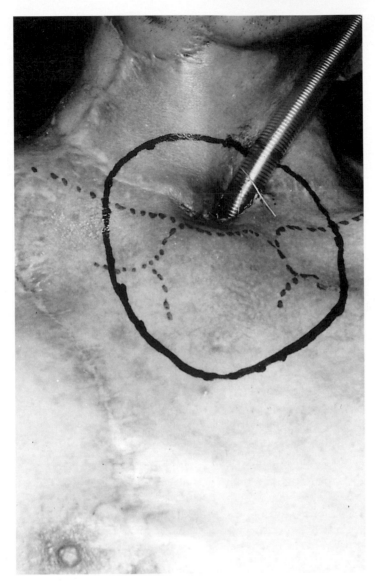

Fig. 31.1   Typical appearance of type A stomal recurrence indicating diffuse, peristomal, subcutaneous induration with slight ulceration of skin. This type probably originated from causes 1 or 4 (Table 3.1); it is necessary to remove the skin which is involved.

they must involve the oesophagus in order to be classified as stage 2; oesophagectomy with primary reconstruction is necessary. Stage 3 lesions are always below the stoma in clock-area nine to three, and the oesophagus is always involved (Fig. 31.5). In addition, the upper mediastinum must not be severely involved, and if the disease extends far down to the carina on bilateral sides of the trachea, the case is evaluated as stage 4. Stage 4 lesions are usually lateral extensions of tumour under the clavicle (Fig. 31.6), and are not resectable because of invasions to major blood vessels or the pleura.

Though clinical experience has shown that the stage of stomal recurrence may be related to the type (which varies, probably as a result of different causes) the stage is essentially different from the type, and it should be considered individually. It is generally accepted that the staging of stomal recurrence should be attempted exclusively on a basis of resectability and prognosis; the author's proposal is summarized in Table 31.2.

TREATMENT

Previously, stomal recurrence was uniformly fatal, and the results of extirpation surgery were miserable until the first successful report by Sisson et al[27] in 1962. These authors introduced the technique of mediastinal dissection, and, since then, many cases have been treated surgically by this technique with an increasing rate of success.

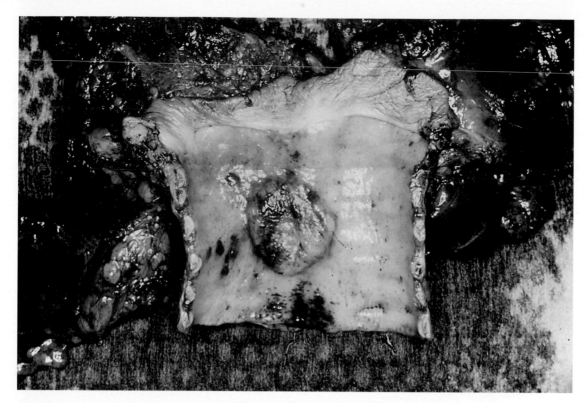

Fig. 31.2   A small tumour in the tracheal wall slightly apart from the mucocutaneous junction of the stoma; it is classified as type C. The disease was resected by mediastinal dissection together with seven rings of trachea.

The most recent data by Sisson[22] in 1989 indicated a 45% survival rate at 42 postoperative months. Though the 5-year survival rate remains low (not better than 20%)[29] it is evident that early diagnosis and radical removal of the disease may provide a much higher success rate. In an attempt to analyse the role of surgical salvage, Gluckman et al[7] in 1987 reported significantly different 5-year survival rates in relation to the stages proposed by Sisson: a 45% 5-year survival with stage 1 and 2 lesions, and 9% survival with stages 3 and 4.

Balm et al[2] in 1986, on the other hand, reported a good result obtained with a combination of cytotoxic regimen and radiotherapy. A synchronous use of chemo-therapy and radiotherapy, then, may be reasonable as a trial prior to definitive surgery if the patient has not been irradiated. However, most patients have had irradiation, and additional radiotherapy is associated with both inordinate morbidity and poor response rates. The author's own experience shows that a great majority of stomal recurrences do not respond well to combinations of chemoradiotherapy, probably because of changes in the biological characteristics of the tumour cells by mutation. Since very few reports on the combined use of chemoradiotherapy are available, it may be reasonable to conclude that, in resectable cases, surgery offers the only realistic chance of cure for this otherwise uniformly fatal disease.[15,19,22,25,27,28]

Operative technique

The immediate morbidity of mediastinal dissection was high, and the survival rate was low at the time of Sisson's first report[27] in 1962, but, nevertheless, the data were encouraging when compared to the previous rate of zero. Since then, solutions to repetitive problems, and ongoing refinements in the ablative and reconstructive techniques, have involved many surgeons.[4,6,11,20,21,23]

By the author's criteria, stage 1 lesions can be operated on satisfactorily by the classical technique of mediastinal dissection. Removal of the sternal manubrium and

Table 31.2   Various stages of stomal recurrence

Stage 1	Small lesions which do not invade any key tissues, including the oesophagus, skin, lower part of trachea near the carina, major vessels in the neck and mediastinum (such as carotid, brachiocephalic, subclavian arteries and veins), and the pleura
Stage 2	Stage 2 lesions are subdivided into two groups:
2A	Lesions that invade the skin neighbouring the tracheal stoma, but no other key tissues
2B	Lesions that invade the oesophagus, but no other key tissues
Stage 3	Lesions that invade both oesophagus and skin, but no other key tissues
Stage 4	Lesions that invade any key tissues other than the oesophagus and skin, and are considered to be unresectable

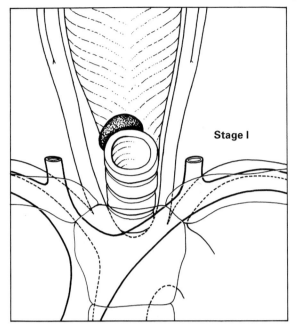

Fig. 31.3 Stomal recurrence classified in Sisson's stage 1.

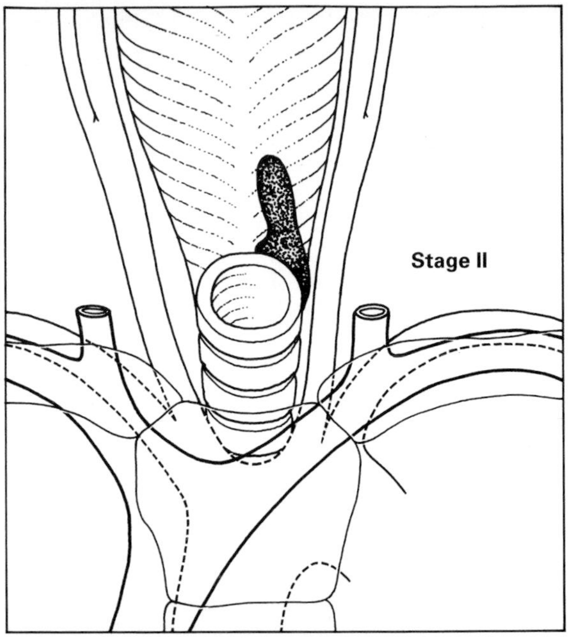

Fig. 31.4 Stomal recurrence classified in Sisson's stage 2.

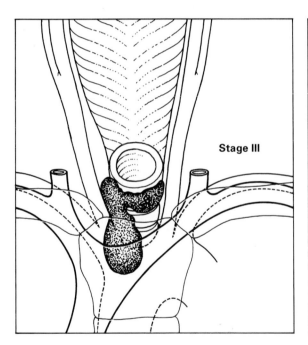

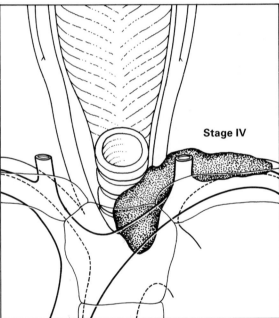

Fig. 31.5 Stomal recurrence classified in Sisson's stage 3.

Fig. 31.6 Stomal recurrence classified in Sisson's stage 4.

bilateral clavicular heads reveals the whole contents of the anterior mediastinum. Dissecting adipose tissue carefully from major vessels, pleura and the oesophageal wall, en bloc resection can be completed so as to include the tracheal stoma and several rings of trachea. The length of trachea to be resected should be decided on the basis of the degree of submucosal invasion; it usually includes five to seven rings. A new tracheal stoma can be created by transpositioning the trachea toward the right side of the brachiocephalic artery and advancement of the anterior chest skin to it (Figs 31.7–31.10).

Stage 2A lesions with skin invasion neighbouring the tracheal stoma inevitably offer problems that arise with the obliteration of anterior space of the mediastinum and the creation of new tracheal stoma because of a large defect in the anterior chest skin (Fig. 31.11). Recon-

structive techniques that bring vascularized muscle bulk and healthy skin to the anterior aspect of the dissection constitute the most important part of the procedure for eliminating fracture of the vessel wall that is the most common fatal complication in the surgical management of stage 2A lesions. Pectoralis major or latissimus dorsi myocutaneous flaps are both good enough for this purpose. When using a pectoralis major myocutaneous flap, the skin paddle is designed so that the nipple is located in the centre of the flap; removal of the nipple creates a hole to which the trachea is sutured (Figs 31.12, 31.13). The vascularized muscular tissues cover the vessels to fill up dead spaces in between them; if postoperative radiotherapy is necessary it will be well tolerated.

Stage 2B and stage 3 lesions with involvement of the oesophagus offer an additional problem relating to the

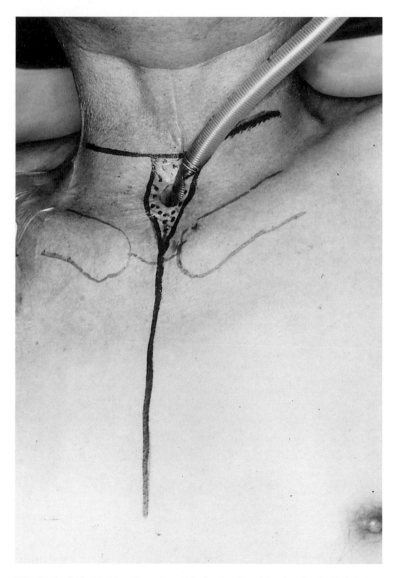

Fig. 31.7 Skin incision for a stage 1 lesion by the author's criteria; it does not involve skin.

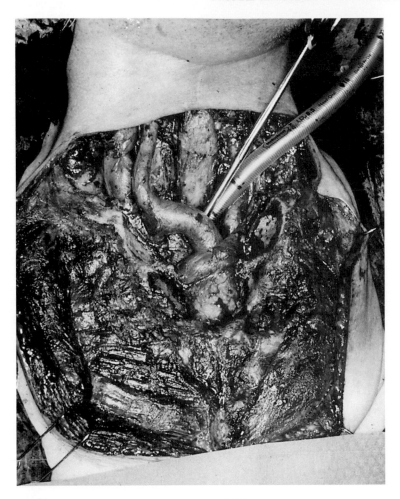

Fig. 31.8   Exposed key tissues after removal of disease.

posterior aspect of mediastinal dissection. Resection of the hypopharynx and oesophagus leaves dead spaces to be obliterated, and dissection of the tracheo-oesophageal party wall may cause a significant complication if the blood supply of the irradiated trachea is compromised. The safest and most effective way of addressing these problems is the blunt, closed, total oesophagectomy with a primary reconstruction by gastric pull-up.[21,30] The stomach provides an excellent, highly vascularized bed for the trachea to prevent possible necrosis, and it also provides bulky tissues for the obliteration of posterior dead spaces. This reconstructive technique requires only one suture line at the base of the tongue; this eliminates

fatal complications originating from a possible salivary fistula in the mediastinum.

Stage 4 lesions with involvement of key tissues in the mediastinum should be considered unresectable. When the disease involves the lower part of the trachea, it may result in an almost total defect of the trachea, which cannot be reconstructed safely. Repair of a part of the vessel wall or the pleura may be established with artificial material (Fig. 31.14), but the total replacement of any major vessels may lead to disasterous complications. Conclusively, patients in this stage should never undergo radical surgery except for short-term airway palliation.

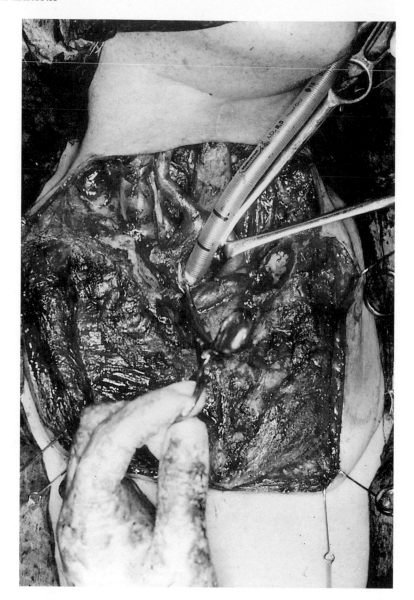

Fig. 31.9 The trachea may be transpositioned to the right of the brachiocephalic artery.

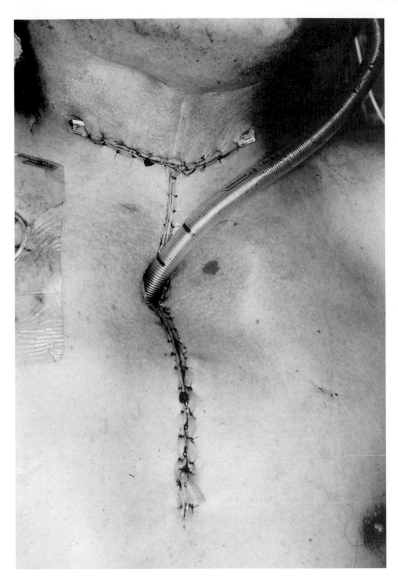

Fig. 31.10 The trachea can be sutured by advancement of skin.

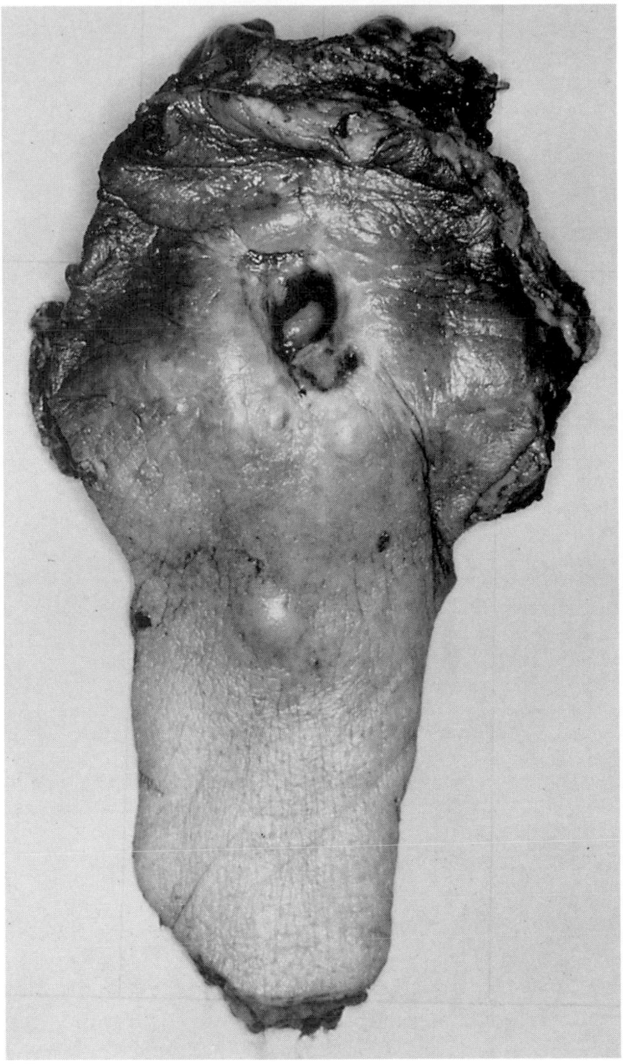

Fig. 31.11 Extirpated stage 2A lesion by the author's criteria; it includes a wider range of anterior chest skin.

COMPLICATIONS

Since the mediastinum is anatomically complicated, and since most patients with stomal recurrence usually have problems of wound healing from previous surgical or radiation therapy, every major complication of head and neck surgery theoretically exists in the surgery for stomal recurrence.[12,14,24,26]

The most frequent — and usually fatal — complication is injury to major blood vessels such as the carotid, subclavian and brachiocephalic arteries and veins, and massive haemorrhage, with subsequent air embolism if veins are involved. The potential for this complication is horrendous, even for experienced surgeons, if these vessels are improperly identified because of scar from previous therapy. Overly aggressive attempts to resect the

lesion often lead to this complication. Prevention depends on meticulous digital or blunt dissections involving careful inspection of the surgical field and anatomical landmarks; these dissections can be accomplished safely only by means of a removal of the sternal manubrium and bilateral heads of the clavicle. This major vessel catastrophe may also occur postoperatively. Where the newly created tracheal stoma is in a lower position, in intimate contact with the brachiocephalic artery, the potential for pressure necrosis of the vessel wall is higher. This is often enhanced by excessive mechanical pressure of a cuffed tracheal cannula for prolonged ventilation, and may result in uncontrollable haemorrhage.

Damage to the pleura is also a frequent intraoperative complication; if undetected it results in pneumothorax. Laceration of the pleura can usually be closed by simple

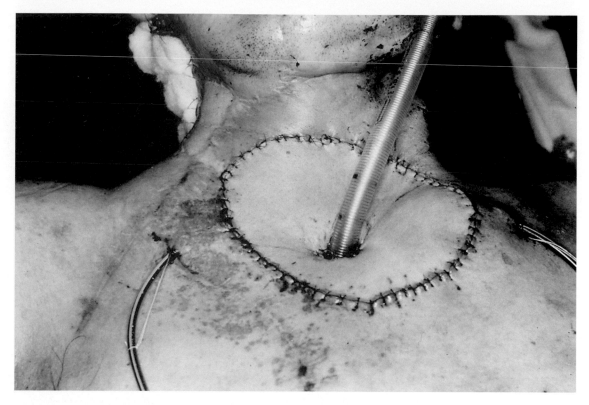

Fig. 31.12 Primary reconstruction of skin defect after removal of stage 2A lesion by pectoralis major myocutaneous flap.

sutures which can be reinforced with the closed-tube thoracotomy.

Chylous leak originates from damage to the thoracic duct; it is often seen in cases of total oesophagectomy. The orientation of the damaged duct may be obscured by scar and blood, but it must be detected and ligated to prevent postoperative chyloma which may compromise suture lines and precipitate electrolyte imbalance.

Infection of the wounds is a major late-postoperative complication which is ascribable to infected haematoma, chyloma, salivary fistula, necrosis of the tracheal party wall or of the muscular tissues that are utilized for reconstruction.

Recently, the pectoralis major or latissimus dorsi myocutaneous flaps have often been utilized for reconstructing anterior chest skin and also for preventing these complications. The vascularized myocutaneous flap is certainly effective, and the incidence of major complications has been decreasing, though minor flap necrosis was reported in about 10% of the patients.[14] The flap necrosis almost always originated from insufficient venous drainage, which may be potentiated by synergistically progressing infections beneath the flap. Continuous

suction drainage, such as haemovacs, certainly diminishes this potential problem due to fluid accumulation, but if active infection is suspected, the wound must be immediately opened, washed daily with saline and drained thoroughly.

Pneumothorax and pulmonary collapse are also fatal postoperative complications which are usually observed in patients in poor general condition. Ineffective cough compromises satisfactory mucous drainage, which must be cleaned by the use of a fibrescope. Closed-tube thoracotomy is mandatory for these complications.

PREVENTION

The morbidity and mortality of mediastinal dissection have certainly been decreasing owing to the refinements in surgical procedure. However, the 5-year survival rate still remains at an unsatisfactory level, which may suggest that the management of stomal recurrence should focus on prevention. In 1984 Komiyama et al[9] reported that the preoperative use of FAR (a combination of 5-FU, vitamin A and radiation) therapy was prophylactically

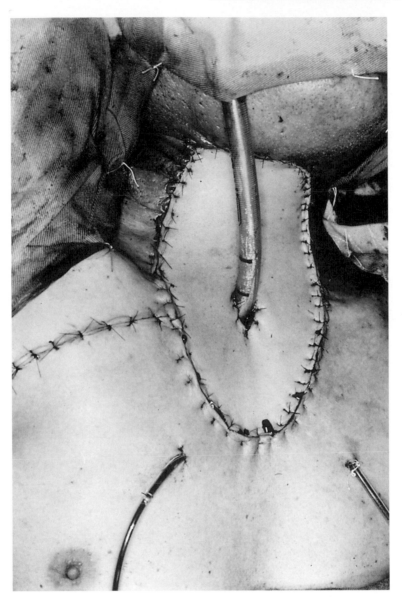

Fig. 31.13   The same type of reconstruction as shown in Fig. 31.12 by latissimus dorsi myocutaneous flap.

effective against stomal recurrence for patients with emergency tracheotomy. In 1988 Breneman et al[5] reported their experience of the treatment of emergency tracheotomies with 20 Gy of prelaryngectomy radiation, in 5 fractions, in an attempt to decrease the incidence of stomal recurrence. They showed a quite acceptable rate of stomal recurrence, but a higher (56%) incidence of overall local recurrence than that reported in most series of similar tumours; they recommended an alternative treatment policy using a planned course of moderate- to high-dose postoperative radiation for sterilizing tumours in the entire locoregional area, including the tracheostoma.

In 1987 Kotwall et al[10] reported that 90% of 387 patients with head and neck carcinomas who died of distant metastasis still had uncontrolled tumour at the primary site or in the neck in spite of having undergone aggressive surgery and radiotherapy for the primary tumour and cervical lymph nodes, and that the second highest incidence of metastases were found in the mediastinal nodes. They suggested these were not true metastases, but instead might represent residual recurrent disease harboured in lymphatic channels between the neck and mediastinum, and they concluded that more mediastinal dissections should be performed at the time of laryngectomy in cases of T3N+ and T4Nx laryngeal carcinomas. Sisson[22] also stated that there is substantial evidence that the mediastinal dissection should be performed in subglottic laryngeal carcinoma when the disease extends 1–1.5 cm below the level of the vocal cord. He recommended preoperative exploration of the mediastinum using

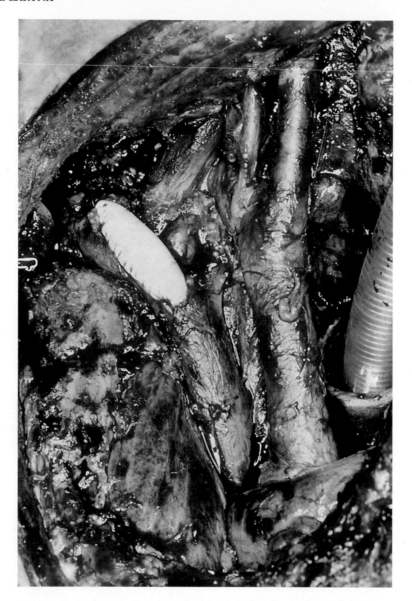

Fig. 31.14 Reconstruction with artificial material after partial removal of the right brachiocephalic vein.

the gated MRI scan and mediastinoscopy. If the results are positive, his treatment policy is a surgical salvage by mediastinal dissection followed by early postoperative radiotherapy.

The surgery for stomal recurrence, by mediastinal dissection, especially in advanced stages, has been fraught with significant morbidity and mortality; however, morbidity and mortality are decreasing owing to refinements in the ablative technique and advances in the reconstructive technique with the use of myocutaneous flaps.

Though the overall prognosis of these patients still remains dismal, the results of surgical salvage for patients at earlier stages have been progressing, and further refinements of treatment modalities are to be expected.

REFERENCES

1. Amatsu M, Makino K, Kinishi M 1985 Stomal recurrence; etiologic factors and prevention. Auris Nasus Larynx 12: 103–110
2. Balm A J, Snow G B, Karim A B, Versluis R J, Njo K H, Tiwari R M 1986 Long-term results of concurrent polychemotherapy and radiotherapy in patients with stomal recurrence after total laryngectomy. Ann Otol Rhinol Laryngol 95: 572–575
3. Barr G D, Robertson A G, Liu K C 1990 Stomal recurrence: a separate entity? J Surg Oncol 44: 176–179
4. Biller H F, Krespi Y P, Lawson W 1980 A one stage flap reconstruction following resection for stomal recurrence. Otolaryngol Head Neck Surg 88: 357–360
5. Breneman J C, Bradshaw A, Gluckman J, Aron B S 1988 Prevention of stomal recurrence in patients requiring emergency tracheotomy for advanced laryngeal and pharyngeal tumors. Cancer 62: 802–805
6. Burnstein F D, Calcaterra T C 1987 The pectoralis major myocutaneous flap: Use in surgery of the lower neck and superior mediastinum. Arch Otolaryngol Head Neck Surg 113: 73–77
7. Gluckman J L, Hamaker R C, Schuller D E, Weissler M C, Charles G A 1987 Surgical salvage for stomal recurrence: a multi-institutional experience. Laryngoscope 97: 1025–1029
8. Keim W F, Shapiro M J, Rosen H 1965 Study of post-laryngectomy stomal recurrences. Arch Otolaryngol 81: 183–186
9. Komiyama S, Watanabe H, Yanagita T, Kuwano M, Hiroto I 1984 Inhibition of stomal recurrence in laryngectomy with preoperative FAR therapy. A statistical evaluation. Auris Nasus Larynx 11: 43–49
10. Kotwall C, Sako K, Razack M S 1987 Metastatic patterns in squamous cell cancer of the head and neck. Am J Surg 154: 439–442
11. Krespi Y P, Wurster C F, Sisson G A 1985 Immediate reconstruction after total laryngopharyngoesophagectomy and mediastinal dissection. Laryngoscope 95: 156–161
12. Krespi Y P, Wurster C F, Wang T D 1985 Hypoparathyroidism following total laryngopharyngectomy and gastric pull-up. Laryngoscope 95: 1184–1187
13. Mantravadi R, Katz A M, Skolnik E M, Becker S, Freehling D J, Friedman M 1981 Stomal recurrence. A critical analysis of risk factors. Arch Otolaryngol 107: 735–738
14. Myers E M 1983 Complications in surgery for stomal recurrences. Laryngoscope 93: 285–288
15. Myers E M, Ogura J H 1979 Stomal recurrences: a clinico-pathological analysis and protocol for future management. Laryngoscope 89: 1121–1128
16. Rockley T J, Powell J, Robin P E, Reid AP 1991 Post-laryngectomy stomal recurrence: tumor implantation or paratracheal lymphatic metastasis? Clin Otolaryngol 16: 43–47
17. Rubin J, Johnson J T, Myers E N 1990 Stomal recurrence after laryngectomy: interrelated risk factor study. Otolaryngol Head Neck Surg 103: 805–812
18. Sato F, Saito H, Hisa Y, Mizukoshi O 1984 Characteristics of 60 laryngeal carcinomas with subglottic extension. Jpn J Otolaryngol 87: 813–816
19. Schuller D E, Hamaker R C, Gluckman J L 1981 Mediastinal dissection: a multi-institutional assessment. Arch Otolaryngol 107: 715–720
20. Sisson G A 1972 Mediastinal dissection for stomal recurrence. In: Conley J J, Dickinson J E (eds.) Reconstruction and obliteration of upper mediastinum. Proceedings of the first International Symposium, 2nd edn. Grune & Stratton, New York
21. Sisson G A 1985 Mediastinal dissection — resectability and curability of stomal recurrence after total laryngectomy. Auris Nasus Larynx 12: 61–66
22. Sisson G A 1989 Ogura memorial lecture: mediastinal dissection. Laryngoscope 99: 1262–1266
23. Sisson G A, Goldman M E 1981 Pectoral myocutaneous island flap for reconstruction of stomal recurrence. Arch Otolaryngol 107: 446–449
24. Sisson G A, Vander Aarde S B 1971 Control of hypoparathyroidism after extensive neck surgery. Arch Otolaryngol 93: 249–255
25. Sisson G A, Bytell D E, Edison B D 1975 Transsternal radical neck dissection (mediastinal approach) (Ch 6). In: Anderson R, Hoopes J (eds) Symposium on malignancies of the head and neck. Saunders, Philadelphia
26. Sisson G A, Edison B D, Bytell D E 1975 Trans-sternal radical neck dissection: postoperative complications and management. Arch Otolaryngol 101: 46–49
27. Sisson G A, Straehly C J, Johnson N E 1962 Mediastinal dissection for recurrent cancer after laryngectomy. Laryngoscope 72: 1064–1077
28. Stell P M, van den Broek P 1971 Stomal recurrence following laryngectomy. J Laryngol Otol 85: 131–140
29. Uchida M, Kawabata K, Shimizu S 1989 Management of stomal recurrences. JOHNS (Tokyo) 4: 1331–1336
30. Ujiki G T, Pearl G J, Poticha S 1987 Mortality and morbidity of gastric pull-up for replacement of the pharyngoesophagus. Arch Surg 122: 644–647

32. Management of complications of surgical intervention

E. N. Myers, A. C. Urquhart

INTRODUCTION

Billroth carried out the first laryngectomy for the treatment of cancer of the larynx 120 years ago. However, even today, cancer of the larynx remains a challenging problem for the patient as well as the surgeon. In recent years, scientific information has helped considerably in our understanding of the aetiology and biological behaviour of these cancers. There has been tremendous activity in the improvement of surgical techniques. Partial laryngeal surgery for conservation of the voice, various procedures for the reconstruction of the pharynx, as well as rehabilitation of the voice following total laryngectomy are relatively recent advances that continue to generate much interest.

Complications of any surgical procedure are detrimental to the patient and disturbing for the surgeon. In any substantial series of cases of laryngeal cancer surgery, complications will occur. There is, however, no doubt that the incidence can be kept to a minimum by good patient selection and meticulous surgical technique. Before discussing these complications and their management, it is important to emphasize certain surgical and oncological principles in the treatment of cancer of the larynx. One may then have a better understanding as to why these complications occur and be in a more favourable position to prevent them.

GENERAL CONSIDERATIONS IN THE PREVENTION OF COMPLICATIONS

Patient selection and assessment

The majority of cancers arising in the larynx are epidermoid or squamous cell carcinomas. These arise from the mucosal surfaces and, as they grow, they may involve different structures in the larynx, producing various symptoms. During the initial visit, a careful and thorough history and physical examination are mandatory and cannot be over-emphasized. Otalgia, dysphagia, voice changes, breathing and articulation problems may all give important clues as to local tumour spread. Direct laryngoscopy, utilizing the operating microscope, allows precise evaluation, particularly of early cancers. Such information is fundamental to precise surgical planning. The use of oesophagoscopy and bronchoscopy in addition to laryngoscopy have been most useful in ruling out synchronous second primary cancers of the air and food passages. Radiological investigations such as MRI and CT scanning, all have their advocates, but none are as important as direct physical, microsurgical examination.

Cancer of the larynx usually occurs in males with a long history of tobacco and, in some patients, alcohol use. Apart from the often poor medical and psychological condition of these patients, the local effect of the cancer may cause chronic aspiration, local pain and difficulty in swallowing and communicating. In the preoperative evaluation, all of these factors need to be carefully considered. The patient's motivation must be evaluated. Many are alcoholics with a poor self-image and a weak support system, and are not candidates for any but the most straightforward surgical procedure with the lowest potential morbidity. The age of the patient should also be considered. Most elderly patients are usually not good candidates for supraglottic laryngectomy due to problems with deglutition and aspiration which follow surgery. The patient's social situation should be evaluated, not only because of the need to comply with all the aspects of the treatment programme, but also for them to attend postoperative follow-up examinations.

Preoperative management of any type of laryngeal surgery should include a careful evaluation of the patient's respiratory function. Most patients with cancer of the larynx have chronic bronchitis and chronic obstructive pulmonary disease secondary to years of cigarette smoking. Patients with compromised respiratory function on physical examination as well as pulmonary function tests, should not be considered for partial laryngeal surgery because of the enormous difficulties they have in rehabilitation.

Many patients are in the older age group and also have associated diabetes mellitus, arteriosclerotic heart disease and cirrhosis of the liver. Hypothyroidism may occur in patients who have had full-course radiation therapy for carcinoma of the larynx, and thyroid function tests should be performed.[23] The patient whose history includes aspirin ingestion, either as an anticoagulant or in the treatment of arthritis, should discontinue taking this medication at least one week prior to surgery because of possible interference with the coagulation mechanism.

Nutrition is a very important aspect of management in cancer of the larynx.[6] As discussed above, many of the patients will present in a malnourished state. Unfortunately, parameters to measure nutrition have not clearly evolved; however, the presence of more than 10–16 pounds of weight loss, a serum albumin of less than 3.2 mg (%) and anergy to skin tests may be present in the severely malnourished patient. The history of weight loss and appearance of the patient are still today the most accurate ways of assessing the patient's state of nourishment. It is very important to correct malnutrition so as to ensure that the patient is in a positive nitrogen balance and therefore optimize wound healing.

The dental examination should be a routine part of the patient's preoperative evaluation. The presence of caries, fractured teeth, or severe periodontal disease should be diagnosed and treated prior to definitive laryngeal surgery. Periodontal disease may predispose to anaerobic wound infections during the postoperative period. Patients with advanced cancers usually require postoperative radiation therapy, and, in order to avoid osteoradionecrosis or radiation caries, the dentition should be in the best possible condition. All extractions should be carried out prior to, or at the same time as, the definitive surgical treatment.

The patient's hearing and communication skills should be evaluated. All patients with laryngeal surgery will be deprived of their speech for some time. We still deal with some illiterate patients who will not be able to communicate postoperatively by writing. Sign boards may be helpful for these patients. It may be worthwhile having a demonstration of the various types of mechanical speaking devices in order to allow the patient to become familiar with these prior to surgery. A visit from a patient who has undergone a laryngectomy and has developed good speech may also be inspiring to the patient about to undergo total laryngectomy.

Surgical technique

Before discussing postoperative complications and their management, we will provide details of the intraoperative techniques we use in order to maximize good results and avoid complications. There can be no doubt that good surgical technique forms an integral part in the prevention of complications.

In all laryngeal surgical procedures, tracheotomy is carried out either under local anaesthetic prior to induction of general anaesthesia or just after general anaesthesia has been induced. The patient is placed in the supine position with a folded towel or blanket under the shoulder in order to extend the neck. Local anaesthetic with epinephrine is injected prior to the prepping and draping in order to allow vasoconstriction to occur. The tracheotomy is carried out through a small transverse incision. In the event that a tracheotomy has been previously performed for partial surgery or for airway distress, the skin surrounding the tracheotomy should be completely excised since this area must be considered potentially contaminated with tumour. Also, an existing tracheotomy is certainly infected and will not heal.

In patients with total laryngectomy, without radical neck dissection, we use a U-shaped flap extending from the lateral aspect of the hyoid bone on each side to the suprasternal notch just medial to the sternocleidomastoid muscle. If a radical neck dissection is included, an incision is made from the mastoid tip, just below the medial border of the trapezius muscle, with the horizontal limb running just above the clavicle as far as the contralateral sternocleidomastoid muscle. When bilateral neck dissections are done with the laryngectomy, an apron flap is fashioned by carrying the above-described incision to the contralateral mastoid tip. The platysma muscle is included in the U-flap for total laryngectomy, but is not included in the neck flaps for radical neck dissections. In the event that there has been previous partial surgery, or when there is tumour fungating through the skin, the skin over the larynx is included with the specimen (Fig. 32.1).

The classical technique for wide-field laryngectomy is well known and will not be repeated here. There are, however, several modifications that may be utilized in order to conserve as much mucosa as possible for closure of the pharynx. If the tumour does not involve the epiglottis, then a great deal of mucosa can be preserved. This is done by identifying the lingual aspect of the epiglottis once the hyoid bone has been excised and the supraglottic musculature transected. The epiglottis is grasped with a tenaculum and the mucosa identified. Dissection is continued until the tip of the epiglottis is identified. At this point, submucoperichondrial dissection is carried down along the laryngeal surface of the epiglottis and the aryepiglottic fold. The mucosa can then be transected and the pharynx entered. This technique provides several additional centimeters of mucosa which can be utilized for pharyngeal closure. Preservation of the mucosa should not, of course, be done at the expense of tumour clearance. If the lesion does not involve the pyriform sinus, then this mucosa should be preserved for pharyngeal closure. When the constrictor muscles are transected, the superior horn of the thyroid cartilage should be identified and the mucosa separated from this, thus preserving pyriform sinus mucosa. Several additional centimetres of mucosa can be preserved by elevation of the mucosa of the hypopharynx at the time the trachea is transected and separated from the cervical oesophagus and pharynx. The dissection should be carried up to the level of the arytenoid cartilages before the mucosa is incised. If the above techniques are utilized, and they usually can be with endolaryngeal lesions, then there is usually adequate mucosa to close in a vertical straight line, without tension, thus helping to ensure primary healing. If there is not sufficient pharyngeal mucosa for a straight line closure, then the usual 'T' closure should be carried out. The pharynx is closed using a 3–0 chromic continuous Connell stitch. An additional layer of closure, continuous or interrupted, is desirable if there is sufficient mucosa. There are some surgeons who do not close the constrictor muscles as an additional layer, feeling that this may leave an inadequate pharyngeal lumen and in some patients with tracheo-oesophageal puncture may predispose to 'spasm' and inadequate voicing. Other surgeons feel, however, that this is essential in order to strengthen the pharyngeal closure and ensure primary healing.[6] The weakest point of the 'T' closure is at the area where the horizontal and vertical limbs come together.[20] If there is sufficient mucosa so that there is no tension in this closure, then primary healing should occur.

Patients with cancer involving the base of the tongue and the hypopharynx often have postoperative healing problems because of closure with inadequate tissue. In such patients, the pharynx is closed primarily under considerable tension and postoperative pharyngocutaneous fistula may occur. The pharynx usually then heals by second intention and scar contracture then provides the patient with complete or partial pharyngeal stenosis with resulting difficulty in swallowing. Two recent innovations have been useful in preventing these complications. Calcaterra[5] has described a transverse flap composed of mucosa and some muscle of the base of the tongue based on the side of the resection of the pharyngeal mucosa. The tissue is transposed into the defect to add additional mucosa for closure. The author has described good results in preventing fistula formation and stenosis. Tucker et al[28] have described the use of a trapezius myocutaneous flap to augment the amount of tissue for closure in patients who have had hypopharyngeal or base of tongue resections.

During total laryngectomy, the lobe of the thyroid on the side of predominant tumour involvement is usually removed and the contralateral lobe is preserved. Every effort should be made to do this, without sacrificing tumour clearance, in order to avoid hypothyroidism.[23] The thyroid lobe should be tacked laterally under the sternocleidomastoid muscle with several sutures so that it is not mistaken in the follow-up phase as an area of tumour recurrence.

A technique for reconstructing the tracheostoma has been published previously.[21] It is important to resect the subcutaneous adipose tissue to a level approximately 3 cm inferior to the tracheostoma in the suprasternal notch area. An ellipse of skin is also excised later, inferior and superior to the stoma to avoid redundant skin. The cartilage should be covered by the skin on the closure to avoid the formation of granulation tissue. We usually utilize 3–0 chromic catgut for tracheostoma closure. These sutures do not need to be removed. Patients who have received preoperative radiation therapy or who will receive postoperative radiation therapy are at risk of developing tracheostoma stenosis. We avoid this by splitting the posterior membranous tracheal wall and transposing a small local flap into the area. This breaks up the circle formed by the tracheostoma and eliminates the possibility of concentric narrowing.[21] This should not be performed in patients undergoing immediate tracheo-oesophageal puncture and is now reserved for patients who later develop stenosis which fails to respond to conservative therapy.

Classically, a nasogastric tube is inserted into the pharynx prior to its closure, in order to provide a means of nourishing the patient in the immediate postoperative period. The wound should be irrigated at the time that meticulous hemostasis has been obtained prior to pharyngeal closure. A second irrigation of the wound should be carried out after the pharyngeal closure has been accomplished and the salivary system has been separated from the clean soft tissue of the neck. Some surgeons have claimed good success with few complications in carrying out cervical oesophagostomy below the level of the pharyngeal closure and bringing the nasogastric tube out through a separate incision.[25] If the tube should fall out prior to complete healing, it should not be re-inserted. The possibility of pushing the tube through the healing pharyngeal suture line may predispose to fistula formation.

We employ clear plastic haemovac suction drains and pressure dressings. We feel that the addition of a pressure dressing is helpful in eliminating flap oedema. In addition, the pressure of the cervical skin against the pharyngeal closure may be useful in some cases in which a pharyngeal seal has not been obtained.

A #8 shiley plastic laryngectomy tube is inserted into the tracheostoma at the end of the procedure, prior to the application of the pressure dressing. This should be a cuffed tube in the event that the patient requires postoperative ventilatory assistance. If the U-shaped flap has been utilized, the usual tracheostomy tapes are securely tied. If, however, a radical neck dissection has been included with the total laryngectomy, the breast plate of the laryngectomy tube is sewn to the skin, using two silk sutures on each side and the tracheotomy tapes are discarded. This is done to avoid pressure necrosis of

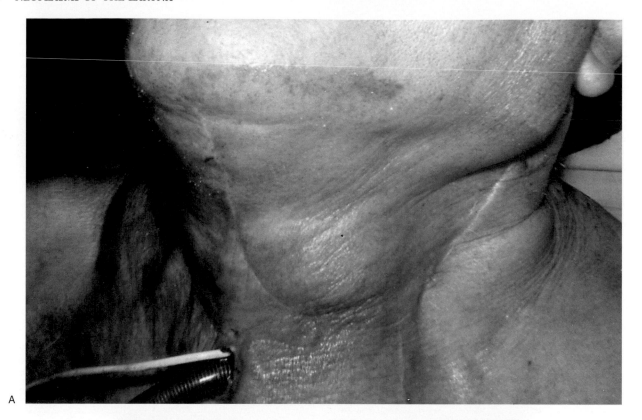

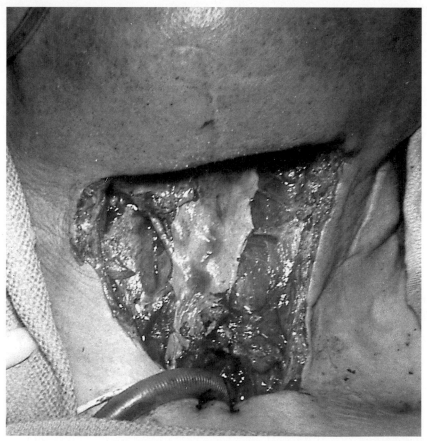

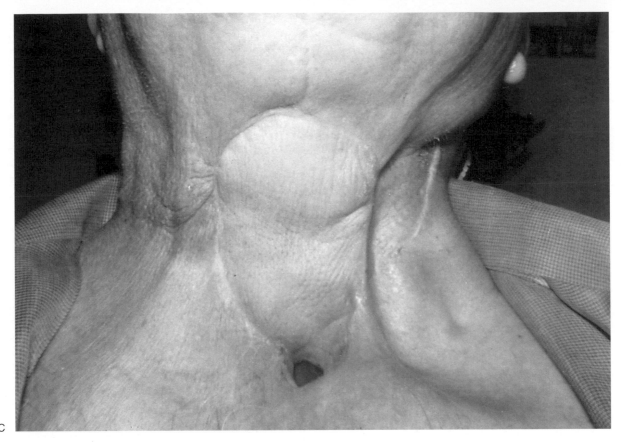

Fig. 32.1 A. (*opposite page, top*) Recurrence of cancer of the larynx following radiation and partial laryngeal surgery and radical neck dissection. B. (*opposite page, bottom*) Patient following laryngectomy and removal of skin overlying larynx. C. (*above*) Appearance of patient following healing of pedicle flap.

the vertical limb of the cervical skin flap by the tapes from the laryngectomy tube. The pressure dressings are applied after the tube has been placed.

Postoperatively, the patient is placed in a sitting position with the haemovac drains attached to wall suction. The pressure dressing is not changed until the haemovac drains are removed, unless there is reason to suspect a complication, either because of the patient's physical examination, or because of the appearance of saliva, purulent exudate, or chyle in the haemovac drains. A high humidification collar should be placed over the laryngectomy tube and frequent suctioning must be carried out.

If there is no evidence of fistula formation, patients who have not previously been radiated are fed by mouth, after removal of the nasogastric tube, on the seventh postoperative day. Those who have been radiated are fed on the tenth or fourteenth postoperative day, since fistula formation may occur later in radiated patients.

Antibiotic prophylaxis is imperative for any contaminated oncological procedure of the head and neck[3,16] and broad-spectrum antibiotics with coverage against anaerobic organisms should be used.[16] The antibiotics should be administered intravenously a few hours prior to surgery and continued until 24 hours after surgery (three doses). Patients undergoing total laryngectomy with partial pharyngectomy or extended supraglottic laryngectomy, when a lot of mucosa is excised, appear to be at an increased risk for wound infection. However, preoperative radiation therapy[4,14] or tracheotomy[4] do not appear to be associated with an increased risk of wound infection in patients undergoing major contaminated head and neck procedures. The most common mechanism leading to wound infection in patients on antibiotic prophylaxis is persistent contamination of the wound with secretions from the oropharynx.[22]

Patients who have more advanced primary disease may require a laryngopharyngectomy. Reconstruction with pectoralis major myocutaneous flaps[1] or pharyngogastric anastomosis[13] is used primarily in some centres. We prefer to use the jejunal free graft, utilizing microvascular anastomosis performed by our plastic surgery colleagues. This provides an excellent pharyngeal lumen.[12] Patients can be fed immediately postoperatively through a feeding jejunostomy. Postoperative radiation therapy seems to be well tolerated by the jejunal interposition grafts.

If the tumour extends into the cervical oesophagus and the resection includes the thoracic oesophagus, jejunal interposition cannot be used. In such cases we utilize a gastric pull-up with pharyngogastric anastomosis. Primary swallowing is achieved in the majority of patients in both gastric pull-ups and jejunal interpositions.[11] Selected patients may also have tracheo-oesophageal (gastric) puncture for voice restoration.

Supraglottic laryngectomy is most successful in those patients with lesions confined to the supraglottic larynx. As mentioned earlier, patients who are to undergo this surgery should be well motivated, have limited lesions, and have reasonably good pulmonary function. Incorrect selection of these patients may make their lives miserable by subjecting them to supraglottic surgery when they would be far more comfortable, have an easier time with rehabilitation, and have excellent tumour clearance with total laryngectomy. The supraglottic laryngectomy is usually carried out in conjunction with bilateral neck dissections. We utilize the same flap as described for total laryngectomy with radical neck dissection, which provides excellent exposure and circulation. Meticulous attention to technique is imperative. It is important to preserve the perichondrium of the thyroid cartilage for later closure. It is almost impossible to dissect the perichondrium from the midline without tearing it, and the remainder of the perichondrial flap should be kept intact. The cartilage cuts should be made with an electric saw. No matter what the location of the lesion, we cut the cartilage at the same level all the way across the entire thyroid cartilage: in males, approximately one-half the distance from the thyroid notch to the cricothyroid membrane, and one-third of the distance in females. The soft tissue cuts should begin just anterior to the vocal process of the arytenoid cartilage on the side of the tumour, with one blade in the previously accomplished cartilage cut. The tip of the epiglottis, when possible, and the aryepiglottic fold should be grasped with a tenaculum and spread so that adequate visualization may be carried out. There may be a temptation to leave the false cords when they are not involved with tumour. This is an error in judgement, however, since leaving the false vocal cords will lead to postoperative oedema and airway problems. Extension of a classical supraglottic laryngectomy to encompass lesions involving the tongue base and the pharynx will require certain modifications of the above technique. If one arytenoid cartilage is taken, then it is mandatory that the vocal cord be sutured into the midline in order to minimize postoperative aspiration and enhance the quality of the voice. Closure should be accomplished by suturing the perichondrium to the base of the tongue and not to the residual mucosa. The mucosa may be draped over the anterior commissure. The second layer should be carried out sewing the strap muscles to the base of the tongue. We always utilize a cricopharyngeal myotomy to minimize aspiration and to assist with the swallowing function. Caution should be exercised to avoid injury to the recurrent laryngeal nerve during this procedure. It takes approximately three weeks for the oedema in the area of the glottis to subside in order for the patient to be decannulated. This varies with the individual and decannulation should await the development of an adequate airway. Once the tracheal fistula closes, the swallowing act is retrained. This requires an adequate cough mechanism, which is a reflection of the patient's pulmonary reserve. This is the primary reason for selecting only those patients with adequate pulmonary reserve for this surgical procedure.

Vertical partial laryngectomy is a very successful surgical procedure which may be applied in carefully selected cases. We try to select those cases of glottic carcinoma which will be predictable failures with radiation therapy. This includes those patients with extension of glottic carcinoma to the vocal process or the anterior commissure, or with subglottic extension less than 10 mm, or patients who have verrucous carcinoma. All of the above patients have mobile cords. If the patient has failed radiation therapy for the above-described lesions, they still remain candidates for vertical partial laryngectomy. We do not perform vertical hemilaryngectomy in patients with fixation of the vocal cord. As stated previously, it is essential to select patients by utilizing meticulous examination with microlaryngoscopy in order to avoid the possibility of having to convert a proposed partial laryngectomy to a total laryngectomy during or after the surgical procedure. If we are quite certain that a partial procedure can be carried out, we utilize a transverse incision in the relaxed skin tension line just overlying the thyroid notch. If we feel there is a possibility for conversion to total laryngectomy at the time of surgery, we utilize a U-shaped flap as described earlier. After undermining the skin flaps, the strap muscles may be split in the midline and undermined in order to expose the thyroid cartilage, or incised at the level of the hyoid bone as is done in a supraglottic laryngectomy. Regardless of this aspect of the technique, the perichondrium overlying the thyroid cartilage is undermined and preserved for later closure. We usually separate constrictor muscles from the thyroid lamina and expose the superior horn of the thyroid cartilage by separating the pyriform sinus mucosa from it. The cartilage cut is made with an electric saw, usually several millimetres off the midline contralateral to the tumour. Transection of the base of the epiglottis superiorly then allows excellent exposure and inspection of the interior of the larynx in order to make the proper soft-tissue cuts. After removal, inspection and frozen section control of the specimen, meticulous haemostasis is obtained. The cut edges of mucosa near the cricoid cartilage are covered with a mucosal flap advanced from the pyriform sinus. This also aids in the later formation of a pseudocord, which makes for a somewhat stronger voice. Primary glottic carcinomas that involve both cords, but in which adequate resection will leave the body of one arytenoid intact, may be reconstructed using epiglottic laryngoplasty (Kambic procedure).[17] It is ideal for reconstruction of an extended frontolateral vertical hemilaryngectomy since the procedure provides structural cartilaginous support and complete epithelial coverage. There are numerous other reconstructive techniques which may be carried out intraoperatively in order to ensure good voice function. The wound is then irrigated both before and after closure of the strap muscles and haemovac drains are placed in the subcutaneous tissue. Antibiotic coverage is utilized and the care of the tracheotomy and nasogastric feedings are as described earlier.

COMPLICATIONS OF SURGICAL INTERVENTION AND THEIR MANAGEMENT

We have emphasized patient selection and assessment as well as surgical technique in the prevention of complications. Unfortunately, no matter how careful and meticulous the surgeon is, complications will occasionally occur. It is difficult to divide these problems into specific groups, but from a practical point of view, some complications will occur earlier than others. There is no specific time frame for this division, but we have grouped complications into 'early' and 'late'. Generally, the early complications are those that occur while the patient is still in the hospital, before discharge, three to ten days after surgery. One must be aware of the possibility of these complications occurring during this period as prompt medical or surgical intervention is often required. Complications occurring later are usually diagnosed during follow-up visits when the patient's well-being and ability to cope are impaired. Careful questioning and patience may be required to elicit these problems in people that are already compromised in their ability to communicate. While 'early' and 'late' complications may well occur in partial laryngeal surgery, a separate note is made regarding problems specific to these procedures.

'Early' complications

Haematoma may be noticed by a mass forming in the neck. Excessive blood in the haemovac drains over the first 24-hour period may also provide evidence of haematoma formation. If a pressure dressing is in place, the combination of excessive blood in the haemovac drains and ecchymosis forming over the upper chest wall are both direct and indirect evidence of haematoma formation. This complication can usually be prevented by meticulous attention to haemostasis during the surgery, using silk suture material and electrocautery. The use of

the Shaw scalpel or cutting cautery with its ability to coagulate bleeding surfaces has also helped in the prevention of haematoma. The treatment of postoperative haematoma requires that the patient be returned to the operating room, the wound opened, and the bleeding area identified and ligated. Very often, no specific site of bleeding is found, but once the clot is evacuated, copious irrigation of the wound must follow in order to prevent postoperative infection. The haemovac and pressure dressing are then replaced. Failure to drain adequately the haematoma may lead to an increased rate of wound dehiscence, major infection and fistula formation.[15]

Flap necrosis occurs more commonly in patients who are poorly nourished or have had postoperative radiation therapy, or both. Knowledge of the blood supply of the neck is important for the design of the skin flap and incisions. The arterial vasculature of cervical skin flaps has been investigated in cadavers using silicone rubber injections.[24] From these studies, it has been stressed that the horizontal limb of an incision should lie between the carotid and subclavian watershed, the upper flap should be larger than the lower flap, and the platysma should remain attached to the flap. In all cases of radical neck dissection, however, we leave platysma on the specimen in order to provide an additional cuff of muscle around tumour but respect the subdermal plexus in order to preserve circulation of the flap. The U-shaped incision described earlier for total laryngectomy is very reliable with little chance of flap necrosis. Trifurcations should be avoided (Fig. 32.2). Sewing in the laryngectomy tube, as described above, in patients who have had neck dissections, is helpful in avoiding partial flap necrosis. Most of these problems require local debridement and wound cleansing with healing by secondary intention. Large defects with possible exposure of vessels may require operative intervention with some form of cover, either a skin graft, a fascia cutaneous or myocutaneous flap (Fig. 32.3).

The formation of an unplanned salivary fistula is the most common cause of prolonged postoperative morbidity following total laryngectomy.[27] Pharyngocutaneous fistula is most commonly caused by closure of the pharyngeal wound under tension due to inadequate tissue for closure due to resection of tumour. The leakage of saliva may contaminate the wound, leading to infection in the area, with the potential for further tissue destruction and enlargement of the fistula. Other predisposing factors in fistula formation include radiation therapy with obliterative endarteritis and lack of good tissue quality, foreign bodies such as silk suture material or devitalized tissue, and persistent tumour.[9] The frequency of fistula formation is, however, directly proportional to compulsive compliance with the highest concept of surgical craftsmanship.[8] If the pharyngeal mucosa is closed properly, there is very little chance that a fistula will

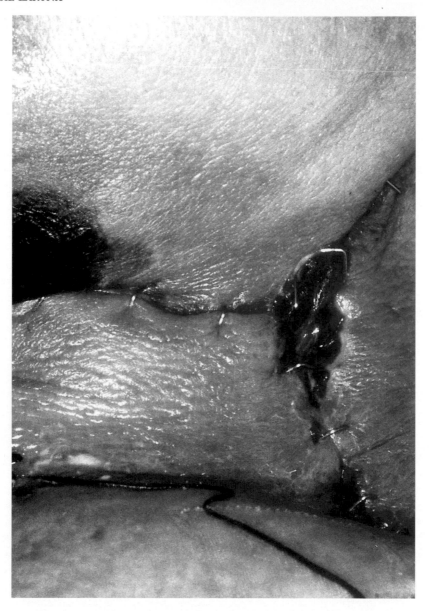

Fig. 32.2 Trifurcations may result in skin necrosis and wound breakdown.

occur. Pharyngocutaneous fistulas occurring very shortly postoperatively are almost all due to errors in technique. The typical fistula will usually occur within one week of surgery. In patients who have been irradiated, fistula may appear up to three weeks following surgery. Fistula formation may first be suspected by the appearance of saliva in the haemovac drains or heralded by the appearance of erythema and oedema in the skin of the anterior neck. Temperature elevation may also be present. This will usually then progress to an infection in the neck which may form an abscess, or may present as leakage of saliva in the area around the superior aspect of the tracheostoma. This is due to saliva tracking down along the anterior aspect of the pharyngeal closure and surfacing at the point of least resistance in the area of the closure of the tracheostoma.

A small pharyngeal fistula will usually close spontaneously within several weeks by simply maintaining gentle pressure with a neck dressing and feeding through a nasogastric tube. However, if there is infection in the neck, the wound must be cultured and the appropriate antibiotics used. If an abscess has formed, it must be drained and treated. If a radical neck dissection has been done in continuity with a total laryngectomy, it is important to prevent infection of the neck because of the potential for carotid artery rupture. Gram-negative and anaerobic organisms are always present, and antibiotics must be utilized. In this situation, a counter-drain in the area of the fistula should be utilized to prevent leakage into the dissected neck. It is sometimes of use to sew the skin to the open pharyngeal mucosa in order to divert the salivary stream onto, rather than under, the cervical skin flaps. In those cases where pharyngeal fistula has formed due to closure under tension with inadequate mucosa, healing by secondary intention will usually provide a certain degree of stenosis that will interfere with the patient's swallowing. This may be further accentuated by postoperative radiation therapy. The development of such problems may be at least partially alleviated by dilatation.

A large pharyngocutaneous fistula, especially when the skin has been sewn to the mucosal edges, must usually be reconstructed by transposing fresh, healthy tissue into the wound.[20] This is done after the infection has subsided and the wound has matured. Various techniques, including the deltopectoral flap and other local flaps have been used in the past. A newer and preferred technique which may be carried out in one stage is that of the pectoralis major myocutaneous flap, in which the skin paddle is split, one half is used for inner epithelial lining and the other for external skin coverage. This flap may also be utilized in those cases requiring excision of cervical skin for tumour clearance. More recently, jejunal interposition may be the best modality for rehabilitation of swallowing in patients with persistent fistula or stricture that fails to respond to traditional management[10] (Fig. 32.4).

Wound infection after head and neck surgery remains a common problem. The incidence varies from study to study, but certainly the use of antibiotic prophylaxis is mandatory. In our laryngectomy patients, prophylaxis is initiated prior to surgery and prolonged administration of antibiotics beyond the first 24 hours is unnecessary, unless there is some other reason to complete a full course of antibiotic therapy. The most common reason for infection is persistent postoperative contamination of the wound with oropharyngeal secretions.[22] The meticulous attention to closure of the pharynx discussed earlier can only be re-emphasized. Usually these cases present after 48 hours of surgery as erythema around the suture line. Postoperative wound infections are usually polymicrobial with aerobic and anaerobic organisms. Suitable antibiotic therapy should be directed towards these organisms.

During laryngeal surgery, one lobe of the thyroid gland is usually preserved, thereby decreasing the chances of hypocalcaemia. If, however, both lobes of the thyroid gland and consequently the parathyroids are removed, hypocalceamia is a real risk. Numbness and tingling around the mouth and fingertips, with muscle spasms in the extremities and face may occur within one to two days of surgery. Tetany requires emergency treatment with a 10% solution of calcium gluconate given slowly intravenously until symptoms are relieved. Calcium levels should be maintained between 7.5 and 9.0 mg/dl. Oral calcium should be started as soon as possible. In addition, a vitamin D analogue may be required together with the oral calcium.

Seroma occurs more commonly when a radical neck dissection has been done in combination with a laryn-gectomy. The exact nature is obscure but it is thought to be a resolving collection of blood undergoing liquification. Usually this collection can be aspirated under sterile conditions with no further sequelae.

In the same way, chylous fistulas are complications found when a neck dissection has been performed. The thoracic duct enters the confluence of the internal jugular and subclavian veins on the left and consequently great care must be taken when dissecting in this area. During surgery, if one is aware that the thoracic duct has been cut, the area should be oversewn to try and stop the flow of chyle. The chylous fistulas usually become apparent when feeding by the nasogastric tube has begun. A white or opalescent type of drainage appears in the haemovac. The skin flaps may bulge and become erythematous. The laboratory analysis of this fluid is positive for fat and protein. A chylothorax may also develop secondary to chyle fistula. Loss of fat, protein, lymphocytes and electrolytes may occur, giving rise to weakness and peripheral oedema. The haemoglobin, electrolytes, calcium, total serum protein, and albumin must be monitored. If the chylous fistula is noticed early, within the first 24–48 hours, the patient should be returned to the operating room and the duct ligated. A pressure dressing alone is usually not sufficient to tamponade the vessels. After several days, it may be difficult to locate the leak; however, if drainage greater than 500 ml per day persists, the wound must be re-explored. In cases recognized late, a pressure dressing and maintenance of the haemovac drain will help the rest of the neck to heal properly. After 7–10 days, the drain may be removed and the pressure dressing maintained. The local tissue pressure will allow the tract to heal. There may be a place for total parenteral nutrition. The use of topical tetracycline powder has been described.[18]

Carotid artery rupture is a grave complication of laryngectomy. Most of these occur in the presence of pharyngocutaneous fistula when a radical neck dissection has been performed in continuity with the laryngectomy, with exposure of the carotid artery. The saliva flowing through tissue has a proteolytic action and together with associated sepsis results in necrosis of cervical skin flap, exposure of the carotid and gradual weakening of the carotid wall with rupture. The use of less than radical neck dissections and the advent of regional myocutaneous flaps and microvascular free flaps have resulted in a decreased fistula rate. In the high-risk patient, these flaps may serve as a substantial protector of the carotid artery. In the event of a fistula and wound infection, every effort should be made to clean and debride the wound and reconstruct the defect with a vascularized flap. A 'sentinel bleed', which often heralds a rupture of the carotid artery, may be a good indicator for emergency ligation of the vessel. However, there is unfortunately a significant morbidity and mortality associated with this complication.

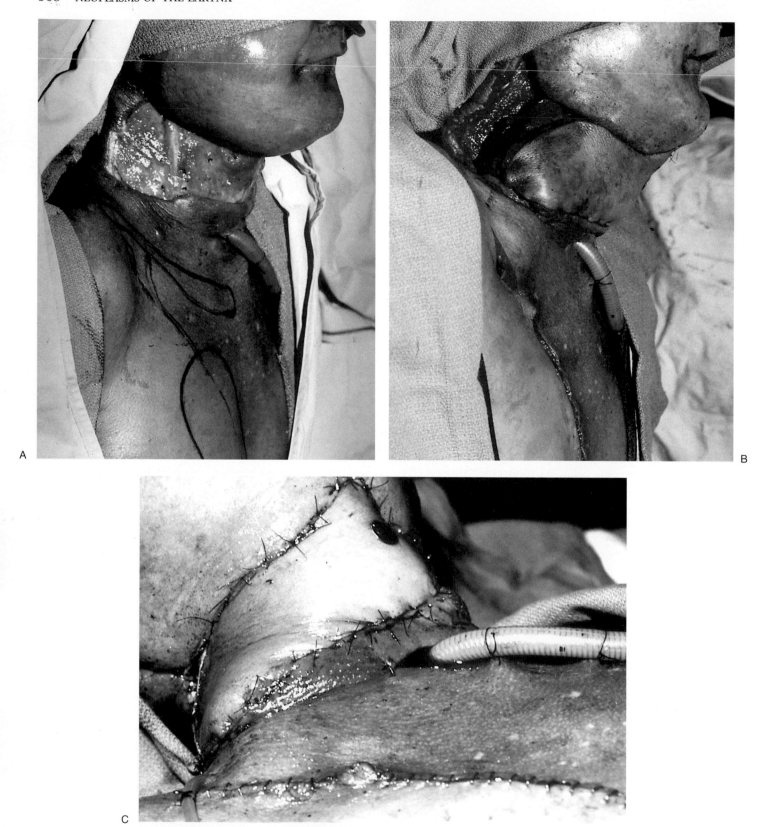

Fig. 32.3   A. (*top, left*) Loss of skin flap with exposure of large vessels. Reconstruction with pectoralis major myocutaneous flap. B. (*top, right*) Pectoralis major myocutaneous flap being sutured into position. C. (*bottom*) Defect repaired with adequate protection.

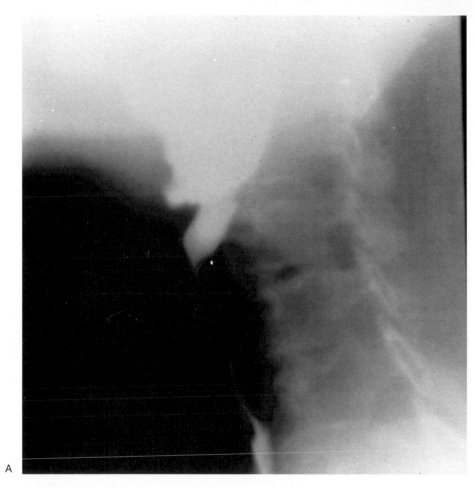

Fig. 32.4 A. Barium swallow demonstrating severe pharyngeal stenosis following laryngectomy.

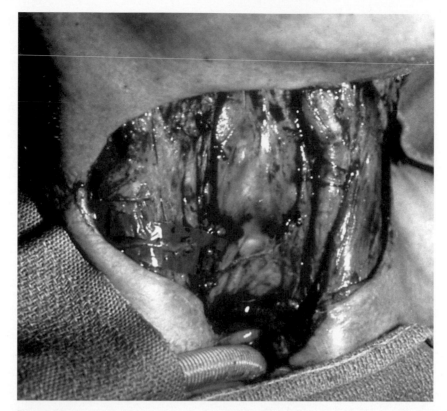

Fig. 32.4B

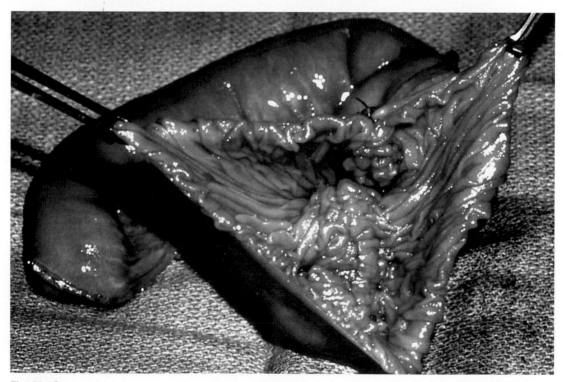

Fig. 32.4C

Fig. 32.4 (*contd*) B. Defect created after completion of pharyngectomy. C. Harvesting of jejunum from the abdomen.

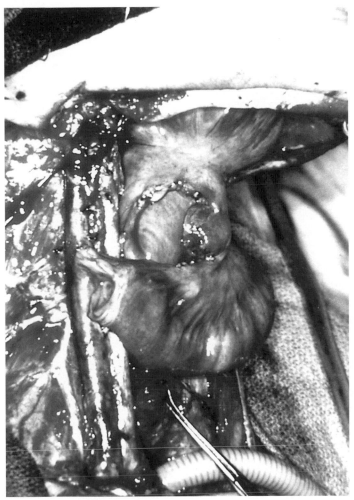

Fig. 32.4D

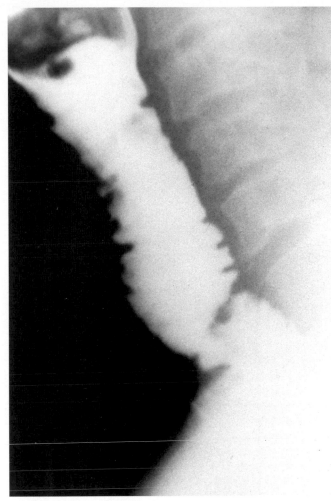

Fig. 32.4E

Fig. 32.4 (*contd*) D. Jejunum being sutured into pharyngeal defect. E. Postoperative barium swallow demonstrating jejunum in position with adequate patency.

In a patient who has undergone laryngectomy, communication is usually compromised. This is made far more severe if one or both of the hypoglossal nerves are damaged and severe loss of tongue movement and articulation occur. The hypoglossal nerve lies deep to the digastric muscle but may dip down below it, making it vulnerable, particularly during skeletization of the hyoid bone. Awareness and good surgical technique should prevent this unfortunate complication occurring.

'Late' complications

Recent studies have shown that hypothyroidism is prevalent in patients who have undergone laryngectomy and even more prevalent in those patients who have undergone total laryngectomy and postoperative radiation therapy, even though at the time of the surgery one lobe of the thyroid gland was preserved.[23] Although it may not be necessary to perform routine thyroid function tests on all patients postoperatively, certainly a high index of suspicion should occur in those patients who show physical findings consistent with hypothyroidism or who experience excessive weight gain. Thyroid replacement therapy after documenting hypothyroidism is satisfactory management for this problem.

Tracheostomal stenosis is a complication which occurs more commonly in patients who have undergone radiation therapy. These patients present with gradual narrowing of the airway with increased difficulty in breathing. Some patients with a relative stomal stenosis occurring fairly soon after surgery may be treated by inserting progressively larger tracheal cannula and then leaving the largest size which can be accommodated in place for a long period of time, or this may be replaced by a plastic tracheostomal button. Myers and Gallia[21] originally described a technique for revision of tracheostomal stenosis. This requires excision of the surrounding scar tissue, the stenotic area, the opening of the tracheostoma, any necrotic cartilage, and the adipose tissue inferior to the stoma. The posterior membranous wall of the trachea

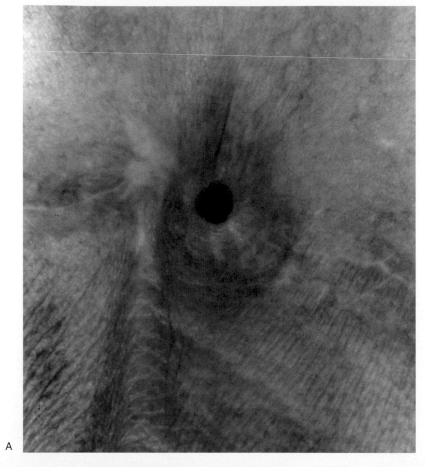

A

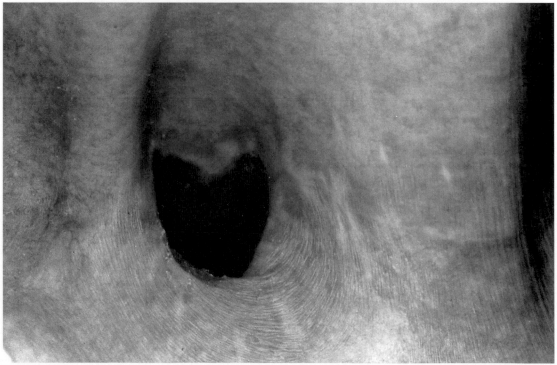

B

Fig. 32.5   A. Patient with tracheostomal stenosis. B. Excision of tracheostomal stenosis and revision using a small local flap.

is split for 1–2 cm and a small flap, based on the skin just above the tracheostoma, is transposed into the tracheostoma. This prevents recurrence of the concentric scarring, which leads to the stenosis (Fig. 32.5).

Pharyngeal stenosis is a problem which usually manifests with progressive dysphagia and weight loss. These patients have usually had resection of at least part of their pharynx (laryngectomy and partial pharyngectomy) resulting in a closure which is too narrow. Also, postoperative pharyngocutaneous fistula with secondary sepsis may result in fibrosis and concentric narrowing of this area. Patients who require more extensive surgery (pharyngolaryngectomy) and are reconstructed with a pectoralis major myocutaneous flap are also at risk of developing pharyngeal stenosis. As mentioned earlier, we utilize the gastric pull-up for pharyngeal reconstruction if the tumour extends into the cervical oesophagus. For all other cases of pharyngolaryngectomy, we use jejunal free grafts. Management of pharyngeal stenosis may require repeated dilatations if not too severe. More severe cases have been treated in the past with some form of local or regional flap in order to increase the surface area of the pharyngeal lumen. We advocate the use of secondary jejunal interposition in these cases as a good option in the management of a difficult problem.[10]

Lack of ability to speak must certainly be considered a complication or at least a sequela of the surgery.[19] Indeed, this is only one aspect of the patient's psychological deprivation that the surgeon may notice. We have excellent results with primary tracheo-oesophageal fistula and use this as our initial modality for voice restoration. There are, however, many patients who are not intelligent enough or motivated enough to learn this technique. In order to accommodate such patients, many varieties of vocal rehabilitation have been described (Ch. 30). It is important to be aware that the patient's world has been drastically altered, and the inability to communicate can only worsen the frustration and depression experienced at this time.

Complications specific to partial laryngeal surgery

Apart from the general complications occurring with total laryngectomy, there are some complications that occur more specifically with partial laryngeal surgery. Partial laryngeal surgery may include vocal cord stripping or laser excision up to a supraglottic or an extended frontolateral vertical hemilaryngectomy. The technique we use for supraglottic and vertical laryngectomy has been discussed. The problems associated with vocal cord stripping, be it with instrumentation or laser, are essentially the same for cancer patients as they are for other vocal cord lesions. Webbing, particularly of the anterior commissure, can be a real problem; occurring when both cords are stripped simultaneously with bare surfaces approximated to each other. This should be avoided.

Supraglottic laryngectomy may be a problem in the older patient, with poor motivation and any compromise in respiratory function. Some degree of aspiration invariably occurs and a motivated patient with excellent postoperative rehabilitation is required. Obviously the patient's preoperative pulmonary status is very important; if any doubt exists, they would probably do better with a total laryngectomy. Management of this problem may be very frustrating. Although good surgical technique is important, correct patient selection is vital for satisfactory results. These patients may develop pneumonia and atelectasis and must be treated with antibiotic therapy and rigorous tracheobronchial toilet. Some patients may not be able to master the swallowing act even after decannulation and may be discharged from hospital with a nasogastric tube in place. Ordinarily, they return within one month able to swallow and the tube may be removed. If aspiration continues to be a problem and the patient develops repeated aspiration pneumonia, conversion to a total laryngectomy may well be required.

Glottic insufficiency due to vocal cord paralysis following surgery may occur. The patients are at significant risk as it is and this will compound the problem. Schramn et al[26] have described the injection of gelfoam into the vocal cords for temporary restoration of glottic sufficiency. Patients may have trouble later on with the formation of a supraglottic web.[19] This may be treated by CO_2 laser carried out through direct laryngoscopy. The formation of such webs is minimized by precise removal of the supraglottis just above the vocal cords. Oedema of the vocal cords may develop when radiation therapy is delivered postoperatively. This may require tracheotomy or re-insertion of the tracheotomy tube on an extended or even permanent basis.

The most common problems attendant upon vertical partial laryngectomy are aspiration, stenosis and inadequate voice.[19] Because of the removal of at least the hemilarynx, an abnormally large glottic chink is present. This promotes wasting of air and a breathy quality to the voice. The use of the Conley skin flap,[7] the Bailey muscle flap,[2] or the flap described above using pyriform mucosa, tends to diminish the breathiness, but few, if any, patients have a normal voice.

The problem of aspiration occurs in those cases when the arytenoid cartilage must be removed. Again, the above-mentioned reconstructive procedures have been helpful in these situations. Even in the absence of such procedures, our personal experience has been that patients will adapt to the problem and rehabilitate themselves without the need for extensive or exotic reconstructive procedures.

Stenosis of the glottis is usually not a problem, unless an extended frontolateral vertical hemilaryngectomy is performed. In this case, reconstruction of the defect using the epiglottic laryngoplasty is used. This reconstruction helps maintain the diameter of the larynx, thereby avoiding stenosis. Care should also be taken in routine vertical partial surgery to avoid taking cricoid cartilage as this certainly predisposes to stenosis.

REFERENCES

1. Beak S M, Biller H F, Krespi Y P, Lawson 1979 The pectoralis major myocutaneous island flap for reconstruction of the head and neck. Head Neck Surg 1: 293–300
2. Bailey B J 1975 Glottic reconstruction after hemilaryngectomy: bipedicle muscle flap laryngoplasty. Laryngoscope 85: 960–977
3. Brand B, Johnson J T, Myers E N, Thearle P B, Sigler B A 1982 Prophylactic perioperative antibiotics in contaminated head and neck surgery. Otolaryngol Head Neck Surg 90: 315–318
4. Brown B M, Johnson J T, Wagner R L 1987 Etiologic factors in head and neck wound infections. Laryngoscope 97: 587–590
5. Calcaterra T L 1983 Tongue flap reconstruction of the hypopharynx. Arch Otolaryngol 109: 750–752
6. Cantrell R W 1978 Pharyngeal fistula: prevention and treatment. Laryngoscope 88: 1204–1208
7. Conley J J 1961 Glottic reconstruction and wound rehabilitation. Arch Otolaryngol 74: 21–24
8. Conley J J 1979 Oropharyngocutaneous fistula. In: Conley J J (ed) Complications of head and neck surgery. Saunders, Philadelphia, pp 92–98
9. Dedo D D, Alonso W A, Ogura J H 1975 Incidence, predisposing factors and outcome of pharyngocutaneous fistula complicating head and neck surgery. Ann Otol Rhinol Laryngol 84: 833–840
10. de Vries E J, Myers E N, Johnson J T et al 1990 Jejunal interposition for repair of stricture or fistula after laryngectomy. Ann Otol Rhinol Laryngol 99: 496–498
11. de Vries E J, Stein D W, Johnson J T et al 1989 Hypopharyngeal reconstruction. A comparison of two alternatives. Laryngoscope 99: 614–617
12. Gluckman J L, McDonough J, Donegan J O 1982 The role of the free jejunal graft in reconstruction of the pharynx and cervical esophagus. Head Neck Surg 4: 360–369
13. Harrison D F N 1979 Surgical management of hypopharyngeal cancer. Particular reference to the gastric pull-up operation. Arch Otolaryngol 105: 149–152
14. Johnson J T, Bloomer W D 1989 Effect of prior radiotherapy on postsurgical wound infection. Head Neck 11: 132–136
15. Johnson J T, Cummings C W 1978 Hematoma after head and neck surgery: a major complication? Trans Am Acad Ophthalmol Otolaryngol 86: 171–175
16. Johnson J T, Yu V L, Myers E N, Muder R R, Thearle P B, Diven W F 1984 Efficacy of two third-generation cephalosporins in prophylaxis for head and neck surgery. Arch Otolaryngol 110: 224–227
17. Kambic V 1977 Epiglottoplasty — New technique for laryngeal reconstruction. Radiologia Iugoslavica (suppl II): pp 33–43
18. Kassel R N, Havas T E, Gullane P J 1987 The use of topical tetracycline in the management of persistent chylous fistulae. J Otolaryngol 16: 174–178
19. Lawson W, Biller H 1981 Cancer of the larynx. In: Suen J Y, Myers E N (eds) Cancer of the head and neck. Churchill Livingstone, New York, pp 434–499
20. Myers E N 1972 The management of pharyngocutaneous fistula. Arch Otolaryngol 95: 10–17
21. Myers E N, Gallia L J 1982 Tracheostomal stenosis following total laryngectomy. Ann Otol Rhinol Laryngol 91: 450–453
22. Newman R K, Weiland F I, Johnson J T, Rosen P R, Gumerman L W 1983 Salivary scan after major ablative head and neck surgery with prediction of postoperative fistulization. Ann Otol Rhinol Laryngol 92: 366–368
23. Palmer B V, Gaggar N, Shaw H J 1981 Thyroid function after radiotherapy and laryngectomy for carcinoma of the larynx. Head Neck Surg 4: 13–15
24. Rogers J H, Freeland A P 1976 Arterial vasculature of cervical skin flaps. Clin Otolaryngol 1: 325–331
25. Saunders W H 1963 Techniques in laryngectomy to minimize postoperative complications and permit immediate feeding. Ann Otol Rhinol Laryngol 72 431–440
26. Schramm V L Jr, May M, Lavorato AS 1978 Gelfoam paste injection for vocal cord paralysis: temporary rehabilitation of glottic incompetence. Laryngoscope 88: 1268–1273
27. Schramm V L, Myers E N 1981 Management of complications in cancer of the head and neck. In: Suen J Y, Myers E N (eds) Cancer of the head and neck. Churchill Livingstone, New York, pp 756–781
28. Tucker H A, Sobol S M, Levine H, Wood B 1982 The transverse cervical trapezius myocutaneous island flap. Arch Otolaryngol 108: 194–198

33. Retreatment

P. M. Stell

INTRODUCTION

We are concerned here solely with squamous carcinoma of the larynx. Only a few such patients—about 5% in the author's series of 1350 patients—are untreatable. Most of the rest have been treated by irradiation, surgery (partial or total) or a combination of these two. A few patients with early disease are now treated by the laser. Chemotherapy is also often used as an adjuvant, although it has been shown repeatedly that it has no effect on survival.[71] This form of treatment is considered in Chapter 29.

There are big differences in the philosophy of treatment throughout the world. In the UK and much of Northern Europe most patients are treated by irradiation, with surgery in reserve for failure. For example, a recent review[58] of 3445 patients recorded in the West Midlands Register showed that only 12.5% of patients were treated initially by surgery. In contrast, in much of the USA and the Latin countries surgery is preferred as the initial treatment. The relative merits of these two philosophies will not be considered here.

RECURRENCE AFTER RADIOTHERAPY

Up to 50% of tumours may recur after treatment by irradiation. The main factor determining recurrence in all series is the original T stage of the tumour. For example, in the author's series the recurrence rate at 5 years varied from 5% for T_1 tumours to 35% for transglottic T_3 tumours.[76]

In the present discussion the important points about a recurrence are its pathology, its diagnosis, and its treatment.

Pathology

The few studies of the pathology of recurrence after radiotherapy have shown that such recurrences are extensive. In the large series reported by the Toronto School, 87% of tumour recurrences after radiotherapy were in stages rpT_3 or rpT_4.[24] No fewer than 59% were in stage rpT_4 due to cartilage invasion. In the author's own series 60% of the tumours were transglottic at recurrence, irrespective of the original site, and over 80% of these were in stage rpT_3 or rpT_4.[76]

Olofsson and van Nostrand stated 'we hoped that, following radiotherapy, the viable tumour would shrink to a small focus that could be more easily and safely resected by the surgeon. This pattern of response was rarely seen'.[52] Kirchner too, emphasized that small but widespread foci of tumour may lie under an intact epithelium in the irradiated larynx.[34] Lederman's concept[37] that tumours shrink and recur in a concentric fashion around the primary site has now been disproved by several pathological studies.[24,34,52,76]

Thus, it is clear on pathological grounds that partial laryngectomy after failed radiotherapy is likely to be dangerous.

Diagnosis

Prerequisites for early detection of recurrent or new tumours after previous treatment of laryngeal carcinomas[53] are:

1. A well-organized follow-up system at oncological centres with necessary expertise and adequate equipment. Patients should be followed by specialists who are able to take care of the patients with recurrent disease.
2. Regular laryngoscopies, with microlaryngoscopy about 3 months after completion of the radiotherapy or after partial laryngectomy for a laryngeal carcinoma. At this time most of the postradiotherapy or postoperative oedema has settled. Biopsies should be taken from all clinically suspect areas but repeated biopsies after previous radiotherapy can introduce infection with the risk of subsequent chondritis.

Of the recurrences, 90% present within the first two years. The check-ups must therefore be more frequent during this period of time. After the initial micro-laryngoscopies later examinations can be done with the mirror or a telescope. If the larynx is difficult to inspect —due, for example, to an overhanging epiglottis—the fibrescope provides an excellent means of close and easy inspection of the laryngeal surface of the epiglottis, the ventricles, vocal cords, anterior commissure and subglottis.

3. Follow-up based on the histopathological findings. The intervals between the laryngoscopies certainly depend on the site and extent of the tumour, but they also depend on histopathological examination of the biopsy specimen and of the surgical specimen. The well-differentiated and diffuse dysplastic lesions are most likely to recur and develop into invasive carcinoma.[29] Patients with carcinoma developing in a chronic laryngitis have an increased risk of further carcinomas in a diffusely changed mucosa after partial surgery or radiotherapy. They often get a longstanding oedema, and a red, swollen, slightly granulated mucosa is common after radiotherapy.

The surgical specimen should be carefully examined. The margins of resection need special attention. However, histologically positive resection margins do not necessarily mean recurrent disease. In a series of 39 patients with cancer at the margin in a hemilaryngectomy specimen, seven (18%) later developed a biopsy-proven local recurrence, whereas four out of 72 patients (6%) with no tumour at the resection margin developed a recurrence.[5]

4. Impaired mobility of the vocal cord after previous endoscopic surgery or radiotherapy should be regarded as indicating recurrent tumour until the opposite is proven.

Repeated radiological examination—soft-tissue plain films and computed tomograms—should be taken. In this situation, a reference, immediate, post-therapeutic, radiological examination may be of great value. Micro-laryngoscopy should be performed and a biopsy taken of the visible tumour. Especially after radiotherapy—but also after partial surgery—there is a risk of a recurrent entirely submucosal tumour. After partial surgery the natural barriers within the larynx are removed and the tumour may spread outside the larynx into the soft tissues.

5. Residual or recurrent carcinoma must be excluded in the presence of persistent oedema. Several authors have drawn attention to the oedematous larynx which appears clinically to harbour a recurrence, but where it is not possible to obtain a positive biopsy. The incidence of laryngeal oedema persisting for more than 3 months after radiotherapy was 15% in the author's series.[76] It increased with original T-stage from 13% for T1 to 21% for T_3 and T_4. Mild, stable oedema limited to the region of the arytenoid cartilages generally requires no treatment other than careful follow-up, whereas progressive oedema, particularly if it is associated with pain or foetor

indicates either persistent carcinoma, chondroradio-necrosis, or both, so that total laryngectomy is indicated. Diagnosis by repeated deep biopsies carries the risk of precipitation of necrosis, although some[22] have not found this to be so. At least half of the larynges will be found to harbour recurrence,[78] despite a negative biopsy before operation. Those larynges that do not contain tumour are often functionally useless, so that the patient seldom suffers great loss.

The salvage rate in these patients is poor—only 25% in one series[78]—emphasizing that the difficulties of diagnosis in these cases leads to delay in treatment.

Treatment

Primary recurrences may be treated by surgery, with a hope of cure, by chemotherapy for palliation, or they may not be treated at all. Chemotherapy is dealt with else-where (Ch. 29). The laryngectomy may be total or partial, and the latter may be vertical or horizontal.

The term vertical hemilaryngectomy will be used here to cover all partial procedures for glottic tumours, such as cordectomy, hemilaryngectomy, frontolateral hemilaryn-gectomy, etc, but not for subtotal laryngectomies.

Total laryngectomy

Radical radiotherapy with total laryngectomy in reserve for failed treatment has been a standard policy, parti-cularly in the UK, for 40 years at least, pioneered notably by Lederman.[37] There have been many papers detailing this treatment, and several devoted specifically to salvage laryngectomy. The results are summarized in Tables 33.1–33.3 for supraglottic tumours, glottic tumours, and tumours described as 'laryngeal'. There were too few reports of subglottic carcinoma to allow meaningful analysis. Sadly, some papers devoted to this topic—for example, that by De Santo et al[17]—had to be omitted because of insufficient data. Furthermore, several papers were omitted because the data were obviously unrepre-sentative—for example, one[60] in which 80% of glottic tumours treated by irradiation recurred. Such an unusual result presumably means that the series was in some way unrepresentative. Furthermore, the control rate of 20% for glottic T_3 carcinomas treated by radiotherapy in another series[16] is much lower than that achieved nowadays, and presumably includes results from an era several decades ago when radiotherapy was not so far advanced.

Tables 33.1–33.3 show that only 77% of patients with a primary recurrence underwent surgery. One of the worrying features of treating most patients with ir-radiation, with surgery in reserve for failure, is the high proportion of patients who are unsuitable for surgery when the tumour recurs, although the tumour was

Table 33.1 Results of salvage total laryngectomy for supraglottic carcinoma

References	Original stage	Number of primary recurrences	Number of recurrences treated	Survival at 5 years
58	$T_{1-4}N_0$	167/458	39/167	12/39
57	I–IV	23/58	11/23	5/11
45	I–IV	30/105	23/30	15/23
48	I–III	12/23	12/12	1/12
4	I–IV	62/199	22/62	7/22
Total		294/843 (35%)	107/294 (36%)	40/107 (37%)

Table 33.2 Results of salvage total laryngectomy for glottic carcinoma

References	Original stage	Number of primary recurrences	Number of recurrences treated	Survival at 5 years
76	T_1–T_3	141/320	123/141	39/100
57	T_{1-4}	28/113	16/28	8/16
20	T_{1-2}	22/212	21/22	13/22
42	$T_{1-2}N_0$	34/143	34/34	22/34
39	T_3N_0	78/141	64/78	33/59
28	T_{2-4}	88/261	70/88	39/66
77	$T_{1-3}N_0$	101/521	80/101	63/90
31	I–IV	26/195	16/26	8/26
79	T_{1-4}	64/247	57/64	49/57
48	I–III	40/125	33/40	15/33
72	I–IV	57/291	28/57	18/28
Total		679/2569 (26%)	542/679 (80%)	293/531 (55%)

Table 33.3 Results of salvage total laryngectomy for 'laryngeal' cancer

References	Original stage	Number of primary recurrences	Number of recurrences treated	Salvage at 5 years
14	T_3T_4	19/58	16/19	8/16
11	T_1–T_4	230/?	230/230	85/230
35	?	178/?	147/178	69/147
12	I–IV	36/126	36/36	20/36
30	I–IV	32/152	32/32	16/32
46	T_{3-4}	60/136	60/60	34/60
Total		147/472 (31%)	521/555 (94%)	232/521 (45%)

presumably operable when the patient was first seen. A review of 3445 patients in the West Midlands of England[58] showed that only 23% of patients with a recurrent supraglottic tumour initially staged $T_{1-4}N_0$ were submitted to salvage surgery. However, in several of the series in Tables 33.1–33.3, all patients with recurrent disease were submitted to surgery. The reasons for these huge differences in operability are not clear.

As is well known, there is a high risk of complications after salvage laryngectomy. Seven of the papers sum-marized in Tables 33.1–33.3 reported complications: 30% of patients developed a pharyngocutaneous fistula, 6% suffered a carotid blow-out, 9% had major skin necrosis, and 7.5% an operative death. More minor complications are not considered here.

Pharyngocutaneous fistulae and carotid rupture have both attracted much attention in the literature.[23]

The best known predisposing factor to a fistula includes previous radiotherapy, although this was not found to be so in one large review.[36] Other factors include a low haemoglobin after operation, and a pre-operative tracheostomy.[36] There are two different pathological types of fistulae: those due to dehiscence of the suture line, and those due to necrosis of tissue. The former almost always heal spontaneously, whereas the latter often require formal repair. Repair should not be undertaken before about six weeks to allow local infection to be overcome.[44] The fistula is then repaired by providing a two-layer closure, one layer on the inside and one on the outside. Depending on the origin of those two layers, fistulae can be divided into three types[69]: I, those where the two surfaces are provided locally, II, those where one surface must be provided from a distance, and III, those where both surfaces must be provided from a distance.

In type I fistulae local flaps are used. In type II the most effective flap for outer cover is a revascularized forearm flap. For type III fistulae the work-horse is the pectoralis major flap with the skin paddle either inside or outside.

The major predisposing cause of carotid rupture is prior radiotherapy. In previously irradiated patients great care should be taken over the choice of the incision, and the carotid sheath should be protected by the sterno-mastoid muscle if still present, by a levator scapuli flap, or by the muscular pedicle of a musculocutaneous flap if such a flap has been used.[68]

Factors influencing cure after total salvage laryngectomy have received little attention. In the author's personal series[76] the main prognostic factors were time to recurrence and T-stage at recurrence. Sex was also just significant, men having a better prognosis.

The survival rate was 35% after salvage surgery for a supraglottic tumour, 55% for glottic tumours and 45% for 'laryngeal' tumours. Presumably the latter were more extensive, transglottic tumours. For glottic cancer, Kaplan et al[31] found that the results of salvage surgery depend on the original stage of the disease. The 5-year survival after salvage surgery for original stages I–II was 47%, compared with only 9% for patients with original stage III–IV. Patients with a mobile vocal cord at the time of recurrence had an 83% chance of surviving a further 5 years, whereas those with a fixed cord at the time of recurrence had only a 44% chance of cure.[77]

Partial laryngectomy

Vertical. The results of salvage vertical hemilaryngectomy for failed radiotherapy are summarized in Table 33.4. The main points are that the morbidity is acceptable: 8% suffered difficulties in swallowing, 11% had delayed decannulation or laryngeal stenosis, and 12% had major infections or fistulae. However, the survival 3 years after salvage surgery was 77%, although 19% of patients submitted to salvage vertical hemilaryngectomy needed a completion laryngectomy for a further recurrence or for an incompetent larynx.

Contraindications to vertical hemilaryngectomy for failed radiotherapy include immobility of the vocal cord, invasion of the arytenoid cartilage and its overlying mucosa, invasion of more than one-third of the opposite cord, evidence of spread above or below the cord, evidence of chondritis and invasion of the cartilages.[61] Others would add to this that the surgeon must have seen the patient before the initial radiotherapy so that he would know that the original tumour had been safe anatomically and pathologically for a hemilaryngectomy,[19] i.e., it was in stage T_1, so that he could confirm that the recurrence correlated with the original tumour.[63] However, one group[39] reported a 100% salvage rate (5/5) for patients with recurrent disease after irradiation of glottic T_3 tumours, a truly remarkable result considering that

these patients were unsuitable for a partial laryngectomy initially.

Horizontal. It is generally agreed that horizontal supraglottic laryngectomy for failed radiotherapy is at best hazardous. Som states that 'conservation surgery may not be the procedure of choice after radiotherapy failure. In fact, delayed healing and perichondritis are to be expected'.[64] The few results available are shown in Table 33.5.

The rate of complications is high; in particular, about three-quarters of these patients have difficulty in swallowing and breathing. One-third have delayed healing with fistulae and carotid rupture. One-quarter develop a further recurrence in the larynx, but the survival at 3 years is 50% after salvage partial laryngectomy.

RECURRENCE AFTER SURGERY

After partial laryngectomy

Vertical hemilaryngectomy

The term 'completion laryngectomy' was coined by Myers and Ogura[49]: 9% of laryngectomies in their series were carried out for removal of the remaining part of the larynx after prior partial laryngectomy. The recurrence rate in their series was 11% after vertical hemi-

Table 33.4   Vertical hemilaryngectomy for failed radiotherapy

Author	Swallowing difficulties	Delayed decannulation	Major infection/ fistula	Survival at 3 years or more	Completion laryngectomy
13	?	5/26	?	12/12	2/26
61	2/23	5/23	1/23	36/54	7/54
73	2/8	?	3/8	4/4	?
66	0/55	0/55	0/55	39/55	16/55
70	?	?	?	6/8	?
15	?	0/16	8/16	12/16	1/16
40	?	3/9	?	5/9	3/9
20	?	?	?	1/1	0/1
39	?	?	?	5/5	0/5
28	?	?	?	6/15	6/15
51	?	1/12	?	10/12	2/12
30	?	?	?	10/12	1/12
7	?	?	?	14/20	4/20
50	?	?	?	8/10	3/13
59	5/28	4/28	4/28	7/10	6/28
1	?	?	?	16/16	4/16

Table 33.5   Horizontal partial laryngectomy for failed radiotherapy

Author	Poor swallowing	Poor breathing	Delayed healing	Survival (3 years or more)	Further recurrence
66	8/10	8/10	4/10	6/10	4/10
61	8/15	?	2/15	5/15	2/15
40	?	?	?	2/2	1/2
50	?	?	?	2/4	?
64	?	3/5	4/5	3/5	?

laryngectomy. All 26 of these patients underwent completion laryngectomy: eight patients developed a stomal recurrence but 18 (69%) were salvaged.

A careful study of 63 partial laryngectomies[40] showed that 13/63 (21%) required completion laryngectomy. These were broken down as follows: 3/9 vertical hemilaryngectomies for failed radiotherapy, 7/21 vertical hemilaryngectomies as primary treatment, 1/2 supraglottic laryngectomies for failed radiotherapy and 2/31 supraglottic laryngectomies as primary treatment. The cure rate after completion laryngectomy for glottic tumours was five out of nine cases.

Guerrier[27] reported 12% of local recurrences in 159 vertical hemilaryngectomies of various types. He stated that small recurrences are treated by irradiation, those of moderate size by subtotal laryngectomy, and large recurrences by total laryngectomy. He gave no further details.

Six of 57 patients in another series[47] with a T_{1-3} glottic tumour submitted to vertical hemilaryngectomy suffered a primary recurrence. All underwent total laryngectomy, and three survived long-term. Of 18 patients undergoing hemilaryngectomy for T_3 glottic tumours, three suffered a primary recurrence: two were controlled by radiotherapy, but one subjected to laryngectomy died.[38]

In summary, completion laryngectomy was carried out in 13% of patients in the above series. It was successful in 64% of cases.

Supraglottic laryngectomy

Primary recurrence after supraglottic laryngectomy is determined, inter alia, by the stage of the original disease. In Bocca's large series of 537 cases the primary recurrence rate increased from 6% for stage I lesions to 33% for stage IV lesions. He does not discuss the further management of those patients with recurrent tumours.[8]

In Myers and Ogura's series, 9/134 patients undergoing horizontal supraglottic laryngectomy suffered recurrence and were subjected to total laryngectomy; four were salvaged.[49]

Vega reported an 11% incidence of primary recurrence after 240 horizontal laryngectomies, the recurrence rate being most common after extended operations for lesions invading the base of the tongue or piriform sinus. Of these, 46% were untreatable, 19% were treated by total laryngectomy and 35% were treated by irradiation. Only 3/26 (11%) of patients with recurrent disease were salvaged.[75]

Soo et al reported 78 patients undergoing supraglottic laryngectomy, 10 of whom developed a recurrence in the larynx.[65] Three patients were not treated radically, one was treated by irradiation, and six were treated by total laryngectomy. Four of the latter patients were alive 5 years after salvage laryngectomy. However, two patients who developed primary recurrence and had nodal recurrences died of their disease.

Thus 10% of patients in these series developed a recurrence within the larynx: only 24% of the patients with recurrence were salvaged.

Subtotal laryngectomy

Subtotal laryngectomy was developed mainly by Pearson.[54] It has several other names—such as 'three-quarter laryngectomy', etc—and is mainly indicated for T_{3-4} laryngeal tumours. It is indicated also for tumours of the piriform fossa, but we are not concerned here with the latter. The principle is that the healthy part of one-half of the larynx is preserved to act as a shunt for air from the trachea to the pharynx. Of 84 patients, five (6%) described in four reports in the literature suffered a local recurrence,[6,18,21,55] an interesting figure considering that the local recurrence rate after *total* laryngectomy for the same disease is of the order of 20%. Even more remarkable are the 48 patients in two series[6,55] none of whom suffered a local recurrence! We are not told of the subsequent fate of those patients in another two series[8,21] who do suffer recurrence.

Piquet is one of the foremost European advocates of subtotal laryngectomy. However, his most recent report of 103 subtotal laryngectomies (crico-hyoidopexy) contains no mention of primary recurrences or their management.[56]

After total laryngectomy

After total laryngectomy local recurrence is, strictly speaking, not possible, since the organ has been entirely removed. However, recurrence is possible in the overlying skin and in immediately adjacent tissue, that is, in the pre-epiglottic space, the muscles of the base of the tongue above, the pharyngeal remnant, and the stoma. Apart from the last, these events have received almost no attention in the literature.

Presumably, recurrence in the base of the tongue is more likely after treatment of supraglottic tumours. However, it is not mentioned in the very large series of 537 supraglottic laryngectomies described by Bocca.[8]

Of the author's total series of 1350 patients with laryngeal cancer, 397 have undergone total laryngectomy, either as primary treatment or for failure of other forms of treatment. Of these, 70 (17.5%) are known to have had local recurrence of their disease. The site and treatment of the recurrence and the fate of the patients are shown in Table 33.6.

Recurrence in the base of the tongue in the author's series was never amenable to treatment, and was always fatal. Recurrence in the skin was also always untreatable, and invariably fatal within 6 months at most.

Table 33.6   Local recurrence after total laryngectomy

Site	Number	Treatment	Survival for treated patients in months (* indicates dead)
Skin	9	Untreated 9	Not applicable
Stoma	35	Untreated 24	Not applicable
		DXRT 3	1*, 2*, 11*
		Sternectomy 8	1*, 1*, 19, 34, 52, 54, 70, 115
Tongue base	11	Untreated 11	Not applicable
Pharynx	15	Untreated 10	Not applicable
		Flap repair 2	5*, 16*
		Jejunum 3	4*, 4, 48
		(One patient had two recurrences)	

Key: DXRT = Deep X-ray therapy.

However, recurrence in the pharyngeal stump could be treated occasionally by pharyngectomy, with repair by a skin flap in earlier years or, more recently, by a free jejunal loop. One-third of patients with recurrence in the pharyngeal stump have been operated on with, sadly, only one long-term survival (Table 33.6).

Stomal recurrence has attracted much attention since Keim et al drew attention to its relationship to tracheostomy.[33] It is better termed 'peristomal recurrence'. It is important to describe the anatomy and pathology of such a recurrence. Stomal recurrence can be divided into four anatomical types: a type I recurrence lies above the stoma, II extends into the oesophagus without inferior extension, III lies superior to the stoma, and IV extends laterally under the clavicles. The first and possibly the second are sometimes treatable; the latter two are not treatable because they usually represent the tip of an iceberg whose main mass lies in the mediastinum entrapping the great vessels. The latter two are thus uniformly fatal.[43] There are at least six different pathological causes of peristomal recurrence: implantation in the track of a prior tracheostomy, incomplete excision of the original tumour, a second primary tumour in the trachea, a metastasis in the paratracheal lymph nodes, tumour in a remnant of the thyroid gland, and tumour tracking down the sheath of the sternomastoid muscle.

Clearly the treatment is determined by the anatomy and pathology of the lesion.

Peristomal recurrences lying above the stoma may be amenable to resection via a sternectomy. The main exponent of this operation has been Sisson et al[62]. Resection of the manubrium was first carried out by Bardenheuer in 1885, for ligation of the subclavian artery, for access to tumours of the mediastinum and for removal of tumours of the manubrium itself.[3] Sisson et al[62] resected the medial end of both clavicles and both first ribs along with the manubrium sterni. In his first few cases the most feared complication was rupture of the great vessels of the mediastinum. To prevent this he inserted pectoralis muscle flaps between the great vessels and the trachea. He reported 28 cases of resection of stomal recurrence. Seven of these patients had major intra-operative complications including pneumothorax, injury to the great vessels, air embolism and cardiac arrest. These were fatal in two patients. A further five patients died in the postoperative phase, making a total hospital mortality rate of 25%. However, the mortality rate improved over this time due to improvements in selection and technique. The 5-year survival after this procedure was 17%. The skin defect must be filled. In earlier times this was done by a pedicled chest flap, as described by Grillo,[26] but nowadays it is done by a pedicled pectoralis major flap, or a free rectus abdominus or latissimus dorsi flap.

Radiotherapy is rarely successful[9] though five out of seven patients were alive at various times beyond 8 months after treatment with a combination of chemotherapy (vincristine, bleomycin and methotrexate) and irradiation.[2]

The author's results are shown in Table 33.6. Two-thirds of patients with a peristomal recurrence were unsuitable for further treatment. Patients treated with irradiation did uniformly badly. However, half the patients submitted to sternectomy were still alive 4 years or more later, despite a hospital mortality rate of 25%.

RECURRENCE AFTER COMBINED RADIOTHERAPY AND SURGERY

Here, further radiotherapy and surgery are scarcely possible because both have already been used to full effect. Many series, for example one of the earliest series by Goldman et al,[25] do not mention recurrence at all. Kazem et al[32] report 17% of local recurrences after combined preoperative radiotherapy and surgery, but give no further details of these patients. In Brandenburg's series of 26 patients, four had local recurrence and none were salvaged.[10] Usually, the most that is possible in these cases is palliative chemotherapy (Ch. 29).

RECURRENCE AFTER LASER TREATMENT

One of the earlier exponents of laser excision of selected small T_1 glottic tumours was Strong in 1975.[74] It appears that none of his first 11 cases suffered a recurrence.

McGuirt and Koufman[41] have recently reported on 14 patients with T_1 glottic squamous carcinoma and nine patients with carcinoma in situ. Four patients have died of their cancer or have been lost to follow-up, with no recurrence in the remaining 19. Six patients have suffered primary recurrence, all controlled by further laser treatment. None have undergone radiotherapy or surgery.

Steiner[67] has been one of the most forceful European advocates of the use of the laser for treatment of more advanced laryngeal carcinomas. Recently he reported 81 patients with T_2–T_4 laryngeal tumours treated by laser. Of these patients, 16% suffered a recurrence at the primary site. Two-thirds of these patients were treated by further laser with or without radiotherapy, but one-third required total laryngectomy. The survival rate in the patients with recurrent disease was 39%.[67]

REFERENCES

1. Ballantyne A J, Fletcher G H 1974 Surgical management of irradiation failures of nonfixed cancers of the glottic region. Am J Roentgenol 120: 164–168
2. Balm A J M, Snow G B, Karim A B M F, Versluis R J J, Njo K H, Tiwari R M 1986 Long-term results of concurrent polychemotherapy and radiotherapy in patients with stomal recurrence after total laryngectomy. Ann Otol Rhinol Laryngol 95: 572–575
3. Bardenheuer 1885 Die Resection des Manubrium Sterni. Dtsch Med Wochenschr 11: 688–690
4. Bataini J P, Ennuyer A, Poncet P, Ghossein N A 1974 Treatment of supraglottic cancer by high dose radiotherapy. Cancer 33: 1253–1262
5. Bauer W C, Lesinski S G, Ogura J H 1975 The significance of positive margins in hemilaryngectomy specimens. Laryngoscope 85: 1–13
6. Biller H F, Lawson W 1984 Partial laryngectomy for transglottic cancers. Ann Otol Rhinol Laryngol 93: 297–300
7. Biller H F, Barnhill F R Jr, Ogura J H, Perez C A 1970 Hemilaryngectomy following radiation failure for carcinoma of the vocal cords. Laryngoscope 80: 249–253
8. Bocca E 1991; Surgical management of supraglottic cancer and its lymph node metastases in a conservative perspective. Ann Otol Rhinol Laryngol 100: 261–267
9. Bonneau R A, Lehman R H 1975 Stomal recurrence following laryngectomy. Arch Otolaryngol 101: 408–412
10. Brandenburgh J H, Rutter S W 1977 Residual carcinoma of the larynx. Laryngoscope 87: 224–236
11. Brugere J, Rodriguez J, Point D, Thanh P 1987 Resultats des interventions de laryngectomie de rattrapage. Ann Otolaryngol Chir Cervicofac 104: 541–544
12. Cleatus S, Steel A 1981 A ten-year survey of laryngeal cancer in a regional hospital. J Laryngol Otol 95: 817–826
13. Croll G A, van Den Broek P, Tiwari R M, Manni J J 1985 Vertical partial laryngectomy for recurrent glottic carcinoma after irradiation. Head Neck Surg 7: 390–393
14. Croll G A, Gerritson G J, Tiwari R M, Snow G B 1989 Primary radiotherapy with surgery in reserve for advanced laryngeal carcinoma. Eur J Surg Oncol 15: 350–356
15. Czigner J 1984 Vertical and horizontal partial resections of the larynx after radiotherapy. In: Wigand M E, Steiner W, Stell P M (eds) Functional partial laryngectomy. Springer-Verlag, Heidelberg, pp 280–284
16. De Santo L W 1984 T3 glottic cancer: options and consequences of the options. Laryngoscope 94: 1311–1315
17. De Santo L W, Lillie J C, Devine K D 1976 Surgical salvage after radiation for laryngeal cancer. Laryngoscope 86: 649–657
18. De Santo L W, Pearson B W, Olsen K D 1989 Utility of near total laryngectomy for supraglottic, pharyngeal, base-of-tongue, and other cancers. Ann Otol Rhinol Laryngol 98: 2–7
19. Ellis P D M 1977 The role of conservation surgery in the management of laryngeal cancer: a review. Proc Roy Soc Med 70: 779–780
20. Fisher A J, Caldarelli D D, Chacko D C, Holinger L D 1986 Glottic cancer. Surgical salvage for radiation failure. Arch Otolaryngol Head Neck Surg 112: 519–521
21. Friedman W H, Katsantonis G P, Siddoway J R, Cooper M H 1981 Contralateral laryngoplasty after supraglottic laryngectomy with vertical extension. Arch Otolaryngol 107: 742–745
22. Fu K K, Woodhouse R J, Quivey J M, Phillips T L, Dedo H H 1982 The significance of laryngeal edema following radiotherapy of carcinoma of the vocal cord. Cancer 49: 655–658
23. Gall A M, Sessions D G, Ogura J H 1977 Complications following surgery for cancer of the larynx and hypopharynx: Cancer 39: 624–631
24. Gilbert R W, Lundgren J A V, van Nostrand A W P, Keane T J 1988 $T_3N_0M_0$, glottic carcinoma — a pathologic analysis of 41 patients treated surgically following radiotherapy. Clin Otolaryngol 13: 467–479
25. Goldman J L, Silverstone S M, Roffman J D, Birken E A 1972 High dosage pre-operative radiation and surgery for carcinoma of the larynx and laryngopharynx. A 14-year program. Laryngoscope 82: 1869–1882
26. Grillo H C 1966 Terminal or mural tracheostomy in the anterior mediastinum. J Thorac Cardiovasc Surg 51: 422–427
27. Guerrier Y 1984 Early detection and management of recurrences after vertical partial laryngectomy. In: Wigand M E, Steiner W, Stell P M (eds) Functional partial laryngectomy. Springer-Verlag, Heidelberg, pp 316–322
28. Harwood A R, Hawkins N V, Beale F A, Rider W D, Bryce D P 1979 Management of advanced glottic cancer. A ten-year review of the Toronto experience. Int J Radiat Oncol Biol Phys 5: 899–904
29. Hellquist H, Lundgren J, Olofsson J 1982 Hyperplasia, keratosis, dysplasia and carcinoma in situ of the vocal cords — a follow-up study. Clin Otolaryngol 7: 11–27
30. Jorgensen K 1974 Carcinoma of the larynx — III. therapeutic results. Acta Radiol Ther Phys Biol 13: 446–464
31. Kaplan M J, Johns M E, Clark D A, Cantrell R W 1984 Glottic carcinoma. The roles of surgery and irradiation. Cancer 53: 2641–2648
32. Kazem I, van Den Broek P 1984 Planned preoperative radiation therapy vs. definitive radiotherapy for advanced laryngeal carcinoma. Laryngoscope 94: 1355–1358
33. Keim W F, Shapiro M J, Rosin H D 1965 Study of postlaryngectomy stomal recurrence. Arch Otolaryngol 81: 183–186
34. Kirchner J A 1989 What have whole organ sections contributed to the treatment of laryngeal cancer? Ann Otol Rhinol Laryngol 98: 661–667
35. Lam K H, Wei W I, Wong J, Ong G B 1983 Surgical salvage of radiation failures in cancer of the larynx. J Laryngol Otol 97: 351–356
36. Lavelle R J, Maw A R 1972 The aetiology of post-laryngectomy pharyngo-cutaneous fistulae. J Laryngol Otol 86: 785–793
37. Lederman M 1970 Radiotherapy of cancer of the larynx. J Laryngol Otol 84: 867–896
38. Lesinski S G, Bauer W C, Ogura J H 1976 Hemilaryngectomy for T3 (fixed cord) epidermoid carcinoma of the larynx. Laryngoscope 86: 1563–1571
39. Lundgren J A V, Gilbert R W, van Nostrand A W P, Harwood A R, Keane T J, Briant T D R 1988 $T_3N_0M_0$ glottic carcinoma — a failure analysis. Clin Otolaryngol 13: 455–465
40. Maceri D R, Lampe H B, Makielski K H, Passamani P P, Krause C J 1985 Conservation laryngeal surgery. A critical analysis. Arch. Otolaryngol 111: 361–365

41. McGuirt W F, Koufman J A 1987 Endoscopic laser surgery. An alternative in laryngeal cancer treatment. Arch Otolaryngol Head Neck Surg 113: 501–505

42. Maipang T, Razack M S, Sako K, Chen T Y 1989 Surgical salvage for recurrent 'early' glottic cancers. J Surg Oncol 40: 32–33

43. Mantravadi R, Katz A M, Skolnik E M, Becker S, Freehling D J, Friedman M 1981 Stomal recurrence. A critical analysis of risk factors. Arch. Otolaryngol 107: 735–738

44. Maw R, Lavelle R J 1972 The management of post-operative pharyngocutaneous pharyngeal fistulae. J Laryngol Otol 86: 795–805

45. Mendenhall W M, Parsons J T, Stringer S P, Cassisi N J, Million R R 1990 Carcinoma of the supraglottic larynx: a basis for comparing the results of radiotherapy and surgery. Head Neck 12: 204–209

46. Meredith A P D'E, Randall C J, Shaw H J 1987 Advanced laryngeal cancer: a management perspective. J Laryngol. Otol 101: 1046–1054

47. Mohr R M, Quennelle D J, Shumrick D A, 1983 Vertico-frontolateral laryngectomy (hemilaryngectomy). Indications, technique and results. Arch Otolaryngol 109: 384–395

48. Morton R P, Chapman P, 1982 The results of treatment of laryngeal cancer in Auckland New Zealand 1965–79. Aust N Z Surg 52: 418–423

49. Myers E M, Ogura J H 1979 Completion laryngectomy. Ann Otol Rhinol Laryngol 88: 172–177

50. Nichols R D, Stine P H, Greenawald K J 1980 Partial laryngectomy after radiation failure. Laryngoscope 90: 571–575

52. Norris C M, Peale A R 1966 Partial laryngectomy for irradiation failure. Arch Otolaryngol 84: 558–562

52. Olofsson J, van Nostrand A W P 1973 Growth and spread of laryngeal and hypopharyngeal carcinoma with reflections on the effect of preoperative irradiation. 139 cases studied by whole organ serial sectioning. Acta Otolaryngol (suppl 308): pp 1–84

53. Olofsson J 1984 Early detection of recurrent tumours after previous treatment of laryngeal carcinomas. In: Wigand M E, Steiner W, Stell P M (eds) Functional partial laryngectomy. Springer-Verlag, Heidelberg, pp 310–314

54. Pearson B W 1981 Subtotal laryngectomy. Laryngoscope 91: 1904–1912

55. Pearson B W 1986 Near total laryngectomy. In: Cummings C W, Frederickson J M, Harker L A, Krause C J, Schuller D E (eds) Otolaryngology — head and neck surgery, Vol 3. Mosby, St Louis, pp 2117–2132

56. Piquet J J, Thill C, Chevalier D 1991 Die subtotale Laryngektomie mit Krikohyoidopexie in der Behandlung der ausgedehnten Tumoren des Larynx. In: Dühmke E, Steiner W, Reck R (eds) Funktionserhaltende Therapie des fortgeschrittenen Larynxkarzinoms. Thieme, Stuttgart, pp 112–116

57. Quayum M A, Glennie J McD, Orr J S 1978 Carcinoma of the larynx — results of primary radiotherapy. Clin Radiol 29: 21–25

58. Robin P E, Rockley T, Powell D J, Reid A 1991 Survival of cancer of the larynx related to treatment. Clin Otolaryngol 16: 193–197

59. Shah J P, Loree T R, Kowaiski L 1990 Conservation surgery for radiation-failure carcinoma of the glottic larynx. Head Neck 12: 326–331

60. Shamboul K, Doyle-Kelly W, Bailey D 1984 Results of salvage surgery following radical radiotherapy for laryngeal carcinoma. J Laryngol Otol 98: 905–907

61. Shaw H J 1991 Role of partial laryngectomy after irradiation in the treatment of laryngeal cancer: a view from the United Kingdom. Ann Otol Rhinol Laryngol 100: 268–273

62. Sisson G A, Bytell D E, Edison B D, Yeh S Jr 1975 Transsternal radical neck dissection for control of stomal recurrences — end results. Laryngoscope 85: 1504–1510

63. Skolnik E M, Martin L, Yee K F, Wheatley M A 1975 Radiation failures in cancer of the larynx. Ann Otol Rhinol Laryngol 84: 804–811

64. Som M L 1970 Conservation surgery for carcinoma of the supraglottis. J Laryngol Otol 84: 655–678

65. Soo K C, Shah J P, Gopinath K S, Gerold F P, Jaques D P, Strong E W 1988 Analysis of prognostic variables and results after supraglottic partial laryngectomy. Am J Surg 156: 301–305

66. Sorensen H, Hansen H S, Thomsen K A 1980 Partial laryngectomy following irradiation. Laryngoscope 90: 1344–1349

67. Steiner W 1991 Transorale, lasermikrochirurgische Behandlung fortgeschrittener Larynxkarzinome als Alternative zur Laryngektomie In: Dühmke E, Steiner W, Reck R (eds) Funktionsershaltende Therapie des fortgeschritten Larynxkarzinoms. Thieme, Stuttgart, 123–130

68. Stell P M 1969 Catastrophic haemorrhage after major neck surgery. Brit J Surg 56: 525–527

69. Stell P M, Cooney T C 1974 Management of fistulae of the head and neck after radical surgery. J Laryngol Otol 88: 819–834

70. Stell P M, Dalby J E 1985 The treatment of early (T1) glottic and supra-glottic carcinoma: does partial laryngectomy have a place? E J Surg Oncol 11: 263–266

71. Stell P M, Rawson N S B 1990 Adjuvant chemotherapy in head and neck cancer. Br J Cancer 61: 779–787

72. Stewart J G, Brown J R, Palmer M K, Cooper A 1974 The management of glottic carcinoma by primary irradiation with surgery in reserve. Laryngoscope 98: 317–320

73. Strauss M 1988 Hemilaryngectomy rescue surgery for radiation failure in early glottic carcinoma. Laryngoscope 98: 317–320

74. Strong M S 1975 Laser excision of carcinoma of the larynx. Laryngoscope 85: 1286–1289

75. Vega M F 1984 Treatment of recurrences after supraglottic horizontal laryngectomy. In Wigand M E, Steiner W, Stell P M (eds) Functional partial laryngectomy. Springer-Verlag, Heidelberg, pp 320–322

76. Viani L, Stell P M, Dalby J E 1991 Recurrence after radiotherapy for glottic cancer. Cancer 67: 577–584

77. Wang C C 1974 Treatment of glottic carcinoma by megavoltage radiation therapy and results Am J Roentgenol 120: 157–163

78. Ward P H, Calcaterra T C, Kagan A R 1975 The enigma of post-radiation edema and recurrent or residual carcinoma of the larynx. Laryngoscope 85: 522–529

79. Woodhouse R J, Quivey J M, Fu K K, Sien P S, Dedo H H, Phillips T L 1981 Treatment of carcinoma of the vocal cord — a review of 20 years' experience. Laryngoscope 91: 1155–1162

34. Prognostic factors

A. Ferlito, B. J. Bailey

INTRODUCTION

Various indicators may predict the clinical course of malignant neoplasms of the larynx. These can be grouped into host factors, tumour factors and treatment factors. Host factors include age, gender, nutritional status, general condition and immunological response.

Tumour factors include T stage, N stage, M stage, oncotype (or histological cell type), grade of malignancy and the presence of another cancer (whether synchronous or metachronous).

Treatment factors include all available types of therapy and various combinations of these modalities.

HOST FACTORS

Age

Data in the literature are controversial concerning the effects of age on survival. Some authors think that the prognosis is better in younger patients, whereas others claim it is better in the more elderly. Stell[40] showed that age and sex are not significant prognostic factors in patients with laryngeal cancer. Though statistical analysis shows that survival is significantly shorter in older versus younger patients,[22, 24] this probably depends on the fact that older patients are also usually affected by other diseases.

Gender

The site of laryngeal carcinoma differs widely according to gender. Women are more likely to have cancer of the supraglottis than of the glottis. In a recent review, the ratio of glottic to supraglottic tumours was 2.12:1 in men and 0.56:1 in women, a highly significant difference.[44]

Nutritional status

This correlates closely with the host's immuno-competence. Patients in negative nitrogen balance have a poorer general condition and respond less well to therapy.[40]

General condition

The patient's performance status is a factor in decisions as to the type of treatment selected. General condition naturally deteriorates with increasing age.[42] The host's general condition is usually evaluated according to three different systems, as outlined below.

Host (AJCC)[2]

H   Physical state (performance scale) of the patient, considering all cofactors determined at the time of stage classification and subsequent follow-up examinations
H0   Normal activity
H1   Symptomatic and ambulatory; cares for self
H2   Ambulatory more than 50% of time; occasionally needs assistance
H3   Ambulatory 50% or less of time; nursing care needed
H4   Bedridden; may need hospitalization

Karnofsky scale: performance status (PS) criteria

Able to carry on normal activity; requires no special care

100   Normal; no complaints; no evidence of disease
 90   Able to carry on normal activity; minor signs or symptoms of disease
 80   Able to carry on normal activity with effort; some signs or symptoms of disease

Unable to work; able to live at home and care for most personal needs; requires varying amount of assistance

 70   Cares for self; unable to carry on normal activity or to do active work
 60   Requires occasional assistance but is unable to care for most of own needs

583

50 Requires considerable assistance and frequent medical care

Unable to care for self; requires equivalent of institutional or hospital care; disease may be progressing rapidly

40 Disabled; requires special care and assistance
30 Severely disabled; hospitalization indicated, although death not imminent
20 Very sick; hospitalization necessary; active supportive treatment is necessary
10 Moribund, fatal processes progressing rapidly
0 Dead

Eastern Cooperative Oncology Group scale (ECOG)

Grade
0 Fully active, able to carry on all predisease activities without restriction (Karnofsky 90–100)
1 Restricted in physically strenuous activity but ambulatory and able to carry out work of a light or sedentary nature — for example, light housework or office work (Karnofsky 70–80)
2 Ambulatory and capable of all self-care but unable to carry out any work activities. Up and about more than 50% of waking hours (Karnofsky 50–60)
3 Capable of only limited self-care, confined to bed or chair 50% or more of waking hours (Karnofsky 30–40)
4 Completely disabled, cannot carry on any self-care, totally confined to bed or chair (Karnofsky 10–20)

Immunological response

Opinions on available immunological parameters of prognostic relevance vary widely.[16] Patients with cancer of the larynx often have immune deficits or abnormal immune reactions, but this altered immunological condition could depend on alcohol abuse in many cases. Lymphocytes and plasma cell infiltration at the edge of the neoplasm can be regarded as an expression of the host's reactive potential against tumour cells.[34] Despite much research, present knowledge of the host's immunological response is rudimentary and requires more intensive investigation.[47] Unfortunately, up to the present moment, the reality has not lived up to the promise with regard to the use of tumour markers to monitor tumour activity and predict treatment outcome in patients with head and neck cancer. A recent review[20] evaluates the potential activity and present status of nine tumour markers, i.e. (i) squamous cell carcinoma antigen; (ii) carcino-embryonic antigen; (iii) serum ferritin; (iv) glycoprotein cancer-associated antigens CA50 and CA19-9; (v) enzymes, phosphohexose isomerase, adenosine deaminase and aliesterase; (vi) immunoglobulins and immune complex; (vii) serum glycoproteins; (viii)

erythrocyte polyamines; and (ix) prostaglandins and prostacyclines. The evidence is that these markers may be of value eventually but no 'ideal' marker has been found so far.

Another aspect that shows potential for providing prognostic information is the *loss of expression of blood-group antigens* as determinants of cellular invasion and survival in patients with head and neck cancer. Carey et al[7] measured the expression of A9 antigen and the loss of blood-group antigens in a series of 37 previously untreated patients with head and neck squamous cell carcinoma. These patients underwent traditional management for their tumours and were followed prospectively for tumour recurrence and death. After a median follow-up time of 22 months, 18 of the patients had relapsed and 18 of them had died (four from unrelated causes). The A9 monoclonal antibody was used to detect an antigen expressed by all of the squamous cell carcinomas tested by this group. They observed that the strong expression of A9 antibody in tumour tissue was associated with tumour recurrence. They also found that the loss of blood group antigen expression is strongly associated with decreased survival.

Bryne et al[6] studied the loss of expression of blood antigen H in association with tumour invasion and spread. They emphasize the difficulty in studying malignant tumours on the basis of the analysis of small samples. They remind us that malignant tumours often have very heterogeneous cell populations and that the sophisticated analysis of a group of cells from the periphery of a malignant neoplasm may be quite different from the findings of a similar analysis on the cell population in the centre of the tumour. Furthermore, the cellular characteristics of the most invasive portions of the carcinoma may be more important for predicting patients' prognosis than characteristics of the cells in other parts of the tumour. These investigators conclude that H antigen staining of the entire tumour did not correlate with the stage of the tumour or its spread, but loss of staining in the most invasive portion of the tumour correlated significantly with the stage of tumour development and the histological grade of malignancy. They feel that these findings support the existence of a linkage between the loss of antigen expression on the deep invasive cell and the prediction of aggressive clinical behaviour of the tumour.

TUMOUR FACTORS

T stage

When the International Union Against Cancer published the document *TNM Classification of Malignant Tumours* in 1987[45] and the American Joint Committee on Cancer followed suit with the same system in 1988,[2] there was agreement for the first time on the TNM classification for laryngeal cancer. The criticism of the new system that subsequently came from laryngologists around the world emphasizes the differences of opinion that are held concerning the prognostic importance of certain biological, biochemical, histopathological and clinical findings. It is important to recognize that the TNM laryngeal cancer classification provides only a standardized group of categories for patients with laryngeal cancer, which is to say that the system allows us to *stratify* patients according to the severity of their illness.[3] We may thus share clinical observations from different parts of the world, confident in the knowledge that we are comparing similar groups of patients. The TNM system provides information on the primary tumour's anatomical location and size and on the presence of regional and distant metastases. Of course, this is useful in predicting survival, and the tumour's precise location within the larynx is a relevant factor influencing prognosis. Patients with supraglottic cancer usually have a worse prognosis than patients with a glottic cancer; in particular, cancers of the aryepiglottic folds present the worst clinical prognosis.[37] Considerable discrepancies can occur between pre-therapeutic classification and the actual extension of the tumour, particularly in the case of the larger lesions. Despite recent advances in imaging techniques (CT and MRI), the tumour's extension and especially its depth of invasion are clinically very difficult to assess.

Stell[41] recently stated that the T stage has very little impact on survival: 'Survival did fall dramatically with an increase in T stage, but this fall is almost entirely due to the increasing incidence of lymph node metastases.' When survival was analysed by multifactorial methods using Cox's regression technique, and taking interactions into account, only N status — and *not* T stage — proved a significant prognostic indicator.[41]

N stage

Treatment and prognosis for patients with laryngeal cancer are determined mainly by nodal status. The most significant single prognostic indicator is the presence or absence of metastatic cancer in cervical lymph nodes. Neck node status is the only factor which significantly predicts *length* of survival in patients who die of their cancer.[41] Squamous cell carcinoma of the larynx tends to metastasize to the cervical lymph nodes in the form of emboli. Few lymph nodes are involved in the great majority of cases. There is generally a relationship between the degree of structural differentiation and the incidence of lymph node metastasis.[29] Poorly-differentiated squamous cell carcinomas prove more aggressive than well-differentiated neoplasms.[14] The level of cervical lymph node involvement is also important: metastases to lymph nodes in the anterior inferior and posterior inferior

cervical triangles worsen the prognosis[35] and so does involvement of the prelaryngeal node.[31] Contralateral involvement, whether synchronous or occurring after primary treatment, is an ominous prognostic finding. Although the number, size and level of invaded nodes is clearly important, these factors are secondary to the overriding prognostic significance of extracapsular spread.[8, 10, 21, 23, 26, 27, 31, 38, 41] Errors in determining the presence and size of occult lymph node metastases have been reduced by the use of ultrasound, ultrasound-guided fine-needle aspiration biopsy, CAT and MRI, which should be used for clinical staging. Application of the AJCC/UICC TNM system provides prognostic information. As observed in other organs, monoclonal antibodies can identify occult micrometastases to the cervical lymph nodes which go undetected by conventional light microscopy.[13] In conclusion, the extent of cervical lymph node metastatic distribution is clearly of paramount prognostic importance.

M stage

Distant metastases in squamous cell carcinoma are usually preceded by lymph node metastases. Blood-borne metastases are uncommon, but widespread dissemination to various viscera may occur in advanced stages of laryngeal cancer. The sites which appear to be most affected by distant metastatic spread are the mediastinal lymph nodes, lungs, liver, pleura, skeletal system, kidney, heart, spleen and pancreas.[37] The cavernous sinus and temporal bones are an unusual site for metastasis. Naturally, distant metastases have been correlated with a poor prognosis. Some tumours, particularly adenoid cystic carcinoma and sarcomas, may metastasize to several viscera, without cervical lymph node metastases.[15]

Histological cell type

The oncotype, or histological cell type, provides a *qualitative* diagnosis of the disease. Approximately 90% of malignant neoplasms of the larynx are squamous cell carcinomas and can be graded as well differentiated (G1), moderately differentiated (G2) or poorly differentiated (G3). Cancers other than squamous cell carcinoma are not considered for the purposes of this analysis, but about 10% of malignant laryngeal tumours do belong to other oncotypes, differing not only in histological findings but also in clinical behaviour. Biological behaviour varies from one type of cancer to another so only similar types are comparable for prognostic implications.

Survival is generally related to specific histological types of laryngeal cancer. It is common knowledge that a small cell neuroendocrine carcinoma metastasizes more frequently than does a squamous cell carcinoma, and that the latter is more malignant than a verrucous squamous cell carcinoma. Each malignant tumour has its own degree of intrinsic aggressiveness strictly correlated with the structure of the neoplasm. Prognosis for such tumours consequently differs enormously (e.g. it is excellent for verrucous squamous cell carcinoma, generally fair for common squamous cell carcinoma and poor for small cell neuroendocrine carcinoma). Five-year survivals are about 60% for squamous carcinoma[2] and 5% for small cell neuroendocrine carcinoma of the larynx,[17] considering all stages of the disease. If we take squamous cell carcinoma as a standard for comparison with other specific histological types of laryngeal cancer, the following are more favourable: verrucous squamous carcinomas, most mucoepidermoid carcinomas and typical carcinoid tumours. The less favourable types include: small cell neuroendocrine carcinoma, basaloid squamous carcinoma and atypical carcinoid tumour. Moreover, the exact identification of the type of laryngeal tumour permits *specific* and *individual tumour staging*, according to the oncotype involved (tumour staging evaluation in verrucous squamous cell carcinoma is not the same as in neuroendocrine carcinomas or lymphomas). The oncotype should be considered as a guide-line for selecting treatment.

Histological grading of malignancy

The variability of a tumour's differentiation in separate areas of a laryngectomy specimen is generally acknowledged and invalidates the grading of biopsy specimens,[16] but the degree of a neoplasm's differentiation should not be confused with its histological grading. Factors allowing for a better assessment of the histological grading of malignancies include: (i) degree of structural differentiation; (ii) cellular anaplasia or pleomorphism; (iii) mitotic activity index (frequency and abnormality of mitotic figures); (iv) expansive or infiltrative growth; (v) inflammatory response to the tumour; (vi) necrosis; and (vii) lymphatic and blood vessel invasion. Multivariate histological analysis is a well-tested method for estimating prognosis.

There has been a great deal of interest in DNA flow cytometry as a prognostic indicator in head and neck cancer, albeit with controversial results.[9, 12, 19, 25, 33] Numerous investigators have concluded that flow cytometry DNA ploidy measurements may eventually provide important prognostic information concerning patients with laryngeal cancer. Goldsmith et al[19] observed that patients with clearly aneuploid primary carcinomas had a significantly better prognosis than those with diploid tumours, and that ploidy was the most significant prognostic variable for the laryngeal group of tumours among several variables that were considered. Kearsley et al[25] studied DNA ploidy and DNA index. They observed that DNA aneuploidy and increased DNA index were significant, independent prognostic factors for both

relapse-free and overall survival. They observed that relapse and death rates among patients with aneuploid cancers were approximately three times as high as those for diploid subjects. Patients with a DNA index greater than 2.11 (hypertetraploidy) were noted to have more than a six-fold higher death rate than patients exhibiting diploid cancer features. Cooke et al[9] measured tumour cellular DNA in 102 patients with advanced head and neck cancer who were being treated with cis-platinum. They found a median survival time of 55 days for patients with aneuploid tumours who did not receive treatment, and 224 days with similar patients who were treated with cis-platinum. By contrast, untreated patients with diploid tumours survived 74 days while those with diploid tumours treated with cis-platinum survived for 118 days. They concluded that ploidy was a significant predictor of survival and therefore could be considered as a prognostic indicator for advanced head and neck cancer.

The relationship between histological features, DNA flow cytometry and the clinical behaviour of squamous cell carcinomas of the larynx was studied intensively by Ruá et al.[33] They performed flow cytometry analysis of the DNA content of primary squamous cell carcinomas in 133 patients who were categorized on the basis of the nature of their primary tumour, regional lymph nodes, tumour grade and keratinization. These features were compared with the form of therapy that was employed as well as the DNA index. All these factors were then analysed in regard to patients' survival. They concluded that ploidy was related to the histological grade of the tumour and noted that in well-differentiated tumours (G1) there was a 42% 4-year survival rate in patients with diploid tumours and a 28% 4-year survival rate in non-diploid tumours. In the subset of patients who had no cervical node metastases (N0) and who underwent surgery for their tumour, the 4-year survival rate was 82% for diploid tumours and 49% for non-diploid tumours. They concluded that ploidy probably provides a new opportunity to estimate the prognosis of a patient with squamous cell carcinoma of the larynx and therefore allows the surgeon to recognize those patients with a more or less favourable prognosis at an early stage of their management.

El-Naggar et al[12] found a high intratumoral heterogeneity of DNA content in laryngeal squamous cell carcinomas and hence variations in prognostic implications. The results of the determination of DNA ploidy in squamous cell carcinoma have remained contradictory to date and have also failed to provide any useful prognostic information in neuroendocrine neoplasms of the larynx.[30]

The presence of another cancer

Another important factor influencing survival is the presence of other, synchronous or metachronous primary cancers, whether in the head and neck area or elsewhere, but especially in the oesophagus, lung and oral cavity. Cancers of the larynx tend to have second primaries in the lung, whereas neoplasms in the oral cavity tend to have second primaries in the oesophagus. The presence of a previous or synchronous cancer halves survival.[41] Patients with cancer are at a higher risk of developing a second primary cancer.

TREATMENT FACTORS

An important factor in the management of cancer of the larynx is the determination whether the carcinoma is in situ, micro-invasive or frankly invasive. 'Minimal laryngeal cancer' defines in-situ carcinoma and micro-invasive carcinoma, and the prognosis is generally favourable. Invasive cancer of the larynx, left untreated, is inevitably a fatal disease: 90% of untreated patients die within 3 years.[36] Surgery and radiation therapy, either alone or in combination, are the conventional modalities for the management of malignant laryngeal tumours. Chemotherapy is also indicated in some rare, non-squamous carcinomas, such as small cell neuroendocrine carcinomas, diffuse lymphomas, etc. Laser surgery is also a valid means of treatment for early malignant neoplasms of the glottis. In squamous cell carcinoma, the role of chemotherapy in conjunction with conventional treatment remains controversial and adjuvant chemotherapy does not usually improve the survival rate achieved by conventional surgery and radiotherapy. In an editorial which appeared in *Clinical Otolaryngology*, Stell[43] claimed that adjuvant chemotherapy for squamous cell carcinoma of the head and neck has even *reduced* survival by 3.5%.

The treatment of laryngeal cancer should be selected according to histological cell type and stage of disease, and the pathologist, whose primary responsibility is to establish an accurate diagnosis, must act as a consultant for the management of patients with cancer of the larynx. The final decision regarding treatment may also be influenced by other factors, including the host's age, general condition and occupation, the physician's experience, treatment centres available, etc. Of course, the choice of treatment is an important parameter influencing not only prognosis but also, more importantly, the patient's *quality of life*. Obviously, prognosis is better if the most suitable therapy is undertaken initially.

Recent reports provide contradictory findings on the effects of blood transfusions on prognosis,[1, 4, 5,46] and although immune suppression due to peri-operative transfusions has been implicated in worsened prognosis after laryngectomy, this remains to be demonstrated conclusively.[11]

CONSIDERATIONS

The TNM system is only an anatomical means of classification which takes into account neither the biological aggressiveness of various neoplasms nor the host's immunological response. It was not developed to serve as a specific guide-line for the management of a particular patient, nor does the system have the ability to predict the outcome of individual patients. However, while physicians are focused on the concept of optimal treatment, patients are interested in their prognosis, and one of the most important tasks is to assess our present ability to predict the probable outcome for a particular patient with laryngeal cancer. Some surgeons feel that we are on the verge of major advances in our search for prognostic indicators, while others have observed that the growing body of scientific literature in the field of laryngeal cancer may represent nothing more than an 'encyclopaedia of ignorance'.[28]

In an editorial by Goepfert and Schantz,[18] several popular criticisms were expressed when they wrote:

> Yet it is widely held that the current staging system for head and neck cancer is limited. For example, the group staging is ambiguous because it includes cancers of different natural behaviour, the possible combinations of T and N classifications grouped under stages III and IV being the most notable deficiency. Two-dimensional definitions that utilize only the size and the location of cancer do not necessarily predict its metastatic potential. Certainly, local spread and distant metastasis have occurred long before they are discernible by clinical examination. . . . We should incorporate the reproducible, sophisticated parameters of both the tumor and host variables in this process. The determination of DNA content and cell cycle kinetics is already being used for the prediction of response to treatment and prognosis. In terms of the cancer cell, the quantification of growth factor receptors could be determined by the initial biopsy, as could the measurements of oncogene expression, presence of viral oncogene promoters, cell cytokine production and the affinity of the cancer cell to grow in particular tissue environments, such as the perineural spaces or distant parenchymas.

The various studies mentioned in this chapter are but a small sampling of the rapidly expanding literature in this exciting field. Each month, there are reports from investigators around the world indicating support for these concepts and suggesting new avenues for scientific investigation. Attempts to incorporate these new proposals into patient care management and patient counselling present a daunting challenge and represent the ultimate in trying to hit a moving target.

The Laryngeal Cancer Association has promoted a worldwide survey to collect expert opinions on the applicability of the TNM system to cancer of the larynx.[3] Of those laryngologists who responded to the survey, only about 10% were entirely satisfied with its practical use. As a consequence, the Association appointed an international Committee on the Classification of Laryngeal Cancer consisting of Byron J. Bailey (Chairman, Galveston, Texas, USA), Lawrence W. DeSanto (Scottsdale, Arizona, USA), Alfio Ferlito (Padova, Italy), Helmuth Goepfert (Houston, Texas, USA), Michael E.

Johns (Baltimore, Maryland, USA), Willy Lehmann (Geneva, Switzerland), Jan Olofsson (Bergen, Norway) and Philip M. Stell (Liverpool, Great Britain). This committee was asked to analyse the current TNM classification system and to explore the opportunities for its correlation with other prognostic features.

One of the useful methods for approaching this type of analysis is to begin by determining the opinions of a specific set of field experts. We therefore devised a questionnaire that listed 38 positive prognostic factors and 55 negative prognostic factors that appear in the literature most frequently. This informal survey was circulated with a request that each member of the committee respond by indicating his current level of enthusiasm for each of these potential prognostic indicators. The overall purpose of the survey is to collect information from a laryngeal cancer study group and organize these opinions, drawing from many decades of clinical and research observation, to see if there is any level of consensus at the present time. This effort is exploratory and preliminary in nature and makes no attempt to make far-reaching conclusions, but we found the responses interesting.

Each respondent was asked to indicate whether he strongly agrees, agrees, is neutral, disagrees or strongly disagrees that each of a series of individual features represents either a favourable or an unfavourable prognostic indicator. The results are summarized in Table 34.1. In analysing the list of positive predictive factors, we used three of these factors as a 'gold standard' in terms of wide acceptance on the basis of inclusion in the TNM system. In general, the most unanimous response of a favourable outcome was felt to be the *absence of metastasis*, a *low T stage* and a *low N stage*. These responses reflect a general acceptance of the value of TNM staging, though it is important to emphasize once again that it is not the primary purpose of the TNM system to predict outcome or direct treatment for individual patients.

The strongest consensus regarding a factor outside the TNM system is expressed in regard to the absence of extracapsular spread of tumour. This is ranked as equivalent to a low T stage or a low N as a predictor of favourable outcome. Next in its predictive value is the clinical finding that a glottic primary is limited to the membranous portion of the true vocal cord. This clinical finding is obviously related to T stage in that all such primaries would be T1 tumours. The high consensus of responders that this represents a predictor of favourable outcome could reflect such opinions as the better prognosis of glottic primaries as opposed to supraglottic or transglottic primaries. The response could also reflect the opinion that small primaries have a better prognosis, even within the T1 category range of tumour sizes and sites.

The next two features in terms of consensus are clear resection margins, as confirmed by histological assessment, and normal true vocal cord mobility (2A rather than 2B glottic cancer).

Table 34.1   Laryngeal panel consensus regarding the most influential favourable and unfavourable prognostic features for laryngeal cancer (in diminishing order of importance)

Favourable features	Unfavourable features
No metastasis	Lymph nodes less-movable to fixed
Low T	Recurrent disease
Low N	Tumour involves overlying skin
No extracapsular spread	Extracapsular spread
Glottic primary limited to membranous portion of true cord	Second malignant primary
Clear resection margins	Continued exposure to carcinogens
Normal vocal cord mobility	Tumour at resection margin
Ceased exposure to carcinogens	Transglottic lesions
Glottic primary	Airway obstruction and emergency tracheotomy
Highly differentiated histology	High tumour volume doubling time
Only unilateral or ipsilateral lymph nodes	Poor performance status
Lesser total tumour volume	Extension to posterior commissure
Lesser depth of invasion	Nerve sheath (perineural) invasion
Lymph nodes easily movable	Neuroendocrine tumours (atypical carcinoid and small cell neuroendocrine carcinoma)
Retain epithelial movement over the vocal ligament	Subglottic extension more than 1 cm
Exophytic growth pattern	Greater tumour volume
Good performance status	More depth of tumour invasion
Histologically 'pushing' tumour margins	Lymph node metastasis in laryngectomy specimen
Smaller lymph nodes size within the range	Impaired vocal cord mobility
Host's good nutritional status	Microscopic vascular invasion
Fewer palpable lymph nodes within stage	'Burrowing' growth pattern
Primary tumour size less than 2 cm	Larger lymph nodes in N stage range
Low tumour volume doubling time	More lymph nodes in N stage

After that, there were three factors felt to be of considerable importance and these are cessation of exposure to carcinogens (a behavioural feature), glottic location of the primary (rather than supraglottic, subglottic or transglottic) and highly differentiated tumour histology. After this, in descending order, were only unilateral or ipsilateral lymph nodes, lesser total tumour volume and lesser depth of invasion.

The list of unfavourable prognostic features in regard to laryngeal cancer consists of the opposite features from the favourable prognosis list in some instances. Other examples of unfavourable features are distinct and independent negative factors on their own. The most unfavourable prognostic features according to these responses is lymph node(s) being from less-movable to fixed in nature. This feature is somewhat outside the TNM staging system but represents a distinction within an already decreased survival category (in that the patient must already have palpable nodes in order to have less-movable to fixed nodes).

The second worst prognostic features were recurrent malignant disease and tumour involving the overlying skin. In the next group, we note the presence of lymph node extracapsular spread, the detection of a second malignant primary tumour and then the patient's continued exposure to carcinogens. After that in the ranking is the presence of tumour at the resection margin.

Three features that tied for the next level of favourable prognosis were transglottic lesions, airway obstruction with the need for emergency tracheotomy and high tumour volume doubling time as measured by cell cycle kinetics.

Next in order were poor performance status, extension to the posterior commissure of the larynx, nerve sheath (perineural) invasion and certain neuroendocrine carcinomas (atypical carcinoid tumour and small cell neuroendocrine carcinoma).

It is timely to consider the possibility of developing a mathematical formula with the appropriate variables that pertain to the visible characteristics of primary tumour, the standard clinical assessment of these patients, new parameters of tumour biology and host response, the impact of different forms of therapy and any additional information that can be gathered from the surgical specimen or any other accessible source.

Our next task would be to weight these dozens of factors according to their predictive power and to vary this weighting as new information is gained. Thereby we would be able to add to the great value of the existing TNM system and what it can accomplish. To take this next step will require a major, coordinated effort to bring basic scientists, clinicians, biostaticians, mathematicians and information scientists together to develop this predictive formula. The time and effort involved in this task is formidable but will be well worth the effort in terms of the benefit that will accrue to our patients.

ACKNOWLEDGEMENTS

The authors would like to express their gratitude to the other members of The Laryngeal Cancer Association's Committee studying the TNM classification system (Lawrence DeSanto, Helmuth Goepfert, Michael Johns, Willy Lehmann, Jan Olofsson, Philip Stell), whose comments and suggestions provided invaluable support in the writing of this chapter. Under the direct control of the Chairman, Dr Bailey, the Committee is currently working on the findings of a questionnaire and planning further steps with a view to ultimately developing a multifactorial predictive formula to guide therapeutic decisions and predict prognosis for patients with laryngeal cancer.

REFERENCES

1. Alun-Jones T, Clarke P J, Morrissey S, Hill J 1991 Blood transfusion and laryngeal cancer. Clin Otolaryngol 16: 240–244
2. American Joint Committee on Cancer 1988 Manual for Staging of Cancer, 3rd edn. Lippincott, Philadelphia
3. Bailey B J 1991 Beyond the 'new' TNM classification. Arch Otolaryngol Head Neck Surg 117: 369–370
4. Böck M, Grevers G, Koblitz M, Heim M U, Mempel W 1990 Influence of blood transfusion on recurrence, survival and postoperative infections of laryngeal cancer. Acta Otolaryngol 110: 155–160
5. Bongioannini G, Vercellino M, Rugiu M G, Ferreri A, Succo G, Cortesina G 1990 Influence of perioperative transfusion therapy on the recurrence potential of locally advanced laryngeal carcinoma. ORL J Otorhinolaryngol Relat Spec 52: 260–264
6. Bryne M, Thrane P S, Dabelsteen E 1991 Loss of expression of blood group antigen H is associated with cellular invasion and spread of oral squamous cell carcinomas. Cancer 67: 613–618
7. Carey T E, Wolf G T, Hsu S, Poore J, Peterson K, McClatchey K D 1987 Expression of A9 antigen and loss of blood antigens as determinants of survival in patients with head and neck squamous carcinoma. Otolaryngol Head Neck Surg 96: 221–230
8. Carter R L, Bliss J M, Soo K C, O'Brien C J 1987 Radical neck dissections for squamous carcinomas: pathological findings and clinical implications with particular reference to transcapsular spread. Int J Radiat Oncol Biol Phys 17: 825–832
9. Cooke L D, Cooke T G, Bootz F, Forster G, Helliwell T R, Spiller D, Stell P M 1990 Ploidy as a prognostic indicator in end stage squamous cell carcinoma of the head and neck region treated with cisplatinum. Br J Cancer 61: 759–762
10. Devineni V R, Simpson R, Sessions D, Spector J G, Hayden R, Fredrickson J, Fineberg B 1991 Supraglottic carcinoma: impact of radiation therapy on outcome of patients with positive margins and extracapsular nodal disease. Laryngoscope 101: 767–770
11. Ell S R, Stell P M 1991 Blood transfusion and survival after laryngectomy for laryngeal carcinoma. J Laryngol Otol 105: 293–294
12. El-Naggar A, Weber R, Luna M, Garsney L, Batsakis J G 1991 Intratumoral heterogeneity of DNA content in laryngeal squamous carcinoma. Am Soc Head Neck Surg, abstract
13. Farrell R W R, Mckenna D M, Clegg R T 1991 Micrometastases from laryngeal carcinoma in cervical lymph nodes: an immunohistochemical study (abstract). Clin Otolaryngol 16: 519–520
14. Ferlito A 1976 Histological classification of larynx and hypopharynx cancers and their clinical implications. Pathologic apects of 2052 malignant neoplasms diagnosed at the ORL Department of Padua

University from 1966 to 1976. Acta Otolaryngol 342: (suppl) 1 –88

15. Ferlito A, Barnes L, Myers E N 1990 Neck dissection for laryngeal adenoid cystic carcinoma: is it indicated? Ann Otol Rhinol Laryngol 99: 277–280

16. Friedmann I, Ferlito A 1988 Granulomas and neoplasms of the larynx. Churchill Livingstone, Edinburgh

17. Gnepp D R 1991 Small cell neuroendocrine carcinoma of the larynx. A clinical review of the literature. ORL J Otorhinolaryngol Relat Spec 53: 210–219

18. Goepfert H, Schantz S P 1990 Is it time for biologic staging of cancer? Head Neck 12: 291–292

19. Goldsmith M M, Cresson D H, Arnold L A, Postma D S, Askin F B, Pillsbury H C 1987 Part I. DNA flow cytometry as a prognostic indicator in head and neck cancer. Otolaryngol Head Neck Surg 96: 307–318

20. Hanna E Y N, Papay F A, Gupta M K, Lavertu P, Tucker H M 1990 Serum tumor markers of head and neck cancer: current status. Head Neck 12: 50–59

21. Hirabayashi H, Koshii K, Uno K, Ohgaki H, Nakasone Y, Fujisawa T, Syouno N, Hinohara T, Hirabayashi K 1991 Extracapsular spread of squamous cell carcinoma in neck lymph nodes: prognostic factor in laryngeal cancer. Laryngoscope 101: 502–506

22. Huygen P L M, van Den Broek P, Kazem I 1980 Age and mortality in laryngeal cancer. Clin Otolaryngol 5: 129–137

23. Johnson J T, Myers E N, Bedetti C D, Barnes E L, Schramm V L, Thearle P B 1985 Cervical lymph node metastases. Incidence and implications of extracapsular carcinoma. Arch Otolaryngol 111: 534–537

24. Katz A E 1983 Immunobiologic staging of patients with carcinoma of the head and neck. Laryngoscope 93: 445–463

25. Kearsley J H, Bryson G, Battistutta D, Collins R J 1991 Prognostic importance of cellular DNA content in head-and-neck squamous cell cancers. A comparison of retrospective and prospective series. Int J Cancer 47: 31–37

26. Kowalski L P, Franco E L, De Andrade Sobrinho J, Oliveira B V, Pontes P L 1991 Prognostic factors in laryngeal cancer patients submitted to surgical treatment. J Surg Oncol 48: 87–95

27. Lefebvre J L, Castelain B, de la Torre J C, Delobelle-Deroide A, Vankemmel B 1987 Lymph node invasion in hypopharynx and lateral epilarynx carcinoma: a prognostic factor. Head Neck Surg 10: 14–18

28. Maran A G D 1990 Head and neck surgery: an encyclopaedia of ignorance. J Laryngol Otol 104: 529–533

29. McGavran M H, Bauer W C, Ogura J H 1961 The incidence of cervical lymph node metastases from epidermoid carcinoma of the larynx and their relationship to certain characteristics of the primary tumor: a study based on the clinical and pathological findings for 96 patients treated by primary en bloc laryngectomy and radical neck dissection. Cancer 14: 55–66

30. Milroy C M, Williams R A, Charlton I G, Moss E, Rode J 1991 Nuclear ploidy in neuroendocrine neoplasms of the larynx. ORL J Othorhinolaryngol Relat Spec 53: 245–249

31. Resta L, Micheau C, Cimmino A 1985 Prognostic value of the prelaryngeal node in laryngeal and hypopharyngeal carcinoma. Tumori 71: 361–365

32. Richard J M, Sancho-Garnier H, Saravane D, Micheau C, Cachin Y 1987 Prognostic factors in cervical lymph node metastasis in upper respiratory and digestive tract carcinomas: study of 1713 cases during a 15-year period. Laryngoscope 97: 97–101

33. Ruá S, Comino A, Fruttero A, Cera G, Semeria C, Lanzillotta L, Boffetta P 1991 Relationship between histologic features, DNA flow cytometry, and clinical behaviour of squamous cell carcinomas of the larynx. Cancer 67: 141–149

34. Sala O, Ferlito A 1976 Morphological observations of immunobiology of laryngeal cancer. Evaluation of the defensive activity of immunocompetent cells present in tumour stroma. Acta Otolaryngol 81: 353–363

35. Sessions D G 1976 Surgical pathology of cancer of the larynx and hypopharynx. Laryngoscope 86: 814–839

36. Shimkin M B 1951 Duration of life in untreated cancer. Cancer 4: 1–8

37. Silvestri F, Bussani R, Stanta G, Cosatti C, Ferlito A 1992 Supraglottic versus glottic laryngeal cancer: epidemiological and pathological aspects. ORL J Otorhinolaryngol Relat Spec 54: 43–48

38. Snow G B, Annayas A A, van Slooten E A, Bartelink H, Hart A A M 1982 Prognostic factors of neck node metastasis. Clin Otolaryngol 7: 185–192

39. Snyderman N L, Johnson J T, Schramm V L Jr, Myers E N, Bedetti C D, Thearle P 1985 Extracapsular spread of carcinoma in cervical lymph nodes. Impact upon survival in patients with carcinoma of the supraglottic larynx. Cancer 56: 1597–1599

40. Stell P M 1988 Prognostic factors in laryngeal carcinoma. Clin Otolaryngol 13: 399–409

41. Stell P M 1990 Prognosis in laryngeal carcinoma: tumour factors. Clin Otolaryngol 15: 69–81

42. Stell P M 1990 Prognosis in laryngeal carcinoma: host factors. Clin Otolaryngol 15: 111–119

43. Stell P M 1990 Adjuvant chemotherapy in head and neck cancer. Clin Otolaryngol 15: 193–195

44. Stephenson W T, Barnes D E, Holmes F F, Norris C W 1991 Gender influences subsite of origin of laryngeal carcinoma. Arch Otolaryngol Head Neck Surg 117: 774–778

45. Union Internationale Contre le Cancer (International Union Against Cancer) 1987 TNM classification of malignant tumours, 4th edn. Springer-Verlag, Berlin

46. Woolley A L, Hogikyan N D, Gates G A, Haughey B H, Schechtman K B, Goldenberg J L 1992 Effect of blood transfusion on recurrence of head and neck carcinoma. Retrospective review and meta-analysis. Ann Otol Rhinol Laryngol 101: 724–730

47. Wustrow T P U 1990 Assessment of immunocompetence for biological staging of head and neck cancer. In: Fee W E Jr, Goepfert H, Johns M E, Strong E W, Ward P H (eds) Head and neck cancer, Vol 2. Decker, Toronto, 108–118

35. Routines for follow-up and the risk of multiple primaries

J. Olofsson

FOLLOW-UP ROUTINES

The routines vary considerably between different oncological centres regarding the follow-up of patients treated for laryngeal and other head and neck carcinomas. Few studies have been performed evaluating our post-treatment follow-up procedures. Boysen et al[9] looked at the value of routine follow-up in patients treated for squamous cell carcinoma of the head and neck. In 20% of the patients with recurrences the diagnosis was made on the basis of symptoms that made the patients contact the hospital between the scheduled appointments. As most recurrences in head and neck carcinomas occur within 2–3 years, Boysen et al[9] concluded that it seems that our routine follow-up procedures for most types of carcinoma may be too extensive and that follow-up beyond 3 years will be of value primarily for the possible detection of second primary malignancies.

Anyhow, most centres have strict routines for their follow-up procedures so that they can detect, as early as possible, locoregional recurrences and—not least—second primaries, on which great interest has been focused, especially during the latter years. To be able to preserve the function, a strict follow-up system is a necessity when dealing with premalignant and malignant laryngeal squamous cell lesions.[25,51]

Many factors have to be taken into account in the follow-up of patients treated for laryngeal carcinoma.

Oncological centres

Patients with head and neck cancer in general should be treated at oncological centres with adequate equipment and necessary expertise available. The number of patients treated should be large enough to provide possibilities for systematized studies to evaluate the treatment results. Computerized registration is more and more becoming an integrated part of the routine work at oncological centres for an easy patient follow-up and for continuous statistical work. The careful initial examination and description is a prerequisite to be able to identify recurrences as early as possible. In many centres in Scandinavia, Great Britain and North America patients are seen in joint ENT–radiotherapy clinics. Under all circumstances the patients are best followed by specialists who are able to manage patients with recurrent disease.

A good photographic documentation of the tumour, preferably as a colour photo in the chart, makes assessment easier.

Examination of the larynx

Microlaryngoscopy should be performed in all patients before the initial treatment. Radiological imaging is also a necessity for the correct classification according to our staging systems.

Previously, all patients had to be examined by microlaryngoscopy 3–4 months after irradiation treatment. Nowadays fibrescopic examination may be enough, at least for minor carcinomas. Smear cytology can be a diagnostic aid, but it is less sensitive after previous radiotherapy.[35,36]

Biopsy specimens should be removed from all clinically suspect areas, and this is best performed at microlaryngoscopy. One has to be careful, however, not to be too aggressive and thereby introduce an infection with the risk of subsequent chondritis in irradiated patients.

Stroboscopy may be useful in the follow-up of patients with vocal cord lesions. After irradiation treatment, glottic waves remain in about 50% of the patients. If these disappear later on, a microlaryngoscopy and biopsy should be performed.

As 90% of recurrences occur within the first 2 years, the follow-up needs to be more frequent during this period of time. Our recommendations are examination every second month during the first year after irradiation therapy, every third month for the following two years, and every fourth month up to five years. After this examination every sixth month will be satisfactory. The 90° optical instruments, the flexible laryngoscope and the stroboscope have markedly improved the possibility of diagnosing early glottic recurrences.

Impaired vocal cord mobility

Impaired mobility or fixation of the vocal cord appearing after previous minor endoscopic surgery or radiotherapy indicates recurrent disease until the contrary is proven. Microlaryngoscopy should be performed and multiple biopsies removed even if there is no visible tumour. After irradiation, but also after partial laryngectomy procedures, there is a risk of recurrent disease entirely under an intact overlying mucosa. After partial surgery the natural barriers within the larynx are removed and the tumours may spread outside the larynx into the soft tissues.

TUMOUR FACTORS

The intervals between laryngoscopic examinations should certainly depend on location and extent of the tumour. A patient with a T3 glottic cancer who has received a full course of radiotherapy needs a more intense follow-up examination, especially if vocal cord mobility is not returning, compared to a patient with a small T1 glottic carcinoma with a normal vocal cord mobility.

Tumours involving the anterior commissure inherit a great risk of subglottic extension. The fibrescope nowadays enables us to make a more detailed examination of the anterior commissure region. The examination can be performed as an outpatient procedure under local anaesthesia.

When dealing with severe dysplasia and carcinoma in situ it is the well-differentiated, diffuse lesions that most often recur and show a progression to invasive carcinoma.[25]

Histological parameters, such as the malignancy grading system introduced by Jakobsson,[32] may be taken into account. For glottic carcinomas, nuclear polymorphism, mode of invasion and total malignancy points were factors of importance for the 5-year disease-free results.

Glanz and Eichhorn[18] set up a simplified four-factor grading system and applied it to surgically treated glottic carcinomas. The malignancy score resulted in a significant prediction of the clinical course, i.e., high-risk patients could be identified and their further treatment and follow-up could be modified accordingly.

Other studies have failed to disclose any differences in malignancy grading between patients with or without recurrence.[16,26,29]

DNA ploidy

Franzén et al,[16] in their series of small glottic carcinomas, found slightly more non-diploid carcinomas in the group which had had recurrences after a full course of radiotherapy than was the case in the group without recur-

rences. The difference however, was not statistically significant.

In a series of 133 squamous cell carcinomas of the larynx Ruá et al[53] found that ploidy was related to histological grade and that the survival rates were 41.7% and 27.7% for diploid and non-diploid carcinomas respectively. In N0 cases that underwent surgery, the 48-month survival rates were 81.8% and 49.2%, respectively, for diploid and non-diploid laryngeal carcinomas.

Walter et al[67] concluded from their study that all aneuploid glottic carcinomas should be treated surgically as all five such carcinomas recurred in a series of 29 irradiated tumours.

Stell[58] reviewed a number of published series involving DNA measurements in head and neck cancer using meta-analysis. In the entire series, survival was better for diploid tumours than for non-diploid tumours. Subgroup analysis showed that this was due to oral cavity carcinomas, whereas ploidy did not affect the outcome for laryngeal cancer. When a tumour recurred after radiotherapy it was more likely to be diploid.

Bromodeoxyuridine cytokinetic studies may provide another possibility for estimating ultimate tumour aggressiveness.[27]

Proliferative cell nuclear antigen (PCNA)

The prognostic factor of proliferative cell nuclear antigen (PCNA) expression has been evaluated in early glottic cancer.[48] Tumours recurring after a full course of radiotherapy displayed lower PCNA activity than did those that were cured.

Epidermoid growth factor receptors (EGFR)

The expression of epidermoid growth factor receptors (EGFR) determined histochemically showed that 80% of small glottic carcinomas recurring after radiotherapy had a higher staining intensity and a higher portion of stained cells than those that did not (39%). The results indicate that EGFR may influence the rate of recurrence of small glottic carcinomas after radiotherapy.[43]

Altered antigen expression

Monoclonal antibody UM-A9 identifies an antigen which is found on the basal surface of epithelial cells and is expressed in squamous cell carcinomas. Strong expression of this antigen or the loss of ABH blood-group antigens and especially a combination with loss of both types of antigen, were bad prognostic indicators.[72]

PATIENT FACTORS

Local and general immune response

Increasing interest is being focused on both local and

general immune response. Cytokines are soluble mediators of inflammation and immune response which have their effect locally through specific receptors on target cells. The roles of cytokines are becoming of great interest for many researchers. Some cytokines have been reported to have a direct cytostatic and/or cytotoxic effect on tumour cells.[11,15,23]

In vitro studies have shown that single agents, IFN-γ regimens, or combinations of IFNs and TNF-α result in cell growth inhibition in most squamous carcinoma cell lines tested.[54]

A considerable number of attempts have been made to correlate immunoglobulin levels, clinical stage and activity of disease in cancer patients. Increased levels of IgA have been found in sera from patients with nasopharyngeal carcinoma and this may reflect a local immune response.[6] Increased IgA levels have also been found in sera and saliva of patients with squamous cell carcinoma of the head and neck.

Serum C1q BM (C1q-binding macromolecules) and serum IgA levels contributed significantly to predict survival in patients with advanced head and neck cancer. Serological analysis did not provide any information in early-stage lesions.[10]

Blood transfusion

Immunosuppression may be brought about by blood transfusion, but this remains unproven. However, there is some evidence which suggests that blood transfusion has a detrimental effect on survival with malignant disease. Alun-Jones et al[2] found a significant difference in survival between transfused and non-transfused patients undergoing laryngectomy; however, it could not be established whether this was a causal relationship.

Ell and Stell[14] did not see any significant effect on survival in their series of patients transfused perioperatively. The survival of patients undergoing neck dissections was also unaffected by blood transfusion. These different conclusions are difficult to explain when an accumulatory weight of evidence indicates a worse outcome for patients receiving blood transfusion. This discrepancy may reflect the fact, as Ell and Stell explain, that blood transfusion is a marker for other risk factors, such as advanced disease, the need for more extensive operations, combined treatment, etc.

Anyhow, these studies should alert the surgeon to the fact that perioperative blood transfusions might have a deleterious effect in cancer patients. All unnecessary blood transfusions should be avoided; this is sound medical practice for many reasons.

All the above-mentioned patient factors have to be considered in the follow-up of patients treated for laryngeal cancer.

Treatment factors

In the follow-up, the treatment modality and its extent has to be taken into account. Has curative therapy been administered, or has the treatment been palliative only?

Radiotherapy

If primary radiotherapy has been administered for a limited glottic primary it is of the utmost importance to have a strict and regular follow-up because further functional procedures—such as endoscopic laser surgery, or a partial vertical laryngectomy—can be performed, saving both airway and voice.

Surgery

If primary functional surgery—with or without pre- or postoperative radiotherapy—has been performed, a total laryngectomy can still be undertaken. In these patients the larynx may sometimes be difficult to evaluate. The best follow-up in these patients is probably performed by the surgeon.

If a primary total laryngectomy has been performed and a recurrence around the stoma occurs, the prognosis is bad, but palliation and, in individual cases, curative multimodality treatment may be elaborated upon.

Lymph nodes

In all these patients the neck has to be carefully observed and palpated. The use of CT and MR is important—as is fine-needle aspiration cytology, perhaps guided by ultrasound (USGFNAC).

If operable neck metastases appear, surgery has to be performed with or without radiotherapy—depending on previous treatment and histopathological results.

Postirradiation problems

Postirradiation oedema may complicate a postradiotherapy examination. A swollen, red and overhanging epiglottis in addition to arytenoid oedema may hide the vocal cords for indirect inspection. The fibrelaryngoscope has proven its value in these instances. In some centres a short-term steroid therapy is employed in these patients before the first post-therapeutic inspection.[71] The major problems are involved in patients receiving a full course of radiotherapy for a glottic T3 carcinoma. The mobility may not return and the hemilarynx stays oedematous and red, but with an intact overlying mucosa. Residual or recurrent disease may be extremely difficult to diagnose in these patients. Deep biopsies may be taken and still be negative, but with the risk of causing chondritis and chondronecrosis. Fine-needle aspiration cytology may also be undertaken. Computed tomography or magnetic resonance imaging often add little information due to postirradiation changes if the laryngeal framework has not become involved.

Sometimes a laryngectomy has to be performed in these patients.[59] Ward et al[68] presented material where persistent oedema 6 months or more after completion of radiotherapy indicated residual carcinoma in over 23 of 43 cases (53%), and only 6 out of these 23 patients were salvaged by total laryngectomy; this indicates the difficulties involved in diagnosing residual or recurrent carcinoma in these patients.

DeSanto et al[12] recognized recurrence after irradiation too late to be able to perform functional surgery.

Irradiation-induced carcinomas are not common, but they may be considered.[1,5,17] Such tumours are often diagnosed decades after irradiation treatment—which means that patients who have undergone radiotherapy have to be followed up for a lifetime.

MULTIPLE PRIMARIES

The risk for second and third primaries has achieved great interest during recent years. Long-term results after improved locoregional control may be reduced by distant metastases and new primaries.

History

In 1869 Theodor Billroth provided the first well-documented case of more than one independent malignant tumour developing in the same patient. The report was not published, however, until some years later.[7] It was not before 1932, when Warren and Gates[69] presented their comprehensive review on this subject, that such development become more familiar and was no longer considered a rarity.

Multicentric tumours, with the original presenting tumour (index tumour) within the upper aero-digestive tract, oesophagus and lungs, are well documented—with an incidence as high as 10–35%.[3,24,30,37,60,61] The second primary in these cases is most commonly found in the upper aero-digestive tract, followed by lung and oesophagus. The second primary is least commonly found in unrelated organs.[8,40,70] The problem of multicentricity thereby presents a major problem when dealing with head and neck carcinomas. It is well known that morphological abnormalities occur in the marginal zone of an invasive carcinoma. Morphological, electron microscopical, abnormalities consistent with those found in malignant neoplasia may be found in random biopsy specimens of macroscopically normal-looking mucosa in patients with a known susceptibility to the development of cancer.[31] These changes may be tobacco- and alcohol-induced, and they may be reversible if the exposure ceases. The ability to demonstrate such early changes during the asymptomatic (silent) period of cancer induction may have several points of usefulness as the mucosa is no longer reported as normal and the changes may be classified as morphological risk factors. The changes may be followed—giving us a better understanding of carcinogenesis and of which changes are reversible.

The phenomenon of multicentricity of squamous cell lesions within the upper aero-digestive tract has led many authors to recommend a more systematic search for additional primary tumours in all patients with one diagnosed squamous cell carcinoma or premalignant lesion within the head and neck.[3,4,8,19,40,41] There are, however, opponents to such a policy; for example, Neel[49] prefers a selection of diagnostic procedures, deferred to prudent clinical judgement based on a careful history of the patient's symptoms, a thorough physical examination, and the findings of preliminary diagnostic tests such as a chest X-ray.

However, detection of a second primary in the lung or oesophagus may be crucial for both management and prognosis of the patient with head and neck cancer, especially before we embark on major head and neck surgical procedures.

Definitions

Warren and Gates[69] laid down their criteria for multiple primary malignancies, and these criteria are still being followed:

1. Each tumour must be microscopically clearly malignant.
2. Each tumour must be geographically separated. There must be no intraepithelial neoplasia connecting them.
3. The possibility that the second tumour represents a metastasis should be excluded.

The temporal sequence was discussed by Moertel et al[44–46] who talked about simultaneous (synchronous) lesions diagnosed within a 6-month period, and interval (metachronous) lesions diagnosed at intervals longer than 6 months.

The original presenting tumour is called the 'index tumour'.

'Multicentric' is a term used to indicate lesions (synchronous or metachronous) that occur in anatomically or functionally allied tissues submitted to the influence of the same exogenic carcinogens.

'Panendoscopy' is a term used synonymously with 'triple endoscopy'; it comprises bronchoscopy, pharyngo-oesophagoscopy using rigid or flexible instruments and microlaryngoscopy. A careful inspection and palpation of the oral cavity is a part of the examination—as is a nasopharyngoscopy with biopsies from suspicious areas.

An individual developing more than one primary tumour in anatomically and functionally unrelated organs may be considered 'cancer-prone'. In these instances genetic factors may play a role, especially if there is a strong family history of cancer.[44–46,61] De Vries et al[62] measured human leukocyte antigens (HLA) and immunoglobulin (Ig) allotypes in 98 patients with single head and neck cancers, and in 51 patients with multiple primary tumours. Immunoglobulin allotype km(1) was present in 4% of patients with multiple primary tumours versus 21% in patients with a single head and neck cancer. The frequency of HLA-B8, HLA-DR3 and HLA-DQW2 in patients with multiple primary tumours, and of HLA-B8 and HLA-B45 in patients with single head and neck cancers, was significantly greater than it was in healthy controls. Next to environmental factors, genetic influences may be of importance for the pathogenesis of multiple primary tumours in head and neck squamous carcinoma patients.

Review of previous reports

Most early reports on multiple primary malignancies with an average of 5% within the head and neck area showed mainly metachronously-occurring second primary tumours.[44–46,50] Recent articles report more synchron-ously-occurring multicentric lesions and a higher total number of second primary malignancies (Table 35.1).

Many factors may explain this rising incidence in reports regarding multiple primaries. There may be increased awareness of the problem which may have promoted a more thorough search for second primary tumours. The use of flexible laryngo-, broncho- and oesophagoscopes has greatly improved our diagnostic procedures and allows the examinations to be performed as outpatient procedures. Better locoregional control with prolonged tumour-free survival has increased the risk for second primary malignancies. In addition, the follow-up may have been prolonged and improved. The incidence of multiple primaries may even be increasing.

In a previous study, Lundgren and Olofsson[35] presented figures regarding second primaries for patients with index carcinoma in the larynx similar to those presented by Wagenfeld and coworkers[65,66] and by Deviri and coworkers.[13]

Gluckman and Crissman[20] reported a significantly worse prognosis for patients with multiple primaries than for those with a single cancer within the head and neck. The second cancer was often located in the lung and oesophagus and was diagnosed late. It is many times more difficult to treat multiple neoplasms effectively — especially after radical therapy of the index tumour.

Table 35.1 Compiled findings in selected series describing multiple primary tumours in the head and neck (adapted and expanded from Lundgren and Olofsson[35])

Series	Number of patients	Study	Number of metachronous tumours	Number of synchronous tumours	Site of second lesion
Weichert and Schumrick[70]	825	Retrospective	35 (4.2%)*	19 (2.3%)*	Head and neck, lung, oesophagus 80%
Vrabec[61]	1518	Retrospective	119 (7.8%)*	56 (3.7%)*	
Gluckman[19]	162	Prospective		15 (9.2%)**	Head and lung, lung
Maisel and Vermeersch[37]	449	Retrospective	21 (4.7%)**	36 (8.0%)**	Lung 47% Oesophagus 11%
McGuirt[40]	100	Prospective		18 (18%)**	Head and neck, lung, oesophagus
Black et al[8]	645	Prospective		58 (9%)**	
	577	Retrospective	85 (14.7%)**	36 (6.2%)**	
	5337	Retrospective	466 (8.7%)**	270 (5.1%)**	
Wagenfeld et al [65,66]	903	Retrospective (larynx)	55 (6.1%)**	13 (1.4%)**	Respiratory tract
Deviri et al[13]	1660	Retrospective (larynx)	70 (4.2%)*	14 (0.9%)*	
Lundgren and Olofsson[35]	295	Retrospective (larynx)	33 (11.2%)**	4 (1.4%)**	Head and neck, lung, oesophagus 74%
Sikhani et al[56]	1961	Retrospective	93 (4.7%)*	97 (4.9%)*	Upper aerodigestive tract 58.5%
Shibuya et al[55]	1429	Retrospective (oral cavity)	103 (7.2%)**	33 (2.3%)**	Oral cavity, pharynx, oesophagus, stomach 63%
Masaki et al[39]	3162	Retrospective	225 (7.1%)* (80 prior carcinoma)	37 (1.2%)*	Head and neck, digestive tract, lung 90%
Panosetti et al[52]	9089	Retrospective	480 (5.3%)* +25 patients with insufficient information	350 (3.9%)*	Head and neck, oesophagus, lung

* Number of patients.
** Number of lesions.

Synchronous tumours have a better prognosis than metachronous ones in general.[20] This may support panendoscopic procedures in all patients with upper aero-digestive tract cancers. Panosetti et al[52] reported, however, a better 5-year survival in metachronous tumours.

Patients with hyperplasia, dysplasia and carcinoma in situ lesions not only have an increased risk for progression into laryngeal cancer; there is also an increased risk for development of independent carcinomas.[34,63] In our series, 19% (51/268) developed a carcinoma elsewhere — located mainly in the head and neck area, bronchi or oesophagus.[34]

In view of the high incidence of multicentric neoplasias in patients with laryngeal carcinoma, and the difficulties not uncommonly associated with their treatment — especially after radical treatment of the primary tumour — it seems logical to include panendoscopy as a primary examination; this should at least give us a chance to detect second primaries earlier. The use of the 'Lugol dye method' at endoscopy may improve diagnostic accuracy for early oesophageal cancer.[57]

The yield of regular fibrescopic examinations of the bronchi and oesophagus in patients treated for one head and neck cancer has to be evaluated, and the cost benefit has to be assessed.

PREVENTIVE MEASURES

Anti-smoking campaign

It is well known that patients who continue smoking are more at risk of developing a second primary than are patients who stop.[47] Therefore, an intensive anti-smoking campaign is warranted for all patients treated for a primary malignancy within the head and neck. It must be realized, however, that the chance of developing a second primary cancer gradually decreases over the following years. Many of the head and neck cancer patients, however, do not stop smoking.

Chemoprevention

Many epidemiological studies show a connection between a low vitamin A intake and certain cancers — such as bronchial cancer in smokers,[33] bladder cancer,[42] laryngeal cancer,[22] and oral cavity carcinomas.[38]

Treatment with retinoids lowers the incidence of squamous metaplasia in the bronchi of smokers and diminishes the extent of leukoplakia in the mucosa of the oral cavity.[21,28]

Positive results with retinol palmitate treatment for patients radically operated on for non-small cell cancer of the lung at the Istituto Nazionale Tumori in Milan initiated the 'Euroscan' programme within EORTC in 1988, using preventive treatment with retinol palmitate and/or N-acetylcysteine to see whether this treatment could prevent second primaries in patients with radically treated index tumours of the larynx, oral cavity and lung.[64]

Hong et al[28] have performed a randomized double-blind study using 13-*cis*-retinoic acid for head and neck cancer patients to prevent recurrence or a new primary. A reduction in new primary tumours was obtained, but the side-effects were marked, and only 67% of the patients could continue with their treatment for 12 months.

CONCLUSIONS

Prerequisites for the early detection of recurrent or new tumours after previous treatment of laryngeal carcinomas are summarized below.

1. A well-organized follow-up system, preferably at oncological centres where they have the necessary expertise available.
2. A regular laryngoscopic examinaton — which can nowadays be performed in many patients using flexible laryngofibrescopes.
3. The value of laryngostroboscopy in assessing vocal cord lesions has been emphasized, especially during latter years, as well as its role for an early detection of recurrence.
4. If a local recurrence is suspected, a microlaryngoscopy and biopsy should be performed and complemented by CT or MR.
5. The follow-up should be based on the initial tumour extent and the histopathology. In addition, follow-up depends on whether or not we can offer the patient another treatment.
6. Until disproven, impaired mobility of the vocal cord following previous radiotherapy or endoscopic surgery indicates recurrent disease.
7. It is often difficult to exclude residual or recurrent disease in a persistent postradiological oedema of the larynx. Microlaryngoscopy with multiple biopsy specimens removed from suspicious areas are often necessary.
8. We have to identify high-risk tumour characteristics such as tumour involvement, malignancy grading, DNA ploidy, EGFR and other tumour markers.
9. We have to identify high-risk patients with genetically determined(?) immunological deficiencies.
10. The risk of synchronous and metachronous multiple primaries must be taken into account. Regular fibre-bronchoscopies and cytological examinations may be undertaken.
11. Preventive measures such as stopping smoking and treatment with retinoids are equally important.

REFERENCES

1. Aanesen J P, Olofsson J 1979 Irradiation-induced tumours of the head and neck. Acta Otolaryngol 360 (suppl): 178–181
2. Alun-Jones T, Clarke P J, Morrissey S, Hill J 1991 Blood transfusion and laryngeal cancer. Clin Otolaryngol 16: 240–244
3. Atkins J P, Keane W M, Young K A, Rowe L D 1984 Value of panendoscopy in determination of second primary cancer. Arch Otolaryngol 110: 533–534
4. Atkinson D, Fleming S, Weaver A 1982 Triple endoscopy. A valuable procedure in head and neck surgery. Am J Surg 144: 416–419
5. Baker D C, Weissman B 1971 Postirradiation carcinoma of the larynx. Ann Otol Rhinol Laryngol 80: 634–637
6. Baskies A M, Chretien P B, Yang C-S et al 1979 Serum glycoproteins and immunoglobulins in nasopharyngeal carcinoma. Correlations with Epstein–Barr virus associated antibodies and clinical tumour stage. Am J Surg 138: 478–488
7. Billroth T 1889 Die allgemeine chirurgische Pathologie und Therapie in 51 Vorlesungen; ein Handbuch für Studierende und Aertzte. 14 Auflage, G Reimer, Berlin, p 908
8. Black R J, Gluckman J L, Shumrick D A 1983 Review. Multiple primary tumours of the upper aerodigestive tract. Clin Otolaryngol 8: 277–281
9. Boysen M, Natvig K, Winther F Ö, Tausjö J 1985 Value of routine follow-up in patients treated for squamous cell carcinoma of the head and neck. J Otolaryngol 14: 211–214
10. Clayman G L, Savage H E, Ainslie N, Liu F J, Schantz S P 1990 Serologic determinants of survival in patients with squamous cell carcinoma of the head and neck. Am J Surg 160: 434–438
11. Clemens M J, McNurlan M A 1985 Regulation of cell differentiation and proliferation by interferons. Biochem J 226: 345–360
12. DeSanto L W, Lillie J C, Devine K D 1976 Surgical salvage after radiation for laryngeal cancer. Laryngoscope 86: 649–657
13. Deviri E, Bartal A, Goldsher M, Eliachar I, Steinitz R, Robinson E 1982 Occurrence of additional primary neoplasms in patients with laryngeal carcinoma in Israel (1960–1976). Ann Otol Rhinol Laryngol 91: 261–265
14. Ell S R, Stell P M 1991 Blood transfusion and survival after laryngectomy for laryngeal carcinoma. J Laryngol Otol 105: 293–294
15. Fidler I J, Heicappell R, Saiki I, Grutter M G, Horisberger M A, Nuesch J 1987 Direct antiproliferative effects of recombinant human interferon alpha B/D hybrids on human tumor cell lines. Cancer Res 47: 2020–2027
16. Franzén G, Olofsson J, Klintenberg C, Brunk U 1987 Prognostic value of malignancy grading and DNA measurements in small glottic carcinomas. ORL J Otorhinolaryngol Relat Spec 49: 73–80
17. Glanz H 1976 Late recurrence or radiation induced cancer of the larynx. Clin Otolaryngol 1: 123–129
18. Glanz H, Eichhorn T 1985 Die prognostische Bedeutung des histologischen 'Gradings' von Stimmlippenkarzinomen. HNO 33: 103–111
19. Gluckman J L 1979 Synchronous multiple primary lesions of the upper aerodigestive system. Arch Otolaryngol 105: 597–598
20. Gluckman J L, Crissman J D 1983 Survival rates in 548 patients with multiple neoplasms of the upper aerodigestive tract. Laryngoscope 93: 71–74
21. Gouveia J, Mathé G, Hercend T et al 1982 Degree of bronchial metaplasia in heavy smokers and its regression after treatment with a retinoid. Lancet i: 710–712
22. Graham S, Mettlin C, Marshall J et al 1981 Dietary factors in the epidemiology of cancer of the larynx, Am J Epidemiol 113: 675–680
23. Haranaka K, Satomi N 1981 Cytotoxic activity of tumour necrosis factor (TNF) on human cancer cells in vitro. Jpn J Exp Med 151: 191–194
24. Healy G B, Strong M S, Uchmakli A, Vaughan C W, DiTroia J F 1976 Carcinoma of the palatine arch: the rationale of treatment selection. Am J Surg 132: 498–503
25. Hellquist H, Lundgren J, Olofsson J 1982 Hyperplasia, keratosis, dysplasia and carcinoma in situ of the vocal cords — a follow-up study. Clin Otolaryngol 7: 11–27
26. Helweg-Larsen K, Græm N, Meistrup-Larsen K-I, Meistrup-Larsen U 1978 Clinical relevance of histological grading of cancer of the larynx. Acta Pathol Microbiol Scand A Pathol 86: 499–504
27. Hirano T, Zitsch R P, Gluckman J L 1991 The use of bromodeoxyuridine cytokinetic studies as a prognostic indicator of cancer of the head and neck. Laryngoscope 101: 130–133
28. Hong W K, Lippman S M, Itri L M et al 1990 Prevention of second primary tumours with isotretinoin in squamous cell carcinoma of the head and neck. New Engl J Med 323: 795–801
29. Hordijk G J 1980 The high-risk group in early glottic carcinoma. Arch Otolaryngol 106: 621–622
30. Hoye R C, Herrold K McD, Smith R R, Thomas L B 1962 A clinicopathological study of epidermoid carcinoma of the head and neck. Cancer 15: 741–749
31. Incze J, Vaughan C W, Lui P, Strong M S, Kulapaditharom B 1982 Premalignant changes in normal appearing epithelium in patients with squamous cell carcinoma of the upper aerodigestive tract. Am J Surg 144: 401–405
32. Jakobsson P 1973 Glottic carcinoma of the larynx. Factors influencing prognosis following radiotherapy. Thesis, Printab, Stockholm
33. Kvåle G, Bjelke E, Gart J J 1983 Dietary habits and lung cancer risk. Int J Cancer 31: 397–405
34. Lundgren J, Gilbert R, Olofsson J, Hellquist H 1990 Precancerous lesions of the vocal cords. Proceeding of the XIV World Congress of Otorhinolaryngology, Head and Neck Surgery, Madrid, Spain, September 10–15, 1989, (eds Sacristán T, Alvarez-Vicent J J, Antoli-Candela F et al) pp 2429–2431, Kugler & Ghedini, Amsterdam, Berkely, Milan
35. Lundgren J, Olofsson J 1986 Multiple primary malignancies in patients treated for laryngeal carcinoma. J Otolaryngol 15: 145–150
36. Lundgren J, Olofsson J, Hellquist H B, Strandn J 1981 Exfoliative cytology in laryngology. Comparison of cytologic and histologic diagnoses in 350 microlaryngoscopic examinations — a prospective study. Cancer 47: 1336–1343
37. Maisel R H, Vermeersch H 1981 Panendoscopy for second primaries in head and neck cancer. Ann Otol Rhinol Laryngol 90: 460–464
38. Marshall J, Graham S, Mettlin C et al 1982 Diet in the epidemiology of oral cancer. Nutr Cancer 3: 145–149
39. Masaki N, Hashimoto T, Ikeda H, Inoue T, Kozuka T 1987 Multiple primary malignancies in patients with head and neck cancer. Jpn J Clin Oncol 17: 303–307
40. McGuirt W F 1982 Panendoscopy as a screening examination for simultaneous primary tumors in head and neck cancer: a prospective sequential study and review of the literature. Laryngoscope 92: 569–576
41. McGuirt W F, Matthews B, Koufman J A 1982 Multiple simultaneous tumors in patients with head and neck cancer. A prospective, sequential panendoscopic study. Cancer 50: 1195–1199
42. Mettlin C, Graham S 1979 Dietary factors in human bladder cancer. Am J Epidemiol 110: 255–263
43. Miyaguchi M, Olofsson J, Hellquist H B 1991 Expression of epidermal growth factor receptor in glottic carcinoma and its relation to recurrence after radiotherapy. Clin Otolaryngol 16: 466–469
44. Moertel C G, Dockerty M B, Baggenstoss A H 1961 Multiple primary malignant neoplasms. I. Introduction and presentation of data. Cancer 14: 221–230
45. Moertel C G, Dockerty M B, Baggenstoss A H 1961 Multiple primary malignant neoplasms. II: Tumors of different tissues or organs. Cancer 14: 231–237
46. Moertel C G, Dockerty M B, Baggenstoss A H 1961 Multiple primary malignant neoplasms. III: Tumors of multicentric origin. Cancer 14: 238–248

47. Moore C 1965 Smoking and cancer of the mouth, pharynx and larynx. JAMA 191: 283–286
48. Munck-Wikland E, Kuylenstierna R, Lindholm J, Fernberg J-O, Auer G 1991 The prognostic value of proliferating cell nuclear antigen (PCNA) expression in early glottic cancer. Eur J Cancer 27 (suppl 3): S81 (abstract)
49. Neel H B III 1984 Routine panendoscopy — is it necessary every time? (Commentary). Arch Otolaryngol 110: 531–532
50. Odette J, Szymanowski R T, Nichols R D 1977 Multiple head and neck malignancies. Trans Am Acad Ophthalmol Otolaryngol 84: 805–813
51. Olofsson J 1984 Early detection of recurrent tumours after previous treatment of laryngeal carcinomas. In: Wigand M E, Steiner W, Stell P M (eds) Functional partial laryngectomy. Conservation surgery for carcinoma of the larynx. Springer, Berlin, pp 310–314
52. Panosetti E, Luboinski B, Mamelle G, Richard J-M 1989 Multiple synchronous and metachronous cancers of the upper aerodigestive tract: a nine-year study. Laryngoscope 99: 1267–1273
53. Ruá S, Comino A, Fruttero A et al 1991 Relationship between histologic features, DNA, flow cytometry, and clinical behavior of squamous cell carcinomas of the larynx. Cancer 67: 141–149
54. Sacchi M, Klapan I, Johnson J T, Whiteside T L 1991 Antiproliferative effects of cytokines on squamous cell carcinoma. Arch Otolaryngol Head Neck Surg 117: 321–326
55. Shibuya H, Hisamitsu S, Shioiri S, Horiuchi J, Suzuki S 1987 Multiple primary cancer risk in patients with squamous cell carcinoma of the oral cavity. Cancer 60: 3083–3086
56. Shikhani A H, Matanoski G M, Jones M M, Kashima H K, Johns M E 1986 Multiple primary malignancies in head and neck cancer. Arch Otolaryngol Head Neck Surg 112: 1172–1179
57. Shiozaki H, Tahara H, Kobayashi K et al 1990 Endoscopic screening of early esophageal cancer with the Lugol dye method in patients with head and neck cancers. Cancer 66: 2068–2071
58. Stell P M 1991 Ploidy in head and neck cancer: a review and meta-analysis. Clin Otolaryngol 16: 510–516
59. Stell P M, Morrison M D 1973 Radiation necrosis of the larynx. Etiology and management. Arch Otolaryngol 98: 111–113
60. Tepperman B S, Fitzpatrick P J 1981 Second respiratory and upper digestive tract cancer after oral cancer. Lancet ii: 547–549
61. Vrabec D P 1979 Multiple primary malignancies of the upper aerodigestive system. Ann Otol Rhinol Laryngol 88: 846–854
62. de Vries N, Drexhage H A, de Waal L P, de Lange G, Snow G B 1987 Human leukocyte antigens and immunoglobulin allotypes in head and neck cancer patients with and without multiple primary tumors. Cancer 60: 957–961
63. de Vries N, Kalter P O, Snow G B 1986 Multiple primary tumors in patients with laryngeal squamous cell hyperplasia. Arch Otorhinolaryngol 243: 143–145
64. de Vries N, Snow G B 1988 Prevention of second primary cancer in head and neck cancer patients: new perspectives. Am J Otolaryngol 9: 151–154
65. Wagenfeld D J H, Harwood A R, Bryce D P, van Nostrand A W P, DeBoer G 1980 Second primary respiratory tract malignancies in glottic carcinoma. Cancer 46: 1883–1886
66. Wagenfeld D J H, Harwood A R, Bryce D P, van Nostrand A W P, DeBoer G 1981 Second primary respiratory tract malignant neoplasms in supraglottic carcinoma. Arch Otolaryngol 107: 135–137
67. Walter M A, Peters G E, Peiper S C 1991 Predicting radioresistance in early glottic squamous cell carcinoma by DNA content. Ann Otol Rhinol Laryngol 100: 523–526
68. Ward P H, Calcaterra T C, Kagan A R 1975 The enigma of post-radiation edema and recurrent or residual carcinoma of the larynx. Laryngoscope 85: 522–529
69. Warren S, Gates O 1932 Multiple primary malignant tumors: a survey of literature and statistical study. Am J Cancer 16: 1358–1414
70. Weichert K A, Schumrick D 1979 Multiple malignancies in patients with primary carcinomas of the head and neck. Laryngoscope 89: 988–991
71. Wey W 1979 Suspicion of persistent or recurrent carcinoma of the larynx after radiation therapy. ORL J Otorhinolaryngol Relat Spec 41: 301–311
72. Wolf G T, Carey T E, Schmaltz S P et al 1990 Altered antigen expression predicts outcome in squamous cell carcinoma of the head and neck. J Natl Cancer Inst 82: 1566–1572

36. Psychological aspects

F. E. Lucente

INTRODUCTION

An essential organ in the communicative process, the larynx is a structure endowed with great psychological significance. Disorders of the larynx can affect a patient's ability to breathe and swallow as well as to speak or to engage in non-verbal forms of communication such as crying and laughing. When the disease affecting the larynx is malignant, it obviously poses a threat to life itself. In reviewing some of the implications of laryngeal diseases and laryngeal surgery (including total laryngectomy), it is important to understand the pathogenesis of laryngeal diseases and the manner in which patients present for treatment.

Understanding the aetiology of laryngeal diseases will help us to appreciate the psychological problems experienced by afflicted patients.[16]

AETIOLOGICAL FACTORS ASSOCIATED WITH LARYNGEAL CARCINOMA

Numerous reports have confirmed an association between smoking and alcohol abuse on one hand and malignant and benign diseases of the larynx on the other. Since psychologists and psychiatrists have suggested that smoking and drinking are self-destructive actions, and since these health-care facts have been liberally publicized throughout the lay media, it can generally be assumed that most patients are aware of the harmful effects of these practices. The persistent use of these carcinogens in the face of strong and frequent warnings from various scientific and public information sources characterizes many laryngeal cancer patients. The implication of these continued abusive practices should be kept in mind in planning any comprehensive care programme. Certainly, patients who are reluctant to change life-threatening social practices are probably not going to be fully compliant with the diagnostic and therapeutic interventions necessary to bring their diseases under control.

PRESENTATION OF LARYNGEAL CANCER

The well-known presenting symptoms of laryngeal lesions, such as hoarseness (or other vocal abnormalities such as breathiness, voice weakness or voice loss), throat pain, dysphagia or odynophagia, haemoptysis and occasionally neck mass, are readily recognized by many affected patients. Unlike various thoracic or abdominal malignancies, in which the first recognizable symptoms may occur late in the disease process and be difficult to associate with the underlying tumour, laryngeal neoplasms frequently present with early and recognizable symptoms. Since rapid diagnosis and prompt institution of care are very influential in the outcome of therapy, it is appropriate to assess the patient's motivation for seeking treatment as well as the patient's understanding of the disease process which brings him to the physician.

INITIAL PHYSICIAN–PATIENT CONTACT

In the initial physician–patient encounters, it is extremely important to attempt to make a thorough evaluation of the entire patient, with particular attention to age, sex, ethnicity, previous medical history, lifestyle and social practices, professional activities, previous experience with diseases or other forms of psychological stress. Since the initial encounter between the patient and physician may have a great impact on the eventual outcome of therapy, it is critical to be sure that this encounter occurs in a relaxed and supportive environment. The office setting or clinic setting in which patients are examined should be tailored to the needs of the patient with a minimum of extraneous factors intruding. Periodic meetings with other members of the health-care team are beneficial in addressing the problems often created by a needlessly stressful environment.

The physician's physical and emotional availability will strongly influence a relationship between him or her and the patient. In the diagnostic and subsequent therapeutic phases of the interaction it is important for the patient to experience a feeling of support and open communication.

In obtaining a history and performing the examination on the patient with laryngeal symptoms, the physician should not allow himself to be interrupted by telephone calls, staff messages or other patient-care matters. The patient and family should receive the physician's undivided attention during the time of the actual examination. Even a brief encounter with a fully-involved and dedicated physician is preferable to a more lengthy encounter in which the physician's attention is simultaneously directed at numerous other problems.

Although all communications should be based on truth, there are certain situations in which it is best not to provide all possible information at the earliest opportunity, especially when the physician receives a direct request from the family or a non-verbal request from the patient in that regard. However, it is not appropriate to mis-state or misrepresent facts, since such practices may adversely affect the creation of a trusting relationship which is critical to the later stages of diseases management.[18]

Great care should be taken in explaining the clinical diagnosis to the patient on the first visit and outlining a proposed plan for further evaluation and therapy. All explanations should be made in terms readily understood by the patient. Repetition of critical elements of the explanation is important. It is often helpful to have family members or other trusted friends present during the explanations and to allow the patient sufficient time to ask questions or to manifest a reaction. Obviously careful attention to the physician's schedule and the provision of a supportive environment will facilitate an initial positive interaction.

INITIAL PATIENT REACTIONS

After learning that he or she has a laryngeal tumour that will require surgery or some other form of therapy, the patient may experience many reactions such as anger, grief or anxiety. The patient usually goes through a period of pre-grief over an expectant loss. Frequently the patient may deal with this period of anxiety by becoming totally dedicated to the physician and endowing that person with god-like powers. The physician might best anticipate this reaction and explain the situation carefully, clearly and promptly to the patient. It is also important to expedite care after this period of explanation since the patient may interpret delays as failures on the part of this respected physician. It is also important for the physician to explain the role of various members of the therapeutic team at this early stage, including resident physicians, nurses, speech therapists, social workers, office and operating room personnel and other oncological staff members.

PREOPERATIVE IDENTIFICATION OF PATIENTS AT HIGH PSYCHOLOGICAL RISK

Although many patients will accept the physician's observation of a laryngeal abnormality which requires further evaluation with a certain amount of equanimity, and consent to the physician's recommendations, other patients may handle this situation less well. Among the patients who have been characterized as more likely to develop emotional complications preoperatively or postoperatively are the following:

1. Patients with a known history of psychotic decompensation or psychiatric therapy.
2. Patients who refuse to cooperate with the proposed plan of therapy by declining to sign a consent form or by threatening to leave the treatment setting.
3. Patients whose relationships with the staff are deteriorating.
4. Patients with extremely unrealistic expectations regarding therapy.
5. Patients whose amount of preoperative concern is disproportionately great or small in comparison to the severity of their illness.[2]

When confronted by these patients, physicians may wish to recommend preoperative counseling in order to help them to deal with the psychological problems that can arise in subsequent oncological therapy.

PREOPERATIVE COUNSELING

One of the most important aspects of treatment of the patient undergoing laryngeal surgery is effective and efficient preoperative counseling. Janis has demonstrated that understanding the therapeutic plan and the anticipated outcome allows the patient to deal with, and adapt to some of the natural concerns about the surgical experience.[10]

Minear and Lucente retrospectively studied 60 patients who had undergone laryngectomy in order to assess their opinions about the nature and extent of preoperative counseling as well as to record their concerns about the problems they were to experience.[20] In the questionnaire part of the study, the patients indicated that their main concern was with the loss of the ability to speak. However, in subsequent direct interviews, they also stated that their principal feeling of concern was the recurrence of cancer and with possible eventual death. In both parts of the study, patients indicated a desire for greater personal participation in their preoperative and postoperative management. When questioned about whether they would like to have had routine preoperative visits with various members of the therapeutic team, including nursing staff, social workers, speech pathologists and members of the ancillary rehabilitative services, the patients generally felt that they would like to be informed in advance that such services were available but did not necessarily wish to have routine visits by all team members.

The patterns of preoperative counseling of laryngectomy patients by members of the American Society for Head and Neck Surgery and by otolaryngological chief residents were studied by Berkowitz and Lucente,[3] who presented 226 members of ASHNS and 68 chief residents that responded to a broadly circulated questionnaire. Each physician was presented with a list of 31 problems that had been observed in laryngectomy patients and was asked whether he or she discussed each problem 'thoroughly', 'superficially', 'not at all', or referred the discussion of the problem to another member of the therapeutic team. The authors noted that a great majority of the responding physicians reported that they discussed 13 problems thoroughly or to a great extent. However, when questioned about the amount of time spent in preoperative counseling, the majority of physicians reported that they spent an average of 30 to 60 minutes for each laryngectomy patient. The authors obviously commented on the disparity between the amount of time spent in counseling and the number of subjects discussed. They also questioned whether the intensity of preoperative counseling as perceived by reporting physicians bore any reliable relationship to the counseling actually offered.

The immediate preoperative preparation of the patient also requires careful attention. It is important not to confuse the benefits of preoperative pharmacological sedation with preoperative psychological counseling and explanations provided by an anaesthesiologist. Egbert and associates have reported that patients given suitable preoperative preparation by an anaesthesiologist require less postoperative analgesia than do patients who have not been similarly prepared.[4,5]

Preoperative counseling allows patients to rehearse,[19] to be desensitized,[22] or to mobilize customary or individualized support systems to reduce preoperative and postoperative distress. Having the patient as an active, informed participant who understands both the procedure and the postoperative course is an obvious goal of optimal preoperative counseling. During this difficult period it is prudent to provide the patient with supportive factual information without focusing on factors which cannot be changed. Also, at this time, despite the self-destructive social habits in which the patient might have engaged, such as smoking, alcohol abuse or other practices, it is not good to instill in the patient a sense of guilt.

HOSPITALIZATION

Many of the psychological problems experienced by the patient with laryngeal lesions, including carcinoma, revolve around the fact that hospitalization is necessary with its attendant denotations and connotations. Hospitalization is a period in which a person enters a depersonalized environment and may be required to submit to authority figures whose role is unclear.[14] Although many patients who previously would have been hospitalized for biopsies are now treated in ambulatory settings, the brevity of the hospitalization experiences does not reduce their potential for provoking anxiety.

The process of entering the hospital itself is frequently the source of concern in that it may involve periods of uncertainty regarding scheduling, arbitrary testing requirements, periods of waiting in unfamiliar surroundings, processing by hospital personnel who may be task-oriented rather than patient-oriented, and eventual deposition in an area in which one must surrender one's personal effects and put on a uniform worn by others with whom one may have little in common.

Strain and Grossman[24] have described the following psychological stresses to which the hospitalized surgical patient is especially susceptible.

1. Basic threat to the sense of self or intactness
2. Strangers and separation anxiety
3. Fear of loss of love and approval
4. Fear of loss of control of developmentally achieved functions (such as swallowing, talking and crying)
5. Fear of loss or injury to body parts
6. Guilt and shame
7. Fear of pain

Although information can allay anxiety, patients vary greatly with regard to the amount of information they would like to have about the details of the hospitalization procedure. Among the various sources of concern noted have been the circumstances surrounding the anaesthetic experience, the identity and role of hospital personnel, the rationale for various diagnostic procedures and the competence of physicians with whom they come into contact. At the present time in the United States, there are pervasive concerns about the safety and security of hospitalization for any potentially risky or invasive procedures, especially procedures which patients interpret as carrying a risk for contracting acquired immunodeficiency syndrome.

The type of hospital to which the patient is admitted can also be a factor in the patient's course. In a study of hospitalization anxiety levels among 408 medical and surgical patients in four hospitals (one large university hospital, one large private hospital, two small community hospitals), Lucente and Fleck demonstrated higher anxiety levels in patients in the university hospital, regardless of disease.[15] Importantly, they also noted a poor correlation between the patient's self-assessment of anxiety and those assessments provided by physicians and nurses involved in the patient's care. These observations suggested that health-care personnel may fail to appreciate the psychological ramifications of the medical problems experienced by the patients studied.

Many authors have cited problems peculiar to teaching hospitals, such as perceptions by patients that they are being used as material for instruction[9] and the adverse psychological impact of ward rounds.[11] In an English study, Barnes observed a prevalent feeling among patients that their physicians and nurses were more oriented toward the treatment of the illness than toward treatment of the patients themselves.[1]

PSYCHOLOGICAL ADAPTATION TO SURGERY

Most patients facing major surgery demonstrate various patterns of response to the attendant stresses and circumstances. Patients facing laryngectomy are no different. Among the responses which have been noted are various degrees of dysphoric mood, anxiety, shame, guilt, and feelings of helplessness. When these unpleasant affects persist, or are particularly intense, the patient may substitute inappropriately pleasant affects and appear euphoric or manic. In attempting to cope with stress, patients may actually demonstrate inappropriate psychological mechanisms such as denial, hyperkinetic activity and paranoid or suspicious relationships with members of their therapeutic staff. Physicians may attempt to deal with these reactions by the use of non-interpretative intervention, strengthening of current ego capacity, clarification of communication, enhancing reality testing and emphasizing positive reinforcement.[7] In planning a programme to assist patients in adapting to the nature and extent of laryngectomy and other illnesses, it is valuable to explore again any previous surgical experiences, the sources of strength in the patient's ego and environmental support such as family and social contacts.[8]

OTHER PROBLEMS SURROUNDING THE OPERATIVE EXPERIENCE

The problem of informed consent has gained much attention in contemporary literature. It is frequently stated that the consent should be obtained in such a manner that the patient is fully and appropriately informed of the nature of the surgery and of all risks, complications and limitations which are to be considered. In many instances this is difficult to obtain without frightening or intimidating the patient to such an extent that essential surgery may be refused. Most physicians are sufficiently trained to provide extensive preoperative counseling before obtaining the permit and to provide all suitable explanations and describe complications. As with the initial patient contact, it is important that the garnering of the permit be conducted in a situation which allows the physician to offer full attention to the patient. It is extremely important that the patient and family members do not feel rushed. Although other members of the health-care team may be available to answer questions about the minor circumstances of hospitalization, it is best for the physician alone to answer all medically significant questions. It may be helpful to offer the patient a photocopy of the consent and to encourage the patient to call with any subsequent questions which may arise. One should be particularly wary of patients who merely give the consent a cursory glance and quickly sign it. With such patients it is helpful to re-read the consent in person and to reinforce the importance of the document.

The prescribing of preoperative medications is usually done by the anaesthesiologist. As mentioned above, it is good to stress with these professional colleagues the request for adequate psychological premedication as well as the use of any pharmacological preparations. In view of the plethora of new medications currently in the anaesthesiologist's armamentarium, it is good for the surgeon to be familiar with them and particularly with their side-effects since the standard operative permit garnered by the surgeon includes permission for anaesthetic medications.

Several seemingly minor details of the operating room experience deserve special comment in an attempt to alleviate possible subsequent postoperative psychological problems:

1. It is helpful for the patient to see the surgeon in the operating room before receiving the anaesthetic agent. Despite previous communications to the contrary, some patients still feel that their surgeon is not actually present.
2. The surgeon should stress with the other operating room staff the need to demonstrate to the patient that he or she is the centre of attention and the most important person in the operating room. Extraneous conversation should be minimized. Discussion of any other patients, particularly by name, is to be discouraged. Patients should be confident that their own anonymity is preserved.
3. It is best to keep surgical instruments covered until the patient is unconscious since observing these instruments may be frightening.
4. If a headlight is to be worn during surgery, it is best to have that worn only by the attending surgeon during the period in which the patient is receiving induction anaesthesia. It is possible that the patient might interpret the wearing of headlights by residents or other surgical assistants as indicating that someone other than the surgeon will actually perform the operative procedure.

POSTOPERATIVE OR INTENSIVE CARE UNIT EXPERIENCE

No amount of preoperative explanation can fully inform the patient of what to expect in the immediate post-anaesthetic and postoperative period. Upon awakening, the patient is likely to experience pain and confusion. The presence of an informed, trained and concerned support staff during this period of fluctuation in consciousness level is extremely important.

Some of the problems which were originally noted in the Intensive Care Unit designed for patients suffering myocardial infarction or open heart surgery are now being seen in units involved in the care of head and neck cancer patients, including those undergoing laryngectomy. The well-documented ICU reactions are most likely secondary to complex and multiple biological, psychological and social factors such as blood loss, electrolyte disturbances, effects of anaesthesia, sensory deprivation, sleep deprivation, changes in body image, fear, presence of strange equipment, and lack of accustomed support systems. It is best to deal with these problems by beginning to re-structure the patient's temporal and spatial environment as soon as possible after surgery. Among the tools which are particularly useful are the following:

1. A clock with a sweep second hand and numbers sufficiently large to be read by the patient
2. A calendar of the type in which each day is listed on a separate page, or each day can be crossed off
3. A window through which the patient is able to observe day and night changes. It is also helpful to have the staff fully informed about the need to participate in this reorientation process.[13]

POSTOPERATIVE PSYCHOLOGICAL DISORDERS

Numerous psychiatric disturbances have been described following surgery — including organic mental disorders, depressive disorders and generalized anxiety reactions. When one considers the total impact of laryngectomy, it is not surprising to note the occurrence of these disturbances after a patient has undergone that procedure. The organic mental disturbances may result from temporary or permanent damage to brain structures precipitated by various processes involved in the surgery itself. Despite the best anaesthetic precautions, it is not possible to have total control over intracranial blood flow and electrolyte changes, which may predispose to disturbances of memory, changes in intellectual capacity, fluctuations in level of consciousness, impairment of judgement and interference with attention levels, capacity for abstract thought and ability to assimilate linguistic signals. The patient may also manifest uncontrolled emotional discharge, agitation, depression, inappropriate fatigue, or apathy. Strain[23] has reported that psychological functions that are most complex and are developed last in the individual's cognitive evolution are the most vulnerable to early disruption, while primitive functions are more enduring.

Although depressive disorders of sufficient severity to require psychiatric intervention or prescription of medication are uncommon, some adjustment disorders manifesting as temporary depression occur frequently. A particular concern surrounds the phenomenon of suicide. It is not unusual for patients who are threatened with the loss of vocal communication to state that suicide would be a preferable alternative — 'I'd rather be dead'. Although such expressions may not be meant seriously, the physician should be particularly concerned about those patients who have demonstrated previous suicide attempts, those who dwell on these thoughts, or those who have family members who have committed suicide. Patients with prolonged or repeated history of substance abuse are also at higher risk of suicide attempts.[18]

In anticipating the various psychological reactions which patients may demonstrate following laryngeal surgery, it is helpful to have a close working relationship with all members of the health-care team. Periodic conferences designed to discuss clinical observations and to formulate plans for all eventualities are useful.

PAIN

Among the most difficult symptoms to treat is post-operative pain. Some patients who indicate that they are experiencing pain are indeed experiencing a genuine physical discomfort for which pharmacological analgesics are required. However, others use the term pain to describe a feeling of psychological distress for which analgesics will offer no relief.

When analgesics are required, they should be prescribed in adequate doses and with sufficient frequency that all reasonable pain can be controlled.[17] It is helpful to determine in advance any excessive tolerance to medications, particularly in patients who may have abused narcotics preoperatively. Since the pain generally does not last longer than seven to ten days, it is important for the physician not to fear making the patient dependent on narcotics simply by offering adequate pain relief. Also, the physician should not view the request for analgesics as a diminution of his or her own role as a healer. A more difficult problem occurs with those patients whose complaints are psychological rather than physically based. In these patients, the use of pharmacological analgesics and their possible attendant depressive side-effects may actually be harmful. One should look carefully for evidence of a pre-existing state of depression which may now be manifesting as pain.

As with other problems related to the psychological reaction to laryngeal surgery, enlisting the assistance of the liaison psychiatrist may be useful in sorting out the complex issues involved.

OTHER POSTOPERATIVE PROBLEMS

The postoperative period can present certain additional problems, especially when the recovery process is slower than predicted by the physician or anticipated by the patient. It is important to anticipate such delays so that their occurrence will not cause the patient to lose faith in the physician or to misunderstand the complexity of the disease process.

The healing of vocal cords following laryngoscopy and biopsy for benign disease may be slow when there is a significant inflammatory component to the disease—such as occurs with gastro-oesophageal reflux and secondary laryngitis. Patients who suffer from this condition may be particularly intolerant of what they presume to be a delayed healing process. The anticipation of such a slow healing process will allow the physician to explain this carefully to the patients preoperatively.

Another important problem is that of patients who manifest uncertainty about their ability to handle their physical and social activities following discharge from the hospital. In the hospitalization anxiety study by Lucente and Fleck,[15] patients who answered positively to the question of whether they thought they were being discharged prematurely tended to have an extremely high overall anxiety level. Some patients may attempt to delay the discharge process by creating factitious fevers, interfering with wound care, refusing to eat, expressing fear or anger or reporting an inability to participate in future rehabilitation.

The laryngectomy patient may manifest frustration when those around him or her do not attend carefully to the efforts at communication. This frustration may present as wild gesticulation, pounding on a table, or creating another noise which brings attention to the patient. In order to deal with this situation, it is important to maintain eye contact with the patient during any encounter. Verbalization is a key mechanism for adaptation, and the loss of this mechanism at a stressful time is a great threat to patients.

The female head and neck cancer patient presents a special challenge to the surgeon. Many of the procedures performed in the head and neck region, including laryngectomy, are particularly defeminizing. They result in significant changes in appearance. Also, the voice acquired by laryngectomy patients is generally a deeper or more masculine voice, even with the most successful oesophageal speech or other techniques.[6,21]

PROBLEMS OF REHABILITATION

Rehabilitation is one of the most important aspects of treatment of head and neck tumours, especially those involving the larynx. The three primary functions of the larynx—respiration, phonation, and protection of the airway—all have their psychological ramifications. Similarly, interference with each of these three functions has psychological consequences. A comprehensive rehabilitation programme may require attention to physical strengthening of neck muscles, assistance with swallowing, overcoming addiction or habituation to smoking or alcohol, restoration of social contacts and re-establishment of an acceptable self-image.

Much attention has been focused on speech rehabilitation, and numerous techniques have been designed to enable the laryngectomy patient to re-acquire verbal communication.[18] Among the techniques currently used are oesophageal speech, tracheo-oesophageal puncture and use of an external electromechanical device to vibrate cervical tissues. Each of these techniques requires participation by a well-trained and highly-motivated patient in order to be successful. In some instances, failure to establish acceptable speech by one or more of these methods is the result of significant anatomical abnormalities or of medical failure. However, in many other instances, it is the result of poor patient compliance. Clearly, the involvement of speech therapists and other health-care personnel, trained in the comprehensive rehabilitation of laryngectomy patients, is advisable.

Other problems experienced in the postlaryngectomy period concern the presence of a permanent tracheal stoma. This can interfere with daily habits such as showering and washing one's hair. Also, changes in self-perception may present as impotence or other impairment of sexual functioning. The treatment of these disorders will clearly involve many members of the health-care team, including physical therapists, speech therapists, nurses, occupational therapists, social workers, psychiatrists and the head and neck surgeons.

DEALING WITH FAMILY MEMBERS AND SOCIAL CONTACTS

Members of the patient's family and social circle can be active and supportive participants in the therapeutic team if they are motivated and if communications with them are carefully structured. In dealing with large families, it is best to identify a key family member who will be the one person to communicate directly, both with the physician and the patient. This will reduce the demands on the physician's time involved in communicating with numerous family members. It will also assist in structuring the format of communications to the family and others involved in patient care.

One must be particularly cautious when family members indicate a desire to withhold vital information from the patient. In that situation it is helpful to explore the reasons for such requests. If they result from the family member's inability to handle the gravity of the diagnosis and therapeutic plan, the physician can assure the family members that he or she will assume that responsibility in dealing with the patient. However, if the family members persist in their desire to withhold information, the head and neck surgeon may wish to enlist the assistance of a psychiatrist or psychologist who can provide additional emotional support as well as explore the complex motives for these requests.

CARE OF THE DYING PATIENT

Since a significant number of laryngeal cancer patients will eventually succumb to their disease, it is appropriate to offer a few comments about terminal care. This can be a particularly challenging problem since the patients have numerous physical and psychological impairments — including behavioural disturbance, voice abnormality, swallowing difficulty and pain.

As soon as the patient's condition is known to be terminal, it is prudent to provide all necessary physical and psychological support as well as to encourage the patient to remain independent for as long as possible. Analgesic use is important for the relief of physical pain. However, as noted above, it is best to look carefully for the source and type of pain in order to provide the best possible therapy. When the pain is real, there is no alternative to the frequent and liberal use of narcotics and other analgesics.[12]

When the patient is unable to remain independent in daily functioning, the physician must readily assume the responsibility for making necessary decisions. He or she may also have to intervene in the earlier stages of terminal illness when the patient's denial of the illness impedes therapy.

Perhaps the most important aspect of terminal care is the physician's actual or perceived availability to the patient and to the family. No sense of abandonment should be conveyed to the patient, even accidentally. This is particularly true when the primary therapy offered is under the direction of a medical oncologist or radiation therapist. The surgeon who was directly involved with earlier management should continue to convey his availability, interest and dedication to the patient.

The recognition that the patient will die should be conveyed to the family members as soon as the terminal situation has been identified. This fact is also profitably repeated on numerous occasions and in different circumstances in order to ensure that the family members have assimilated the gravity of the situation.

The patient's death is naturally distressing to the physician as well as to the patient's family. For the physician, it may represent technical failure, human and medical inadequacy, or simply the personal loss of a patient in whom he or she has invested a tremendous amount of time, effort and knowledge. This patient's death reminds the physician of his or her own mortality. The assignment of taking care of the dying patient has been compared to the job of the harp player who must develop 'a callus on the tip of each finger so that he may pluck the strings without bleeding. And yet, despite this, he must have a sure and delicate touch and a consummate sensitivity to all the nuances of the strings'.[25]

ROLE OF LIAISON PSYCHIATRY

Psychiatry can offer several types of service to otolaryngologists or head and neck surgeons in dealing with the psychological aspects of laryngeal cancer. In some instances, direct referral of the patient to the psychiatrist for consultation is the best choice. At other times, the physician may prefer to discuss the patient's problems with the psychiatrist himself or herself in order to get advice on handling them — rather than ask the psychiatrist to see the patient directly. A third alternative is the use of the services of a liaison psychiatrist who participates directly in patient care throughout treatment. Wallack and colleagues have described the interactions between liaison psychiatry and otolaryngology/head and neck surgery with particular focus on the use of a routine weekly multidisciplinary patient conference approach.[26] They noted that these conferences improved patient care and heightened staff awareness of the psychosocial factors involved in head and neck disease processes. They also assisted the staff in dealing with the stresses precipitated by the illness and hospitalization of cancer patients.

In conclusion, laryngeal cancer and other laryngeal disorders have numerous psychological ramifications that require a thorough diagnostic evaluation and well-planned therapy if the best results are to be obtained. Attention to these problems will be most beneficial in preparing comprehensive and effective patient-care plans.

REFERENCES

1. Barnes E 1961 People in hospital. Macmillan, London
2. Baudry F, Weiner A 1975 The surgical patient. In: Strain J J, Grossman S (eds). Psychological care of the medically ill: a primer in liaison psychiatry. Appleton-Century-Crofts, New York
3. Berkowitz J F, Lucente F E 1985 Counseling before laryngectomy. Laryngoscope 95: 1332–1336
4. Egbert L D, Battit G E, Turndoff H, Beecher H K 1963 The value of preoperative visits by the anesthetist. JAMA 185: 553–555
5. Egbert L D, Battit G E, Welch C E, Bartlett M K 1964 Reduction of postoperative pain by encouragement and instruction of patient. N Engl J Med 270: 825–827
6. Gardner W H 1966 Adjustment problems of laryngectomized women. Arch Otolaryngol 83: 31–42
7. Hackett T P, Weismann A D 1960 Psychiatric management of operative syndrome. Psychosom Med 22: 356–372
8. Holland J C, Mastrovito R 1980 Psychologic adaptation to breast cancer. Cancer 46: 1045–1052
9. Hugh-Jones P, Tanser A R, Whitby C 1964 Patients' view of

admission to a London teaching hospital. Br Med J 2: 660–664

10. Janis I L 1958 Psychological stress: psychoanalytic and behavioral studies of surgical patients. Wiley, New York

11. Kaufman M R, Fransblau A N, Kairys D 1956 The emotional impact of ward rounds. J Mt Sinai Hosp 23: 782–803

12. Lucente F E 1972 Thanatology. Trans Am Acad Ophthalmol Otolaryngol 76: 334–339

13. Lucente F E 1973 Psychiatric problems in otolaryngology. Ann Otol Rhinol Laryngol 82: 340–346

14. Lucente F E 1973 Psychological problems in otolaryngology. Laryngoscope 83: 1684–1689

15. Lucente F E, Fleck S 1972 A study of hospitalization anxiety in 408 medical and surgical patients. Psychosom Med 34: 304–312

16. Lucente F E, Strain J J 1988 Psychological implications of laryngeal disease and laryngectomy. In: Fried M P (ed) The larynx: a multidisciplinary approach. Little Brown, Boston pp 615–623

17. Marks R M, Sachar E J 1973 Undertreatment of medical inpatients with narcotic analgesics. Ann Intern Med 78: 173–181

18. Mathieson C M, Stam H J, Scott J P 1990 Psychosocial adjustment after laryngectomy: a review of the literature. J Otolaryngol 19: 331–336

19. Meichenbaum D, Turk D, Burstein S 1975 The nature of coping with stress. In: Sarason I G, Spielberger C D, (eds). Stress and anxiety, Vol 2, Wiley, New York

20. Minear D, Lucente F E 1979 Current attitudes of laryngectomy patients. Laryngoscope 89: 1061–1065

21. Shanks J 1979 Development of feminine voice and refinement of esophageal voice. In: Keith R, Darley F (eds) Laryngectomee rehabilitation. College Hill Press, Houston, pp 367–378

22. Shipley R H, Butt J H, Horwitz B, Farbry J E 1978 Preparation for a stressful medical procedure: effect of amount of stimulus pre-exposure and coping style. J Consult Clin Psychol 46: 499–507

23. Strain J J 1978 Psychological interventions in medical practice. Appleton-Century-Crofts, New York

24. Strain J J, Grossman S 1975 Psychological care of the medically ill: a primer in liaison psychiatry. Appleton-Century-Crofts, New York

25. Wahl W 1962 The physician's management of the dying patient. In: Masserman J H (ed). Current psychiatric therapies. Grune and Stratton, New York

26. Wallack J J, Lucente F E, Biller H F, Strain J J 1982 Liaison psychiatry-otolaryngology rounds. Laryngoscope 92: 125–127

Index